Leading & Managing Occupational Therapy Services

An Evidence-Based Approach

Second Edition

Leading & Managing Occupational Therapy Services

An Evidence-Based Approach

Second Edition

Brent Braveman, PhD, OTR/L, FAOTA

Director, Department of Rehabilitation Services
MD Anderson Cancer Center
Houston, Texas

F.A. Davis Company • Philadelphia

F. A. Davis Company
1915 Arch Street
Philadelphia, PA 19103
www.fadavis.com

Printed in the United States of America

Last digit indicates print number: 10 9 8 7 6 5 4 3 2 1

Senior Acquisitions Editor: Christa Fratantoro
Director of Content Development: George W. Lang
Developmental Editor: Andrea Edwards
Art and Design Manager: Carolyn O'Brien

As new scientific information becomes available through basic and clinical research, recommended treatments and drug therapies undergo changes. The author(s) and publisher have done everything possible to make this book accurate, up-to-date, and in accord with accepted standards at the time of publication. The author(s), editors, and publisher are not responsible for errors or omissions or for consequences from application of the book, and make no warranty, expressed or implied, in regard to the contents of the book. Any practice described in this book should be applied by the reader in accordance with professional standards of care used in regard to the unique circumstances that may apply in each situation. The reader is advised always to check product information (package inserts) for changes and new information regarding dose and contraindications before administering any drug. Caution is especially urged when using new or infrequently ordered drugs.

Library of Congress Cataloging-in-Publication Data

Braveman, Brent, author.
Leading & managing occupational therapy services : an evidence-based approach / Brent Braveman.—Second edition.
    p. ; cm.
  Leading and managing occupational therapy services
  ISBN 978-0-8036-4365-9—ISBN 0-8036-4365-9
  I. Title.   II. Title: Leading and managing occupational therapy services.
  [DNLM: 1. Occupational Therapy—organization & administration.
2. Evidence-Based Medicine.   3. Leadership.   WB 555]
  RM735.4
  615.8'515068—dc23

2015032642

I would like to dedicate this book to all of the leaders who have inspired me to listen, reflect, learn, and strive to be a better leader myself in order to make a difference. In particular I want to acknowledge the following:

Gary Kielhofner, DrPH, OTR/L, FAOTA
Carolyn Baum. PhD, OTR, FAOTA
Florence Clark, PhD, OTR/L, FAOTA
Charles Christiansen, EdD, OTR (C), FAOTA
Virginia Stoffel, PhD, OT, BCMH, FAOTA

My sincere appreciation also goes out to all of the occupational therapy volunteers and professionals who demonstrated patience and grace as I have worked to develop my skills as a manager and occupational therapy leader.

Finally, I dedicate this book to my sweetie and the love of my life—Michael Paul Appleman. Thank you for sharing your life and your passion with me. Thank you for living out our story together.

Preface

I am very happy to present the second edition of this textbook, *Leading & Managing Occupational Therapy Services: An Evidence-Based Approach*. The first edition of the text was well received; however, I have both updated information and added new content in response to feedback and in response to changes in the social, political, financial, legislative, and professional environments in which occupational therapy practitioners operate. One of the challenges faced in designing the original text was to provide students and new managers with the breadth and depth of information needed to support their practice while not providing detail that might quickly become outdated. This challenge became even more difficult in the second edition given the fast-changing landscape in our health-care and organizational systems; however, the contributors and I have done our best to provide useful and practical information for entry-level managers that will remain current and relevant for quite some time.

Once again I began preparations for the text by reviewing management literature in other fields and disciplines and found that, regardless of the field or discipline in which they are based, entry-level texts on management often begin by pointing out that managers complete commonly recognized functions for organizations. The functions most commonly identified include (a) planning, (b) organizing and staffing, (c) controlling, and (d) directing. There are sometimes variations because some authors may pull the function of "staffing" out from that of organizing and present five rather than four categories. Nonetheless, a discussion of leadership and the basic functions of management and their relationship to leading and

managing evidence-based practice is a logical place to begin.

Chapters have been reordered in this edition; the first chapter is on leadership to emphasize the importance of using leadership theory and evidence no matter what your professional role. Other content has been reorganized and relabeled to make the traditional management functions more easily identified. There is increased emphasis and content on strategic planning, business knowledge, financial planning, and financial management. New content has been added on interprofessional teams, interprofessional collaborative practice, and interprofessional competencies.

This text is now organized in four sections with 18 chapters that are as follows:

Section I: Introduction to Leadership and Evidence-Based Management

Chapter 1: Leadership: The Art, Science, and Evidence
Chapter 2: Engaging in Evidence-Based Management

Section II: Leading and Managing in Context

Chapter 3: Understanding Health-Care Systems and Practice Contexts
Chapter 4: Understanding and Working Within Organizations
Chapter 5: Communicating Effectively in Complex Environments

Section III: Managerial Skills, Responsibilities, and Competencies

Section IV: Leading Evidence-Based Practice and Professional Considerations

The focus of this text is the management of occupational therapy services. As such, every chapter within the text relates to content, functions, or issues that lie within the domain of concern for occupational therapy managers. The overarching theme for this text is how occupational therapy managers can utilize theory, data, information, and other forms of evidence to become more effective. For this reason, particular topics and content have been chosen upon which to focus entire chapters. The topics of leadership, the roles and functions of the manager, and the roles and functions of the supervisor are addressed in three different chapters. Some occupational therapy managers work in jobs where they are only responsible for the oversight of occupational therapy services. However, it is becoming more common for managers in health care to be asked to manage several disciplines; therefore, the interprofessional manager has been emphasized throughout the text.

The key features of this text are focused on enhancing usability for the readers. A glossary has been added at the start of each chapter to identify key terms. The "Real-Life Management" and "Real-Life Solutions" features remain, and case examples and vignettes are used for emphasis. Text boxes and tables are used liberally to focus on important knowledge. Each chapter concludes with a list of additional resources to help readers expand their knowledge base or to find additional information for class projects or for use to support day-to-day practice. A selection of multiple-choice questions has been added to each chapter to stress key points and to help readers assess their understanding.

A final comment on the content chosen for inclusion in this text is warranted. As an occupational therapy professional who has been involved in clinical practice in some way for over three decades, I have found that I have continually benefited from reliance on the combination of paradigmatic occupational therapy knowledge and related knowledge from multiple other disciplines. As a professional who has also held leadership and management roles for much of that same time, I have found the same benefit from looking both within our profession and outside to other disciplines for knowledge and insight. As a teacher of management, I try to highlight the uniqueness of occupational therapy while stressing the benefit of collaborating with our peers from physical therapy, nursing, medicine, psychology, case management, educational administration, social work, and other disciplines. I am confident that this text will lend itself to that approach in both the classroom and in practice.

Contributors

Patricia Bowyer
EdD, MS, OTR, FAOTA
School of Occupational Therapy
Texas Woman's University
Houston, Texas

Regina F. Doherty
OTD, OTR/L, FAOTA, FNAP
Department of Occupational Therapy
MGH Institute of Health Professions
Boston, Massachusetts

Marcia Finlayson
PhD, OT Reg (Ont), OTR
School of Rehabilitation Therapy
Queen's University
Kingston, ON, Canada

Gail Fisher
MPA, OTR/L, FAOTA
Department of Occupational Therapy
University of Illinois at Chicago
Chicago, Illinois

Gayle Harper
MSW
Department of Clinical Support Services Administration
University of Texas
MD Anderson Center
Houston, Texas

Brenda Koverman
MBA, MS, OTR/L
Department of Occupational Therapy
Rush University Medical Center
Chicago, Illinois

Alanna Motzi
LCSW
Department of Clinical Support Services Administration
University of Texas
MD Anderson Center
Houston, Texas

Lauro Munoz
OTR, MOT, CHC
Department of Rehabilitation Services
University of Texas
MD Anderson Center
Houston, Texas

Julie Ann Nastasi
ScD, OTD, OTR/L, SCLV, FAOTA
Department of Occupational Therapy
The University of Scranton
Scranton, Pennsylvania

Elizabeth W. Peterson
PhD, OTR/L, FAOTA
Department of Occupational Therapy
University of Illinois at Chicago
Chicago, Illinois

Shawn Phipps

PhD, MS, OTR/L, FAOTA

Chief Quality Officer & Associate Hospital Administrator

Rancho Los Amigos National Rehabilitation Center

Vice President

American Occupational Therapy Association

Adjunct Assistant Professor of Clinical Occupational Therapy

University of Southern California

USC Chan Division of Occupational Science & Occupational Therapy

Los Angeles, California

Maureen Triller

MPA, DrPH

Department of Clinical Support Services Administration

University of Texas

MD Anderson Center

Houston, Texas

Reviewers

Amanda Cline
OTR/L
Adjunct Faculty/Program Manager at Laclede Groves
Saint Louis University and Laclede Groves
St. Louis, Missouri

Elizabeth Deluliis
OTD, OTR/L
Academic Fieldwork Coordinator, Assistant Professor
Duquesne University
Pittsburgh, Pennsylvania

Pamela K. Evans
OTR, MBA, DBA
Doctor
Brenau University
Norcross, Georgia

Cecilia Fierro
OTR, OTD
Clinical Assistant Professor
University of Texas at El Paso
El Paso, Texas

Valley O. McCurry
MBA, OTR/L
Assistant Professor
University of Alabama at Birmingham
Birmingham, Alabama

Shirley O'Brien
PhD, OTR/L, FAOTA
Professor
Eastern Kentucky University
Richmond, Kentucky

Debora Oliveira
PhD, CRC, OTR/L
Interim Director
Florida A&M University
Tallahassee, Florida

Linda L. Orr
MPA, OTR/L
Professor, Program Coordinator
Lewis and Clark Community College
Godfrey, Illinois

Ingrid Provident
EdD, OTR/L
Assistant Professor
Chatham University
Pittsburgh, Pennsylvania

Charlotte Brasic Royeen
PhD, OTR/L, FAOTA
Professor
Saint Louis University
St. Louis, Missouri

Jennifer L. Womack
MS, MA, OTR/L SCDCM, C/PH, CAPS, FAOTA
Associate Professor
University of North Carolina–Chapel Hill
Chapel Hill, North Carolina

Acknowledgments

I would like to thank the following persons for their support, consultation, and guidance in conceptualization of this text and in my daily practice as an occupational therapy leader and manager:

Christopher Bluhm
Chief Operating Officer
American Occupational Therapy Association

Christina Metzler
Chief Public Affairs Officer
American Occupational Therapy Association

Virginia Stoffel, PhD, OT, BCMH, FAOTA
Associate Professor
University of Wisconsin, Madison

Frank Tortorella, MBA, JD, FACHE
Vice President of Clinical Support Services
University of Texas
MD Anderson Cancer Center

I also wish to extend thanks to the following who are directors at the University of Texas MD Anderson Cancer Center Division of Clinical Support Services:

- Carol Frankmann, Clinical Nutrition
- Gayle Harper, Clinical Support Services Administration
- Gale Kennebrew, Chaplaincy and Pastoral Education
- Daniel Kowalczyk, Dining Services
- Connie Longuet, Patient Access
- Margaret Meyer, Social Work
- Pamela Douglas-Ntagha, Patient Resources
- Cesar Palacio, Language Assistance
- Donna Ukanowicz, Case Management

Contents

CHAPTER 13
Continuous Quality Improvement, 327

Maureen Triller, MPA, DrPH
Alanna Motzi, LCSW
Gayle Harper, MSW

CHAPTER 14
Marketing Occupational Therapy Services, 357

Brent Braveman, PhD, OTR/L, FAOTA
Julie Ann Nastasi, ScD, OTD, OTR/L, SCLV, FAOTA

CHAPTER 15
Developing Evidence-Based Occupational Therapy Programming, 375

Brent Braveman, PhD, OTR/L, FAOTA

SECTION IV
Leading Evidence-Based Practice and Professional Considerations, 411

CHAPTER 16
Introducing Others to Evidence-Based Practice, 413

Marcia Finlayson, PhD, OT Reg (Ont), OTR
Brent Braveman, PhD, OTR/L, FAOTA

CHAPTER 17
Turning Theory Into Practice: Managerial Strategies, 439
Lauro Munoz, OTR, MOT, CHC
Patricia Bowyer, EdD, MS, OTR, FAOTA
Brent Braveman, PhD, OTR/L, FAOTA

CHAPTER 18
Responsible Participation in a Profession: Fostering Professionalism and Leading for Moral Action, 467
Regina F. Doherty, OTD, OTR/L, FAOTA, FNAP
Elizabeth W. Peterson, PhD, OTR/L, FAOTA

About the Author

Dr. Brent Braveman is the director of the Department of Rehabilitation Services at the University of Texas MD Anderson Cancer Center. The department employs nearly 100 occupational therapy and physical therapy practitioners, treats 20,000 patients each year, and had a gross revenue of over $24 million in fiscal year 2015.

Dr. Braveman earned his BS in Occupational Therapy in 1984 from the University of New Hampshire, an MA in Education and Human Development from the George Washington University in 1992, and a PhD in Public Health from the University of Illinois at Chicago in 2002.

He has been an author on 38 refereed journal articles and book chapters, has presented at numerous national and international conferences, and is the author of two occupational therapy textbooks, *Leading & Managing Occupational Therapy Services: An Evidence-Based Approach* and *Work: Occupational Therapy Intervention to Promote Participation and Productivity*.

He has served on multiple national expert panels providing consultation on issues related to work disability and employment, HIV and AIDS, and oncology rehabilitation for groups including the American Cancer Society, the Institute of Medicine, and the National Institutes of Health. He has been a coinvestigator on $1.2 million of federally funded research grants.

Dr. Braveman has a long history of volunteer service in state and national association activities, including serving as a state association president, a member of American Occupational Therapy Association's (AOTA's) Roster of Accreditation Evaluators, the chairperson of AOTA's Administration and Management Special Interest Section, the AOTA Special Interest Section Council Chairperson, speaker of the AOTA Representative Assembly, and secretary of AOTA. Dr. Braveman has a passion for occupational therapy, leadership development, and social justice; he is committed to the promotion of the profession and to helping occupational therapy practitioners to meet society's occupational needs.

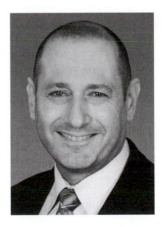

Introduction to Leadership and Evidence-Based Management

CHAPTER 1

Leadership: The Art, Science, and Evidence

Brent Braveman, PhD, OTR/L, FAOTA

■ Real-Life Management

Christi recently relocated from a large city to a smaller suburban town after accepting a position at an acute care facility that is also associated with a skilled nursing facility. The facility employs 14 occupational therapy and physical therapy practitioners and one rehabilitation technician. Christi has 14 years of experience and is commonly recognized as a clinical expert in a number of areas by many of her peers. Christi was originally asked to act as interim director for the position of director of rehabilitation, which has been vacant for several months; now she has been offered the position on a permanent basis. She is excited about the promotion and the opportunity but is also nervous about moving into the role of department director. She is questioning her leadership skills because she feels comfortable interacting on a one-on-one basis but is not as comfortable when leading groups.

Christi shared her reservations about taking on a formal leadership role with Carole, the division director who would be her new boss. Carole was empathetic to Christi's concerns and committed to her that, if Christi accepted the position, she would mentor her to develop her leadership skills. Christi appreciated the offer but now has the following questions:

1. Can an individual develop skills as a leader, or are leadership skills something with which one is born?

2. What sort of leader does Christi want to be? She respects both Carole and her former boss, Steve, but they seem to have very different styles of leadership.

3. If it is possible to develop skills as a leader, what specific steps can she take to do so?

Christi decided to go to the local bookstore to see if there were any resources on leadership skills that would be helpful. She was surprised to find a large number of books, and they seemed to approach leadership from many different perspectives. After scanning a few books, she also noted that a number of different theories and models were mentioned. She decided to make a visit to the local university library and do some more investigation to find out if any of the theories or models mentioned in the "popular press" books in the bookstore had been validated by research.

Critical Thinking Questions

As you read this chapter, consider the following questions:

- Are leadership skills innate traits with which we are born or are they skills that can be learned and developed over time?

- How can an understanding of theories of leadership and the evidence on these theories assist in examining your current skills and interpersonal tendencies in order to identify areas for development?

- How can leadership theories classified as supervisory or as strategic be used in combination to be most effective as a leader?

- What is the relationship of leadership to traditionally recognized management functions such as planning, organizing, directing, and controlling?

Glossary

- **360-degree feedback:** receiving feedback on performance from subordinates, peers, and supervisors or those higher in an organizational structure.
- **Charisma:** ability to instill pride, faith, and respect in subordinates by transmitting a sense of mission that is effectively articulated.
- **Contingent rewards:** rewards and recognition exchanged for accomplishment of assigned work duties or reaching organizational objectives.
- **Individualized consideration:** delegates projects to stimulate the learning and growth of employees, coaches and teaches employees, and treats each employee with respect.
- **Intellectual stimulation:** arousing followers to think in new ways and emphasizing problem-solving and the use of reason before acting.
- **Leadership:** a process of creating structural change wherein the values, vision, and ethics of individuals are integrated into the culture of a community as a means of achieving sustainable change.
- **Management:** the process of guiding an organization by planning for future work obligations, organizing employees into functional units, directing employees in the process of completing daily work tasks, and controlling work processes and systems to assure adequate quality of work output.
- **Management by exception:** type of management in which leaders follow work performance closely to identify mistakes and intervene or give directions to correct actions during the work process (active management by exception) or may wait until work is completed and provide an employee with a negative evaluation, hoping that future performance will be improved (passive management by exception).
- **Mindfulness:** approaching communication in a thoughtful and conscious manner in each interaction and avoiding the appearance that communication and leader behavior have become routine.
- **Transaction:** in Transactional Leadership Theory, occurs whenever the leader promises rewards and benefits to subordinates for their fulfillment of agreements and their contributions to goal achievement.

Introduction

Occupational therapy practitioners have the opportunity to take on various formal leadership roles in both paid and volunteer positions. Examples include the roles of supervisor, department director, or elected volunteer leader in state professional associations or at the national level in the American Occupational Therapy Association (AOTA). Practitioners also have the opportunity to assume informal leadership roles such as acting as a resource person for less experienced students or practitioners, functioning as a thought leader on a task force or committee (e.g., as an expert or authority leading innovations) as it completes its work, or being a lead voice in a community of practitioners. Peter Northouse (2013), the author of a widely read text on leadership, refers to people who are leaders because of their formal position in an organization as "assigned leaders" and those who are leaders because of the way others respond to them as "emergent leaders." Whether you are in a formal assigned leadership role or lead others because of a natural affinity to share your knowledge, skills, and experiences with them, you can benefit from learning and applying theory and evidence on leadership. Just as you would use an "evidence-based" approach to applying any clinical skill set with your clients and patients, using an evidence-based approach to leadership will help you be more effective.

Leadership is a topic that permeates every aspect of management. Whether we are involved in planning a new program, organizing staff for daily work, directing personnel on how to complete their assignments, or controlling output and services by measuring and improving quality, we can function as leaders and have an impact on how others in the organization view the organization and their work.

Leadership has been a topic of interest and scientific investigation in sociology, psychology, organizational development, and business administration—and in the popular press—for decades. Much of the literature has focused on the qualities of effective leaders, including in-depth explorations of what has made some of our most notable public figures effective as leaders. Examples include biographies of famous public figures such as Eleanor Roosevelt and Mahatma Gandhi, politicians such as William Jefferson Clinton and George Walker Bush, and successful business leaders such as Steve Jobs, Bill Gates, and Warren Buffet (Bush, 2010; Clinton, 2004; Gerber & Burns, 2002; Isaacson, 2011; Loomis, 2012; Rogak, 2012; Rudolph & Rudolph, 1983). Leadership has also become a topic of great interest in health care as the costs of providing care have skyrocketed. In addition, there has been wider political debate about health care surrounding the adoption of the Patient Protection and Affordable Care Act in 2010 (U.S. Department of Health and Human Services, 2013). Books on the application of leadership have been written in the fields of nursing, case management, and occupational therapy (Dunbar, 2009; Gilkeson, 1997; Grohar-Murray & Dicroce, 2002; Marshall, 2011; Powell, 2000).

Health-care organizations today are in a constant state of flux and are influenced by rapidly evolving government policies such as the Patient Protection and Affordable Care Act (e.g., Obamacare), economic conditions, shrinking reimbursement, increased competition, and heightened scrutiny by consumers who have become more sophisticated in managing their own health care. Because of an increase in managed care, tighter compliance regulations for payment, and increased competition for both public and private funding, the management structure of most health-care organizations and community-based organizations has "flattened." As a result of this flattening, many managers who used to lead discipline-specific departments have been asked to accept formal managerial responsibility for other disciplines. It is commonplace today for directors of rehabilitation or similar departments to have responsibility for oversight of multiple disciplines, including occupational therapy, physical therapy, and speech-language pathology, as well as technical staff, including transportation or business staff.

It is clear that the topic of leadership has warranted much attention, but it is easy to understand how, as an occupational therapy student or entry-level practitioner, you might ask, "I just want to treat my patients so why should I care about leadership at this point?" It is easy to appreciate that new practitioners might be most concerned with the patient care issues that they expect to confront on a day-to-day basis. However, given the dynamic health-care environment, occupational therapy students and new graduates may find themselves in both formal and informal leadership roles much sooner than they expect or perhaps desire.

Leadership Versus Management

It is helpful to begin a practical discussion of leadership by differentiating between the concepts of leadership and management. One conceptualization of the relationship between leadership and management is that the leader's role is to guide change, whereas the manager's role is to maintain stability. For example, Zaleznik described leaders as developing fresh approaches to long-standing problems and open issues to new options but described managers as acting to limit choices to solve problems (Zaleznik, 2004). He further stated, "A managerial culture emphasizes rationality and control. Whether his or her energies are directed toward goals, resources, organization structure, or people a manager is a problem-solver. The manager asks: 'What problems have to be solved and what are the best ways to achieve results so that people will continue to contribute to this organization?'" (Zaleznik, 2004, p. 75). Similarly, Beech (2002) suggested that managers tend to rely primarily on strategy, structure, and systems, whereas leaders are inclined to use style, staff, skills, and shared goals to yield desired results.

These conceptualizations of the relationship between leadership and management may be unnecessarily narrow, however. In fact, one may be a leader, a manager, or both. As noted by Schruijer and Vansina (2002, p. 872), "Such splitting obscures the complexity of life. Leaders often face environmental change and stability simultaneously; organizations may need change in some domains yet stability in others." Distinguishing between leadership and management has a functional implication for new managers and is not simply an academic exercise. By thoughtfully distinguishing between the constructs of leadership and management, we may more successfully identify the skills and behaviors associated with each so that they can more easily be practiced and incorporated into our daily behavior. To this end, the following definitions of leadership and management will be used:

- **Leadership** is a process of creating structural change wherein the values, vision, and ethics of individuals are integrated into the culture of a community as a means of achieving sustainable change.
- **Management** is the process of guiding an organization by planning for future work obligations, organizing employees into functional units, directing employees in the process of completing daily work tasks, and controlling work processes and systems to assure adequate quality of work output.

Understanding Leadership

To begin to understand leadership, it is important to distinguish between the act or process of leading (i.e., leadership) and the individuals who are in the position of guiding others (i.e., leaders). It is problematic to attempt to define and investigate leadership, and in particular strategies for developing skills in the process of leading others, by solely focusing on descriptions of effective leaders. If leadership is a process, then it, like all processes, will have results. Reflecting on the definition of leadership provided, leadership is a process of change whereby we hope to impact others in some sustainable manner and have lasting impact on the function of a department or organization. The definition of leadership provided also implies that the focus of this process of change is specifically on individuals and that these individuals are part of a larger community. This means that when examining the process of leading, we must consider the impact on individual workers and on the larger work community (e.g., the occupational therapy department, our clients, members of other departments in our organization).

Theory and evidence on leadership has greatly evolved and is still evolving. The majority of research can be found in the business and psychology literature, although some can be found in the health-care literature as well. In a review of health and business literature from 1970 to 1999, only 4.4% of 6,629 articles reviewed were data based, indicating the continued need for evidence-based research on the topic of leadership effectiveness (Vance & Larson, 2002). By 2009 Avolio, Walumbwa, and Weber noted that,

Today, the field of leadership focuses not only on the leader, but also on followers, peers, supervisors, work setting/context, and culture, including a much broader array of individuals representing the entire spectrum of diversity, public, private, and not-for-profit organizations, and increasingly over the past 20 years, samples of populations from nations around the globe. Leadership is no longer simply described as an individual characteristic or difference but rather is depicted in various models as dyadic, shared, relational, strategic, global, and a complex social dynamic. (Avolio et al, 2009, p. 422)

New models, theories, and methods of examining leadership such as servant leadership continue to be introduced. In fact, the number and variety of leadership theories is such that not all can be discussed in this chapter. Leadership scholars most consistently agree upon one thing: Leaders are supposed to motivate followers to accomplish organizational goals. How leaders accomplish this task can be explained and may depend on the theory or theories of leadership on which they base their behavior.

Leadership Theories: An Overview

An Early Focus on Traits

Early studies of leadership focused on identification of the common traits of effective leaders, or what Thomas Carlyle referred to as "Great Men" or natural leaders in the 19th century (Carlyle, 1888). Smith and Kreuger (1933) provided an early review of the literature and organized traits into the categories of personality traits (e.g., alertness), social traits (e.g., sociability), and physical traits (e.g., height). Stogdill (1948, 1974) conducted two surveys of leadership traits that contributed much to the relationship between individuals' traits and how they became and performed as leaders. Other researchers, including Kirkpatrick and Locke (1991), completed various studies later that identified a considerable range of traits and characteristics that contribute to effective leadership. Many of the traits commonly thought to be associated with effective leaders are presented in Box 1-1.

However, as early as the mid-20th century, some challenged the trait approach and questioned the universality of leadership traits (Northouse, 2013). Trait identification can contribute to understanding how a particular leader might be perceived, but there has been relatively little recent research to validate Trait Theory as effective in linking leaders with leadership outcomes; therefore, these theories will not be addressed further in this chapter.

Early research on leadership also often sought to answer the question, "Are great leaders born or made?" Answering this question provides much insight into whether or not training in leadership is effective and a valuable investment of resources. However, little emphasis is placed on this question today because evidence now seems to support that many factors may influence the effectiveness of leaders, including skills, knowledge, work experience, and personality. Although we may not be able to change some of our basic personality traits, it seems clear that over time, we can seek the types of experiences (e.g., practice in solving novel problems and working with different sorts of groups in various environments) that may contribute to becoming a more effective leader.

Knowledge and skills may be gained over time, and the problems encountered by leaders often become more complex and long term as these individuals rise higher in organizations, which allows for the existence of leaders at all levels of organizations. Leadership development initiatives often attempt to address intrapersonal competence through efforts that include training in self-awareness (e.g., emotional awareness), self-regulation (e.g., self-control, trustworthiness), self-motivation (e.g., commitment, initiative, optimism), social awareness (e.g., empathy, service orientation), and social skills (e.g., collaboration and cooperation, conflict management) (Day, 2001; Lussier, 2010).

BOX 1-1

Traits Commonly Associated With Being an Effective Leader

Intelligence	Persistence	Drive	Honesty
Integrity	Dominance	Self-Confidence	Cognitive Ability
Openness	Initiative	Sociability	Achievement

Leadership in the Occupational Therapy Literature

A review of the occupational therapy literature reveals attention to the topic of leadership in most occupational therapy textbooks on management and, to a more limited extent, in the research literature. For example, a chapter of the 2011 edition of *The Occupational Therapy Manager*, Fifth Edition, is devoted to leadership development. In this text, Snodgrass (2011) compared the responsibilities of leaders and managers, identified the two main types of leaders as transformational and transactional, and presented a review of the evidence on leadership. Several recent articles describe the perception of, or self-perception of, various leadership groups in occupational therapy, including managers and directors of academic programs. For example, Fleming-Castaldy and Patro (2012) examined the leadership characteristics of 53 occupational therapy clinical managers. A demographic measure and a self-inventory of leadership behaviors were collected in a nonexperimental survey. No significant associations were found between the demographics and the scores on the inventory. Snodgrass, Douthitt, Ellis, Wade, and Plemons (2008) conducted a study that investigated the relationship between faculty perceptions of occupational therapy program directors' leadership styles and outcomes of leadership and the effects of moderating demographic and institutional characteristics. They reported that, in general, transformational leadership had a significant ($p < 0.001$) positive predictive relationship with the leadership outcomes, whereas transactional leadership had a significant ($p < 0.001$) negative predictive relationship. Findings from this study indicated that overall, transformational and transactional leadership styles are associated with leadership outcomes. More recently, leadership development has been a focus of AOTA, which has implemented programs for academic leaders, middle managers, and emerging leaders (AOTA, 2014). AOTA President Virginia Stoffel made leadership the focus of her 2013 Inaugural Presidential Address titled, "From Heartfelt Leadership to Compassionate Care" (Stoffel, 2013).

Categorizing Theories on Leadership

Boal and Hooijberg (2001) differentiated between what they described as theories of leadership *within*

organizations (supervisory leadership theories) and theories of leadership *of* organizations (strategic leadership theories). Supervisory leadership theories, including the Path-Goal Theory of Leadership and the Transactional Leadership Theory, draw from Expectancy Motivation Theory. Expectancy Motivation Theory supposes that a subordinate's performance is related to the extent to which he or she believes that his or her actions will lead to specific outcomes. Strategic leadership theories, including the Charismatic Leadership Theory, Transformational Leadership Theory, and Situational Leadership Theory, draw from the study of organizational behavior and the notion that leaders are able to motivate followers to commit to and realize performance that exceeds their own expectations. Leadership within these latter theories has been likened to the process of empowerment. The end result of empowerment is a change in organizational culture that helps subordinates generate a sense of meaning in their work and a desire to challenge themselves to experience success (Bennis & Nanus, 1985). Servant leadership, which is also described in this chapter, does not fit neatly into either the supervisory or strategic category of theories. Northouse (2013, p. 219) described servant leadership as a "paradox—an approach to leadership that runs counter to common sense" and asked, "How can leadership be both service *and* influence?"

Table 1-1 provides a brief overview of the classification of six theories of leadership chosen for presentation in this chapter and their major foci. These theories were chosen because of their inclusion in the occupational therapy literature and because of their applicability to leadership in health-care settings.

A Few Words About Leadership Theories and Evidence

Before beginning an exploration of the theories of leadership to be discussed in this chapter and the evidence related to each theory, it will be helpful to make a few comments about the nature of empirical investigations in this area. In Chapter 2 you will be introduced to the process of conducting a search for evidence; a critical step in this process is to develop a question to guide selection of evidence. In regard to leadership theory and corresponding behavior of leaders who adopt a particular theory, what we might be most interested in knowing is whether behaviors

TABLE 1-1
Overview of Leadership Theories

Supervisory Theories of Leadership

Theory	Primary Focus
Path-Goal	Leaders increase personal payoffs for subordinates for goal attainment and make the path to these payoffs easier to travel by reducing obstacles, thereby improving performance.
Transactional	Leaders promise rewards and benefits to subordinates for meeting work goals, and leaders and subordinates agree through transactions on what will lead to reward and how to avoid punishment.

Strategic Theories of Leadership

Theory	Primary Focus
Charismatic	Stresses the personal identification of followers with the leader, who formulates an inspirational vision and impression that the leader's mission is extraordinary.
Transformational	Leaders achieve change by expressing the value associated with outcomes and by articulating a vision of the future resulting in commitment, effort, and improved performance on the part of subordinates.
Situational	Leaders should adopt a leadership style that best fits the developmental level of their subordinates' competence and commitment.

Servant Leadership: Supervisory or Strategic?

Leaders should be attentive to the concerns of followers and empathize and nurture them by first empowering them and helping them to develop their personal capacities.

guided by one theory result in better performance on the part of subordinates than when a leader uses behavior guided by a different theory. In other words, "Do behaviors guided by a particular leadership theory result in higher perceived effectiveness as measured by indicators of subordinate perception or by organizational measures of leader performance (e.g., peer reviews or performance appraisals)?" These questions may be difficult to answer because well-designed empirical investigations of the direct impact of leader behavior on subordinate performance and results are relatively rare. This dynamic exists primarily for two reasons. First, outside of contrived laboratory situations (i.e., studies of leader behavior with college students who volunteer for a study), relatively few experimental studies examine leaders in real-time and real-life situations. It is easy to appreciate that not many organizations are going to allow their employee leaders to be manipulated (e.g., to change their style of leadership for the purpose of study) because of

worry over financial and performance costs to the organizations. Second, when we try to answer the question of whether a particular approach to leadership results in improved subordinate performance, things get cloudy very quickly. This is true because so many other things besides leadership behavior can influence performance of subordinates, such as the organization's culture, the subordinates' skills and experiences, and the relationship of subordinates or work units to other subordinates or work units in the organization.

Recent research on issues such as the mediating effects of subordinate trust in leaders or the congruence of subordinates' values with a leader's values may shed valuable light on why some leaders are effective (Zhu, Newman, Miao, & Hooke, 2013). However, such research is not as well developed as that related specifically to the direct impact of leader behavior. For this reason, evaluating evidence in regard to leadership theory and behavior may be a sticky situation.

However, as a student or new occupational therapy practitioner who may be assuming his or her first leadership role, you may be perfectly happy to find an answer to the question, "If I adopt behaviors guided by a particular leadership theory, am I more likely to be perceived as effective?" The next section of this chapter presents four well-established theories of leadership and two less researched—but often cited—leadership theories, as well as a summary sample of evidence on each theory.

Leadership Theories

Path-Goal Theory of Leadership

The genesis of the Path-Goal Theory of Leadership lies in the work of the Institute for Social Research at the University of Michigan. The theory was developed primarily to reconcile prior research findings on the effects of leader–task orientation (the extent to which leaders focused on completing work tasks) and leader–person orientation (the extent to which leaders focused on the emotional and psychological needs of subordinates) on subordinate satisfaction and performance (House, 1996). The initiation of research on the Path-Goal Theory represented a shift in research from a focus on task and person orientation to a focus on leader effectiveness.

The Path-Goal Theory was initially developed as a dyadic theory of supervision concerning relationships between formally appointed supervisors and subordinates in their day-to-day functioning. As such, it did not address leadership of groups, leadership of change, or leadership related to strategic planning or whole organizations; rather, it dealt with the effect of leader behavior on individuals. However, in 1996, R. J. House presented a "reformulated" theory that he described as a theory of work unit leadership addressing the effects of leaders on the motivation and abilities of immediate subordinates and the effects of leaders on work unit performance. This reformulated theory included a focus on "unconscious" motives of subordinates and the "valence" of leadership behaviors (i.e., the strength of the attractiveness of outcomes to the followers). The primary propositions of the Path-Goal Theory are included in Box 1-2.

The function of a leader as explained in the Path-Goal Theory is to "use a leadership style that best meets subordinates' motivational goals" (Northouse,

---

BOX 1-2

Primary Propositions of Path-Goal Theory of Leadership

- Leader behavior is viewed as positive to the extent that subordinates see the behaviors as an immediate source of satisfaction or key to future satisfaction.
- Leader behavior will improve employee performance to the extent that it
  - Enhances the motivation of members of work units, enhances the relevant abilities of employees, provides guidance, and removes obstacles and provides resources.
  - Makes satisfaction of employee needs and employee rewards contingent on performance, makes work tasks and goal attainment intrinsically satisfying, and complements the work environment by providing structure, support, and rewards necessary for good performance.
  - Enhances employee work tasks in a way that promotes collaborative working relationships among employees and between employees and the organization, ensures that the requisite resources are available to work units, and enhances the need for the work unit in the eyes of the rest of the organization.
  - Serves as a role model for learning relevant task behavior.

Based on concepts from House, R. J. (1996). Path-Goal Theory of Leadership: Lessons, legacy and a reformulated theory. Leadership Quarterly, 7, 323–352.

2013, p. 137). This is done by increasing personal payoffs to subordinates for achieving the workplace goals, targets, and outcomes established by management. Leaders make the paths to these payoffs easier to travel by reducing roadblocks and helping subordinates choose behaviors that are most appropriate for the situation and problems at hand. The Path-Goal Theory is basically a "functional" approach to leadership, calling for a diagnosis of functions that need to be fulfilled in subordinates' work environments for them to be motivated, perform at high levels, and be satisfied (Schriesheim & Neider, 1996).

The reformulated 1996 Path-Goal Theory of Leadership identifies 10 classes of leader behaviors that are theoretically acceptable, satisfying, and motivational for employees. These behavior classes and examples of each are listed in Table 1-2.

In addition to a leader's characteristics, the Path-Goal Theory also considers characteristics of the subordinates and of the task. Subordinate characteristics include needs for affiliation, preferences for structure, desires for control, and self-perceived level of task

TABLE 1-2	
Classes and Examples of Leadership Behavior According to Path-Goal Leadership Theory	
Leader Behavior	**Examples**
Clarifying	• Setting clear performance goals and how to achieve them • Setting clear standards for performance in job descriptions and everyday assignments • Clarifying from whom the employee should and should not take direction • Using rewards and punishment with restraint and only in response to work performance
Supportive	• Expressing concern about the welfare of employees • Creating a friendly work environment • Listening to employees' complaints
Participative	• Asking for suggestions on how to proceed • Including employees in decision-making using formal and informal means
Achievement oriented	• Setting challenging goals • Showing confidence in the ability of employees to perform well • Emphasizing excellence in performance
Work facilitation	• Planning, scheduling, and organizing work tasks effectively to promote employee performance • Mentoring, guiding, and coaching employees • Assisting employees to develop needed knowledge and skills
Interaction facilitation	• Assisting employees to resolve conflicts • Assuring that minority opinions are heard • Using team-building activities to promote close and satisfying relationships
Group-oriented decision process	• Encouraging all members of the work unit to participate in discussions • Preventing individuals from dominating discussions • Waiting to select options until the entire team has had the opportunity to give input
Representation and networking	• Advocating for the work unit throughout the organization • Presenting a positive view of the work unit to superiors • Obtaining resources to facilitate work • Participating in organization-wide social functions
Value-based behavior	• Use of "envisioning" activities with employees • Showing passion and self-sacrifice to achieve a described vision • Frequent positive evaluation of employees as a group • Communicating high performance expectations and confidence in employee ability to meet the expectations
Shared leadership	• Promoting interdependence among employees • Delegating leadership visibly to various employees for different tasks

Based on concepts from House, R. J. (1996). Path-Goal Theory of Leadership: Lessons, legacy and a reformulated theory. Leadership Quarterly, 7, 323–352.

ability. Characteristics of the task include the design of the subordinate's task, the formal authority system of the organization, and the primary work group of subordinates.

Evidence for the Path-Goal Theory of Leadership

The Path-Goal Theory of Leadership has been the focus of considerable research; however, most leadership scholars agree that the theory still has not been adequately tested and that empirical validation of the theory as a whole has proved difficult (Knight, Shteynberg, & Hanges, 2004). Some hypotheses of the theory have been well supported, whereas others have not. For instance, relationships between leader behavior and follower performance are more consistently found than are relationships between leader behavior and follower satisfaction. Several early meta-analyses found support for the basic propositions of the Path-Goal Theory, including strong support for the role that leaders may play in developing organizational

structures that promote goal attainment by employees and an overall positive relationship between leader consideration and subordinate job satisfaction (Fisher & Edwards, 1988; Indvik, 1986; Wofford & Liska, 1993). Most research on the Path-Goal Theory has relied on various versions of the Leader Behavior Description Questionnaire (LBDQ) to measure leader behaviors. Yet, scholars have repeatedly noted the inappropriateness of this instrument in investigating the relationships posited by the Path-Goal Theory, arguing that the scale does not adequately tap the proposed constructs. Ayman and Adams (2012) recently provided an overview of the Path-Goal Theory consistent with the mixed findings about the theory. They noted that, "Path-Goal Theory can be seen as an important development in leadership theory that encouraged the evolution of new leadership conceptualizations" and that "although the empirical support for the model is mixed, it helped drive new thinking about leadership" (Ayman & Adams, 2012, p. 227).

Table 1-3 summarizes selected evidence on the Path-Goal Theory of Leadership.

TABLE 1-3

Summary of Selected Evidence on Path-Goal Theory of Leadership

Author	Study Type	N (Sample Size)	Level of Evidence	Results
Dixon & Hart (2010)	Survey	260 manufacturing workers in 20 work groups	Fair	Path-Goal leadership styles have significant positive relationships with diverse work group effectiveness.
Schriesheim, Castro, Zhou, & DeChurch (2006)	Questionnaire	295 state social services agency employees	Good	Main element of theory contradicted because no evidence found that contingent reward negatively moderates the relationship between transformational leadership and outcomes (job satisfaction and performance).
Wofford & Liska (1993)	Meta-analysis	120 studies	Strong	Positive relationship between leader consideration (behaviors aimed at increasing subordinate job satisfaction) and job satisfaction.
Fisher & Edwards (1988)	Meta-analysis	12 studies	Strong	Positive relationship between leader consideration and job satisfaction.
Indvik (1986)	Meta-analysis	48 studies with 11,862 respondents	Strong	Analyzed prior "mixed" results and found overall sufficient support for basic propositions of the theory to warrant continued investigation.

Transactional Leadership Theory

James MacGregor Burns published a major work on leadership in 1978 and introduced two types of leadership. In Transactional Leadership, leaders focus on the relationship between the leader and follower, and in Transformational Leadership, leaders focus on the beliefs, needs, and values of their followers. He defined leadership as "inducing followers to act for certain goals that represent the values and the motivations—the wants and needs, the aspirations and expectations—of *both leaders and followers*" (Burns, 1978, p. 19).

Bass (1985) used the work of Burns and developed a model that included both transactional elements and transformational elements. The theories are discussed separately in this chapter for clarity, but recent scholars have encouraged researchers to use the full range of the theory presented by Bass. Little recent research has been conducted on Transactional Leadership Theory alone (Antonakis & House, 2002). Most research focuses on the combination or additive effect of transformational leadership and transactional leadership.

The Transactional Leadership Theory is based on examining the transactions or exchanges between a leader and his or her subordinates. A **transaction** occurs whenever the leader promises rewards and benefits to subordinates for their fulfilment of agreements and their contributions to goal achievement (Bass, 1990). Ideally, the leader and his or her subordinates agree on what the subordinates need to do to get rewards or to avoid punishment. For example, a rehabilitation services manager might assign a senior therapist the task of documenting a standard of care for a particular intervention as part of the annual performance goals established each year. If the therapist is successful in completing this task according to expected standards, the accomplishment is noted in the therapist's annual performance evaluation; this contributes to the therapist's merit increase (e.g., a raise).

Transactional leadership consists primarily of two factors or sets of strategies—**management by exception** and **contingent rewards** (Bass, 1985). Managing by exception is when leaders follow work performance closely to identify mistakes and intervene or give directions to correct actions during the work process (active management by exception) or wait until work is completed and provide an employee a negative evaluation, hoping that future performance will be improved (passive management by exception). A leader who utilizes managing by exception may fall into the background at times when things are going well and only assert his or her presence when there is a need to intervene and provide corrective criticism.

Contingent rewards are rewards and recognition exchanged for accomplishment of assigned work duties or reaching organizational objectives. The more directly that a reward or recognition is tied to a specific behavior, the more impact the reward is likely to have on promoting the desired behavior. The leader who uses contingent rewards approaches subordinates with an eye toward exchanging one thing for another. For example, a leader may make it clear that high levels of productivity are necessary to be considered for an average or above-average merit increase in salary. Another example of a contingent reward might be recognizing staff with praise and friendly interaction when duties such as documentation are completed in a timely manner and meet expectations for completeness and accuracy but withholding such interaction with staff members who are not performing up to par.

Evidence for the Transactional Leadership Theory

Studies on the impact of the two primary factors identified by the Transactional Leadership Theory (management by exception and use of contingent rewards) have generally shown positive effects on subordinate performance, although it has been hypothesized in some studies that these effects were mediated by other variables such as the trust placed in the leader by subordinates. A review of the literature shows that contingent rewards appear to have been studied more than the behavior of managing by exception, perhaps because it is easier to introduce a new behavior in organizations and measure the direct impact of rewards and recognition.

It is difficult to find recent studies that focus on transactional leadership strategies alone. For example, Zhu, Sosik, Riggio, and Yang (2012) examined the underlying processes through which transformational and active transactional leadership styles affect followers' organizational identification in a survey study. Their findings suggest that transformational leadership compared with active transactional leadership has a stronger positive relationship with followers' psychological empowerment and organizational identification. In their analysis, they stated, "Not surprisingly, these findings, again, show that transformational leadership seems to be a superior and a more effective leadership style than transactional leadership and add new evidence of the augmentation effect of transformational leadership over transactional leadership" (Zhu, Sosik, Riggio, & Yang, 2012, p. 207).

Jung and Avolio (2000) found that transactional leadership had only indirect effects on performance when mediated through followers' trust and value congruence. Other studies, such as that by Gellis (2002), found direct correlations between contingent rewards and measures of leader effectiveness as perceived by subordinate satisfaction and the willingness of subordinates to extend extra effort to achieve organizational

goals. Table 1-4 includes a summary of selected evidence on Transactional Leadership Theory.

Transformational Leadership Theory

Early researchers on Transformational Leadership Theory, including Downton (1973) and Burns (1978), focused on leaders who build more effective relationships with their subordinates and express the importance and values associated with desired outcomes in ways that are easily understood by those they lead. Transformational leaders are seen as distinct from transactional leaders whose leadership actions are not easily explained by the way traditional workplace

TABLE 1-4

Summary of Selected Evidence on Transactional Leadership Theory

Author	Study Type	N (Sample Size)	Level of Evidence	Results
Groves & LaRocca (2011)	Multiple survey	580 leaders and their direct reports from 97 organizations	Fair	Only transformational and not transactional leadership was associated with follower beliefs in the stakeholder view of corporate social responsibility (CSR).
Bono & Judge (2004)	Meta-analysis	26 studies	Strong	Examination of the personality–Transactional leadership relationships indicated that, in general, ratings of transactional leadership behaviors were less strongly related to personality than were ratings of transformational leadership behaviors. Agreeableness was the strongest predictor of contingent reward.
Gellis (2002)	Cross-sectional questionnaire	187 social workers	Good	Contingent rewards (rewards based upon meeting certain conditions) were significantly correlated with the leader outcomes of effectiveness, satisfaction, and extra effort by subordinates.
MacKenzie, Podsakoff, & Rich (2001)	Cross-sectional correlational	477 sales agents	Good	Although both transformational and transactional leader behaviors were effective, transformational behaviors were more effective than transactional behaviors in influencing extra effort.
Jung & Avolio (2000)	Experimental with randomization	194 students	Strong	Indirect effects on followers' performance were mediated through followers' trust and value congruence.

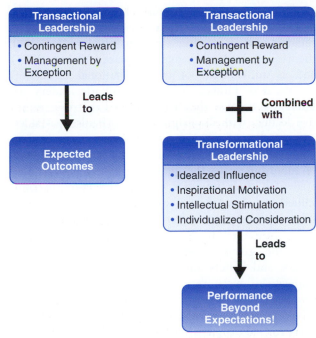

Figure ■ 1-1 Additive Effect of Transformational Leadership.

exchanges had been defined. Burns (1978) and Bass (1985) promoted the view that transactional and transformational leadership are not contradictory styles but instead are complementary, a view that has been widely accepted in most recent research. It is common to find references to the additive effect of transactional leadership when used with transformational leadership. This additive effect can be represented in various ways; however, the take-home message is that when you combine strategies based on transactional leadership with those based on transformational leadership, you can obtain performance that exceeds expectations! This effect is illustrated in Figure 1-1.

Bass and Avolio (1994) initially identified four classifications of behaviors associated with transformational leaders: inspirational motivation, individualized consideration, intellectual stimulation, and idealized influence. They developed a measure (the Multifactor Leadership Questionnaire [MLQ]) for the complementary elements of transactional leadership (e.g., management by exception and contingent rewards) and the primary elements of transformational leadership. Factor analysis indicated that the four characteristics of transformational leaders could be measured

by three scales (Box 1-3) that had acceptable reliabilities; as a result, inspirational motivation and idealized influence were combined into a single construct of "*charisma*."

In summary, the transformational leader can be described as a leader who does the following:

- Articulates a vision of the future that can be shared with peers and subordinates, stimulates their intellect, and pays high attention to individual differences among people (Yammarino & Bass, 1990)
- Realizes that the group's goals are expected to transcend the individuals who comprise it and to result in the achievement of significant change in team effectiveness
- Seeks new ways of working, seeks opportunities in the face of risk, prefers effective answers to efficient answers, and is less likely to support the status quo (Avolio & Bass, 1988)
- Makes tasks and the mission of the work group outcomes appealing to followers, and generates commitment, effort, and greater performance on the part of followers (Conger, 1999)

Evidence for the Transformational Leadership Theory

Research on the impact of the Transformational Leadership Theory has included studies that examine the impact of transformational leader behavior both

---

BOX 1-3

Characteristics of Transformational Leaders

- **Charisma:** Instills pride, faith, and respect in subordinates by transmitting a sense of mission that is effectively articulated
- **Individualized consideration:** Delegates projects to stimulate the learning and growth of employees, coaches and teaches employees, and treats each employee with respect
- **Intellectual stimulation:** Arouses followers to think in new ways and emphasizes problem-solving and the use of reason before acting

on subordinate perception of leader effectiveness and subordinate satisfaction, and on subordinates' objective performance. In general, evidence supports that the transformational leader behaviors of charisma, individualized consideration, and intellectual stimulation promote higher levels of subordinate satisfaction, higher perceptions of leader effectiveness, and, in some cases, higher levels of subordinate performance.

Wang, Oh, Courtright, and Colbert (2011) published a meta-analytic study demonstrating that transformational leadership was positively related to individual-level follower performance, with a stronger relationship for contextual performance than for task performance across most study settings. In addition, transformational leadership was positively related to performance at the team and organization levels. A study by Elenkov (2002) showed that transformational leader behavior had a direct impact on the performance of Russian companies and positively influenced group cohesiveness. In an experimental study, Levy, Cober, and Miller (2002) documented that transformational leader behavior correlated with feedback-seeking behavior of subordinates so that subordinates were more likely to seek feedback on their performance, facilitating behavior change and improved performance. Other studies by McColl-Kennedy and Anderson (2002), Gellis (2002), and Dvir, Eden, Avolio, and Shamir (2002) found positive but varying levels of relationships between transformational leader behavior and subordinate performance, extra effort by subordinates, and perceived satisfaction. Table 1-5 provides a summary of selected evidence on transformational leadership.

Charismatic Leadership Theory

Hearing the word *charisma* brings to mind famous historical leaders such as President John F. Kennedy or Martin Luther King. Charismatic leaders have been portrayed as those who have been able to move followers to overcome great obstacles or to create vision, drive, and enthusiasm among followers in difficult times. John Antonakis (2012, p. 265) stated that, "Charismatic leaders communicate symbolically, use imagery, and are persuasive in communicating a vision that promises a better future. In this way, they create an intense emotional attachment with their followers."

The model of charismatic leadership was first introduced by Max Weber in 1946 and has been referred to both as a framework in which more recent theories of leadership may be placed (Jones, 2003) and as an element of transformational leadership (Jacobsen & House, 2001). Charismatic leaders are influential because they are perceived as strong, effective leaders with appealing visions (Paulsen, Maldonado, Callan, & Ayoko, 2009). Charismatic leaders are those who are successful in tying the self-concepts of subordinates to the goals and experiences associated with their missions so that the latter become valued aspects of the subordinates' self-concepts (Shamir, House, & Arthur, 1993). As a result, subordinates are likely to develop a stronger identification with the group, strengthening behavioral norms, values, and beliefs and enabling a unified effort to achieve the mission's goals. Charismatic leaders also provide a strong vision for the future by providing direction and meaning, communicating high expectations for subordinate performance, and focusing on building the self-confidence and personal development of subordinates.

It has been hypothesized that charismatic leaders transform subordinate self-concepts through at least four mechanisms (Conger, 1999); these mechanisms are listed in Box 1-4. If this hypothesis is accurate, it then may be assumed that leader behaviors that result in subordinates being more likely to examine their values or beliefs or that "access" their self-concepts may correspond with higher perceptions of leader effectiveness; in fact, this has been a focus of recent research (Conger, Kanungo, & Menon, 2000; Paul, Costley, Howell, Dorfman, & Trafimow, 2001).

Far fewer empirical studies are found in the last decade that focus solely on the Charismatic Leadership Theory unrelated to Transformational Leadership Theory; therefore, the primary constructs related to charisma and its associated strategies remain an important element of the literature on leadership (Dinh et al, 2014; Dionne et al, 2014). Dinh et al (2014) completed a search of 10 journals known for publishing leadership research that also have high impact factors and regularly appear at the top of journal ranking lists in the field of organizational behavior. They noted that between 2000 and September 2012, "Neo-charismatic theories, which emerged historically from Charismatic Leadership Theory, received the most attention from scholars in the new millennium (total 294 instances),

---

TABLE 1-5

Summary of Selected Evidence on Transformational Leadership Theory

Author	Study Type	N (Sample Size)	Level of Evidence	Results
Wang, Oh, Courtright, & Colbert (2011)	Meta-analysis	113 primary studies	Strong	Transformational leadership was positively related to individual-level follower performance as well as performance at the team and organization levels. Transformational leadership had an augmentation effect over transactional leadership (contingent reward) in predicting individual-level contextual performance and team-level performance.
Bono & Judge (2004)	Meta-analysis	26 studies	Strong	In a study of personality characteristics and elements of transformational leadership, extraversion was positively linked and neuroticism was negatively linked to all three transformational leadership dimensions.
Elenkov (2002)	Cross-sectional questionnaire	253 senior managers and 498 immediate subordinates	Good	Transformational leadership directly and positively predicted organizational performance of Russian companies. Group cohesiveness was positively related to the ratings of transformational leaders.
Levy, Cober, & Miller (2002)	Experimental laboratory with randomization	132 students	Strong	Transformational leadership style was significantly related to feedback-seeking behavior.
McColl-Kennedy & Anderson (2002)	Cross-sectional questionnaire	121 sales representatives	Good	Significant but indirect effect of transformational leadership on subordinate performance mediated by the emotions of frustration and optimism.
Gellis (2002)	Cross-sectional survey	187 social workers	Good	Using the MLQ, all transformational leadership factors were significantly correlated with leader outcomes of effectiveness, satisfaction, and extra effort.

BOX 1-4

Mechanisms by Which Charismatic Leaders Transform Follower Self-Concepts

- Change the perceptions of the work itself
- Offer a positive future vision
- Develop a strong collective identity among all followers
- Heighten individual and group self-efficacy

with transformational leadership and charismatic leadership, respectively, representing the dominant forms of interest" (p. 39).

As with each of the theories presented in this chapter, specific strategies or leader behaviors can be identified that flow from the theory's primary premises. Examples of the primary strategies most often used by charismatic leaders are summarized in Box 1-5.

- Help subordinates "reframe" behavior and expectations so that they begin to question the status quo by challenging current social conventions
- Engage the self-concept of subordinates so that it becomes cognitively difficult for them to act in ways that do not support the mission of the organization
- Role-model innovation by taking risks and trying new strategies and approaches while maintaining a willingness to change course based upon results
- Use inclusive language (i.e., "we," "us") to build an association between hesitant subordinates and those who are on board with a new vision

Evidence for the Charismatic Leadership Theory

As with other theories of leadership, the empirical evidence related to charisma includes laboratory studies of perceived effectiveness of charismatic leaders or the correlation between charismatic leader behavior and subordinate traits such as openness to accessing their self-concept when responding to a charismatic leader. These studies have sometimes been conducted with college students, who may be responding to tapes of speakers, to trained actors portraying various leadership styles and behaviors, or to those reading a prepared manuscript. These types of studies have inherent limitations associated with their design and biases that may come with utilizing college students as subjects. However, there have been field studies in which superiors or subordinates of leaders rated characteristics of leaders in question, and these ratings were correlated with perceived effectiveness of the leaders. Although there is a range of findings from relatively weak to strong, evidence overall suggests that leaders who show higher levels of charisma are perceived as more effective than less charismatic leaders and may be more effective in contexts in which subordinates are particularly demoralized or where there has been a lack of prior vision or strong leadership.

Although research does indicate a correlation between charismatic behavior and perceived effectiveness, the relationship between charisma and other leadership theories presented in this chapter should be remembered. Charisma has often been associated with historical figures who are especially memorable. The evidence on charismatic leadership should not be mistaken to mean that only leaders with charisma are effective. Rather, the evidence on transformational leadership suggests that strategies such as delegating projects to stimulate the learning and growth of employees, personal coaching of employees, and emphasizing problem-solving and the use of reason before acting are leader behaviors that may be used by those who feel "less outgoing." Table 1-6 summarizes selected evidence on the Charismatic Leadership Theory.

Situational Leadership

As with all other theories, a leadership theory provides an explanation of how or why a particular phenomenon (in this case, leading others) occurs and how that phenomenon might be influenced. Theories are often composed of both general concepts that refer to larger segments of reality and specific concepts that refer to the factors that make up these segments. Thus, the key element of a theory is explanation—that is, giving a plausible account for how something works (Kielhofner, 2004). In contrast, leadership style refers to the elements of leading, such as the ordering and temporal spacing of leadership behaviors, and can be defined as "a pattern of emphases, indexed by the frequency or intensity of specific leadership behaviors or attitudes placed on different leadership functions" (Casimir, 2001). It has been suggested most recently that effective leaders vary their style because different situations may require different styles.

Leaders also must manage the tasks to be accomplished as well as the relationship between themselves and followers. Task behaviors include goal setting, organizing work and workers, establishing deadlines and project timelines, directing work, and providing feedback on the quality of performance (i.e., controlling as a management function). Relationship behaviors include engaging in two way communication,

TABLE 1-6

Summary of Selected Evidence on Charismatic Leadership Theory

Author	Study Type	N (Sample Size)	Level of Evidence	Results
Wilderom, van den Berg, & Wiersma (2012)	Survey	1,214 bank employees	Good	Charisma increased financial performance; however, organizational culture did not.
Sosik, Juzbasich, & Chun (2011)	Comparison of self-, superior, and subordinate ratings	377 upper- and lower-echelon managers	Good	Upper-echelon managers at conventional and postconventional levels of moral reasoning agreed with their subordinates and superiors that their charismatic leadership ratings exceed those in lower management but are lower than those of leaders who possess preconventional moral reasoning.
Sosik, Avolio, & Jung (2002)	Multisource field data	83 managers, 249 subordinates	Good	Charismatic leadership predicted manager and work unit performance.
De Cremer (2002)	Experimental laboratory (with students)	183 students	Strong	Self-sacrificing leaders were perceived as more charismatic and were able to motivate decision-makers to cooperate more.
Paul et al (2001)	Laboratory, read statements in a hypothetical situation	379 students	Good	Charismatic and integrative leadership messages from a leader resulted in higher follower collective self-concept accessibilities than did routinized messages.

listening, providing support, and facilitating leader behavior (Center for Leadership Studies, 2006). Striking the appropriate balance between focus on task behaviors and relationship behaviors can be tricky. At times, a leader may need to exhibit high focus on task and lower focus on relationship, such as when operating under a deadline in which available time is short and the work to be done is clear. At other times, a leader may need high focus on the relationship behaviors and lower focus on task behaviors. This might be appropriate when a follower is struggling with his or her performance and is exhibiting low confidence and the situation allows the leader to take the time to support and mentor the follower. There are also times when task demands or relationship demands are both low or both high.

The Situational Leadership Theory, originally developed by Hersey and Blanchard in 1969, has been refined over the decades; most recently, it was presented by Hersey, Blanchard, and Johnson (2012).

This theory suggests that the most effective leaders are those capable of using different leadership styles and behaviors in response to the demands of the situation and the fluctuating maturity levels of their subordinates. The four styles of leadership identified by this theory are directing, coaching, supporting, and delegating (Box 1-6).

According to the Situational Leadership Theory, the most effective leadership style will depend very much on the readiness of the person being led, or the follower. Leader behaviors include directive (task) behaviors and supportive (relationship) behaviors (Northouse, 2013). The model has been extended to include the follower's developmental level, and the performance readiness levels of followers are presented in Table 1-7. According to the model, the leader's style should be driven by the follower's competence and commitment. Four distinct categories of director and supportive behaviors have also been identified, as illustrated in Table 1-8.

The developmental levels of subordinates are also situational. A subordinate might be generally skilled, confident, and motivated in his or her job, but might drop to a lower developmental level when faced with a task requiring skills that he or she does not possess. For example, a subordinate who normally functions at a higher developmental level when dealing with day-to-day familiar tasks might drop to the lowest level when confronting an ethical issue that overchallenges his or her comfort level and for which he or she lacks the skill and motivation to rise to the challenge.

According to the Center for Leadership Studies (2006), there are three steps to using the Situational Leadership Model:

1. Identify the specific job, task, or activity.
2. Assess current performance readiness of the follower to which the task will be assigned.
3. Match your response to the needs of the task and the follower.

Applying the model to specific situations involves identifying the level of follower readiness (e.g., R1, R2, R3, or R4) and responding with "influence behaviors" that match according to the four quadrants (S1, S2, S3, or S4).

As noted, despite limited empirical support, Situational Leadership Theory continues to be highly popular in the leadership literature and in leadership training programs. Northouse (2013) pointed to four strengths that can explain its continued use and investigation:

1. It is widely used in training programs.
2. It is received as a practical approach that is easily understood.

BOX 1-6

The Four Styles of Situational Leadership

- *Directing* leaders define the roles and tasks of the followers and supervise them closely. Decisions are made by the leader and announced, so communication is largely one way.
- *Coaching* leaders define roles and tasks but seek ideas and suggestions from the followers. Decisions remain the leader's prerogative, but communication is much more two way.
- *Supporting* leaders pass day-to-day decisions, such as task allocation and processes, to the followers. The leader facilitates and takes part in decisions, but control is with the followers.
- *Delegating* leaders are still involved in decision-making and problem-solving, but control is with the followers. The followers decide when and how the leader will be involved.

TABLE 1-7

Performance Readiness Developmental Levels of Followers According to the Situational Leadership Theory

Level	Mix of Competence and Commitment	Follower Characteristics
4	High competence, high commitment (able, confident, and willing)	Experienced at the job and comfortable with his or her own ability to do it well; may even be more skilled than the leader
3	High competence, variable commitment (able but insecure or unwilling)	Experienced and capable but may lack the confidence to go it alone or the motivation to do it well or quickly
2	Some competence, low commitment (unable but confident or willing)	May have some relevant skills but will not be able to do the job without help; task or situation may be new to him or her
1	Low competence, low commitment (unable and insecure or unwilling)	Generally lack the specific skills required for the job at hand and lack any confidence or motivation to tackle it

TABLE 1-8

Four Leadership Styles as Characterized by the Situational Leadership Theory

S1 High Directive–Low Supportive (Directing—high task and low relationship)	Leader is focused on communication and goal achievement, with less use of supportive behaviors. Careful instructions are given about how to do work and accomplish goals.
S2 High Directive–High Supportive (Coaching—high task and high relationship)	Leader is focused on communication regarding achieving goals and meeting the subordinate's socioemotional needs. Encouragement is given and input from the subordinate is sought.
S3 High Supportive and Low Directive (Supporting—high relationship and low task)	Leader is not focused on goals but on behaviors that elicit the subordinate's skills, including listening, praising, asking for input, and giving feedback.
S4 Low Supportive and Low Directive (Delegating—low relationship and low task)	Leader focuses less on task input and support and boosts the subordinate's confidence and motivation. The subordinate has more control over how to do his or her work.

3. It includes a prescriptive approach to improving leader effectiveness.
4. It stresses that there is not one best style of leadership and emphasizes flexibility.

Evidence for the Situational Leadership Theory

There has been limited research to establish the credibility of the Situational Leadership Theory. Thompson and Vecchio (2009, p. 837) noted that, "Although it is among the most widely-known theories in the domain of managerial leadership, Situational Leadership Theory (SLT) remains among the less well-substantiated models. Although popular management textbooks routinely include SLT in their leadership chapter, they seldom critique the absence of empirical support for the theory." The authors provided a review of four empirical studies between 1987 and 2006 and suggested that the model may be more predictive for employees with low or moderate levels of readiness and not as predictive for employees with moderate or higher levels of readiness.

Still, Silverthorne and Wang (2001) found moderate but not statistically consistent support for the hypotheses that highly adaptive leaders are more successful than less adaptive peers and that nonadaptive leaders are generally less successful. They found a clear relationship between being more adaptive in leadership style and higher employee productivity.

Lee-Kelly (2002) examined the leadership style of program managers responsible for projects with changing project boundaries and multiple interfaces with other projects. Observations and conclusions of the study that were useful to the project sponsor as well as the project manager were that they might seek either to select situations that would best match the project manager's inclination or style or to avoid projects that were likely to present him or her with situations that were counter to his or her preferred style.

The applicability of the Situational Leadership Theory to leaders from different cultures has been questioned because managers in some cultures may wish to avoid a particular leadership style. This is especially true of the directive style, even after managers received training and stated that they saw the relevance and usefulness of all four leadership styles. It should also be noted that several authors have questioned the internal consistency of concepts included in the Situational Leadership Theory (Avery & Ryan, 2002).

A summary of selected evidence on Situational Leadership Theory is presented in Table 1-9.

Servant Leadership

Servant leadership was introduced by Robert Greenleaf in his text *The Servant as Leader* in 1970 and

TABLE 1-9

Summary of Selected Evidence on Situational Leadership Theory

Author	Study Type	N (Sample Size)	Level of Evidence	Results
Rabarison, Ingram, & Holsinger (2013)	Case study	1 public health agency	Weak	Situational Leadership Theory was successfully applied to guide a public health agency through the process of preparing for accreditation.
Thompson & Vecchio (2009)	Self- and subordinate ratings and focus groups	357 subordinates and 80 supervisors in 8 Norwegian financial firms	Fair	In general, support was not found for the original, revised, or a proposed model of Situational Leadership Theory.
Vecchio, Bullis, & Brazil (2006)	Questionnaires	860 military cadets	Good	Results did not yield clear evidence of a predicted interaction among leader style and follower attributes, suggesting the theory may have little practical utility.
York (2003)	Cross-sectional survey	250 social workers in leadership and clinical positions	Good	Found support for propositions of the theory related to "delegation" but not to "support"; these differences were not related to performance ratings, suggesting only partial support of the theory.
Avery & Ryan (2002)	Cross-sectional survey	17 trainees in situational leadership	Good	Subjects did not find it difficult to assess subordinate developmental level, found situational leadership easy to apply, but were more apt to be supportive and wished to avoid directive leadership.
Silverthorne & Wang (2001)	Cross-sectional questionnaire	79 managers and 234 subordinates	Good	The more adaptive the leaders were in style, the more productive the organization was likely to be.

has gained increasing attention in the last decade (Greenleaf, 1970). Until recently, however, little empirical research was published in peer-reviewed journals on this concept, and writings were more prescriptive in describing how leaders "should be" than descriptive in describing what servant leadership is in practice (Northouse, 2013). For example, Parris and Peachey (2013) completed a systematic literature review of 39 studies and papers on servant leadership. They noted that over 20 of these papers present narrative examples of how servant leadership was being used in organizational settings and that the primary limitation of much of the servant leadership literature is that it is anecdotal in nature instead of empirical.

The philosophical basis of servant leadership has been described as serving others first rather than leading others first and to act as a servant and a steward rather than a leader or owner (Sendjaya & Sarros, 2002). According to Greenleaf, servant leaders are those who put the needs and interests of others above their own (Greenleaf, 1977). The servant leader is "primus inter pares" (i.e., first among equals); the leader does not use his or her power to get things done but tries to persuade and convince staff. A servant leader may be thought of as operating within the role of a steward who holds the organization in trust (Reinke, 2004).

Greenleaf (1970, p. 15) defined servant leadership as follows:

> *Servant leadership begins with the natural feeling that one wants to serve, to serve first. Then conscious choice brings one to aspire to lead. The difference manifests itself in the care taken by the servant—first to make sure that other people's highest priority needs are being served. The best test is: do those served grow as persons; do they while being served, become healthier, wiser, freer, more autonomous, more likely themselves to become servants? And, what is the effect on the least privileged in society? Will they benefit, or at least not further be harmed?*

Smith, Montagno, and Kuzemenko (2004) noted that because of the similarity of some of the theoretical basis for servant leadership and transformational leadership, what each theory contributes on its own can be questioned. They suggest that servant leaders' motivation to lead arises from an underlying attitude of egalitarianism where all organizational members are of equal value and create organizational cultures that are focused on the members' personal growth. The transformational leader is motivated by "a sense of mission to recreate the organization to survive in a challenging environment" (p. 86). For the transformational leader, individual development must be related to the organization's success in the external environment.

In the last 2 decades, there have been a number of attempts to further delineate and define the tenants of Servant Leadership Theory, including the characteristics of a servant leader. Larry Spears (2002) listed 10 characteristics that represent the behavior of a servant leader: (1) listening, (2) empathy, (3) healing, (4) awareness, (5) persuasion, (6) conceptualization, (7) foresight, (8) stewardship, (9) commitment, and (10) building community. Van Dierendonck (2011, p. 1232) noted that "Regretfully, Spears never took his characteristics to the next step by formulating a model that differentiates between the intrapersonal aspects, interpersonal aspects, and outcomes of servant leadership." Van Dierendonck identified six key characteristics of servant leadership behavior as experienced by followers. Servant-leaders (1) empower and develop people, (2) show humility, (3) are authentic, (4) accept people for who they are, (5) provide direction, and (6) are stewards who work for the good of the whole.

A number of scholars have developed various measures on Servant Leadership Theory over the years (Barbuto & Wheeler, 2006; Dennis & Bocarnea, 2005; Laub, 1999; Liden, Wayne, Zhao, & Henderson, 2008; Page & Wong, 2000; Sendjaya, Sarros & Santora, 2008; Van Dierendonck, 2011) but they failed to develop comprehensive measures, because each of these instruments was shown to reflect only some of the six key characteristics of servant leaders. Recently Van Dierendonck and Nuijten (2011) found more success in developing a scale with solid internal consistency. The Servant Leadership Survey (SLS) includes 30 items in eight dimensions: (1) standing back, (2) forgiveness, (3) courage, (4) empowerment, (5) accountability, (6) authenticity, (7) humility, and (8) stewardship. Reed, Vidaver-Cohen, and Colwell (2011) also introduced a scale, noting that although a number of scales to measure servant leadership have appeared in the literature, none has focused specifically on the conduct of top executives. They identified 55 items to measure key dimensions of servant leadership, modifying these items to target top executive behavior specifically. Through confirmatory factor analysis, they identified a second-order factor of executive servant leadership associated with five first-order factors, reflecting essential servant leadership attributes identified originally by Greenleaf. The five first-order factors were (1) interpersonal support, (2) building community, (3) altruism, (4) egalitarianism, and (5) moral integrity. The focus of this instrument on executive leaders appears unique among the instruments developed thus far.

Evidence on Servant Leadership

As discussed in the introduction to this theory, there has been a lack of solid empirical evidence to date. Van Dierendonck (2011) noted that despite its introduction 4 decades ago and empirical studies that started more than 10 years ago, there is still no consensus about a definition and theoretical framework of servant leadership. More recently, studies have begun to be published examining servant leadership across cultures and examining servant leadership as a moderating factor on process and goal clarity (Hu & Liden, 2011; Mittal & Dorfman, 2012). Parolini, Patterson, and Winston (2009) published a study confirming that servant leaders are perceived as more concerned with the individual than with the organization. Systematic

TABLE 1-10

Summary of Selected Evidence on Servant Leadership Theory

Author	Study Type	N (Sample Size)	Level of Evidence	Results
Parris & Peachey (2013)	Systematic literature review	39 studies	Good	The synthesis of these empirical studies revealed: (a) there is no consensus on the definition of servant leadership; (b) Servant Leadership Theory is being investigated across a variety of contexts, cultures, and themes; (c) researchers are using multiple measures to explore servant leadership; and (d) servant leadership is a viable leadership theory that helps organizations and improves the well-being of followers.
Mittal & Dorfman (2012)	Survey completion via the GLOBE research program	12,681 cases spread across 59 societies	Good	Findings indicate that servant leadership is perceived as important for effective leadership in all societies. Although different cultures differ in the degree of their endorsement of four component dimensions of servant leadership, the moral integrity dimension of servant leadership seems to be equally endorsed as important in all cultures.
Hu & Liden (2011)	Rating by team members on six scales	304 employees of Chinese banks working on seven teams	Good	Servant leadership moderated the relationships between both goal and process clarity and team potency, such that the positive relationships between both goal and process clarity and team potency were stronger in the presence of servant leadership.
Parolini, Patterson, & Winston (2009)	Completion of 19 semantic scales	511 persons working in different types of organizations	Good	Compared with transformational leaders, servant leaders are perceived as focusing more on the needs of the individual; their allegiance lies more with the individual than with the organization, whereas the opposite indeed holds for transformational leaders.

reviews continue to call for more focused empirical research to be conducted (Table 1-10).

Gender and Leadership

Considerable study exists of the relationship between gender, leadership style, and perceived leadership effectiveness. Although not related to any specific theory of leadership, this body of evidence may be of particular interest to new practitioners in the profession of occupational therapy, a profession still dominated by women. In its 2010 Member Compensation Survey, AOTA noted that the ratio of women to men in occupational therapy positions has remained substantially unchanged since 1990, with 91.9% of the membership being women and 8.1% men for both occupational therapists (OTs) and occupational therapy assistants (OTAs) (AOTA, 2010).

Some have hypothesized that, because of the interaction between role expectations of leaders in organizations and gender roles in society, men and women may be perceived differently even when using the same style or leadership approach, and there is some evidence supporting this belief. Substantial evidence produced more than 2 decades ago suggests that when women are given the opportunity to lead, they tend to employ leadership styles similar to those used by men (Eagly & Johnson, 1990). Van Engen, van der Leeden, and Willemsen (2011, p. 13) completed a meta-analysis and found that "there is no justification for claims that female leaders are underrepresented in a leadership role because they lack appropriate leadership styles."

Various leadership styles and behaviors have been characterized as being associated with masculine or feminine characteristics. Koenig, Eagly, Mitchell, and Ristikari (2011) completed a meta-analysis examining three common research paradigms related to gender and leadership (e.g., think manager–think male paradigm, agency-communion paradigm, and masculinity-femininity paradigm). They concluded that, "All three paradigms showed that stereotypes of leaders are decidedly masculine. Specifically, people viewed leaders as quite similar to men but not very similar to women, as more agentic than communal, and as more masculine than feminine" (Koenig et al, 2011, p. 634). The stereotypical feminine leadership style has been characterized by nurturing of interpersonal relationships, whereas the stereotypical male leadership style has been characterized by a focus on task completion and goal attainment (Eagly & Johannesen-Schmidt, 2001; van Engen et al, 2001). These stereotypes may be explained by examining research related to how leadership traits have been "gendered" (associated with the male or female gender). Research has shown that traditional managerial roles are gendered as masculine, meaning that characteristics deemed necessary to be a successful manager have thus far been stereotypically associated with men (Kawakami, White, & Langer, 2000). If women demonstrate characteristics associated with strong leadership and traits considered to be stereotypically male, they may be seen as performing outside of socially defined female roles and be viewed in a negative manner (Neubert & Palmer, 2004).

Kawakami et al (2000) noted that women can use leader behaviors that have been stereotyped as masculine while still being perceived as genuine and not as incongruent with gender expectations. Their suggestion is that women can increase the extent to which they are perceived as effective leaders by using what they refer to as **mindfulness.** Mindfulness refers to approaching communication in a thoughtful and conscious manner in each interaction and avoiding the appearance that communication and leader behavior have become routine. By assuming a conscious approach to communication and behavior, it is assumed that others will perceive the speaker or leader as acting in a genuine and novel way, so less attention will be paid to whether behavior is consistent with behaviors stereotypically associated with the speaker's gender. Although it is unfortunate, in today's world in which our standards and expectations have been influenced primarily by male role models, a female leader may have to exert effort beyond that of her male counterparts to be conscious of how she is perceived when demonstrating the same behavior. Initial research suggests that a mindful approach may indeed allow a woman to use a wider range of leader behaviors while remaining effective.

Vinkenburg, van Engen, Eagly, and Johannesen-Schmidt (2011) examined whether gender stereotypes about the transformational, transactional, and laissez-faire leadership styles constitute an advantage or an impediment for women's access to leadership positions in organizations. Inspirational motivation was perceived as more important for men than women and especially important for promotion to chief executive officer (CEO). In contrast, individualized consideration was perceived as more important for women than men and especially important for promotion to senior management. Consistent with these stereotypical beliefs about leadership, women interested in promotion may be well advised to blend individualized consideration and inspirational motivation behaviors.

Stereotypes of male and female leadership styles have been challenged, however, since the feminist movement began and particularly in the last 3 decades as the role of women in the workforce has continued to change and women have become more visible in leadership roles in the full range of contexts in Western society. Notable female leaders of the past 2 decades include Supreme Court Justices Sandra Day O'Connor and Ruth Bader Ginsberg; Secretaries of State Hillary Clinton, Condoleeza Rice, and Madeline Albright; and German Chancellor Angela Merkel, who all assumed leadership roles in labor functions not typically associated with women. In 2012, Hillary Clinton made a now famous observation in her concession speech at the end of her bid to become the president of the United States about the "glass ceiling" that women have faced, stating, "Although we weren't able to shatter that highest, hardest glass ceiling this time, it's got about 18 million cracks in it."

Indeed, women are making substantial progress breaking the glass ceiling and closing the gender gap in leadership. For example, the American College of Health Care Executives noted in 2006 that "In contrast to the earlier reports, women appear to have moved up the organizational hierarchy within their current firms at nearly the same rate that men have." Comparing one's first job to current job in the same employing firm showed that 30% of men and 25% of women were promoted from vice president to chief operating officer (COO) or CEO positions. About 20% of both men and women who began as COOs/senior vice presidents/associate administrators were in CEO positions in 2006 (American College of Health Care Executives, 2006). In November 2012, a record 98 women—20 in the Senate and 78 in the House—took their place in the new 113th Congress (Parker, 2013). In 2013, women held 4.2% of *Fortune 500* CEO positions and 4.6% of Fortune 1000 CEO positions according to Catalyst, a nonprofit organization with a mission of expanding opportunities for women (Catalyst, 2013).

Ely, Ibarra, and Kolb (2011, p. 475) concluded that "organizational research on the causes of women's persistent underrepresentation in leadership positions has thus shifted away from a focus on actors' intentional efforts to exclude women to consideration of so-called second-generation forms of gender bias, the powerful yet often invisible barriers to women's advancement that arise from cultural beliefs about gender, as well as workplace structures, practices, and patterns of interaction that inadvertently favor men."

Ely et al (2011) provided suggestions for effective strategies for women and for leadership development for women. These strategies include:

1. Participate in **360-degree feedback** and coaching programs.
2. Develop active leadership networks.
3. Become skilled in everyday negotiation.
4. Develop the capacity to effectively lead change.
5. Successfully manage career transitions by shedding old identities and developing new ones that are more fitting for a new role.

As we move forward in the 21st century, researchers will need to continue to examine the assumption that leader behaviors can be either masculine or feminine in the context of changing gender roles, especially the worker role, in our society.

Evidence on Leadership and Gender

Evidence on gender and leadership presents some contradictions. Koenig, Eagly, Mitchell, and Ristikari (2011) concluded in their meta-analysis that three historical research paradigms showed that stereotypes of leaders are decidedly masculine. As noted earlier, people often view "leaders as quite similar to men but not very similar to women, as more agentic than communal, and as more masculine than feminine" (Koenig, et al, 2011, p. 634). Vinkenburg, van Engen, Eagly, and Johannesen-Schmidt (2011) also noted results consistent with stereotypical beliefs about leadership and suggested that women interested in promotion may be well advised to blend individualized consideration and inspirational motivation behaviors found in the Transformational Leadership Theory. Kawakami et al (2000) noted that the apparent contradictions in evidence may place female leaders in what they describe as a "double bind." The double bind is that effective leadership has been associated with characteristics that are stereotypically associated with maleness, yet women acting outside of the stereotypical feminine gender role have often been evaluated unfavorably. Billing and Alvesson (2000) noted that there is considerable evidence, including comparative studies of men and women, concluding that there are modest if any differences between male and female leaders who are perceived as effective. The one noted difference was in an earlier study by Eagly and Johnson (1990) in which some support for differences is found, with women being more participation oriented than men.

Although the research conducted to date does appear to support the notion that if women adopt behaviors that are stereotypically perceived as masculine, they may be perceived as less effective, we must also examine the context of this evidence. Much of the evidence suggesting that women should adopt leader behaviors that are different from those effective for men was produced during the same time frame during which dramatic shifts in the roles of women in the workplace and in our larger society occurred. Although most would likely agree that workplace discrimination based on gender and concepts such as a glass ceiling for women in many fields are still relevant, progress has been made. There is no doubt that the roles of women in the workforce and in other public leadership arenas, including politics, is evolving, albeit slowly. For example, according to the U.S. Census Bureau (2011), the gap between wages earned by men and women for full-time work narrowed as we approached the new millennium, with the female-to-male earnings ratio increasing from approximately 60% in 1960 to 77% in 2011 (DeNavas-Walt, Proctor, & Smith,

2012). Still, the Center for American Progress reported that progress in closing the income gap may have stalled. In 2010, women who worked full-time, year round, still only earned 77% of what men earned. The median earnings for women were $36,931 compared with $47,715 for men, and neither real median earnings nor the female-to-male earnings ratio has increased since 2009 (U.S. Census Bureau, 2011).

Evidence on gender and leadership may begin to show different results over the next decades as women achieve true equality in the workplace. Table 1-11 provides a summary of selected evidence on gender and leadership.

TABLE 1-11

Summary of Selected Evidence on Gender and Leadership

Author	Study Type	N (Sample Size)	Level of Evidence	Results
Koenig, Eagly, Mitchell, & Ristikari (2011)	Meta-analysis	40, 22, and 7 studies related to three research paradigms	Strong	All three paradigms showed that stereotypes of leaders are decidedly masculine and more agentic than communal.
Vinkenburg, van Engen, Eagly, & Johannesen-Schmidt (2011)	2 studies using a questionnaire	271 randomly assigned business travellers	Fair	Consistent with stereotypical beliefs about leadership, women interested in promotion may be well advised to blend individualized consideration and inspirational motivation behaviors.
Kawakami et al (2000)	Laboratory, view of videotape	42 male business leaders	Good	Male businessmen perceived a woman who chose a "mindfully adopted" style typically associated with men to be a better leader than a woman who did not.
Eagly, Karau, & Makhijani (1995)	Meta-analysis	76 studies	Strong	Men were substantially more likely than women to be assessed as effective in male-dominated contexts (e.g., military), but women were moderately more likely to be assessed as effective in contexts including education, government, and service domains.
Eagly, Makhijani, & Klonsky (1992)	Meta-analysis	114 studies	Strong	Female leaders who were perceived as having stereotypically masculine styles were less positively evaluated and seen as more threatening than male leaders.

Real-Life Solutions

Christi visited her local university library and conducted a review of the theories and evidence related to leadership. The readings and the evidence clarified several issues for her. Based on her review of the literature, Christi decided that with conscious effort and perhaps some training and experience, she could improve her leadership skills and abilities and could take actions to be perceived as a more effective leader. Using what she had learned by reviewing the evidence, Christi decided to accept the position of department director and to do the following:

- Implement strategies based on multiple theories, because evidence provides at least partial support for each of the theories of leadership, suggesting that the use of more than one leadership approach may be effective.

- Structure work assignments and tasks to establish a clear connection between performance and rewards to influence subordinates' perceptions of work goals and make the paths to goal attainment clearer.

- Combine the use of transactions to set expectations and establish the relationships between behavior and reward and punishment with methods such as delegating projects to stimulate the growth of employees.

- Help subordinates reframe behavior and expectations by modeling innovation, taking risks, trying new strategies and approaches, and using inclusive language to build an association with a new vision.

- Adopting a "mindful" approach to communication, especially in times of high stress or conflict, but not avoiding any specific behavior just because it has typically been stereotyped as masculine.

Christi also decided to continue to closely observe other leaders in her organization to identify the strategies that they adopted in different situations and how others in the organization perceived these behaviors. After her review of the theories and evidence on leadership, Christi felt more encouraged about taking on the new challenge of accepting the position as director of occupational therapy.

Chapter Summary

This chapter has provided an introduction to leadership, including a definition of leadership and the relationship between leadership and management. The development of leadership theory was reviewed and six common theories of leadership were discussed. Evidence on each of the theories of leadership was presented, as were methods for translating the tenets of each theory into behavior. Because of the large percentage of women within the profession of occupational therapy and because of the dramatic shift in women's roles in the workplace, evidence related to gender and leadership was also reviewed.

Although the evidence on each of the leadership theories continues to evolve, it seems clear that leaders who adopt behaviors based on multiple theories and who choose strategies and behaviors to fit the situation may be most effective. More importantly, the limited amount of research on personality traits of effective leaders in the last few decades suggests that effective leadership behavior can be adopted or learned and that novice managers would benefit from conscious evaluation of their leadership skills in order to pursue strategies for becoming more effective leaders.

Study Questions

1. **One often-cited difference between leadership and management mentioned in this chapter is:**
   a. Leaders are born, whereas managers are made.
   b. Leaders focus on strategic change, whereas managers focus on the "status quo."
   c. Leadership has been researched in depth, whereas little research exists on management.

d. Leadership skills are a distinct set of skills used at particular times, whereas management skills are broad skills used in almost every situation.

2. **Which of the following would be most accurate in regard to current thinking about the relationships between human traits and leadership effectiveness?**

    a. Human traits are predetermined at birth and there is little ability to change them as we develop.
    b. Trait Theory is a new development in leadership research; although there is limited empirical evidence, the research to date appears promising as an explanation for leader effectiveness.
    c. Traits may help us understand how a particular leader might be perceived, but there is little recent research to validate Trait Theory as effective in linking leaders with leadership outcomes.
    d. The connection between traits and leader outcomes has only been shown to have a strong correlation in strategies related to Transactional Leadership Theory.

3. **Which of the following pairs includes two theories of leadership that could both be categorized as *supervisory* theories of leadership?**

    a. Path-Goal Theory of Leadership and Servant Leadership Theory
    b. Transactional Leadership Theory and Charismatic Leadership Theory
    c. Transformational Leadership Theory and Transactional Leadership Theory
    d. Path-Goal Theory of Leadership and Transactional Leadership Theory

4. **A theory of leadership that focuses on identifying the relationship between task characteristics and employee readiness and matching a supervisory response is best called:**

    a. Servant Leadership Theory.
    b. Path-Goal Theory of Leadership.
    c. Transformational Leadership Theory.
    d. Situational Leadership Theory.

5. **Two leadership theories that were developed separately but are recognized as most effective when they are combined are:**

    a. Transactional Leadership Theory and Transformational Leadership Theory.
    b. Situational Leadership Theory and Servant Leadership Theory.
    c. Charismatic Leadership Theory and Servant Leadership Theory.
    d. Path-Goal Leadership Theory and Situational Leadership Theory.

6. **In regard to the additive effect of transformational leadership and transactional leadership, which of the following is generally accepted as true?**

    a. Transactional leadership and transformational leadership are not contradictory styles but instead are complementary and can be used together.
    b. The impact of transformational leadership on follower satisfaction is limited and only shown to occur when strategies are added to transactional leadership strategies.
    c. There is no additive effect, as transformational leadership and transactional leadership have been proven to be contradictory in nature.
    d. There is no relationship between transformational leadership and transactional leadership because one is a strategic approach and the other is a supervisory approach.

7. **When comparing Servant Leadership Theory and Transformational Leadership Theory, which of the following best describes the motivation of the leaders?**

    a. Transformational leaders are concerned about work groups only and typically do not consider the development of the individual, whereas servant leaders focus only on the individual.
    b. Servant leaders tend to see all persons as equal and valued, whereas transformational leaders value individuals but more in relation to helping the organization succeed.
    c. Servant leaders and transformational leaders are both thought to have a strong orientation toward the individual rather than consideration of the organization's success.

d. Servant leaders and transformational leaders are both thought to have a strong orientation toward the success of the organization rather than toward the individual.

8. **One accurate summary statement about what we know about the evidence on gender and leadership would be:**

   a. Women are typically perceived as more effective leaders than men as long as they present themselves as stereotypically female.
   b. Men have consistently shown to be more effective leaders than women.
   c. Men and women are perceived as more effective as leaders when the approaches they use match their presentation as more "masculine" or "feminine" as perceived by followers.
   d. Evidence on gender and leadership has established that there is essentially no difference in how male and female leaders are perceived.

Resources for Learning More About Leadership

Journals That Often Address Leadership

The Leadership Quarterly

http://www.journals.elsevier.com/
the-leadership-quarterly/

This journal brings together a focus on leadership for scholars, consultants, practicing managers, executives, and administrators, as well as those numerous university faculty members across the world who teach leadership as a college course. It provides timely publication of leadership research and applications and has a global reach. It also focuses on yearly reviews of a broad range of leadership topics on a rotating basis and emphasizes cutting-edge areas through special issues.

Journal of Management Development

http://www.emeraldgrouppublishing.com/products/
journals/author_guidelines.htm?id=jmd

The *Journal of Management Development* covers a broad range of topics in its field, including competence-based management development, developing leadership skills, developing women for management, global management, the new technology of management development, team building, organizational development and change, and performance appraisal.

Journal of Leadership and Organizational Studies

http://jlo.sagepub.com

The *Journal of Leadership and Organizational Studies* is published quarterly for all who teach, study, or practice leadership. The journal is intended as a forum for the expression of current thought and research (although not for the presentation of empirical research data). The stated goal of the journal is to bring together a recurring reference work designed to appeal to a national base of individuals seeking the latest materials, thoughts, sources, and networking opportunities in leadership education.

Journal of Organizational Behavior

http://www.wiley.com/WileyCDA/WileyTitle/
productCd-JOB.html

The *Journal of Organizational Behavior* is dedicated to the study of how organizations impact people and how people shape organizations. It publishes information on worldwide work-related issues, including leadership and leadership development. The editorial staff encourages both theoretical and empirical inquiry from a diversity of perspectives, methods, and national cultures.

Journal of Applied Psychology

http://www.apa.org/journals/apl.html

The *Journal of Applied Psychology*, published by the American Psychological Association (APA), emphasizes the publication of original investigations that contribute new knowledge and understanding to fields of applied psychology. The journal's focus is on empirical and theoretical investigations of interest to psychologists doing research that fosters an understanding of the psychological and behavioral phenomena of individuals, groups, or organizations in settings such as education and training, business, government, health, or service institutions, and that may be in the private or public sector, or for-profit or nonprofit.

Associations That Are Concerned With Leadership

The American Society of Association Executives

http://www.asaenet.org/

The American Society of Association Executives, known as the "association of associations," is considered the advocate for the nonprofit sector. The primary mission of this association is to advance the value of voluntary associations to society and to support the professionalism of the individuals who lead them.

The Center for Creative Leadership

http://www.ccl.org/

The mission of the Center for Creative Leadership is to advance the understanding, practice, and development of leadership for the benefit of society worldwide. The center's stated role is to help address the leadership component of both business and organizational challenges. The center was founded 30 years ago in Greensboro, North Carolina, and is today one of the largest institutions in the world focusing solely on leadership. It seeks to generate and disseminate knowledge about leadership and leadership development.

Useful Websites on Leadership

Robert K. Greenleaf Center for Servant Leadership

www.Greenleaf.org

The Robert K. Greenleaf Center for Servant Leadership is an international nonprofit organization that serves individuals and organizations seeking to be better servant leaders. The center's website provides descriptions of those services and other resources on servant leadership.

Psychology.Com

http://psychology.about.com/cs/lead/

Resource links include leadership article assessment tools, studies, styles, theory, training and consulting services, development programs, book reviews, student leadership, and world-famous leaders.

Reference List

American College of Health Care Executives. (2006). *A comparison of the career attainments of men and women healthcare executives December, 2006.* Retrieved from http://www.ache.org/pubs/research/gender_study_full_report.pdf

American Occupational Therapy Association. (2010). *Occupational therapy compensation and workforce study.* Bethesda, MD: Author.

American Occupational Therapy Association. (2014). *Advance your career.* Retrieved from http://www.aota.org/Education-Careers/Advance-Career.aspx

Antonakis, J. (2012). *The nature of leadership.* Thousand Oaks, CA: Sage Publications, Inc.

Antonakis, J., & House, R. (2002). An analysis of the full-range leadership theory: The way forward. In B. J. Avolio & F. J. Yammarino (Eds.), *Transformational and charismatic leadership: The road ahead* (pp. 3–34). Amsterdam, The Netherlands: JAI.

Avery, J. C., & Ryan, J. (2002). Applying situational leadership in Australia. *Journal of Management Development, 21,* 242–262.

Avolio, B. J., & Bass, B. M. (1988). Transformational leadership, charisma and beyond. In J. G. Hunt, B. R. Baglia, H. P. Dachler, & C. A. Schriesheim (Eds.), *Emerging leadership vistas* (pp. 185–201). Lexington, MA: Lexington Books.

Avolio, B. J., Walumbwa, F. O., & Weber, T. J. (2009). Leadership: Current theories, research, and future directions. *Annual Review of Psychology, 60,* 421–449.

Ayman, R., & Adams, S. (2012). Contingencies, context, situation and leadership. In D. V. Day & John Antonakis, *The nature of leadership* (2nd ed., pp. 218–255). Thousand Oaks, CA: Sage Publications, Inc.

Barbuto, J. E., & Wheeler, D. W. (2006). Scale development and construct clarification of servant leadership. *Group & Organization Management, 31*(3), 300–326.

Bass, B. (1985). *Leadership and performance beyond expectations.* New York, NY: Free Press.

Bass, B. M. (1990). *Transformational leadership: Theory, research, and managerial applications.* New York, NY: Free Press.

Bass, B. M., & Avolio, B. J. (1994). *Improving organizational effectiveness through transformational leadership.* Thousand Oaks, CA: Sage.

Beech, M. (2002). Leaders of managers: The drive for effective leadership. *Nursing Standard, 16,* 35–36.

Bennis, W. G., & Nanus, B. (1985). *Leaders: The strategies for taking charge.* New York, NY: Harper & Row.

Billing, Y. D., & Alvesson, M. (2000). Questioning the notion of feminine leadership: A critical perspective on the gender labeling of leadership. *Gender, Work and Organization, 7,* 144–157.

Boal, K. B., & Hooijberg, R. (2001). Strategic leadership research: Moving on. *Leadership Quarterly, 11*, 515–549.

Bono, J. E., & Judge, T. A. (2004). Personality and transformational and transactional leadership: A meta-analysis. *Journal of Applied Psychology, 89*(5), 901–910.

Burns, J. M. (1978). *Leadership*. New York, NY: Harper & Row.

Bush, G.W. (2010). *Decision points*. New York, NY: Broadway Paperbacks.

Carlyle, T. (1888). *On heroes, hero-worship and the heroic in history*. New York, NY: Fredrick A. Stokes & Brother.

Casimir, G. (2001). Combinative aspects of leadership style: The ordering and temporal spacing of leadership behaviors. *Leadership Quarterly, 12*, 245–278.

Catalyst. (2013). *Women CEOs of the Fortune 1000*. Retrieved from http://www.catalyst.org/knowledge/women-ceos-fortune-1000

Center for Leadership Studies. (2006). Situational leadership: The core. In *Participant workbook* (Version 3.0). Escondido, CA: Author.

Clinton, B. (2004). *My life*. New York, NY: Alfred A. Knopf Publisher.

Conger, J. A. (1999). Charismatic and transformational leadership in organizations: An insider's perspective on these developing streams of research. *Leadership Quarterly, 10*, 145–169.

Conger, J. A., Kanungo, R. N., & Menon, S. T. (2000). Charismatic leadership and follower effects. *Journal of Organizational Behavior, 21*, 747–767.

Day, D. V. (2001). Leadership development: A review in context. *Leadership Quarterly, 11*, 581–613.

De Cremer, D. (2002). Charismatic leadership and cooperation in social dilemmas: A matter of transforming motives? *Journal of Applied Social Psychology, 32*, 997–1016.

DeNavas-Walt, C., Proctor, B. D., & Smith, J. C. (2012). Income, poverty, and health insurance coverage in the United States: 2011 (U.S. Census Current Population Report P60-243). Washington, DC: U.S. Government Printing Office.

Dennis, R. S., & Bocarnea, M. (2005). Development of the servant leadership assessment instrument. *Leadership & Organization Development Journal, 26*(8), 600–615.

Dinh, J. E., Lord, R. G., Gardner, W. L., Meuser, J. D., Liden, R. C., & Hu, J. (2014). Leadership theory and research in the new millennium: Current theoretical trends and changing perspectives. *Leadership Quarterly, 25*, 36–62.

Dionne, S. D., Gupta, A., Sotak, K. L., Shirreffs, K. A., Serban, A., Hao, C., . . . Yammarino, F. J. (2014). A 25-year perspective on levels of analysis in leadership research. *Leadership Quarterly, 25*(1), 6–35.

Dixon, M. L., & Hart, L. K. (2010). The impact of Path-Goal Leadership styles on work group effectiveness and turnover intention. *Journal of Managerial Issues, 22*(1), 52–69.

Downton, J. V. (1973). *Rebel leadership: Commitment and charisma in a revolutionary process*. New York, NY: Free Press.

Dunbar, S. B. (2009). *An occupational therapy perspective on leadership: Theoretical and practical dimensions*. Thorofare, NJ: Slack.

Dvir, T., Eden, D., Avolio, B. J., & Shamir, B. (2002). Impact of transformational leadership on follower development and performance: A field experiment. *Academy of Management Journal, 45*, 735–744.

Eagly, A. H., & Johannesen-Schmidt, M. C. (2001). The leadership styles of women and men. *Journal of Social Issues, 57*, 781–797.

Eagly, A. H., & Johnson, B. T. (1990). Gender and leadership style: A meta-analysis. *Psychological Bulletin, 108*, 233–256.

Eagly, A. H., Karau, S. J., & Makhijani, M. G. (1995). Gender and the effectiveness of leaders: A meta-analysis. *Psychological Bulletin, 117*, 125–145.

Eagly, A. H., Makhijani, M., & Klonsky, B. (1992). Gender and the evaluation of leaders: A meta-analysis. *Psychological Bulletin, 111*, 3–22.

Elenkov, D. S. (2002). Effects of leadership on organizational performance in Russian companies. *Journal of Business Research, 55*, 467–480.

Ely, R. J., Ibarra, H., & Kolb, D. (2011). Taking gender into account: Theory and design for women's leadership development programs. *Academy of Management Learning & Education, 10*, 474–493.

Fisher, A. C., & Edwards, I. E. (1988). Consideration and initiating structure and their relationships with leader effectiveness: A meta-analysis. In *Best papers: Proceedings of the Academy of Management meeting* (pp. 201–205). Briarcliff Manor, NY: Academy of Management.

Fleming-Castaldy, R. P., & Patro, J. (2012). Leadership in occupational therapy: Self-perceptions of occupational therapy managers. *Occupational Therapy in Health Care, 26*(2–3), 187–202.

Gellis, Z. D. (2002). Social work perceptions of transformational and transactional leadership in health care. *Social Work Research, 25*, 17–26.

Gerber, R., & Burns, J. M. (2002). *Leadership the Eleanor Roosevelt way: Strategies from the first lady of courage*. Upper Saddle River, NJ: Prentice Hall.

Gilkeson, G. E. (1997). *Occupational therapy leadership: Marketing yourself, your profession, and your organization*. Philadelphia, PA: F.A. Davis.

Greenleaf, R. K. (1970). *The servant as leader*. Westfield, IN: The Greenleaf Center for Servant Leadership.

Greenleaf, R. K. (1977). *Servant leadership: A journey into the nature of legitimate power and greatness*. New York, NY: Paulist Press.

Grohar-Murray, M. E., & Dicroce, H. R. (2002). *Leadership and management in nursing* (3rd ed.). Upper Saddle River, NJ: Prentice Hall.

Groves, K. S., & LaRocca, M. A. (2011). An empirical study of leader ethical values, transformational and transactional leadership, and follower attitudes toward corporate social responsibility. *Journal of Business Ethics, 103*, 511–528.

Hersey, P., & Blanchard, K. H. (1969). *Management of organizational behavior: Utilizing human resources*. Englewood Cliffs, NJ: Prentice Hall.

Hersey, P., Blanchard, K., & Johnson, D. E. (2012). *Management of organizational behavior: Utilizing human resources* (7th ed.). Englewood Cliffs, NJ: Prentice Hall.

House, R. J. (1996). Path-Goal Theory of Leadership: Lessons, legacy and a reformulated theory. *Leadership Quarterly, 7*, 323–352.

Hu, J., & Liden, R. C. (2011). Antecedents of team potency and team effectiveness: An examination of goal and process clarity and servant leadership. *Journal of Applied Psychology, 96*(4), 851–862.

Indvik, J. (1986). Path-Goal Theory of Leadership: A meta-analysis. In *Best papers: Proceedings of the Academy of Management meeting* (pp. 189–192). Briarcliff Manor, NY: Academy of Management.

Isaacson, W. (2011). *Steve Jobs*. New York, NY: Simon & Schuster.

Jacobsen, C., & House, R. J. (2001). Dynamics of charismatic leadership: A process theory, simulation model and tests. *Leadership Quarterly, 12*, 75–112.

Jones, H. B. (2003). Magic, meaning and leadership: Weber's model and the empirical literature. *Human Relations, 54*, 753–771.

Jung, D. I., & Avolio, B. J. (2000). Opening the black box: An experimental investigation of the mediating effects of trust and value congruence on transformational and transactional leadership. *Journal of Organizational Behavior, 21*, 949–964.

Kawakami, C., White, J. B., & Langer, E. J. (2000). Mindful and masculine: Freeing women leaders from the constraints of gender roles. *Journal of Social Issues, 56*, 49–63.

Kielhofner, G. (2004). *Conceptual foundations of occupational therapy* (3rd ed.). Philadelphia, PA: F.A. Davis.

Kirkpatrick, S. A., & Locke, E. A. (1991). Leadership: Do traits matter? *Academy of Management Executive, 5*, 48–60.

Knight, A. P., Shteynberg, G., & Hanges, P. J. (2004). Path-Goal analysis. In J. M. Burns, G. R. Goethals, & G. J. Sorenson (Eds.), *Encyclopedia of leadership* (pp. 1164–1169). Thousand Oaks, CA: Sage.

Koenig, A. M., Eagly, A. H., Mitchell, A. A., & Ristikari, T. A. (2011). Are leader stereotypes masculine? A meta-analysis of three research paradigms. *Psychological Bulletin, 137*(4), 616–642.

Laub, J. A. (1999). Assessing the servant organization; Development of the Organizational Leadership Assessment (OLA) model. *Dissertation Abstracts International, 60*(02), 308A (UMI No. 9921922).

Lee-Kelly, L. (2002). Situational leadership: Managing the virtual project team. *Journal of Management Development, 21*, 461–476.

Levy, P. E., Cober, R. T., & Miller, T. (2002). The effect of transformational and transactional leadership perceptions on feedback-seeking intentions. *Journal of Applied Social Psychology, 32*, 1703–1720.

Liden, R. C., Wayne, S. J., Zhao, H., & Henderson, D. (2008). Servant leadership: Development of a multidimensional measure and multi-level assessment. *Leadership Quarterly, 19*(8), 161–177.

Loomis, C. J. (2012). *Tap dancing to work: Warren Buffett on practically everything, 1966–2012*. New York, NY: Penguin Group Publishers.

Lussier, R. (2010). *Human relations in organizations: Applications and skill building* (8th ed.). Whitby, Ontario, Canada: McGraw-Hill Ryerson.

MacKenzie, S. B., Podsakoff, P. M., & Rich, G. A. (2001). Transformational and transactional leadership and salesperson performance. *Journal of the Academy of Marketing Science, 29*, 115–134.

Marshall, E. S. (2011). *Transformational leadership in nursing*. New York, NY: Springer Publishing Company.

McColl-Kennedy, J. R., & Anderson, R. D. (2002). Impact of leadership style and emotions on subordinate performance. *Leadership Quarterly, 13*, 545–559.

Mittal, R., & Dorfman, P. W. (2012). Servant leadership across cultures. *Journal of World Business, 47*, 555–570.

Neubert, M. J., & Palmer, L. D. (2004). Emergence of women in healthcare leadership: Transforming the impact of gender differences. *Journal of Men's Health and Gender, 4*, 383–387.

Northouse, P. G. (2013). *Leadership: Theory and practice* (6th ed.). Los Angeles, CA: Sage Publications Inc.

Page, D., & Wong, T. P. (2000). A conceptual framework for measuring servant-leadership. In S. Adjibolosoo (Ed.), *The human factor in shaping the course of history and development* (pp. 69–109). Lanham, MD: University Press of America.

Parker, A. (2013). Day of records and firsts as 113th Congress opens. *The New York Times*. Retrieved from http://www.nytimes.com/2013/01/04/us/first-day-of-113th-congress-brings-more-women-to-capitol.html?_r=0

Parolini, J., Patterson, K., & Winston, B. (2009). Distinguishing between transformational and servant leadership. *Leadership and Organization Development Journal, 30*, 274–291.

Parris, D. L., & Peachey, J. W. (2013). A systematic literature review of servant leadership theory in organizational contexts. *Journal of Business Ethics, 113*, 377–393.

Paul, J., Costley, D. L., Howell, J. P., Dorfman, P. W., & Trafimow, D. (2001). The effects of charismatic leadership on followers' self-concept accessibility. *Journal of Applied Social Psychology, 31*, 1821–1844.

Paulsen, N., Maldonado, D., Callan, V. J., & Ayoko, O. (2009). Charismatic leadership, change and innovation in an R&D organization. *Journal of Organizational Change Management, 22*, 511–523.

Powell, S. K. (2000). *Case management: A practical guide to success in managed care* (2nd ed.). Baltimore, MD: Lippincott Williams & Wilkins.

Rabarison, K., Ingram, R. C., & Holsinger Jr., J. W. (2013, August). Application of situational leadership to the national voluntary public health accreditation process. *Frontiers in Public Health, 1*, 1–4.

Reed, L. L., Vidaver-Cohen, D., & Colwell, S. R. (2011). A new scale to measure executive servant leadership: Development, analysis and implications for research. *Journal of Business Ethics, 101*(3), 415–434.

Reinke, S. J. (2004). Service before self: Towards a theory of servant-leadership. *Global Virtue Ethics Review, 3*, 30–57.

Rogak, L. (2012). *Impatient optimist: Bill Gates in his own words*. Evanston, IL: Agate Publishing.

Rudolph, S. H., & Rudolph, L. I. (1983). *Gandhi: The traditional roots of charisma*. Chicago, IL: University of Chicago Press.

Schriesheim, C. A., Castro, S. L., Zhou, X., & DeChurch, L. A. (2006). An investigation of Path-Goal and Transformational Leadership Theory predictions at the individual level of analysis. *Leadership Quarterly, 17*, 21–38.

Schriesheim, C. A., & Neider, L. L. (1996). Path-Goal Leadership Theory: The long and winding road. *Leadership Quarterly, 7*, 317–321.

Schruijer, S. G., & Vansina, L. S. (2002). Leader, leadership and leading: From individual characteristics to relating in context. *Journal of Organizational Behavior, 23*, 869–874.

Sendjaya, S., & Sarros, J. C. (2002). Servant leadership: Its origin, development and application in organizations. *Journal of Leadership and Organizational Studies, 9*(2), 57–64.

Sendjaya, S., Sarros, J. C., & Santora, J. C. (2008). Defining and measuring servant leadership behaviour in organizations. *Journal of Management Studies, 45*(2), 402–424.

Shamir, B., House, R. J., & Arthur, M. B. (1993). The motivation effects of charismatic leadership: A self-concept based theory. *Organization Science, 4,* 584.

Silverthorne, C., & Wang, T. H. (2001). Situational leadership style as a predictor of success and productivity among Taiwanese business organizations. *Journal of Psychology, 135,* 399–412.

Smith, B. N., Montagno, R. V., & Kuzmenko, T. N. (2004). Transformational and servant leadership: Content and contextual comparisons. *Journal of Organizational Studies, 10*(4), 80–91.

Smith, H. L., & Kreuger, L. M. (1933, Spring). A brief summary of the literature on leadership. *Bulletin of the School on Education,* 3–80.

Snodgrass, J. (2011). Leadership development. In K. Jacobs & G. L. McCormack (Eds.), *The occupational therapy manager* (5th ed., pp. 265–280). Bethesda, MD: AOTA Press.

Snodgrass, J., Douthitt, S., Ellis, R., Wade, S., & Plemons, J. (2008). Occupational therapy practitioners' perceptions of rehabilitation managers' leadership styles and the outcomes of leadership. *Journal of Allied Health, 37*(1), 38–44.

Sosik, J., Avolio, B. J., & Jung, D. I. (2002). Beneath the mask: Examining the relationship of self-presentation attributes and impression management to charismatic leadership. *Leadership Quarterly, 13,* 217–242.

Sosik, J., Juzbasich, J., & Chun, J. U. (2011). Effects of moral reasoning and management level on ratings of charismatic leadership, in-role and extra-role performance of managers: A multi-source examination. *Leadership Quarterly, 22,* 434–450.

Spears, L. C. (2002). Tracing the past, present, and future of servant leadership. In L.C. Spears & M. Lawrence (Eds.), *Focus on leadership: Servant-leadership for the 21st century* (pp. 1–16). New York, NY: John Wiley & Sons.

Stoffel, V. C. (2013). From heartfelt leadership to compassionate care (Inaugural Presidential Address). *American Journal of Occupational Therapy, 67,* 633–640.

Stogdill, R. M. (1948). Personal factors associated with leadership: A survey of the literature. *Journal of Psychology, 25,* 35–71.

Stogdill, R. M. (1974). *Handbook of leadership: A survey of theory and research.* New York, NY: Free Press.

Thompson, G., & Vecchio, R. P. (2009). Situational Leadership Theory: A test of three versions. *Leadership Quarterly, 20,* 837–848.

U.S. Census Bureau. (2011). *Income, poverty and health insurance coverage in the United States: 2011.* Retrieved from http://www.census.gov/prod/2011pubs/p60-239.pdf

U.S. Department of Health and Human Services. (2013). *Affordable Care Act and the Title X Program.* Retrieved from http://www.hhs.gov/opa/affordable-care-act/index.html

Van Dierendonck, D. (2011) Servant leadership: A review and synthesis. *Journal of Management, 37*(4), 1228–1261.

Van Dierendonck, D., & Nuijten, I. (2011). The Servant Leadership Survey: Development and validation of a multidimensional measure. *Journal of Business Psychology, 26,* 249–267.

van Engen, M. L., van der Leeden, R., & Willemsen, T. M. (2001). Gender, context and leadership styles: A field study. *Journal of Occupational and Organizational Psychology, 74,* 581–598.

Vance, C., & Larson, E. (2002). Leadership research in business and health care. *Journal of Nursing Scholarship, 34,* 165–171.

Vecchio, R. P., Bullis, R. C., & Brazil, D. M. (2006). The utility of Situational Leadership Theory: A replication in a military setting. *Small Group Leadership, 37,* 407–424.

Vinkenburg, C. J, van Engen, M. L., Eagly, A. H., & Johannesen-Schmidt, M. C. (2011). An exploration of stereotypical beliefs about leadership styles: Is transformational leadership a route to a woman's promotion? *Leadership Quarterly, 22,* 10–21.

Wang, G., Oh, I., Courtright, S. H., & Colbert, A. E. (2011). Transformational leadership and performance across criteria and levels: A meta-analytic review of 25 years of research. *Group Organizational Management, 36,* 223–270.

Wilderom, C. P. M., van den Berg, P. T., & Wiersma, U. J. (2012). A longitudinal study of the effects of charismatic leadership and organizational culture on objective and perceived corporate performance. *Leadership Quarterly, 23*(5), 835–848.

Wofford, J. C., & Liska, L. Z. (1993). Path-Goal theories of leadership: A meta-analysis. *Leadership Quarterly, 19,* 857–876.

Yammarino, F. J., & Bass, B. M. (1990). Long-term forecasting of transformational leadership and its effects among naval officers: Some preliminary findings. In K. E. Clark & M. B. Clark (Eds.), *Measures of leadership* (pp. 151–169). West Orange, NJ: Leadership Library of America.

York, R. O. (2003). Adherence to Situational Leadership Theory among social workers. *Clinical Supervisor, 14,* 5–24.

Zaleznik, A. (2004). Managers and leaders: Are they different? *Harvard Business Review, 82*(1), 74–81.

Zhu, W., Newman, A., Miao, Q., & Hooke, A. (2013). Revisiting the mediating role of trust in transformational leadership effects: Do different types of trust make a difference? *Leadership Quarterly, 24,* 94–105.

Zhu, W., Sosik, J. J., Riggio, R. E., & Yang, B. (2012). Relationships between transformational and active transactional leadership and followers' organizational identification: The role of psychological empowerment. *Institute of Behavioral and Applied Management.* Retrieved from http://www.ibam.com/pubs/jbam/articles/vol13/no3/Zhu_Sosik_Riggio_Yang.pdf

CHAPTER 2

Engaging in Evidence-Based Management

Marcia Finlayson, PhD, OT Reg (Ont), OTR
Brent Braveman, PhD, OTR/L, FAOTA

■ Real-Life Management

Dan is an occupational therapy student who is completing his final fieldwork placement at a community facility serving older adults. When Dan started his placement, he expected to be treating clients seen through the outpatient rehabilitation and homecare programs. He was surprised to find out that he was also going to be working with Elena, the director of occupational therapy, to prepare a proposal to expand the occupational therapy services in the facility's respite, community outreach, and educational wellness programs. The occupational therapy staff had previously not been involved in these aspects of the facility's services. As Dan works with Elena, he is struck by the range of information Elena draws on to argue her case for expansion—theory, clinical and marketing research, census data about the community, and data from third-party payers. The list seems endless. Dan wonders how Elena is going to make sense of all of the information they have gathered. How is she going to decide if it is relevant? How is she going to put the information together to use it? Then there seem to be so many aspects to the proposal itself. Elena explains that it has to address a diversity of issues related to the management of occupational therapy services: staff supervision, communication, leadership, program development, continuous quality improvement, and funding, as well as the decision-making processes about space, equipment, and other resources. Dan feels overwhelmed. Elena explains that occupational therapy managers use theory, models, and evidence to make decisions about, plan, implement, and evaluate all facets of occupational therapy programming and services in much the same way that Dan is learning to use theory, models, and evidence to plan, implement, and evaluate intervention decisions with individual clients. Dan asks the simple question, "How do we get started?"

Critical Thinking Questions

As you read this chapter, consider the following questions:

- What types of tasks and activities are included in the wide range of work completed by occupational therapy managers and supervisors?

- What are examples of common questions and dilemmas faced by occupational therapy managers and supervisors in the course of their daily work?

- How is the process of finding and evaluating diverse forms of evidence to determine the best course of action to respond to management questions and dilemmas similar to solving clinical questions?

- How can you use an evidence-based approach to management and administration of occupational therapy services to engage in a knowledge-to-action process to address issues and resolve problems?

Glossary

- **Critical appraisal:** the process of judging the quality of a piece of information and determining the extent to which its design and conduct are accurate and free from bias.
- **Critical appraisal matrix:** a tool used to record the key characteristics, findings, strengths, and limitations of the materials that have been uncovered and appraised during a search in a compact and manageable format.
- **Evidence:** includes data, information, research results, program descriptions, and the opinions of clinical experts and consumers that can be used to guide managerial decision-making and inform the development and provision of occupational therapy and other health-care services.
- **Evidence-based management:** using the best available evidence and information to guide action in response to the daily questions, problems, and dilemmas encountered when performing the management functions of planning, organizing and staffing, controlling, and directing.

- **Evidence-based practice (EBP):** the process of identifying and defining a practice-related problem, formulating a question consistent with this problem, and then seeking and evaluating information that will help to answer the question and guide a clinical decision.
- **Grey literature:** papers, reports, and other documents from government, the academy, business, and industry that are not controlled by commercial publishers but are a valid form of evidence. Examples include progress reports, technical briefs, market research reports, conference proceedings, theses and dissertations, and commercial documentation (The New York Academy of Medicine, n.d.).
- **Levels of evidence:** indicate the relative strength of a form of evidence such as randomized control trials, nonrandomized studies, qualitative studies, or case examples, as well as other types of data, information, and evidence.

Introduction

Today's occupational therapists (OTs) and occupational therapy assistants (OTAs) are constantly challenged to offer the best and most effective interventions possible to individual clients. At the same time, occupational therapy managers are challenged to create and maintain practice environments that enable these interventions to be delivered within the constraints of available resources, including people, money, space, equipment, and time. The challenges faced by all of these occupational therapy practitioners come from a number of sources, one of which is the push in health care to ensure that activities and decisions are *evidence-based*.

When most occupational therapy personnel think about **evidence-based practice (EBP),** they tend to think about using research findings to help them make decisions about what type of intervention has the greatest probability to work with a given client in a specific situation, considering their own clinical experience and knowledge, as well as the client's preferences and support networks. Rarely does EBP conjure up the image of an occupational therapy manager making decisions about program development, staffing patterns, equipment and space distribution, continuous quality improvement programs, or the style of leadership that he or she wishes to adopt. Yet, given the impact of each of these decisions on the operations and effectiveness of occupational therapy services overall, it is critical for managers to engage in **evidence-based management,** which draws on many of the same processes that individual occupational therapy practitioners use to select an intervention approach for a client. The key difference is that the manager is often making decisions about interventions that will occur at a systems level rather than at the level of an individual client. For example, managers must make decisions about issues such as what staffing patterns are most likely to reduce turnover, or what departmental layout will maximize patient safety. These decisions should not be based on historical practices, fears or fads, or guesswork. They should be informed by the best available **evidence** and then translated into actions that fit the local situation, for example, by developing or changing policies, procedures, or other aspects of organizational operations and culture.

The purpose of this book is to overview the primary functions of an occupational therapy manager and to provide strategies for using theory and evidence related to a wide range of occupational therapy knowledge and knowledge from related fields to guide performance as a manager. Therefore, the purpose of this chapter is to further set the stage for this book by:

1. Reviewing principles and processes of evidence-based management, which often requires translating and mobilizing knowledge into system-level changes
2. Highlighting the need for evidence-based management for occupational therapy services
3. Identifying the types of evidence that can be used by occupational therapy managers as they perform various tasks and activities
4. Explaining a step-by-step process for finding, evaluating, and translating evidence into the management of occupational therapy services

Evidence-Based Practice and Evidence-Based Management: Reviewing the Basics

Evidence-based practice has dominated thinking about health-care delivery since the early to mid-1990s. The practice emerged in response to efforts in medicine and other disciplines to be more conscientious and explicit about the process of making clinical care decisions for individual clients. The basic EBP process involves identifying and defining a practice-related problem, formulating a question consistent with this problem, and then seeking and evaluating information that will help to answer the question and guide a clinical decision. The impetus for the EBP movement can be traced back to the influential book by Archie Cochrane, *Effectiveness and Efficiency: Random Reflections on Health Services*, which was published in the United Kingdom in 1972. In the 40 years since Cochrane's book was published, three important changes have transpired to solidify the place of EBP in the context of health care and support its expansion into specific areas such as *evidence-based management*.

First, a number of groups have responded to Cochrane's reflections by developing processes, practices, and specific tools to enable health-care professionals to find, evaluate, and use evidence to inform their clinical decisions. Some of these groups include the Cochrane Collaboration, which has centers internationally (http://www.cochrane.org), the Campbell Collaboration (http://www.campbellcollaboration.org/), and the Joanna Briggs Institute (http://joannabriggs.org/). In occupational therapy, key examples are the Evidence-Based Practice Research Group at McMaster University in Canada (http://srs-mcmaster.ca/research/evidence-based-practice-research-group) and OTseeker in Australia (http://www.otseeker.com). There are also specific resources to guide policy makers and health-care managers as they make evidence-based decisions (e.g., http://archive.ahrq.gov/policymakers/measurement/decisiontoolbx/index.html).

Second, access to evidence has exploded over the past several decades because of the Internet and open-access publishing. Increased access has made it more and more important to use rigorous and replicable strategies for finding and selecting sources of information, evaluating it, and then deciding whether or not it can inform decision-making. Issues of relevance, quality, and applicability are paramount. EBP has provided a range of rigorous and replicable strategies that health-care professionals and managers can use so that their decisions are defensible to patients, families, payers, and others.

Finally, the training of and accountability expectations for health-care professionals have increased in many jurisdictions. Many professions, including occupational therapy, now require graduate-level education in places such as the United States and Canada. In addition, serious discussions are also occurring about the need for and role of advanced practice, specialty, and doctoral-level education in our profession. Even without these discussions, the organizations that accredit occupational therapy education programs around the world require that graduates are competent in EBP processes for entry-level practice. Educational programs emphasize that EBP is a lifelong process of self-directed, problem-based learning that can inform their decision-making and enable them to justify their decisions to key stakeholders (Law & MacDermid, 2013).

Together, these three changes demonstrate that EBP is here to stay. Being evidence-based—as both a practitioner and manager—carries with it some important responsibilities, which are discussed next and summarized in Box 2-1.

To be evidence-based, you must work constantly to stay up-to-date with literature that is relevant to the

---

BOX 2-1

Responsibilities Stemming From an Evidence-Based Approach

- Staying up-to-date with the sources of information that may have an impact on the decisions you will make in practice
- Using sound judgment based on accepted practices and approaches about the information you have gathered by critically evaluating its quality
- Communicating with others about what you have learned from synthesizing information
- Recognizing that translating evidence into everyday practice will not be easy and will also require the application of evidence-based strategies

---

type of work that you do and decisions you must make. Whenever possible, focusing on already synthesized evidence such as systematic reviews, meta-analyses, and meta-syntheses can overcome common EBP barriers such as time, access to evidence, and confidence in search and evaluation skills. Staying up-to-date does not imply that you will read everything in your field—that would be impossible. What it does mean is that you need to be aware of the journals, programs, researchers, and other resources that can inform the tasks and activities that make up your practice. For occupational therapy managers, this means information from within the discipline of occupational therapy, but also from other disciplines and fields including health services research, business administration, organizational development, and psychology. Frequently, evidence will come from the research literature, but, as you will see later in this chapter, there are different kinds of data and information that an occupational therapy manager may want to use. All of these types of information may be considered to be *evidence*.

Being evidence-based also requires that you use sound judgment based on accepted practices and approaches about the information you have gathered to answer your question. *Judgment* refers to the responsibility to recognize that not all data, information, and evidence are created equal. Some sources of evidence have questionable reliability and validity, cannot be confirmed by other sources, are not generalizable to the situation in which you work, or are based on studies that have not been conducted ethically (Law & MacDermid, 2013). Part of using an evidence-based approach is using good judgment about the specific sources of evidence you select to guide your decisions.

Being evidence-based also means that you have a responsibility to share what you have learned with the people who will be affected by any decisions you make based on the evidence you have selected and evaluated. Decision-making about health-care options and their delivery is not the sole responsibility of one person—it is shared. Using an evidence-based approach means that you must be able to communicate well with your clients, whomever they may be—an individual patient, a family, the staff members you supervise as a manager, or the board of directors to whom you are accountable.

Despite the solid place of EBP in today's health-care systems, *using* available evidence can still be challenging as it often requires changes in long-standing routines and processes, or development of entirely new ones, whether for specific individuals or at broader levels of the organization. For managers, these changes must often occur at the system level, which means changing routines and processes that are used by and affect many different groups of people, including therapy staff, patients, families, professional peers, upper management, and others. Even a relatively small change—for example, deciding to stagger the work hours of a small number of practitioners to increase access to therapy services—may have ripple effects throughout the department and organization. Learning about the barriers to research implementation and knowledge mobilization—for example, knowledge, skills, beliefs about capabilities and consequences, reinforcement, and environmental resources (Cane, O'Connor, & Michie, 2012)—as well as ways to overcome them will enable managers to move knowledge into action. Strategies for overcoming these barriers and others include training, role modeling, incentivisation, and environmental restructuring, to name a few (Michie, van Stralen, & West, 2011). Occupational therapy managers need to recognize that they are catalysts for EBP because they are able to set the tone for an evidence-based culture, role model evidence-based decision-making, and develop organizational infrastructure to support and sustain EBP overall (Fisher & Robertson, 2007; Smith & Woods, 2003).

The Need for Evidence-Based Management of Occupational Therapy Services

As you know, this book is about managing occupational therapy services. You have probably scanned through the table of contents by now, and have seen that the topics that will be covered are broad—leadership, communication, program development and evaluation, continuous quality improvement, budgeting, and many others. The tasks and activities that an occupational therapy manager performs are numerous, and yet many of the fundamentals of occupational therapy practice can be seen in the work of an occupational therapy manager. For example, a manager must evaluate the client and the client's situation; identify problems, concerns, and priorities; and develop an intervention plan, implement it, and then evaluate the outcomes. Table 2-1 provides a few examples of the types of clients an occupational therapy manager might have, and how the occupational therapy process might look when applied to these clients from the manager's perspective.

Although the examples in Table 2-1 might make a lot of sense, the discerning reader should be asking, "How does the occupational therapy manager know that his or her approach is the best one? What is the evidence that choosing that particular intervention or way of proceeding is the most likely to lead to the desired outcomes? How does a manager move evidence into action at a systems level?" The answer to these questions should be, "Because the manager used an evidence-based management approach to make a decision, evaluated barriers to implementation, and applied strategies to overcome these barriers to implement the decision." As the example of Dan at the beginning of this chapter points out, occupational therapy managers perform a wide range of tasks and activities, and have to make many different types of decisions every day. Their choices and decisions can have a major impact on the overall functioning of occupational therapy services, and thereby on clients, families, practitioners, support staff, other

TABLE 2-1			
The Occupational Therapy Process Applied to the "Clients" of an Occupational Therapy Manager			
	An Individual Therapist Having Difficulty Fulfilling the Demands of the Job	**The Hospital Unit Staff Feels That the Occupational Therapy Services Are Not Meeting the Staff's Needs**	**A Board of Directors That Is Thinking About Cutting the Occupational Therapy Budget**
Evaluate Client and Situation	New graduate is overwhelmed with job demands of working at a busy neurology service that has high-need clients.	Staff on an orthopedics unit has seen a 30% increase in clients with hip replacements, but there has been no increase in therapy services. Staff is being pushed to discharge earlier, but this can't be done without the aftercare input of occupational therapy staff.	The organization is experiencing drops in income, and has to cut budgets throughout the system. Members of the board of directors question the size of the occupational therapy budget.
Identify Problems, Concerns, and Priorities	Therapist lacks confidence and has not connected with a mentor in the department. She came seeking help to improve performance.	There are only two OTs assigned to this unit, and no OTAs. The OTs work regular 8-to-4, Monday-to-Friday hours. The unit staff wants services more responsive to the unit's needs.	Members of the board are unfamiliar with occupational therapy services and what is involved in providing them. They want to have a better understanding of the department's resource needs.
Select and Implement Appropriate Intervention	Manager decides to provide closer supervision and to connect therapist with another senior therapist for mentoring about managing workload demands.	Manager decides to reassign an OTA to assist on the unit half-time and to restructure occupational therapy work hours to provide part-time coverage on Saturdays.	Manager pulls together lay descriptions of occupational therapy, and brief case examples of the work in the facility that includes information about the resources used during the cases. She also gathers stories from clients about the impact of occupational therapy services on their lives. This information is provided to the board members in a formal presentation, followed by a question-and-answer period.
Evaluate Outcomes	Therapist's confidence is increasing, and she feels more able to manage her job demands.	Unit staff senses that occupational therapy services are better meeting the unit's needs, and the increased patient load and discharge schedule.	The board evaluates the extent of the cut to the occupational therapy budget.

professionals, the organization, and potentially the broader community in which the occupational therapy services are offered. Because of these system-level impacts, there is a critical need for evidence-based management of occupational therapy services. Like the individual occupational therapy practitioner, the occupational therapy manager must carry out his or her job tasks and activities in an appropriate, responsible, ethical, and professional way in the ever-changing world of health care.

Types of Evidence Used by Occupational Therapy Managers

As Table 2-1 suggests, the types of interventions that an occupational therapy manager might employ are very diverse. Consequently, the types of evidence that might be necessary to guide his or her decisions are equally diverse. It is important to think broadly about the concept of evidence for management tasks and activities. But what are those tasks and activities? Some of the most common ones are listed in Table 2-2, together with the chapters in which they are discussed in this book and the types of evidence that might be used by a manager during the process of performing them.

As Table 2-2 shows, research and theory are critical to the occupational therapy manager as he or she goes about making decisions and performing various tasks and activities. As in other areas of occupational therapy practice, it is important for the manager to draw on related knowledge to perform his or her job—theories on leadership, communication, change management, and organizational development and behavior are critical. In addition, health services research that addresses issues such as the impact of different organizational structures and processes, staffing patterns, and service configurations on the health outcomes of clients served is extremely important for the occupational therapy manager to read, evaluate, and apply to his or her work. This related knowledge will have to be used in conjunction with knowledge specific to occupational therapy in order for the manager to function in an evidence-based way. But what exactly does this mean? What are the specific steps involved in managing occupational therapy services from an evidence-based approach?

BOX 2-2

The Evidence-Based Management Process

Step 1: *Frame* a question related to a decision that needs to be made.
Step 2: *Acquire* evidence that may contain information relevant to the question.
Step 3: *Assess* the evidence for accuracy, comprehensiveness, applicability, and actionability.
Step 4: *Present* the evidence to those who must act on it.
Step 5: *Apply* the evidence to the decision.
Step 6: *Evaluate* the results.

Process of Finding, Evaluating, and Using Evidence in Occupational Therapy Management

Using an evidence-based approach to management involves following six basic steps (Evashwick & Rundall, 2010). These steps are outlined in Box 2-2. Over the next few pages, we describe each of these steps in detail. We have woven an example into these steps to illustrate the process more clearly.

Frame the Question

The first and most important step in evidence-based management is identifying or *framing* a question. This step requires the manager to identify the decision he or she must make, as well as what needs to be known to ensure that the decision is well informed (http://archive.ahrq.gov/policymakers/measurement/decisiontoolbx/index.html). Because the decisions made by managers are often complex and have several components, it may be necessary to frame a series of questions to inform the decision-making process. Question(s) need to be direct, clear, and focused on a single information gap. A good question will identify the intervention (i.e., decision), the outcome, and the type of setting, time frame, and population. For more guidance about developing a good question, we suggest you visit one of the Internet resources provided in the

TABLE 2-2

Sample Management Functions or Tasks

Common Tasks and Activities of Managers	Chapter	Types of Evidence That Might Be Used to Inform Manager as He or She Performs Tasks and Activities
• Mentoring • Motivating others • Staff development	Chapter 1: Leadership: The Art, Science, and Evidence	• Research on effective leadership styles and strategies • Theory on leadership and mentoring • Performance reviews of manager • Performance of staff under manager's supervision • Statistics on staff retention
• Strategic planning • Information gathering and staying informed about rules • Deciding on billing • Staffing patterns and plans	Chapter 3: Understanding Health-Care Systems and Practice Contexts	• Organizational theory • Research on the impact and effectiveness of different staffing structures, patterns, and mix on patient outcomes • Statistics on billings outcomes • Internal administrative data on admissions, discharges, average length of stay, etc.
• Hiring • Firing • Mentoring • Motivating others • Staffing patterns and plans	Chapter 7: Roles and Functions of Supervisors	• Research on the impact and effectiveness of different staffing structures, patterns, and mix on patient outcomes • Theory on supervision styles • Workload statistics • Internal administrative data on admissions, discharges, average length of stay, etc. • Productivity statistics • Statistics on staff retention • Performance reviews of staff • Staff recognition within facility and outside of it
• Writing reports • Doing verbal presentations • Interacting with staff, upper management, public, and third-party payers	Chapter 5: Communicating Effectively in Complex Environments	• Research on effective communication styles • Theory on communication • Feedback on reports and presentations • Extent of responsiveness from those with whom manager is communicating
• Designing processes (e.g., referrals, assessment, documentation) • Setting criteria for performance of staff and programs • Monitoring performance of processes, staff, and programs	Chapter 13: Continuous Quality Improvement	• Research on the impact of different processes on the efficiency of an organization • Data collected within the organization on a process • Benchmarking • Satisfaction surveys of clients
• Needs assessment • Program planning • Program implementation • Program evaluation	Chapter 15: Developing Evidence-Based Occupational Therapy Programming	• Research on existing programs and their effective components • Theory on program development • Census information on potential clients • Marketing research • Satisfaction surveys of clients attending program

Resources list at the end of this chapter. In addition to these resources, you may find it valuable to review information on conducting effective literature searches, which is commonly found on the library websites of many university libraries; this will be helpful in the process of developing an effective question to guide your search.

For our example, imagine being an occupational therapy manager who is about to complete annual staff performance appraisals. At a weekly staff meeting, you announce that appraisals will begin next month. Staff members at the meeting express the concern that the current appraisal process is not useful because it is only used to determine merit pay. They want a process that also helps them meet their needs for professional growth and development. As the manager, you decide to review the process and see if there are alternative ways of doing performance appraisals that will also meet the staff's needs. You set the following question:

What methods of performance appraisal facilitate professional development over a 1-year period for professionals in a hospital setting?

In this question, you have been clear, direct, and focused. The population of interest has clearly been defined as "professionals." Although this is a broad population, it is often wise to start this way and then narrow the population as your search and evaluation of evidence proceeds. Your question has also clearly identified the intervention: performance appraisals and the outcome: facilitation of professional development. You have also identified the time frame (1 year) and setting (hospital).

Acquiring Evidence

Once your question has been set, the next step in the evidence-based management process is to find the evidence needed to answer your question. As Table 2-2 demonstrates, there is a wide spectrum of evidence that an occupational therapy manager might use in the course of his or her day-to-day work. Finding these potential sources of evidence can involve a number of different processes, for example, reviewing internally available administrative data (e.g., reasons for referral, average number of visits, number of cancellations); searching the Internet for government reports,

publicly available data, and other "grey literature"; or searching electronic bibliographic databases such as PubMed, CINAHL, or Wilson Business. **Grey literature** refers to papers, reports, and other documents from government, the academy, business, and industry that are not controlled by commercial publishers but are a useful and valid form of evidence. Examples include progress reports, technical briefs, market research reports, conference proceedings, theses and dissertations, and commercial documentation (The New York Academy of Medicine, n.d.).

It is important to distinguish between searching the Internet and searching electronic bibliographic databases. Electronic bibliographic databases are compilations of published research, scholarly articles, books, newspaper articles, and other recognized sources of information. There is a wide range of different databases, many of which have a disciplinary focus such as medicine, psychology, or education. For example, PubMed is a compilation of medically related publications, CINAHL focuses on publications from the allied health professions, and Wilson Business focuses on business and economics.

In comparison to an electronic bibliographic database, searching the Internet will not limit you to published articles and reports. Although you may find a journal article in the course of an Internet search, you will also find all sorts of other information that may have no direct relevance to the question or problem you are trying to address. Narrowing your search on the Internet can be very challenging, particularly because there are no set key terms or search words to use. In addition, much of what you will find will be of questionable credibility. Anyone can create a website or a Web page, as long as he or she has Internet access. Therefore, it is important to have strict criteria for selecting sites to review if you are going to use the Internet to find evidence. More information on appraising websites is provided later in this chapter. Generally speaking, it is a good idea to limit your Internet searches initially to government, university, and professional association websites. Ultimately, searching electronic bibliographic databases is probably going to be the most focused and productive option for finding information and evidence to support decision-making in management of occupational therapy services.

Regardless of the sources of information you seek to answer your question, it is critical that your search be systematic and reproducible. It is important to clearly document your search and, if possible, save your search to be replicated at a later date if you need to update the evidence. Most electronic bibliographic databases offer features such as "Save search history." The question you have posed will also assist you in making your search systematic and reproducible. Identify the key words and phrases in your question and use them to build your search strategy. The best way to start is by writing down the terms that correspond to the intervention, outcomes, population, and setting identified in your question. It will often not be possible to search by time frame; you may need to pull out this information from identified evidence sources during Step 3 of the evidence-based management process. From the example we introduced earlier, we would write down "performance appraisal" and "professional development" to start. During an actual search, these words and phrases are linked together using Boolean terms such as "AND," "OR," and "NOT" to focus the search and find the best and most relevant information. Using the "OR" term results in the largest number of citations by identifying any citation that includes any of the linked key words. Using the "AND" term limits citations to those including *all* key words. Using the "NOT" term eliminates citations including key words you do not wish to include in your search.

Next, you need to select appropriate electronic bibliographic databases (e.g., PubMed, CINAHL, ProQuest Business) for your search. Determining if a database is appropriate can be done by reviewing its focus (e.g., health) and content (e.g., names of journals included). This information is typically available through the "Help" or general information section of a database. In the example we presented earlier, our question focuses on methods of performance appraisal that facilitate professional development. Given that performance appraisals are a task for managers, it is likely that databases addressing management and business-related topics will be the most relevant. When we looked for databases that had these foci, we found PsycINFO, ProQuest Business, and CINAHL.

Once you have selected databases, it is a good idea to cross-reference the key words and phrases with the index terms in the database you decide to use, if possible. For our example, we started with the key words "performance appraisal." In the PsycINFO database, this term mapped to 11 different terms. We chose to narrow our search by focusing on the terms "job performance," "personnel evaluation,"

and "feedback." Finding the evidence that matches your questions is a process of initiating the search, making modifications to your search terms as necessary, and documenting your search and related decisions as you go. It is best to record the search words and phrases you use, and identify the combinations of terms that you use. The search can be limited or expanded as necessary. Ways of limiting your search include focusing on research articles only, or focusing on particular publication years. Expanding your search can be accomplished by using synonyms for your key words, and connecting these synonyms together with the Boolean search term "OR." Regardless of the way your search develops, it is critical to document it as you go, so that you can replicate it later if need be.

For our question, when we were using the PsycINFO database, the terms that we used ("performance appraisal" AND "job performance" OR "personnel evaluation" OR "feedback") resulted in 19,294 citations. We then chose to limit the search by combining our results with the term "professional development." These actions reduced the number of citations to 110. For our last limit, we focused on "health professional," and ended with 5 resources, all of which were directly relevant to the question. A similar search process in the ProQuest Business database identified 124 related citations, and in the CINAHL database, 24 related citations. In some cases, you may have to go back and expand your search by using other key words or be willing to accept data, information, or other forms of evidence that are not as focused on your question as you might have hoped if directly related literature is not found.

Once you have identified a manageable number of sources from your search, you can review what you have found to determine if they are, in fact, relevant to your question. Typically, this review starts with the title and abstract, if one is available. This information is examined to decide whether or not to obtain a full copy of the specific source for further and more thorough review.

Because of the diversity of tasks and activities that the occupational therapy manager performs, searching the literature for evidence to assist in decision-making will necessarily have to involve looking for all sorts of publications, such as books, journals, and, if it is appropriate, newspaper articles, government documents, and websites. It will be critically important to search the literature from disciplines other than occupational therapy. Once you have completed your search, your next step is to assess what you have found.

Assessing the Evidence

Once evidence has been located, the next step is to assess it. As a manager, you must assess the evidence for its accuracy or quality, as well as its comprehensiveness, applicability, and actionability. In EBP more broadly, evidence assessment involves three components—the quality of the evidence, the level of the evidence, and the overall strength of the evidence (Jones, 2010). For the evidence-based manager, all of these aspects should be considered when assessing the evidence that will ultimately be used to guide a decision.

Quality of Evidence

Evaluating the quality of the evidence requires you to conduct a *critical appraisal*. **Critical appraisal** is the process of judging the quality of a piece of information and determining the extent to which its design and conduct are accurate and free from bias. Critical appraisal also considers the extent to which the findings are applicable to your setting. To assist with this evaluation process, one can draw on a large number of books, journal articles, and appraisal guidelines to learn about what to look for and evaluate across a wide variety of potential sources of evidence. For example, the occupational therapy EBP group at McMaster University has published guides for evaluating different types of research designs. In addition, there are a series of appraisal questions that managers can use on the online resource The Informed Decisions Toolbox (http://www.ahrq.gov/policymakers/measurement/decisiontoolbx/), which was specifically designed for health-care decision-makers. Other sources, such as the University of California at Berkeley Library (http://www.lib.berkeley.edu/Help/tutorials.php#eval), have produced tutorials and guides for evaluating information that is available through websites. Additional resources for evaluating information found on websites are provided at the end of the chapter.

Essentially what all of these different resources provide is a list of questions to ask yourself as you read an article or review a resource that has the potential to inform your decision-making process. Some of the questions are specific to the study's design and conduct,

whereas other questions address issues related to the study's comprehensiveness, as well as the extent to which it is applicable to your situation (e.g., similar population, setting, context) and could be acted upon in your environment. Examples of some key questions that are asked in these guides are presented in Tables 2-3, 2-4, and 2-5.

Critical appraisal is a crucial step in the process of evidence-based management. It is one thing to be able to locate evidence, but unless you can evaluate its quality and determine its utility for informing decisions, the evidence-based management process will break down. Therefore, after reviewing the evidence you have found and answering the appraisal questions, it will be necessary to look across all of the material and decide what is worth keeping for further consideration and what should be filtered out. To aid in this process, it is a good idea to determine the level of evidence of the evidence you have uncovered, compare and contrast the various sources, determine whether any obvious choices are emerging, and determine whether the strength of the evidence supports action. You will need to decide whether the evidence you have gathered will allow you to make a clear decision, identify concrete strategies for implementation, and anticipate possible consequences (http://archive.ahrq.gov/policymakers/measurement/decisiontoolbx/index.html).

Level of Evidence

There are many different typologies for determining the **levels of evidence** of a resource you are appraising. The majority of these typologies focus on quantitative types of research such as randomized controlled trials, systematic reviews, meta-analyses, and quasi-experiments. Often, there is limited room within these typologies to consider the role or value of qualitative research, theoretical pieces, government or organizational reports, or administrative data (e.g., reports produced through aggregating discharge summary information). Some allow for the testimony of expert committees or the opinions of respected authorities, but these types of evidence are usually rated as the weakest form.

Although there are variations in the approaches used by different scholars and sources, most use similar approaches to assigning a level to the evidence that is being examined. Table 2-6 includes three such typologies. It is important to note that these are only

TABLE 2-3

Basic Appraisal Questions for Research Articles

Area for Review	Questions to Guide the Appraisal Process
Study significance	Is the reason for doing the study well developed? Do the authors convince you that doing this study was important?
Purpose of research	Is the purpose of the study clear?
Design	What is the design of the study? Does it match the purpose of the study?
Sampling procedure	What is the sampling procedure? Does it correspond well to the question and the design? What are the strengths and limitations of the procedure with respect to being able to answer the question?
Sample	What are the characteristics of the sample? Are there any potential biases inherent in the makeup of the sample that might interfere with the ability to answer the question?
Data collection procedures and measures	How were data collected for this study? What measures were used? What do you know about the methods and measures (consider reliability, validity, who developed it, for what purpose, pretesting or pilot testing, etc.)?
Intervention (if applicable)	What was the intervention? Is the intervention adequately described? Is the intervention conceptually congruent with the outcomes chosen?
Results	What were the findings? Overall, do you feel that they are free of bias? If not, why not? Do the results include information about the estimates of intervention effects (if applicable)?
Conclusions	Do you agree with the conclusions? What are the strengths and limitations of the study overall? Do you feel that the purpose of the study has been addressed (i.e., is the question answered)?
Other considerations	Does the study setting and context match well with your setting? Does the study provide information that informs your decision? Could you replicate the intervention in your setting? Does the study address its limitations? Does the study provide a complete and balanced viewpoint? Does the study list or raise questions about potential conflicts of interest?

examples. There are numerous typologies available. Which one will best meet your needs will depend on the types of questions you are asking and the nature of the evidence that is best suited to answer them.

The first typology included in Table 2-6 is provided by the Centre for Evidence-Based Medicine (Oxford Centre for Evidence-Based Medicine, 2011), which is a resource for evidence-based reviews in medicine. Within this resource, there are typologies for reviews of interventions, diagnostic tests, economic evaluations, and treatment harms. Only the typology for interventions is provided in Table 2-6. The second typology is that used by the American Occupational Therapy Association's (AOTA's) Evidence-Based Literature Review Project. The third typology was presented by Dr. Margo Holm in her Eleanor Clarke-Slagle Lecture entitled "Our Mandate for the New Millennium: Evidence-Based Practice" (Holm, 2000). As previously noted, you will find that there is more of an emphasis in these typologies on quantitative research using traditional experimental designs, but that some recognition of other forms of evidence is included.

How do you evaluate the level of evidence if the materials you have located are not research studies? The answer has already been provided to some extent in Table 2-4. In this table, you were given a set of basic appraisal questions for non–research-related reports

TABLE 2-4

Basic Appraisal Questions for Review Articles and Non–Research-Related Reports and Documents

Area for Review	Questions to Guide the Appraisal Process
Purpose	Is the purpose of the material clear? What are the key points or messages?
Main messages	How reliable do you feel the key points or messages are? Consider number, type, and age of citations; expertise of author(s); where material is published (e.g., peer-reviewed journal, professional magazine, etc.); consistency with other materials you have read.
Population addressed	To what populations are the key points or messages relevant? How well do these populations correspond to the population(s) that you are interested in planning or making decisions for?
Interventions, processes, and structures addressed	What types of interventions, processes, and structures are addressed? To what extent might they apply in your setting?
Outcomes addressed	What types of outcomes are addressed? Consider micro-, meso-, and macro-level outcomes. How relevant are these outcomes to your setting?
Overall credibility	Overall, do you believe what is in this resource? Why or why not? What questions do you have remaining after reviewing this resource?

TABLE 2-5

Basic Appraisal Questions for Websites

Area for Review	Questions to Guide the Appraisal Process
Reliability	To what extent can you count on the information provided at this site? Is the source trustworthy? How did the site's creators come up with the information listed here? Do they cite sources? Did they follow good research procedures? Do they have a bias? A reason to distort? Is this advertising?
Accuracy	Are these real numbers and facts? Do they match reality? How do you know they are real and on target?
Currency	How recent are the facts and figures? Does the site tell you? Does it matter? Might reported rates such as crime or employment have changed since the data were posted to the site?
Authority	Do the site's creators have any credentials to be providing this information? Any evidence of training or professional skill? Do they identify the author or provider by name? Who did this work?
Fairness	Have the site's creators presented the material selectively or in an unbalanced manner? Is there bias or slanting in the reporting? Did they leave some information out? Did they focus only on the positive? The negative?
Adequacy	Do the site's creators tell you enough? Do they provide sufficient data or evidence? Do they go into enough detail and depth?
Efficiency	Can you find what you need at this site relatively quickly, or is it loaded down with graphics and elements that prolong your visit and your searching unnecessarily?
Organization	Is the information laid out in a logical fashion so that you can easily locate what you need without wandering around and wasting time?

TABLE 2-6

Strategies for Classifying Levels of Evidence

Level of Evidence	Centre for Evidence-Based Medicine	The American Occupational Therapy Association*	Moore, McQuay, and Gray (from Holm, 2000)
Strongest	I—Systematic reviews of randomized trials or n-of-1 trials	I = Randomized controlled trial	I = Some evidence from at least one systematic review of multiple well-designed randomized controlled studies
Weakest	II—Randomized trial or observational study with dramatic effect	II = Nonrandomized controlled trial, two groups	II = Strong evidence from at least one properly designed randomized controlled trial of appropriate size
	III—Nonrandomized controlled cohort or follow-up study	III = Nonrandomized controlled trial, one group with pretest and posttest	III = Evidence from well-designed trials without randomization, or single-group pre and post, cohort, time series, or matched case-control studies
	IV—Case-series, case-control studies, or historically controlled studies	IV = Single-subject design	IV = Evidence from well-designed nonexperimental studies from more than one center or research group
	V—Mechanism-based reasoning	NA = Narratives and case studies	

Note that some typologies, such as that used by the American Occupational Therapy Association's Evidence-Based Literature Review Project, assign separate ratings for the study design, internal and external validity, and sample size.

---

and documents. To expand on Table 2-4, we have developed a suggested typology for use in rating review articles, program descriptions, and non–research-related reports and documents. This typology is provided in Table 2-7.

Throughout this book, you will be presented from time to time with sample data, information, and other forms of evidence related to a variety of managerial topics. Because of the diversity of topics included in this book, choosing a single typology or method to categorize the level of the evidence proved difficult. In practice, we would recommend that you choose a typology that best fits the type of evidence that matches the question you are exploring. However, we were also concerned that continually shifting from one typology to another would be very confusing. For that reason, we have developed a simple typology that will be used throughout the book, regardless of the type of evidence being evaluated. This typology is presented in Box 2-3.

Once you have appraised the evidence you have uncovered and assigned each source a level of evidence rating, the next step is to summarize so you can decide how to proceed. Summarizing the evidence will require you to have some systematic way of comparing the relative strengths and weaknesses of all of the sources of evidence you have appraised. You will need a way to examine patterns and consistencies across articles to determine the overall strength of the evidence you have. This need to compare and summarize across articles is particularly important when you are drawing from a large body of literature in which materials contradict each other. This is where evaluating the overall strength of the evidence you have found comes into the process.

Strength of Evidence

When you are using an evidence-based approach, you will most likely identify several useful sources of

TABLE 2-7

A Suggested Typology for Rating Review Articles, Program Descriptions, and Non–Research-Related Reports and Documents

Level of Evidence	Characteristics
Strong	• Widely used and recognized material. • Numerous other citations or examples of use are provided. • Discussions across the multiple citations or examples are consistent with each other. • Was developed specifically for use by occupational therapy practitioners or other practitioners in the setting in which you intend to use it. • Presented by an author, group, or resource with well-documented expertise in the relevant subject matter. • Presented by an author with clearly documented and relevant training and education. • Documented in a manner that clearly highlights the strengths, weaknesses, advantages, and disadvantages of the strategy, model, or approach. • Presented in a peer-reviewed publication or resource.
Good	• Generally recognized by individuals familiar with the literature, but its use may be restricted to certain geographic regions or be associated with a particular setting or school. • Some other citations or examples of use are provided. Discussions across these citations or examples are generally consistent with each other, although some variability exists. • Was developed specifically for use by occupational therapy practitioners or other practitioners in a setting that is closely related to where you intend to use it. • Presented by an author, group, or resource with some documented expertise in the relevant subject matter, but length of expertise may be limited. • Presented by an author with related training and education. • Documented in a manner that allows the reader to extract the strengths, weaknesses, advantages, and disadvantages of the strategy, model, or approach. • Presented in a peer-reviewed publication or resource.
Weak	• Somewhat familiar, but not generally recognized even among individuals familiar with the literature. • Only one or two other citations or examples of use are provided. • Was developed for use by occupational therapy practitioners or other practitioners in a setting that has a few similarities to the one in which you intend to use it. • Presented by an author, group, or resource for which very limited information is available about expertise in the relevant subject matter. • Presented by an author with very limited training or education that is relevant. • Documented in a manner that makes it difficult for the reader to identify the strengths, weaknesses, advantages, and disadvantages of the strategy, model, or approach. • Presented in a trade or professional magazine that is reviewed by editors only.
Poor	• Being introduced for the first time and no other citation or example of use is provided. • Was developed specifically for use by another discipline or other practitioners in an unrelated setting. • Presented by an author, group, or resource for which no documentation of expertise in the relevant subject matter is provided. • Presented by an author whose training and education is not relevant or not documented. • Discussion is limited to application only, with no mention of the strengths, weaknesses, advantages, and disadvantages of the strategy, model, or approach. • The source or date of the publication cannot be determined. • No indication of any peer or editorial review.

BOX 2-3

A Simple Typology for Evaluation of Level of Evidence Throughout This Text

- **Level I—Strong:** Well-designed quantitative or qualitative research with larger sample sizes; systematic reviews, meta-analyses, or well-designed replications of other studies
- **Level II—Good:** Quantitative or qualitative research with limited sample size but with acceptable validity and credible recognition of limitations
- **Level III—Weak:** Descriptive program evaluations including participant summaries and some outcome data, in-depth program evaluations with outcome data,* description or analysis of multiple cases, or research-focused literature reviews
- **Level IV—Poor:** Recommendations of experts, single-case descriptions or program descriptions with limited outcome data,* or non–research-focused literature reviews

As is noted in Tables 2-4 and 2-7, when evaluating a program description or non–research-related article, the extent to which the evidence directly relates to your population or program of concern may strengthen or weaken your evaluation of the evidence.

---

evidence. Some of them will be of high quality, whereas others will not. Some will provide higher ratings for level of evidence than others. One of the challenging steps in the evidence-based process is synthesizing across a body of evidence, examining similarities and differences in findings, and determining how to consider and weight the information you have uncovered. This is what we mean by the *strength* of the evidence. A body of evidence that is strong will be made up of several high-quality studies that have consistent results. A weak body of evidence will either have few high-quality studies or inconsistent results or both. Only strong bodies of evidence will make the manager's decision easier to make. When a body of evidence is somewhere in the middle between strong and weak, decision-making will be challenging; therefore, decision-makers will have to consider other factors such as experience and feedback from others.

In the example we have been using to illustrate the steps of the evidence-based process, we reviewed the abstracts of the articles from each database that appeared relevant to our question after narrowing the search results. We uncovered several articles that addressed our initial question about the methods of performance appraisal that facilitate professional development over a 1-year period for professionals in a hospital setting. One way of summarizing the evidence that you have found in order to consider if and how to use it is to construct what is called a **critical appraisal matrix**. A critical appraisal matrix that includes three of the articles we found for our question is provided in Table 2-8.

Critical appraisal matrices provide an opportunity to record the key characteristics, findings, strengths, and limitations of the materials that have been uncovered and appraised during a search in a compact and manageable format. The organization of these matrices will depend on the topic of the search, how the information is going to be used, and what pieces of information we need to answer our question. In our example, we wanted to know about methods of performance appraisal. Therefore, including a column on "strategies" in the matrix is prudent. In addition, we might want to include information on how the strategies were identified (i.e., methods), how many and what type of employees were being considered in the source of evidence, what the nature of the employment was (e.g., health or business), and what we thought of the overall quality of the material.

Once all of this information is extracted into the matrix, it is then possible to scan across the sources easily and quickly, looking for similarities and differences. From here, you determine the overall strength of the evidence and determine if there is enough evidence to support a particular decision or to rule out other possibilities for your specific context. According to Guyatt and colleagues (2008), several factors should reduce your confidence in a body of evidence: study limitations, inconsistent findings across studies, indirectness of evidence for your specific situation or context, imprecise measurement, and publication bias. This group also identified three factors that should increase your confidence in a body of evidence: the findings across the studies show large effects, there is a dose–response relationship (i.e., the more you do, the better the results), and there are controllable factors that could make the findings even better in

TABLE 2-8

Sample Critical Appraisal Matrix

Author	Level of Evidence	Design	Purpose	Method of Appraisal	N (Sample Size)	Results or Findings
Finlay & McLaren, 2009	Weak	Cross-sectional postal survey	Examine whether appraisal has an impact on learning, practice, and continuing professional development.	Self-guided, annual appraisal using a Web-based interface	276 general practice physicians	Over half of respondents reported that the appraisal process supported their professional development by identifying and prioritizing learning needs and supporting documentation of learning.
Salvatori, Simonavicius, Moore, Rimmer, & Patterson (2008)	Good	Pilot project	Describe how a chart-stimulated recall (CSR) peer-review process and interview tool was revised, implemented, and evaluated to assess the clinical competence of occupational therapy staff at a large urban health center.	CSR peer-review and interview. Note: evaluation criteria and scoring provided in article.	14 pairs of OTs; 7 were interviewed and 7 were reviewed	The appraisal process was able to discriminate the levels of clinical competence among therapists and identify areas of concern that could be targeted for professional development. Participants found the process helpful.
Capan, Ambrose, Burkett, Evangelista, Flook, & Straka (2013)	Weak	Surveys conducted before and after the review process	Determine if the use of an electronic nursing portfolio helped nurse managers and direct-care staff nurses validate professional development during annual performance reviews.	Electronic portfolio with an annual face-to-face review	149 direct care staff nurses; 8 nurse managers	Managers found the portfolios useful for validating nurses' attendance at conferences and community service. Staff nurses found the portfolio useful for validating honors and awards and participation in committees.

some situations. Preparing a matrix and a brief written summary of what you have learned can help you synthesize the evidence and set the stage for broader dialogues, if the decision you are making will necessitate more input.

Present the Evidence to Those Who Must Act On It

As a manager, the decisions you make will affect many people—OTs, OTAs, departmental support staff, individuals in other departments (e.g., nursing, physical therapy, medicine, etc.). For this reason, there will be times when it will be crucial to engage others in your evidence-based management process. Engaging others early in the process will facilitate the implementation of the decisions you make. For example, when involved in the process of developing new programs (see Chapter 15) you may benefit from engaging upper management, staff, and customers in the design process by sharing how evidence will translate to program elements. This will assist you with getting their buy-in to the program and give them opportunities to help you improve the program as you design it.

There are several ways that you can present the evidence to those who must act on it, and which way you use will depend on your overall objectives. There will be times when you simply wish to explain your decision and why you are making it to others. In these situations, you may want to prepare a short written summary of the evidence and how it supports the choice you have made.

There will be other times, particularly when the evidence is less clear or when the clear decision will require significant changes in routines and practice patterns, that you will need additional input to inform your decision. Bringing together key stakeholders to discuss the evidence, pros and cons of different options, what is feasible in your setting, and what barriers might exist to implementation may be warranted. To ensure that all stakeholders are familiar with the evidence available, providing an evidence brief in preparation for the meeting will be valuable.

Regardless of whether you present your evidence to others to justify your decision or to obtain additional input to inform your decision, the evidence-based manager needs to be thinking about the next step—implementation of whatever decision is finally made, based on available evidence.

Apply the Evidence to the Decision

As a manager, you may find that implementing your evidence-based decision may lead you to write new policies or procedures, change a process, develop a new program, or take some other step. If the evidence to make your decision was not clear, your decision may involve a short pilot test of different options so that you can have better information to move forward. Other chapters in this book provide guidance on each of these options. For example, the process of continuous quality improvement described in Chapter 13 often calls for piloting potential solutions and measuring the change or impact of the solution to assure that it is effective before permanently putting the solution in place. In the process of developing and implementing new programs (see Chapter 15), you may pilot program elements and involve staff and consumers in the evaluation of the elements and the program as a whole in order to make improvements. Regardless of the final product of your decision, it is important to map out the steps to get to the endpoint, set clear criteria for what will constitute success, and consider facilitators and barriers to overall implementation. Strategies should be put in place to overcome any barriers you expect, for example, planning staff training sessions so they are clear about new processes or procedures.

Evaluate the Results

Being an evidence-based manager not only means seeking and applying evidence from other sources, it also means ensuring that you are generating your own information and evidence to guide your decision-making processes. When you make a decision based on evidence, it is important to follow up and determine whether the choice you made led to the results you expected. If we go back to our example of methods of performance appraisal that facilitate professional development, you would want to design a way of gathering input from the therapy staff about new methods you decide to trial or put in place. Chapters 13 and 15 also provide information on the process of evaluating programs and assessing program outcomes. Finally, the process of assessing staff competencies described in Chapter 12 will help you determine if the strategies suggested by the evidence are being implemented effectively.

Challenges of Using an Evidence-Based Approach

Most readers will have some familiarity with some or all of the steps of the evidence-based approach that we have just reviewed and described. Even if you have great skills in writing clear questions, searching the literature, and appraising and summarizing what you have found, challenges will still emerge. For the occupational therapy manager, the key challenges include getting access to facilities for searching, finding too much or not enough during a search, actually obtaining the materials that you have found, keeping up-to-date with relevant materials in the field, and actually implementing the evidence-based decisions you have made. Let's explore each of these challenges a bit more.

The challenge for many occupational therapy managers is that they may not have easy access to electronic bibliographic databases if the facility they work in does not have a library that purchases subscriptions to these services, or alternatively, does not have access to a university-based library. A good alternative for many people is PubMed, which is freely available through the National Library of Medicine (http://www.ncbi.nlm.nih.gov/pubmed/). For occupational therapy managers who are members of AOTA, OTSearch is also freely available (http://www1.aota.org/otsearch/index.asp). For members of the Canadian Association of Occupational Therapists, OTDBASE is a free member service (http://www.caot.ca/). Another option for occupational therapy personnel is OTseeker, freely available online at http://otseeker.com/. The National Board for Certification in Occupational Therapy (NBCOT) provides ProQuest to certificants in good standing. ProQuest provides "direct links to more than 7 million citations, 875 full-text titles and 12,000 full-text dissertations sourced from hundreds of renowned publications

in the fields of science, medicine and technology (National Board for Certification in Occupational Therapy, 2014).

Managers who begin to use an evidence-based approach to decision-making will find that sometimes the amount and variety of evidence can seem overwhelming. Although results can be narrowed using the strategies described earlier, another useful strategy is to focus on materials that have already been appraised, synthesized, and published by someone else. These resources include systematic reviews, meta-analyses, meta-syntheses, and, in some cases, practice guidelines and decision-making algorithms.

At other times, very little information will be found or the evidence that is found may seem only generally related to your managerial question. For example, a substantial amount of research on leadership styles and their effectiveness exists, but little of it directly addresses leadership specifically within occupational therapy services. In such situations, an occupational therapy manager may need to read material from other fields and evaluate its applicability to his or her situation. For example, much of the research conducted on the effectiveness of transformational, transactional, and other theories of leadership presented in Chapter 1 were conducted in areas such as banking, manufacturing, and even the military. Although evidence from these areas may not seem directly relevant to leading occupational therapy services, it is often important and necessary to read these related materials carefully. Depending on their focus and purpose, they can often hold some insights that the occupational therapy manager can reflect on and draw from in his or her daily work.

Nevertheless, in situations in which the evidence is thin or the relevance is not direct, it may be difficult to make decisions about how to use the information that has been uncovered. This reality means that a manager needs to be prepared for the possibility that there may be no clear answer to the question he or she was trying to address. An example is the task of finding a model to guide the steps of developing a new occupational therapy program. For managerial questions such as this, the only evidence that you may be able to find will be program descriptions or the opinions of subject matter experts. It is unlikely that you will find research equivalent to a "clinical trial" in which the effectiveness of the use of one model is compared with the effectiveness of the use of another. However, there are still strategies that can be used for evaluating the quality of evidence, such as a description of the application of a program development model, which we presented in Table 2-7.

Another common challenge that faces occupational therapy managers who are trying to use an evidence-based approach is actually obtaining the materials that they have found and want to appraise for further consideration and use. If this is a problem for you, check to see if the library at your facility has an inter-library loan agreement with a university library in the area. You can also check the websites of local university libraries to determine whether or not they carry subscriptions to the journals or materials you are seeking. Fortunately, many new journals are open-access, which means that they are freely available on the Internet.

Even for the manager who is regularly searching the literature for evidence to aid decision-making, keeping up-to-date with new materials that are coming out can be challenging. Many resources are now available to reduce this problem. For example, many journals have *electronic table of contents (ETOC)* alerts in which the table of contents of the most recent issue of a journal is e-mailed to you free of charge. Another resource is medical news services that provide concise abstracts about recent publications, advances, and media coverage of medical subjects. One example of such a service is CNN Health (http://www.cnn.com/health/). Finally, some federal agencies and nonprofit associations provide e-mail services through which information about current events, conferences or other learning opportunities, key research results, or updated demographic information is sent to you on a regular basis. For example, the Centers for Disease Control and Prevention (http://www.cdc.gov/) has a number of statistical reports on various health problems that are available through its website, and you can sign up to be notified by e-mail when updated reports are available.

Even in their best application, it is unlikely that the strategies suggested in this chapter or by other resources on evidence-based management will eliminate all of your decision-making difficulties. However, it is likely that following the guidelines and suggestions that have been presented in this chapter will help to reduce some of your confusion and stress, and the product of your work will be of higher quality.

Chapter Summary

Today's OTAs, OTs, and occupational therapy managers are constantly challenged to offer the best and most effective interventions possible. Practicing from an evidence-based approach provides the foundation to act in a professional, responsible, and ethical manner. As explained in the introduction, the purpose of this book is to overview the primary functions of an occupational therapy manager and to provide strategies for using theory and evidence related to a wide range of occupational therapy knowledge and knowledge from related fields to guide performance as a manager. To set the foundation for the contents of this book, this chapter has reviewed the basics of EBP and evidence-based management; described the relevance of evidence-based principles to management of occupational therapy services; identified the types of evidence that can be used by an occupational therapy manager as he or she performs various tasks and activities; and explained a step-by-step process for finding, evaluating, and using evidence in occupational therapy management.

Useful Resources for Applying Evidence-Based Practice to Management of Occupational Therapy Services

As this chapter has explained, EBP is here to stay, and its principles and processes are relevant to management of occupational therapy services. Entire books have been dedicated to different aspects of EBP, or the applications of its processes by different disciplines or in different settings. It is not possible to cover all that is known about EBP or management in this chapter, or to explain its steps in the level of detail that some readers might like. Therefore, in the final section, we have outlined some of the resources that we have found to be the most useful in the learning and application of EBP, particularly for management of occupational therapy services. You will notice that, at the end of each chapter, similar resources such as journals, organizations or associations, or other types of resources related to the chapter focus are provided.

■ Real-Life Solutions

After Elena explained to Dan the importance of using theory, models, and evidence to plan and implement the different facets of occupational therapy programming and services, Dan felt more comfortable. He especially appreciated how Elena was able to explain that a manager uses the same evidence-based process for answering a "practice-related" question as does a clinician. From his schoolwork, Dan knew about how to write answerable questions, search the literature, and evaluate what he had read. Although the materials that he would need to use to help Elena prepare the proposal to expand the occupational therapy services at the facility would come from many different sources and consist of a variety of types of evidence, Dan felt more prepared to engage in the process.

Dan worked with Elena to identify the types of demographic data they wanted to review related to their potential customers as well as data about the location of existing services and estimated needs. They utilized local and state government databases and websites to find this type of evidence. They identified the clinical questions related to the wellness services they envisioned developing and conducted searches of literature databases to identify the most current and relevant evidence; then they began to categorize it and evaluate the strength and quality of the evidence they found. They also visited numerous websites of various organizations around the country and began to evaluate the strength of program descriptions and other types of qualitative data found on these sites.

As Dan worked with Elena on gathering and evaluating the evidence, he realized that he now needed to turn his attention to learning about the specific issues related to administering and managing occupational therapy services, including staff supervision, communication, leadership, program development, continuous quality improvement, and funding, as well as decision-making processes about space, equipment, and other resources.

Study Questions

1. **Which of the following have contributed to the proliferation of evidence-based practice and evidence-based management?**

   a. The development of processes, practices, and specific tools to enable health-care professionals to find, evaluate, and use evidence to inform their clinical decisions
   b. A dramatic increase in the access to evidence over the past several decades because of the Internet and open-access publishing
   c. Higher expectations for the training and skills of occupational therapy practitioners
   d. All of the above

2. **Which of the following best describes the approach you should take to finding and evaluating evidence related to management questions?**

   a. Only use evidence obtained through searches on well-established and recognized search tools such as PubMed.
   b. Search using multiple sources and strategies, considering all forms of evidence, but carefully evaluate the quality and strength of the evidence that you use.
   c. Limit your search and use of data to the field or discipline (e.g., occupational therapy) to exclude evidence from other fields or disciplines that may not be directly related to your question.
   d. Limit your search to only consider evidence developed through the strongest experimental methods such as randomized control designs.

3. **In assessing the evidence you are considering, which of the following would be least likely to impact your decision?**

   a. Country of origin of the evidence
   b. Strength of the evidence
   c. Quality of the evidence
   d. Level of the evidence

4. **Which of the following is the best description of *grey literature*?**

   a. Papers, reports, and other documents from private industry that often may be biased because of private funding
   b. Papers, reports, and other documents referred to as grey because of the weak evaluation of their accuracy and usefulness
   c. Papers, reports, and other documents controlled by commercial publishers that have passed the highest levels of review and academic scrutiny
   d. Papers, reports, and other documents from government, the academy, business, and industry that are not controlled by commercial publishers but are a valid form of evidence

5. **All of the following were identified as challenges to using an evidence-based approach to management by occupational therapy managers *except*:**

   a. Access to electronic journals and scientific forms of evidence.
   b. Time to find and carefully assess the evidence.
   c. Little evidence exists on management-related questions.
   d. The amount of evidence available can be overwhelming.

6. **Which of the following is most accurate regarding the typologies you might select to evaluate evidence related to management questions?**

   a. Because using an evidence-based approach to occupational therapy management is so new, there have not been any appropriate typologies for evaluating related evidence identified.
   b. Although there are variations in the approaches used by different scholars and sources, most use similar approaches to assigning a level to the evidence that is being examined.
   c. There is wide variation in the approaches used in various typologies for evaluating evidence and they have little in common.
   d. There is a single universal typology for evaluating all forms of evidence that has been identified for use with the occupational therapy management literature.

7. **Which of the following is most accurate regarding involvement of key stakeholders in the EBP process?**

   a. You may present an evidence brief or summary to key stakeholders to discuss the evidence, pros and cons of different options, what is feasible in your setting, and what barriers might exist to implementation.
   b. It is best not to discuss evidence with key stakeholders because many have not been exposed to or properly trained in EBP approaches.
   c. Key stakeholders should only be involved in identifying the questions to be answered through an EBP process.
   d. Key stakeholders may be a useful source of data, information, and other forms of evidence but you must be extremely careful of the bias this introduces to answering evidence-based management questions.

8. **Which of the following is the best strategy for occupational therapy managers who do not have easy access to electronic bibliographic databases to find evidence?**

   a. Return to graduate school for an advanced degree in order to access relevant databases.
   b. Access free databases such as PubMed or ProQuest, which are accessible with membership or certification through occupational therapy organizations.
   c. Rely on articles and evidence found on the Internet through Internet search engines.
   d. Rely only on data and other forms of evidence published in the public domain by commercial publishers.

Resources for Learning More About Evidence-Based Practice

Journals That Are Likely to Include Evidence Relevant to Management of Occupational Therapy Services

The Milbank Quarterly

http://www.milbank.org/the-milbank-quarterly

The *Milbank Quarterly* has been published for over seven decades and features peer-reviewed original research and articles that review health-care policy and provide analysis of current and evolving policy. Other content includes commentary from a range of professionals representing academicians, practitioners, researchers, and policy makers. Articles and commentary found in this journal represent multidisciplinary perspectives on empirical research as well as the application of research and policy in a variety of settings. Social, legal, and ethical issues are addressed.

Journal of Health Services Research & Policy

http://hsr.sagepub.com

The *Journal of Health Services Research & Policy* includes articles presenting results of qualitative and quantitative multidisciplinary research from a wide variety of disciplines. In addition to the reporting of empirical results, articles also address current and evolving debates in the scientific, methodological, and empirical arenas.

Health Services Research

http://www.hsr.org/hsr/abouthsr/journal.jsp

The journal *Health Services Research* provides researchers, policy makers and analysts, and health-care administrators and managers with access to empirical findings as well as articles addressing policy and methodological issues. Readers interested in health-care financing, the organization or delivery of health services, or the evaluation of health delivery outcomes will find *Health Services Research* a useful resource. The journal provides a forum for the exchange of practices related to individuals, health systems, and communities.

Professional Organizations Relevant to Management of Occupational Therapy Services

American College of Healthcare Executives

http://www.ache.org

The American College of Healthcare Executives (ACHE) is an international professional society of health-care executives working in a variety of settings, including hospitals, health-care systems, and other health-care organizations. The ACHE is known for its credentialing and educational programs. The annual Congress on Healthcare Management is a nationally recognized and widely attended event. The ACHE publishes the *Journal of Healthcare Management*, and a magazine titled *Healthcare Executive*.

General Information on Finding and Evaluating the Literature

- Cochrane Collaboration and the Cochrane Library (http://www.cochrane.org/index0.htm)
- Health Information Research Unit at McMaster University (http://hiru.mcmaster.ca/)
- Database of Abstracts of Reviews of Effects (DARE) (http://community.cochrane.org/editorial-and-publishing-policy-resource/database-abstracts-reviews-effects-dare)

Occupational Therapy–Specific Resources on Evidence-Based Practice

- OTseeker (http://www.otseeker.com/)
- AOTA Evidence-Based Practice Project (http://www.aota.org/)
- Center for Evidence-Based Rehabilitation at McMaster University (http://fw4.bluewirecs.ca/ResearchResourcesnbsp/ResearchGroups/CentreforEvidenceBasedRehabilitation/tabid/543/Default.aspx)
- National Board for Certification in Occupational Therapy—ProQuest (http://www.nbcot.org/proquest)

Government-Related Websites and Documents

- Centers for Disease Control and Prevention (http://www.cdc.gov/)
- National Center for Health Statistics (http://www.cdc.gov/nchs/)
- Agency for Health Care Research and Quality (http://www.ahcpr.gov/)
- Centers for Medicare and Medicaid Services (http://cms.hhs.gov/providers/edi/default.asp)

Other Useful Resources for the Evidence-Based Manager

- AcademyHealth: http://www.academyhealth.org
- Canadian Health Services Research Foundation: http://www.chsrf.ca/
- Center for Evidence-Based Management: http://www.cebma.org/
- Center for Health Management Research: http://www.nsf.gov/pubs/2002/nsf01168/nsf01168tt.htm
- Cochrane Collaboration Effective Practice and Organization of Care Group: http://www.epoc.uottawa.ca/
- Informed Decisions Toolbox: http://www.ahrq.gov/policymakers/measurement/decisiontoolbx/
- Institute for Healthcare Improvement: http://www.ihi.org/
- The Robert Wood Johnson Foundation Synthesis Project: http://www.rwjf.org/en/library/collections/the-synthesis-project.html

Resources on Evaluating Information Found on Websites

- Beck, S. (2009). Evaluation criteria. In *The good, the bad & the ugly: Or, why it's a good idea to evaluate Web sources*. Retrieved from http://lib.nmsu.edu/instruction/evalcrit.html
- The University of California Berkeley Library (http://www.lib.berkeley.edu/TeachingLib/Guides/Internet/Evaluate.html)

Reference List

Cane, J., O'Connor, D., & Michie, S. (2012). Validation of the theoretical domains framework for use in behaviour change and implementation research. *Implementation Science*, 7–37. Retrieved from http://www.implementationscience.com/content/7/1/37

Capan, M., Ambrose, H., Burkett, M., Evangelista, T., Flook, D., & Straka, K. (2013). Nursing portfolio study. *Journal for Nurses in Professional Development* [serial online], *29*(4), 182–185.

Cochrane, A. (1972). *Effectiveness and efficiency: Random reflections on health services*. London, UK: Nuffield Provincial Hospitals Trust.

Evashwick, C., & Rundall, T. (2010, January–February). No better time: The effects of the recession make evidence-based management all the more compelling for health care leaders. *Health Progress*, Jan–Feb, 37–41.

Finlay, K., & McLaren, S. (2009). Does appraisal enhance learning, improve practice and encourage continuing professional development? A survey of general practitioners' experiences of appraisal. *Quality in Primary Care*, *17*(6), 387–395.

Fisher, B., & Robertson, D. (2007). Is evidence-based management right for you? Chances are it will help your organization—if you have time to implement it. *Information Outlook*, *11*(12), 10–15.

Guyatt, G. H., Oxman, A. D., Kunz, R., Vist, G. E., Falck-Ytter, Y., Schunemann, H. J., and the GRADE Working Group. (2008). What is "quality of evidence" and why is it important to clinicians? *British Medical Journal*, *336*, 995–998.

Holm, M. (2000). Our mandate for the new millennium: Evidence-based practice. *American Journal of Occupational Therapy*, *64*, 575–585.

Jones, K. R. (2010). Rating the level, quality, and strength of the research evidence. *Journal of Nursing Care Quality*, *25*(4), 304-312.

Law, M., & MacDermid, J. (2013). *Evidence-based rehabilitation: A guide to practice* (3rd ed.). Thorofare, NJ: Slack.

Michie, S., van Stralen, M. M., & West, R. (2011). The behaviour change wheel: A new method for characterising and designing behaviour change interventions. *Implementation Science*, *6*, 42. Retrieved from http://www.implementationscience.com/content/6/1/42

National Board for Certification in Occupational Therapy. (2014). Professional development tools. Retrieved from http://www.nbcot.org/proquest

Oxford Centre for Evidence-Based Medicine. (2011). *Levels of evidence*. Retrieved from http://www.cebm.net/wp-content/uploads/2014/06/CEBM-Levels-of-Evidence-2.1.pdf

Salvatori, P., Simonavicius, N., Moore, J., Rimmer, G., & Patterson, M. (2008). Meeting the challenge of assessing clinical competence of occupational therapists within a program management environment. *Canadian Journal of Occupational Therapy*, *75*(1), 51–60.

Smith, K. P., & Woods, J. (2003). The healthcare manager as catalyst for evidence-based practice: Changing the healthcare environment and changing experience. *Healthcare Papers*, *3*(3), 54–57.

The New York Academy of Medicine. (n.d.). *What is grey literature?* Retrieved from http://www.greylit.org/about

Leading and Managing in Context

CHAPTER 3

Understanding Health-Care Systems and Practice Contexts

Gail Fisher, MPA, OTR/L, FAOTA
Brent Braveman, PhD, OTR/L, FAOTA

■ Real-Life Management

Andrea is an occupational therapist (OT) who has been working in an outpatient clinic in a suburban area for 5 years. She has just accepted a position in a small-town hospital in a semirural area. The hospital has only had part-time contractual occupational therapists and she is the first full-time employee. More doctors have recently been requesting occupational therapy services for their patients.

During the first week at her new job, Andrea, as both the director of occupational therapy and the only OT, knew she had her work cut out for her. She needed to review and establish charges for services, determine what occupational therapy services would be reimbursable by Medicare, figure out what documentation each payer required, and determine unmet needs that occupational therapy

could address. She noticed that the hospital was not fully compliant with the Americans With Disabilities Act, and wanted to assist it in correcting these deficiencies. She also wanted to begin planning for hiring another practitioner within the next year to assist her, and needed to find out about the supply of occupational therapy personnel in her state and local area.

Andrea already had been contacted by the local school district, which was interested in contracting for occupational therapy services from the hospital. Rather than feeling overly challenged, Andrea knew that there were multiple resources to guide her as she analyzed the larger systems that impacted on her new role and her potential success. Andrea decided to start by networking with other managers who had faced similar challenges and to begin to collect data, information, and other forms of evidence to guide her decision-making.

Critical Thinking Questions

As you read this chapter, consider the following questions:

- How is being knowledgeable about the contexts within which we practice essential to succeed as an occupational therapy manager?

- What types of data, information, and other forms of evidence exist to assist managers to learn about payment, legislation, trends, and other relevant subjects?

- What strategies for staying up-to-date regarding policies and other changes in the environment can you use as data, information, and forms of evidence are constantly updated?

- How will scanning the environment for indicators of future trends keep you one step ahead in anticipating changes that will affect your practice and your organization?

Glossary

- **Accountable care organizations (ACOs):** groups of providers associated with a defined population of patients that are accountable for the quality and cost of care delivered to that population.

- **Dualism:** term that has been used to reflect the involvement of both government (at the national, state, and local levels) and private industry in the health-care system.

- **Free-market system:** term used to describe the type of economic system characterized by the principles of supply and demand, competition, and free choice based on information.

- **Health maintenance organization (HMO):** company that uses a managed care approach to limit use of unnecessary health care by requiring the insured person to choose from a selected panel of physicians, and to get approval from his or her primary care provider for desired specialty services, including therapy.

- **Managed care:** method of controlling utilization of health care by requiring approval of hospitalizations and specialty services, as well as by negotiating reduced fees with providers and promoting efficient health-care delivery.

- **Medicaid:** state-run program for people who have limited income or high medical expenses. Eligibility for the limited income cohort is based on the family income and size in relation to the national poverty level, although states can expand eligibility.

- **Medicare:** federal program for people over 65 years and some individuals with chronic disabilities.

- **Mixed economy:** term that reflects the type of economic system found in the United States and elsewhere where there is both individual ownership and individual freedom but also a significant component of the economy is controlled by the government.

- **Patient-centered medical homes (PCMHs):** primary care model based on patient-centered, coordinated, team-driven care and supported by strong health information technology (HIT).

- **Post-acute care bundling:** uses a single payment for all services related to a specific treatment or condition (e.g., a stroke), possibly spanning multiple providers in multiple settings. A single episode of care might include initial hospitalization; rehospitalization; post-acute care; and physician and other services, such as occupational therapy.

- **Preferred provider organization (PPO):** manner of organizing the payment for health services by placing limits on where an insured person can obtain his or her health care and controlling costs by negotiating discounts with providers.

- **Triple aim of health care:** the aim of seeking to improve population health, improve health care, and reduce costs.

Introduction

An understanding of the larger systems within which you work is essential for managers. In Chapter 2, you were introduced to the different types of evidence and strategies for evaluating evidence. In particular, you learned to think more broadly about evidence and understand that, as an occupational therapy manager, you will rely on evidence beyond results of clinical research. Although other types of data and information (e.g., demographic trends or information about unmet needs of a population) might not fit perfectly with a researcher's conceptualization of evidence, the effective occupational therapy manager must be able to locate, evaluate, and integrate disparate types of information quickly. Learning to adapt the basic process of evidence-based practice introduced in Chapter 2 will aid you in making sound decisions based on the best available information.

In this chapter, evidence is discussed in relation to staying up-to-date on the larger health-care system and service delivery context as it evolves. Finding and using evidence about payment, legislation, practice requirements, personnel, licensure, and future trends will allow you to make better informed decisions and plans in your role as a manager or even in your role as an occupational therapy practitioner. This chapter introduces you to a variety of sources and strategies for locating data, information, and other forms of evidence to help you make managerial decisions.

ing the organizations in which occupational therapy personnel most often work. One way of classifying organizations is by "setting" or naming organizations according to the function they serve in society. These settings may be placed along a continuum from those that are the most closely aligned with the medical model to those that are the least like the medical model (Box 3-1). Regardless of where it falls on this continuum, an organization may have other characteristics, such as being for-profit or not-for-profit, or being part of a large network of providers, that influence how the organization interacts in the larger health-care system.

The health-care system in the United States is unique among nations. The United States is the only industrialized country that does not have health care funded by or provided by the government to all of its citizens, although it is clear that our government does play a large role in our health-care system (the details follow later in this chapter). The U.S. economic system is commonly classified as a **mixed economy**. It does have a high degree of private ownership and individual freedom, but a significant component of the economy is controlled by the government. In fact, current estimates indicate that federal government spending accounts for up to one-third of our economy (BB&T Program on Capitalism, Markets, and Morality, 2014). Mixed economies do include many principles of the free-market system, which are reflected in our health-care system with a large part of the system

Health-Care Systems and Occupational Therapy Service Delivery Settings

Despite recent changes in health-care policy such as the Patient Protection and Affordable Care Act (ACA) of 2010, the term *health-care "system"* is a misnomer, but one that is commonly used to describe the larger service delivery context. What we have in the United States is a cobbled-together network of loosely connected pieces, including hospitals, long-term care facilities, outpatient centers, private offices of physicians and therapists, primary care clinics, home care agencies, and community-based, not-for-profit agencies. Schools and early intervention (EI) centers are also part of the network, because they provide therapy and other health-related services. In Chapter 4, you will be introduced to various typologies for categoriz-

---

BOX 3-1

Continuum of Occupational Therapy Delivery Settings (Most to Least Medically Oriented)

- Hospital
- Long-term care facility
- Primary care clinic
- Outpatient therapy center
- Home health and hospice
- Early intervention (EI)
- Industrial or work rehabilitation
- School system
- Community or social service agency

oriented toward making a profit. There are also some not-for-profit segments of the system, such as many community-based agencies and some hospitals, long-term care facilities, and home care agencies. Because the government is also involved in financing and regulating health care, there is built-in interaction between the government and the service providers (Sandstrom, Lohman, & Bramble, 2014).

Dualism is a term that has been used to reflect the involvement of both government (at the national, state, and local levels) and private industry in the health-care system (Sandstrom et al, 2014). Both advantages and disadvantages can be identified related to a dualistic system. Having the government involved in oversight of aspects of health care through accreditation, licensing, and certification systems may be seen as a safeguard to protect the public. Federal and state financing of some health care through systems such as Medicare and Medicaid provides access for a portion of our population that might not otherwise be able to afford care. However, governmental systems are often characterized as overly bureaucratic, slow to change, and relatively inflexible in administering policies and procedures in a way that allows for individual needs and situations.

The involvement of private industry and individuals in the system has contributed to innovation in care, as well as competition that typically is thought to act to keep costs lower, and provides for much greater choice and, in some cases, improved access for consumers. Yet great reliance on private providers makes oversight of quality and standardization of care very difficult, has allowed for fraud and abuse of payment structures, and contributes to an abundance of some types of providers and shortages of providers in other, less lucrative specialties. For example, lucrative medical specialties such as plastic surgery have attracted a larger number of medical residents, whereas primary care delivery has received less attention from medical students entering the field. Moreover, relying on private providers for a substantial portion of delivery of health care in our country results in potential conflict of interest for the providers. These providers have a mandate to make a profit for the company's shareholders and must balance what is good for their financial "bottom line" with what is in their patients' best interest.

Health-care economics is tremendously complex, but having an understanding of basic economic principles and their relationship to the health-care system is useful for the occupational therapy manager if for

no other reason than to help you understand the dynamic tensions faced by health-care providers, payers, and consumers and why the health-care system is so volatile. Further, it sometimes seems that a never-ending role for occupational therapy managers is to interpret limitations and demands within organizational systems for those we supervise. Those who intend to move into roles in higher organizational administration or who desire to start and operate their own business would benefit from a more detailed investigation of health-care economics. However, the scope of the discussion here will be limited to an overview of key concepts.

A basic economic principle to understand is that the goal of any economy is to *allocate limited resources* (Mansfield, 1980). Regardless of the type of economy within a given country or the health of an economy at a given time, there simply is a limited amount of human, financial, and capital resources that must be divided among competing needs. For example, Medicare is still the primary payment source for much of the occupational therapy intervention that is reimbursed by a third party in the United States. Yet we know that there is a limited Medicare budget that is under constant scrutiny as our federal government tries to manage growing budget deficits, and that there is competition for Medicare funds to pay for services ranging from prescription drugs to rehabilitation. Even in countries where "universal" health care provides health coverage for every citizen, limits are placed on who qualifies for various types of care and how long they must wait to receive it. For example, in Canada, although all citizens are insured and have access to health care, in 2013 Canadians faced an average wait time of 9.3 weeks for treatment by a specialist after referral by a general practitioner, which was longer than other countries with universal health care (National Center for Policy Analysis, 2014).

Earlier it was mentioned that the U.S. health-care system is based upon principles including those of the **free-market system**. Three key principles underlie free-market economies. The first key principle is that of *supply and demand*. Simply stated, as supply and demand diverge, the price of products should respond accordingly such that, when supply exceeds demand, costs to the consumer should go down, and when demand exceeds supply, costs to the consumer should go up. A second key principle of a free-market economy is that of *competition*. In many industries, competition helps to assure that consumers get higher-quality products at lower prices. Consider, for example, electronics or communication devices and the familiar phenomenon that occurs when new technology is introduced (e.g., smartphones). Initially, as availability of new technology is limited, quality expectations may be lower and prices are higher. However, as the number of companies producing a product increases and competition for buyers' attention grows, quality often improves while prices decrease. The third key principle of free-market economies is that of *free choice* based on information. However, a sometimes unrecognized assumption of a free-market economy is that consumers have access to information, the ability to gather information, and the ability to make informed choices when more than one provider is available. Further, it is typically assumed that economies work best when people are free to make what they want, buy what they want, and work where they want (Drafke, 2002; Mansfield, 1980).

When considering health care in the United States, however, application of principles from the free-market system is imperfect and affects health care in complex ways. Let's briefly examine the application of the principles of supply and demand, competition, and free choice to the health-care market in the United States to identify how this market functions differently from markets for other goods or services. Supply and demand and competition are principles that interact in most markets. Often, as manufacturers, providers, or entrepreneurs note that there is growing demand for a product or service, they will move into that market. Production will increase eventually, increasing competition and supply, which in turn promotes quality and lowers prices. However, these principles do not function in the same manner in health care because of the complex interactions between availability and access to services (e.g., supply), need (e.g., demand), and the involvement of third parties in the payment for many services.

The involvement of third-party payers and **managed care** in the health-care market limits the effects of supply and competition in a number of ways. For example, some forms of insurance limit access to providers and therefore limit competition to some extent (e.g., use of a **preferred provider organization [PPO]**). The intent of such a structure is to control costs by negotiating discounts with providers if those who are insured are forced to choose from a designated list of providers. However, we need to ask what

can happen to quality when consumer choice is limited. For example, if persons are essentially forced into choosing a particular hospital system because of severe financial penalties if they go "outside of the PPO," how does the consumer know that all care delivered in that system is the best available? Although a given hospital might provide excellent cardiology services, it might not provide similarly effective orthopedic services. Yet the demand to improve these services that typically comes from a fully competitive free-market system is lessened by the restrictions on consumer choice. A second example of the limits that health insurance places on competition is the **health maintenance organization (HMO)**, which uses "gatekeepers" to control access to specialists by requiring that the decision to pursue specialty services such as a consultation with a dermatologist must first be approved by a general practitioner, a physician assistant, or a nurse. If approved, referral will be made to a specialist in the HMO's network of providers, thus denying the free choice of the person seeking services.

Competition in health care is limited in some ways as a result of both legal structures and to some extent societal values. Some aspects of competition are restricted by governmental regulation, such as the *certificate of need* process whereby a state typically requires health-care providers to obtain permission for activities including construction of new health-care facilities, acquisition of some types of major medical equipment (e.g., a new magnetic resonance imaging device), changes in ownership, or the addition of new services. Certificates of need are usually limited to major changes or additions, yet there is no doubt that to some extent they limit the ability of some providers to compete with others, and this means that the principle of supply and demand cannot be fully applied to health care.

Advertising in health care is common, especially among hospitals and pharmaceutical companies. However, it is rare that prices for health-care services are openly discussed in public formats so the costs of one provider might be compared to another, as is typical with most other products. The suggestion to compare prices of various providers for the same procedure or services has become more common, but it can be difficult to access this information. Yet without access to all of this information, it is challenging for consumers to be fully informed, a prerequisite for making free choices. Additionally, when considering the relationship between cost and quality for most products, consumers will often choose to pay a lower price, knowing that it also means accepting a lower level of quality. Yet, when making health-care choices for oneself or one's family, who is willing to make a comparable decision? Consumers of health services typically expect and assume that they will get the best care possible regardless of the fee charged.

Supply-and-demand and free-choice principles have become more consequential in the health-care system with the rise in the number of individuals with high-deductible health plans. High-deductible plans require the consumer to pay more out-of-pocket, typically $2,000 to $5,000 per year, before insurance begins to cover any health-care charges. The proportion of employees covered by this type of plan rose from 4% to 19% from 2004 to 2012 (Kaiser Family Foundation, 2012), and the majority of the plans purchased on the ACA health insurance exchanges have a high deductible, with many also having a high copayment for each visit to a physician or therapist. The implications are that individuals will have to pay more out-of-pocket for therapy; therefore, the therapist will have to convince the client that therapy is worth paying for by explaining the potential benefits of therapy and the risks of not receiving therapy, as well as by achieving excellent outcomes. Therapy consumers are more likely to compare prices and outcomes if they are paying directly for the services, thus driving competition. This competitive environment may drive innovation, customer service enhancements, and increased quality. The higher out-of-pocket payments and potential decrease in clients may make it more challenging for therapist-owned private practices to make a substantial profit.

The assumption that information for health care decision-making is readily accessible and understandable by all is false. For example, in today's society access to information is clearly easier for those who also have Internet access and the skills and experiences to take advantage of it. To some degree, persons of lower socioeconomic status or education attainment may have more difficulty obtaining information than those with more resources. A growing amount of information is available through the Internet to assist consumers in making health-care decisions. For example, at www.Medicare.gov, consumers can access quality comparison data on nursing homes, hospitals, and home health agencies. One can do a side-by-side comparison of several hospitals in one's

community on patient satisfaction, outcomes and readmission rates across major diagnostic categories, and number of patients served with specific diagnoses. For nursing homes, one can access a star rating system to learn about overall rating, health inspections, staffing, and quality measures. Drilling down provides details on health inspection citations across domains, including a rating of potential harmfulness to the residents, and full inspection and complaint reports. Data on physicians and therapists is primarily a listing of providers in a specified geographic area, but availability of quality data for therapists will expand as the data from the Physician Quality Reporting System (PQRS), which includes data from private therapy practices, is posted. Providing this data in an easy-to-follow format increases transparency of provider outcomes and will assist educated consumers and discharge planners in seeking higher-quality services, therefore driving demand for quality providers and providing lower-ranked providers with incentives to improve their processes and outcomes.

Even if outcome and quality information is accessible and understandable, making informed health-care choices can be incredibly complex when you add payment as a consideration. Terminology that health-care professionals use routinely, such as PPOs, deductibles, copayments, or out-of-pocket maximums, may be confusing to consumers, especially as our population becomes more diverse and a growing percentage of Americans have a language other than English as their first language. Finally, obtaining factual information about an illness or disease, the usual treatment, alternative treatments, and risks and benefits from busy providers may be difficult, especially if you are not skilled in advocating for your needs. For all these reasons, being an informed consumer and making a "free choice" is much more difficult in the health-care market than for most other products or services.

The complexity of our health-care system and its inherent conflicts make enhancing cost, access, and quality across all elements of the system challenging. Raising costs to the consumers of the service may mean that fewer people can access the services they need. Service providers that cut costs to payers to appear more competitive may feel pressure to decrease the quantity or quality of services provided to the consumer. Reducing costs without reducing access to services or quality of services is a significant challenge that our elected officials, providers, payers, and employers grapple with daily. Most changes to the system are incremental in nature—increasing access here, cutting costs there—and building in incentives for quality and efficiency wherever possible. This is an evolving system that is continually changing. For that reason, the focus of this chapter is to point you to the relevant sources of data, information, and other forms of evidence. Rather than providing you with extensive details about specific payment or legislation that may quickly become outdated, this chapter focuses on strategies for obtaining current data, information, and other forms of evidence on an ongoing basis. What is most important is for you to learn the skills to scan the environment for current information and future trends, and to stay abreast of developments relevant to your setting.

In addition to the health-care system, occupational therapy practitioners practice in many other contexts, such as school systems, EI programs, and community agencies. Similar to the health-care system, these practice settings are also influenced by changes in legislation, funding, and training requirements. The focus of relevant legislation may be different, but the need to be informed remains the same.

Evidence, Health Systems, and the Occupational Therapy Manager

A variety of data, information, and other forms of evidence is available to assist you in better understanding the segment of the health system in which you work, and for planning and implementing programs in health-care, educational, or other types of settings. The type of evidence with which you are most likely familiar is evidence gained through empirical investigations. Common approaches to gathering empirical evidence are listed in Box 3-2. In addition to their use in research, these general approaches may be used to collect data (another form of evidence) to answer questions you will have as a manager. The type(s) of approach chosen will depend upon the question(s) you are trying to address.

However, at times it may be difficult to find formally published data, information, or evidence specific to your setting and your situation. At those times, you may rely more on informal evidence, such as interviewing others in a similar position, online communication through social media or professional sites such as OTConnections provided by the American Occupational Therapy Association (AOTA), informal

---

BOX 3-2
Common Approaches for Gathering Data

- **Quantitative:** Numerical data
  - *Example of data obtained:* Mail survey, which includes a rating scale, sent to parents of children receiving special education to determine if they desire summer therapy programs at an outpatient clinic, followed by an analysis of the numerical data obtained.
- **Qualitative:** In-depth interviewing and observing
  - *Example of data obtained:* Key informant interview with the director of the local senior citizens center to determine the need for a health promotion program delivered by occupational therapy students, followed by an analysis of interviews conducted with a number of key informants to determine common themes.
- **Retrospective observational research:** Database approaches
  - *Example of data obtained:* Demographic statistics and trends in the incidence of stroke affecting people age 50 years and younger and the health-care services that they utilized.
- **Participatory research:** Involving practitioners and consumers in the generation of knowledge or in the generation of knowledge and taking action to improve services (the latter is Participatory Action Research)
  - *Example of data obtained:* Town hall meeting with consumers who have received occupational therapy to help plan for a new outpatient therapy center, followed by an analysis of the relevant comments.

networking at conferences, and gathering information from colleagues or former classmates. In considering the value of this type of evidence, you should apply one of the appropriate typologies for evaluating evidence that were introduced in Chapter 2. In the next section of this chapter, we briefly review common types of data, information, and other forms of evidence of use to the occupational therapy manager and how and where you might find it.

Common Types of Data, Information, and Other Forms of Evidence Used by Occupational Therapy Managers

Payment and Reimbursement

Who is paying for occupational therapy services and how much they are paying is core knowledge for managers. Several therapy-oriented texts provide a detailed analysis of payment sources and how they operate (Jacobs & McCormack, 2011; Lohman, 2014; Sandstrom et al, 2014). There are also websites that have up-to-date information for managers (see Resources section at the end of this chapter). Because the specifics of what various payers reimburse can change frequently, rather than discussing "who pays for what," it is more valuable to focus on understanding the long-standing facets of payment in our health-care system. If the payment source is the government, there are official documents that detail the rules about what is covered and what is excluded (e.g., Medicare guidelines, eligibility for the State Children's Health Insurance Program [SCHIP]).

Deciding on rates for therapy services (i.e., what you will charge consumers for the services they receive) requires researching the relevant sources of payment as well as market influences and the population served. Determining a specific fee for a service can be difficult at times. You may be able to obtain information from your peers or request information from other providers of service, and some service providers or payers may be willing to share their charge or payment structures. You must be careful, however, because the process of agreeing with another service provider to set costs together at a determined level (thereby removing competition) is known as *price fixing* and is illegal. Box 3-3 details information that managers need to know about sources of payment as part of the process of setting rates for therapy services as well as determining potential sources of revenue.

For example, occupational therapy for Medicare patients will only be reimbursed if the payer determines that services are *"reasonable and necessary,"* and that a *"skilled"* service is required (i.e., not services that can be provided by an aide or family member) (AOTA,

---

BOX 3-3

What Managers Need to Know About Potential Sources of Reimbursement or Payment

- What target populations are of concern to the payment source (e.g., age, income level, medical condition, employment status)?
- What services are included and excluded for payment (e.g., occupational therapy evaluation and treatment, treatment focused on sensory integration, driver evaluation, adaptive equipment for the bathroom)?
- Are there restrictions on payment or conditions that need to be met for payment to occur (e.g., doctor must provide a written statement of medical necessity; client can only be seen by an occupational therapist)?
- Is certification or provider status necessary for obtaining payment for services (e.g., hand therapy covered only if provided by a certified hand therapist [CHT], or industrial rehabilitation services covered only if provided by a Commission on Accreditation of Rehabilitation Facilities [CARF]–approved agency)?
- Is a physician referral required for evaluation or treatment?
- What documentation is required (e.g., daily notes versus weekly or monthly summary)?
- Does the payer require additional information such as codes that indicate the reasons for therapy, the extent of the disabling condition, and the areas targeted for improvement?

2014b; Centers for Medicare and Medicaid Services, 2014d). Payment rates change and are influenced by legislative and presidential decision-making, fluctuation in the costs of providing care, the gross national product, the state of the economy, and shifts in the number of Medicare beneficiaries and of people paying into the system through payroll taxes. Payment for occupational therapy may also be influenced by payment changes for other professions. For example, because occupational therapy payment for outpatient services is tied to physician payment through a governmental cost containment measure known as the

BOX 3-4

Who Pays for Health Care and Occupational Therapy?

- **Medicare:** A federal program for people over 65 years and some individuals with long-term disabilities.
- **Medicaid:** A state-run program for people who have limited income or high medical expenses. Eligibility for the limited income cohort is based on the family income and size in relation to the national poverty level, although states can expand eligibility.
- **Workers' compensation:** A state-administered program for workers injured on the job that provides temporary and permanent disability income as well as coverage of medical and rehabilitation expenses.
- **Rehabilitation services administration:** A federal agency that funds state vocational rehabilitation and independent living support services, including therapy.
- **Commercial insurance:** Privately owned companies that provide indemnity insurance, HMOs, or PPOs.
- **Out-of-pocket payment:** Recipients pay for services in cash either because they don't have insurance or they have insurance with a large deductible that must be paid by the recipient before the insurance starts covering expenses.

sustainable growth rate, their lobbying and advocacy work may have indirect benefits for occupational therapy practitioners and vice versa. AOTA provides payment updates to practitioners through its publications and electronic communications (see www.aota.org).

A few of the major payment sources for health care are listed in Box 3-4, and a brief description of each is provided in the following sections of the chapter.

Medicare

Medicare has been and continues to be the largest payer of health-care services in the United States, and

also the largest payer of occupational therapy services (Lassman, Hartman, Washington, Andrews, & Catlin, 2014; Radomski & Trombly-Latham, 2008; Sandstrom et al, 2014). Medicare is managed and funded by the federal government, and administered by the Centers for Medicare and Medicaid Services (CMS) of the Department of Health and Human Services. There are specific guidelines for eligibility, covered services, and payment. Payments to hospitals primarily follow a model of prospective payment, identifying amounts that will be paid in advance based on patient characteristics, service needs, and facility characteristics. Outpatient services are reimbursed using a resource-based relative value scale (RVU), which takes into account the technical ability, knowledge, and skill of the provider; overhead and malpractice cost factors; and a local cost index (CMS, 2014c). Therapists in private practice must apply to be an approved Medicare provider before payment is allowed.

CMS contracts out vital program operational functions (i.e., claims processing, provider and beneficiary services, appeals, etc.) to a set of contractors known as Medicare administrative contractors (MACS). MACS are contracted for a period of 5 years to process Medicare claims (CMS, 2013).

These organizations develop coverage guidelines that may include descriptions of what they are looking for in documentation and exclusions of coverage. Medicare contractors can be found through an interactive map at the Medicare.gov website (http://www.cms.gov/Research-Statistics-Data-and-Systems/Monitoring-Programs/Medicare-FFS-Compliance-Programs/Review-Contractor-Directory-Interactive-Map/). Contractors may post frequently asked questions, recommendations for documentation, and information on enrolling as a provider. The Office of the Inspector General of the federal government periodically evaluates service provision. In the past, it has evaluated whether occupational therapy delivered in skilled nursing facilities (SNFs) was medically necessary and met all the requirements of Medicare. "According to the U.S. Department of Health & Human Services, Office of Inspector General's (OIG's) recent report, skilled nursing facilities (SNFs) improperly billed Medicare in one-quarter of all claims submitted in 2009, costing Medicare $1.5 billion in inappropriate payments. After reviewing the medical records supporting 499 claims submitted to Medicare in 2009, OIG found that a large percentage of the inappropriate charges resulted from upcoding attributable to claims for "ultrahigh" therapy in SNFs (Peterson, 2012). The well-informed manager will be familiar with the facts that a payer has collected and how those facts are influencing its funding rules.

Because Medicare is administered by the federal government, passage of legislation can have a direct and dramatic impact on payment for services. For example, in 1997, the U.S. Congress passed the Balanced Budget Act (BBA). This brought SNFs under prospective payment rather than fee-for-service billing, and dramatically changed the payment to facilities. In addition, a $1,500 annual limit per person, or cap, was placed on occupational therapy services provided under Medicare Part B in outpatient settings or SNFs (hospital outpatient services were initially exempted from the cap). The resulting downsizing of assistant (OTA) and occupational therapist (OT) jobs due to implementation of the caps was significant (Fisher & Cooksey, 2002). As therapy personnel were laid off from SNFs, they moved into other settings and created a ripple effect in the job market, leading to a period of surplus of occupational therapy personnel in many regions of the country that lasted several years (Fisher & Keehn, 2007). It was critical for the occupational therapy managers who remained in the SNFs to understand the new rules for payment and to reconfigure the services delivered to fit the new payment model. These rules included the actual funding changes that based payment on the intensity of therapy and nursing services needed, implementation dates, case mix and length-of-stay implications, payment changes, personnel requirements, treatment implications (i.e., group vs. individual therapy), and the outpatient therapy cap. The cap was fully implemented in 1999, placed on moratorium in 2000, and an exception process to the cap was put in place in March 2006. The exception process allowed the therapist to justify continuing therapy services beyond the cap if the therapy recipients met certain requirements. The amount of the cap is adjusted for medical inflation and was $1,920 in 2014. In 2013, an additional requirement was imposed for a manual medical review of any Medicare beneficiary that received over $3,700 per calendar year for therapy. Every year, legislation must be passed to extend the exception process. At the time of this writing, the cap had not been permanently repealed, although AOTA and the

other therapy associations worked together for repeal. When changes of this nature occur, the best resources are AOTA federal affairs and payment specialists, the AOTA website, and AOTA publications. Although the job market has since rebounded and there is a current shortage of OTs and OTAs, the BBA is an example of why it is important for occupational therapy managers to be continually scanning the environment, including the legislative environment.

An example of how legal decisions can affect therapy practice is the *Jimmo v. Sebelius* case that was decided in 2013. In January 2011, five national groups filed a class action lawsuit against the Department of Health and Human Services about a Medicare policy that required a beneficiary to exhibit "demonstrable improvements" to qualify for skilled nursing care and physical, speech, and occupational therapy. This criterion was perceived as discriminating against people with progressive conditions such as Parkinson disease and multiple sclerosis. A settlement was reached with the Department of Health and Human Services and Department of Justice, stipulating that skilled services to maintain an individual's condition or prevent or slow his or her decline are covered by Medicare and that the so-called "improvement standard" that Medicare had been employing is illegal. It was clarified that Medicare coverage hinges on whether the skilled services of a health-care professional are medically necessary, not whether the beneficiary will "improve." Medicare can no longer deny care to patients on the grounds that their condition is stable, chronic, or not improving. The CMS implemented a nationwide education campaign for all who make Medicare determinations to ensure that beneficiaries with chronic conditions are not denied coverage for critical services because their underlying conditions will not improve (AOTA, 2014a).

Before the *Jimmo* case, therapists would discharge clients who were no longer making improvements, due to anticipated lack of payment for clients whose progress had plateaued. Or, therapists may have attempted to continue to provide services with a justification that the therapy was preventing functional decline, with a subsequent denial of payment by the MACS due to lack of progress. As a result of the *Jimmo* case, if the therapist can document that skilled occupational therapy is necessary to maintain function or prevent decline, there will not be the automatic denial of payment that existed before the *Jimmo* case was settled (AOTA, 2014a). However, the outpatient therapy cap described previously still applies and may now be considered to be the primary factor limiting extensive ongoing outpatient therapy services under Medicare Part B.

Medicaid

Medicaid is jointly funded by the federal government and the states. Each state determines what Medicaid will pay for and who is eligible, providing at least the minimum required by federal law. Therefore, coverage for occupational therapy varies from state to state. You can often find details on Medicaid coverage on your state government website and on the Medicaid portion of the U.S. government's CMS website (http://www.medicaid.gov). Some states require prior approval of occupational therapy treatment for all diagnoses, whereas others waive the prior approval requirement for certain diagnoses, and still others do not require prior approval for treatment. Rates vary from state to state, and are prone to change depending on a state's fiscal situation.

In 1997, as part of the BBA, Congress created a new children's health insurance program called the SCHIP. This program gave each state permission to offer health insurance for children who are not already insured to address the growing problem of children without health insurance. The SCHIP was designed as a federal–state partnership, similar to Medicaid, with the goal of expanding health insurance to children whose families earn too much money to be eligible for Medicaid, but not enough money to purchase private insurance. The SCHIP was the single largest expansion of health insurance coverage for children since the initiation of Medicaid in the mid-1960s. In 2014 the program provided health coverage to nearly 8 million children. The ACA of 2010 maintained the SCHIP eligibility standards in place through 2019 and extended funding until 2015, when the federal matching rate increases to 93% (Centers for Medicare and Medicaid, 2014b).

With the passage of the ACA in 2010, opportunities were made available to the states to expand Medicaid coverage to additional individuals who had not previously qualified, with the majority of expansion costs covered by the federal government. Some states chose not to expand, creating an inequity in Medicaid eligibility across the states. Although the payment rate for

Medicaid patients is typically lower than other payers, it provides a safety net for those who do not have other insurance coverage.

Workers' Compensation

Workers' compensation is mandated by the federal government and exists in all 50 states. In addition to paying wage replacement after a worker injured on the job has been off of work for 3 days, workers' compensation funds medical services, including therapy that is ordered by a physician. Each state has an industrial commission that determines payment and rules about what the employer or the employer's insurance company must cover. Because each state has its own industrial commission, the process of referral to and payment for therapy varies state by state. For example, some states are using a managed care model with tight case management practices. The rules about the employees' right to choose their own doctors also vary and influence where you would market your work rehabilitation services. State industrial commissions may have data related to work injury rates, the most common work injuries, typical time off work, percentage of workers' compensation clients returning to work, and the percentage receiving rehabilitation or vocational services. These data will help you to ascertain the need for a new program or expansion of an existing program. When considering any type of insurance (e.g., Medicare, Medicaid, workers' compensation, or private insurance), it is critical that you consider what services are traditionally covered by the insured's "policy" and the extent to which you can negotiate payment for a service that is not covered. For example, it is very difficult to negotiate for services typically not covered by Medicare or Medicaid even if providing the services might result in an overall cost savings to the federal or state government. It is much more likely that you can negotiate payment for services on a case-by-case basis with a private insurer or with a workers' compensation insurer if you can demonstrate that covering the service will result in savings for the insurer.

Rehabilitation Services Administration

What about local vocational and rehabilitation service agencies? This often-overlooked source of referrals and payments exists in every state. Through joint federal and state funding, the Rehabilitation Services Administration state-level agencies provide funding for vocational and independent living services for teens and adults with disabilities. A list of the state agencies and their websites can be found at the U.S. Department of Education website by using the states and territories list at http://wdcrobcolp01.ed.gov/Programs/EROD/org_list_by_territory.cfm.

Relevant information that you need to know includes requirements for providers, criteria for payment for occupational therapy, referral mechanisms, and payment rates. Because these are state-run agencies, each agency differs in how it operates. Gathering this information in person from the local vocational rehabilitation office may provide an opportunity to make personal contact with a referral source. Your state government website should have information on where these local offices are and how to make contact.

Self-Pay

Another payment source to consider is out-of-pocket payment, which is sometimes referred to as "self-pay." More providers are making the decision to collect fees for services, and then the client or client's family can collect from their insurance company if able to do so. Trends in the use of alternative medicine, much of which has been paid for out of pocket, have demonstrated that people are willing to pay for something themselves if they think the benefits will be worth the cost (Frass et al, 2012). The National Center for Complementary and Alternative Medicine (NCCAM) reported that, "According to the 2007 National Health Interview Survey (NHIS), U.S. adults spent an estimated $33.9 billion out-of-pocket on complementary health approaches in the previous 12 months. They spent about two-thirds ($22.0 billion) on self-care costs (i.e., products, classes, and materials), and the remaining one-third ($11.9 billion) on visits to complementary health practitioners. The $33.9 billion represented approximately 1.5 percent of total health-care spending but 11.2 percent of total out-of-pocket health care spending in the United States" (NCCAM, 2013). However, some clients would not be able to receive services if out-of-pocket payment was the only option. If you are considering moving to an out-of-pocket payment system, gathering data before making the decision is crucial. How

many of your current clients would continue if you switched to this method of payment? What would people be willing to pay for out-of-pocket? You must make sure you are able to articulate the value of your services and what people can expect when they foot the bill. You must be able to describe occupational therapy's distinct value to your clients. This marketing approach also applies to therapy recipients with high-deductible health plans, since they pay such a large portion of initial costs out-of-pocket.

Legislation

In addition to legislation related to payment, other laws are passed that directly affect our profession, our employers, and the people with whom we work. The most relevant pieces of legislation are listed in Box 3-5 and described in more detail in the next section.

Patient Protection and Affordable Care Act (ACA) of 2010

The ACA was signed into law on March 23, 2010. Implementation was staged over several years with most of the elements of the law enacted by 2014. Despite this timeline, changes to the law to improve effectiveness and in response to legal challenges have continued to evolve. It is anticipated that the law will continue to be refined in the future, since it was such an ambitious piece of legislation, and unanticipated consequences will need to be addressed. The following are major components of the law that were part of the original ACA of 2010 and implemented by 2014.

Individual Mandate for Health Insurance

Almost all U.S. citizens and legal residents must have qualifying health coverage. Those without coverage pay a tax penalty that is phased in over 3 years starting at $95 or 1.0% of taxable income in 2014, or $325 or 2.0% of taxable income in 2015 and increasing to $695 or 2.5% of taxable income in 2016. After 2016, the penalty will be increased annually by the cost-of-living adjustment. Exemptions will be granted for financial hardship, religious objections, American Indians, those without coverage for fewer than 3 months,

---

BOX 3-5

Key Legislation Affecting Occupational Therapy Practice and People With Disabilities

- **Patient Protection and Affordable Care Act of 2010 (ACA):** Enacted in 2010 and phased in over 4 years, the ACA significantly changes health care in the United States through a range of health insurance and health-care reforms. Citizens are mandated to have health coverage that can be obtained through health insurance exchanges; the law mandates coverage of essential health benefits and extends coverage through the elimination of denials for preexisting conditions and other mandates. The ACA includes incentives for providing higher-quality and more efficient care and penalties for readmissions and inefficient, lower-quality care.

- **Americans With Disabilities Act (ADA):** Enacted in 1990 and amended in 2008, this act provides for equal access for people with disabilities in employment, public transportation, private businesses, government services, and telecommunications.

- **Rehabilitation Act:** Enacted in 1973, this act requires affirmative action hiring policies for federal agencies, nondiscrimination in hiring people with disabilities when the employer receives federal funding, and access to government buildings and services.

- **Individuals With Disabilities Education Act (IDEA):** Enacted in 1997; earlier version (Education for All Handicapped Children) passed in 1975. Provides for free and appropriate education for children with disabilities in the least restrictive environment. Includes requirements for the states to develop EI programs.

---

undocumented immigrants, incarcerated individuals, those for whom the lowest-cost plan option exceeds 8% of an individual's income, and those with incomes below the tax filing threshold (in 2009 the threshold for taxpayers under age 65 was $9,350 for singles and

$18,700 for couples) (U.S. Department of Health and Human Services, 2014).

Health Insurance Exchanges

The ACA called for the creation of state-based American Health Benefit Exchanges and Small Business Health Options Program (SHOP) Exchanges, administered by a governmental agency or nonprofit organization, through which individuals and small businesses with up to 100 employees can purchase qualified coverage. It also called for states to allow businesses with more than 100 employees to purchase coverage in the SHOP Exchange beginning in 2017. The law envisioned that most states would set up and run their own online exchanges, but that if states opted not to form an exchange, a federally run exchange would be put in place. Initially only 16 states and the District of Columbia formed their own exchanges and seven more partnered with the federal government to operate their exchanges. In the other 27 states, people without insurance used federally managed exchanges to shop for coverage (Kaiser Family Foundation, 2013).

Essential Health Benefits

The ACA established a set of health-care service categories that must be covered by certain plans, starting in 2014. Health plans offered in the individual and small group markets, both inside and outside of the Health Insurance Marketplace, must offer a comprehensive package of items and services, known as essential health benefits. Essential health benefits must include items and services within at least the following 10 categories: (1) ambulatory patient services, (2) emergency services, (3) hospitalization, (4) maternity and newborn care, (5) mental health and substance use disorder services including behavioral health treatment, (6) prescription drugs, (7) rehabilitative and habilitative services and devices, (8) laboratory services, (9) preventive and wellness services and chronic disease management, and (10) pediatric services, including oral and vision care. Insurance policies must cover these benefits in order to be certified and offered in the Health Insurance Marketplace. States expanding their Medicaid programs must provide these benefits to people newly eligible for Medicaid.

Because the exact coverage is determined in each state using the state's benchmark health plan as a guide, there will still be variations in the extent of coverage. This presents both opportunities and challenges for the profession of occupational therapy, such as working to help define what services are covered under essential benefit categories such as habilitation.

New Mandates for Employers

Employers with over 50 full-time equivalent (FTE) employees must provide health insurance for their full-time employees, or pay a per-month *Employer Shared Responsibility Payment*" on their federal tax return. The employer mandate was originally set to begin in 2014 but was delayed until at least 2015 or 2016. Small businesses with 50 to 99 FTE employees are expected to be required to start insuring workers by 2016, employers with 100 or more employees are expected to start providing health benefits to at least 70% of their FTE employees by 2015 and 95% by 2016. Health-care tax credits have been retroactively available to small businesses with 25 or less FTE employees since 2010 (http://www.obamacare.com).

Changes to Insurance Regulation

New regulations were imposed on all health plans that will prevent health insurers from denying coverage to people for any reason, including health status and pre-existing medical conditions, and from charging higher premiums based on health status and gender. Annual and lifetime limits on coverage were eliminated, and young adults can remain on their parent's health insurance until age 26 (U.S. Department of Health and Human Services, 2014).

Medicaid Expansion

The ACA sought to expand Medicaid to all non-Medicare-eligible individuals under age 65 (children, pregnant women, parents, and adults without dependent children) with incomes up to 133% of the federal poverty level. All newly eligible adults were to be guaranteed a benchmark benefit package that meets the essential health benefits available through the Exchanges. To finance the coverage for the newly eligible, states were to receive 100% federal funding for 2014 through 2016, 95% federal financing in 2017, 94% federal financing in 2018, 93% federal financing

in 2019, and 90% federal financing for 2020 and subsequent years. This aspect of the law was challenged in the courts; the Supreme Court ruling on the constitutionality of the ACA upheld the Medicaid expansion, but limited the ability of the Department of Health and Human Services to require that states implement it, making the decision to expand Medicaid optional for states. As of August 2014, 26 states and the District of Columbia had chosen to expand their Medicaid programs, and two states were debating whether to expand (Kaiser Family Foundation, 2014).

Post-Acute Care Bundling

Post-acute care bundling is a pilot program that uses a single payment for all services related to a specific treatment or condition (e.g., a stroke), possibly spanning multiple providers across settings. A single episode of care might include initial hospitalization; rehospitalization; post-acute care; and physician and other services, such as occupational therapy (CMS, 2014a). The CMS is considering several bundling options for both Medicare and Medicaid, including a retrospective and prospective model for payment, and is conducting pilot programs to test the bundling options through the CMS Innovation Center (http://innovation.cms.gov/).

According to the CMS website, "The Bundled Payments initiative is comprised of four broadly defined models of care, which link payments for multiple services beneficiaries receive during an episode of care. Model 1 includes an episode of care focused on the acute care inpatient hospitalization" (CMS, 2014a). It is further explained on the website that, "Models 2 and 3 involve a retrospective bundled payment arrangement where actual expenditures are reconciled against a target price for an episode of care. Model 4 involves a prospective bundled payment arrangement, where a lump sum payment is made to a provider for the entire episode of care." For example, in Model 4, a provider could get a lump sum payment that would cover the acute hospital stay as well as all post-acute care for 60 days after discharge, including SNFs, home health, and outpatient services.

Although the future of bundled payments is undetermined, if implemented, this would have a major impact on therapy providers. Hospital occupational therapy departments will need to convince whoever is holding the bundled payment why therapy services are warranted. If the acute care hospital receives the bundled payment, there will be incentives for hospitals to partner with post-acute care providers who will limit rehospitalizations while providing high-quality and efficient care. For example, a hospital may assign its own nurses or case managers to work in a local SNF to ensure that residents receive needed services to facilitate their recovery, but not unnecessary services. These hospital personnel working within the nursing home can potentially reduce hospital readmissions from the nursing home, which will both cut into the hospital's profits as well as possibly result in readmission penalties for the hospital. These new incentives for hospitals to work more closely with post-acute care providers would influence therapists in both settings to work more closely together during the transition from one level of care to the other.

Accountable Care Organizations (ACOs)

Accountable care organizations (ACOs) are groups of providers associated with a defined population of patients that are accountable for the quality and cost of care delivered to that population. Examples of ACOs may include a hospital, a group of primary care providers, specialists, and possibly other health professionals who share responsibility for the quality and cost of care provided to patients as care is provided across multiple settings (e.g., acute care hospital, SNF, and the patient's home). ACOs that are able to address rapidly rising health-care costs and related inefficiencies (e.g., acute readmissions, duplication of services) while meeting quality standards will be financially rewarded with a share of the savings. Occupational therapists can play an integral role in an ACO by providing cost-effective care that improves health outcomes, such as chronic disease self-management and fall prevention to reduce hospital admission (AOTA, 2012).

Patient-Centered Medical Homes

Patient-centered medical homes (PCMHs) focus on coordination of care in the medical home and are led by a personal physician with the patient serving as the focal point of all medical activity. The medical home model promotes an interdisciplinary team-based approach to care of a patient through a spectrum of disease states, including behavioral health challenges, and across the various stages of life. According to AOTA, the PCMH

> *is a primary care model based on patient-centered, coordinated, team-driven care and supported by strong health information technology (HIT). Although the ACO structure houses many practices under one umbrella, the Medical Home is centered on a single practice. Each patient is assigned to a physician-directed practice and a personal physician, and the two are jointly held accountable for providing and coordinating the entire spectrum of that patient's care needs, including physical and mental health, prevention and wellness, acute care, and chronic disease and disability management (AOTA, 2012)*

AOTA has taken a lead role in establishing occupational therapy's role in primary care and medical homes through publishing descriptions of the primary care setting and occupational therapy's role in this setting (Metzler, Hartmann, & Lowenthal, 2012; Muir, 2012). For example, occupational therapists can screen patients for depression or arthritis-related functional problems and recommend resources and approaches to improve functional status. Therapists can provide developmental screenings that are paired with well-child care. Teaching chronic disease self-management and addressing barriers to occupational participation are important contributions that occupational therapists can provide to assist primary care medical homes in broadening their role beyond acute medical care (Metzler et al, 2012).

Implications of the ACA for Occupational Therapy

The ACA presents both opportunities for and threats to the occupational therapy profession. Although it is tempting to focus on the threats, the implementation of the ACA provides what are likely some one-time opportunities for occupational therapy to demonstrate its distinct value by demonstrating how occupational therapy can contribute to the **triple aim of health care** (Berwick, Nolan, & Whittington, 2008) by helping to improve population health, improve health care, and reduce costs (AOTA, 2013). Braveman and Metzler (2012) provided a summary of the opportunities for promoting and expanding the role of occupational therapy within the health-care system as a result of the ACA. Their observations included:

- Recognition of the occupational therapy practitioner as an integral member of the primary care team within reform strategies such as medical homes and ACOs
- Increased involvement of occupational therapy in prevention and wellness activities and interventions
- Promotion of occupational therapy services through the inclusion of rehabilitation and habilitation services as a required category in the mandatory benefits package
- Increased involvement in mental health and substance abuse disorder services in all points of the care continuum including *behavioral health treatment* as a required category in the mandatory essential benefits package
- Demonstrating the distinct value of occupational therapy through involvement in the coordination of services in medical homes, ACOs, and the promotion of cost-effective care management
- Demonstrating that occupational therapy can be an essential part of health-care systems by providing interventions and expertise on self-management

In addition, the ACA shapes provider behavior by providing bonuses for high-quality and efficient care and penalties for poor outcomes or care delivery. These payment strategies include a reduction of Medicare payments to hospitals with hospital-acquired conditions and readmissions that exceed expected rates. Beginning in October 2012, Medicare's Hospital Readmission Reduction Program (HRRP) imposed a financial penalty on hospitals with excess Medicare readmissions. The HRRP applies to all general hospitals paid under the Medicare IPPS (James, 2013).

This creates an opportunity for hospital-based therapy personnel to demonstrate how they can reduce the risk of hospital-acquired conditions such as falls, decubiti, and blood clots (Roberts & Robinson, 2014). Occupational therapy personnel who assist hospitals in reducing readmission by screening for deficits in cognition and health literacy, promoting smooth transitions to the next level of care postdischarge, and providing expanded patient and family education will be of great value due to the payment incentives for reducing readmission (Fisher & Friesema, 2013).

Undoubtedly, the ACA has presented challenges to the profession of occupational therapy and these challenges may become threats if the profession does not mobilize in response. Possible threats to the profession as a result of implementation of ACA include:

- Decreased direct payment for services under evolving payment mechanisms that focus on paying for episodes of care. This may be especially true if outcomes and quality of services are not a primary focus of these payment structures.
- Being excluded as members of the interprofessional team as strategies such as medical homes are implemented and we do not successfully define our roles and the contributions that occupational therapy can make to objectives such as cost-effectiveness, health promotion and disease prevention, full recovery, full return to productivity, and societal and population health levels of health care.
- Missing out on the opportunities as other disciplines step forward and establish themselves as key players in rehabilitation, habilitation, mental health, prevention and wellness, chronic illness management, and long-term care.
- Not being perceived as contributing to the hospital's ability to prevent hospital-acquired conditions and readmissions, both of which can result in significant loss of revenue if the hospital has more than the expected proportion.
- Decreased jobs in hospitals as the system reshapes to limit initial and repeat hospitalizations and relies more on decentralized, community-based care.

Americans With Disabilities Act

One example of disability-related civil rights legislation is the Americans With Disabilities Act (ADA) of 1990, which was amended in 2008. This law built on the Rehabilitation Act of 1973 and intended people with disabilities to have equal opportunity to participate fully in society. It resulted in a number of changes in both physical and programmatic access for people with disabilities in the workplace, government buildings, community, and transportation arenas, although there is still much work to do. Managers should be familiar with this law because we are in a key position to provide education and resources to our clients, particularly people with newly acquired disabilities. Information on the ADA itself, accessible design standards, recent court cases, regional technical assistance centers, and the process for filing a complaint can be found on the ADA website at http://www.ada.gov/.

The ADA may affect how services are delivered at your setting. For example, the ADA specifies that all deaf patients have the right to interpreter services. New construction or renovation has requirements for bathroom accessibility, door width, height of drinking fountains, and availability of text telephones (TTYs). The ADA has guidelines regarding accommodations that employees or students can request. An excellent resource for finding information on the ADA is the ADA National Network at http://adata.org/national-network. The ADA National Network website states that the network "consists of 10 regional centers and an ADA Knowledge Translation Center. The regional centers are distributed throughout the United States to provide local assistance and foster implementation of the ADA. Funded by the National Institute on Disability and Rehabilitation Research (NIDRR), the ADA National Network provides information, guidance and training on the Americans with Disabilities Act (ADA), tailored to meet the needs of business, government and individuals at local, regional and national levels" (ADA National Network, 2014).

How should a manager respond when a therapist with a hearing impairment requests a sign language interpreter for staff meetings? Is it reasonable for a therapist to request not to do transfers of patients over 120 pounds because of an old neck injury? Can you create a revenue source by screening job applicants for the hospital maintenance department to identify those who may be at risk for back injury? Consulting the ADA, accompanying resources, and technical assistance centers will provide the evidence you need to make legally sound decisions that also are consistent with your facility's policies. Published studies that report the outcomes and cost-benefit ratios of preemployment screenings and environmental adaptation can be used to guide decision-making in this area (Littleton, 2003).

Learning about the ADA or other new legislation may also be advantageous when considering consultation roles either as part of a practice or as a special area of practice. Roles can include consulting with employers on reasonable accommodation requests and return-to-work issues, with architects on universal design and access guidelines, with planners on playground design and community access to public spaces, with attorneys on discrimination cases, and with local government regarding how to make programs accessible, particularly for persons with learning disabilities, intellectual disabilities, or other nonvisible impairments. AOTA provides a number of networking opportunities such as the "Home Modifications Network," which is part of the Home and Community Health Special Interest Section (www.aota.org). There are a number of discussion forums on the networking site sponsored by AOTA (www.OTConnections.aota .org), including discussions specifically on the ADA. Centers for independent living, which are run by people with disabilities, often provide ADA consultation and assist consumers with community access challenges. They exist in every state and can be located at http://www.ilusa.com/links/ilcenters.htm. Best practice in the area of ADA consultation is for therapists to partner with people with disabilities to provide a consumer as well as a professional perspective for clients.

Disability-related legislation also includes laws and funding to support individuals moving out of nursing homes into community living, such as *Money Follows the Person* (Medicaid, 2014b), and long-term supports to prevent institutionalization, such as the *Home and Community-Based Waiver Services* provided by Medicaid (Medicaid, 2014a). Familiarity with the rights of people with disabilities and related policies and programs can assist therapy practitioners to be more client-centered and client-driven, and to respect the client's right to self-determination, choice, and control (Hammel, Charlton, Jones, Kramer, & Wilson, 2014).

Individuals With Disabilities Education Act

Another example of a piece of legislation that has had far-reaching effects is the Individuals With Disabilities Education Act (IDEA). Congress enacted the Education for All Handicapped Children Act (Public Law 94–142) in 1975 to support states and localities in protecting the rights of, meeting the individual needs of, and improving the results for infants, toddlers, children, and adolescents with disabilities and their families. This landmark law is currently enacted as the IDEA, last reauthorized in 2004 (National School Boards Association, 2014; U.S. Department of Education, 2012). Reauthorization of the act was scheduled for 2011 but continues to be delayed.

This law provides for free and appropriate education for students with disabilities. If you work with children, you may get questions on the IDEA from patients or clients, family members, teachers, and other therapists. Understanding how occupational therapy fits within the larger educational system requires that you look beyond your immediate environment to understand the law that is responsible for the presence of occupational therapy in the schools. Checking the website (http://www.ideapartnerships.org) is a great way to get up-to-date information. Consulting AOTA official documents and networking with other managers can yield information on caseload, best practices, consultation roles, and billing practices. Resources also exist that provide evidence to support decision-making regarding eligibility for occupational therapy, use of assessment data, and intervention models and can found in the practice section of the AOTA website (www.aota.org). Conducting a literature search on billing practices in schools, for example, will provide information on the pros and cons of schools' billing of insurance or Medicaid for therapy services, as they are allowed to do.

The policy on billing at your local school district will influence expectations for documentation, goals, and the need for physician referral. Other evidence can be obtained from analyzing data on the number of children served under the IDEA in your district or region, the most common categories of disability classification used, the number of children receiving self-contained versus resource services, how many children have a one-on-one aide in the classroom, and so forth. As a manager, these data will help you to anticipate needs, have the appropriate number and type of personnel, and determine where and when your supervisory services will be most needed.

Clinical Practice Requirements

When you are practicing in a particular setting, or contemplating practicing in that setting, learning the requirements for evaluation, documentation, treatment protocols, data collection, and discharge decision-making is essential for survival. Each setting is unique, but there are common requirements that cross a number of settings. One good place to start your search for this information is with AOTA official documents such as position papers, standards for practice, or other documents that are written by AOTA

representatives. It is critical to keep in mind that AOTA official documents represent a consensus opinion of volunteer experts and paid staff on behalf of AOTA and the profession. They are not legal documents and are almost always superseded by federal or state legislative acts—or sometimes by payer guidelines. You should also remember that not all occupational therapy practitioners are members of AOTA and may not be aware of the existence or content of these documents. Table 3-1 details the types of official documents available from AOTA, and a full list of current official AOTA documents can be found at http://www.aota.org/.

The next place to look is guidelines from the payers in a particular setting. For example, in several settings, Medicare requires that data be collected and reported before payment. In some settings, these data must also be collected on non-Medicare beneficiaries. These requirements minimally apply in hospitals, SNFs, home health agencies, and inpatient rehabilitation facilities (IRFs). Table 3-2 provides a sample of settings in which Medicare payment is prevalent, the system used by Medicare for payment, required assessments used to gather data, and the implications for occupational therapy. Information on required assessments is also available in various manuals for different settings (e.g., SNF, IRF) on the CMS website at http://www.cms.hhs.gov/manuals/. The outpatient and private practice settings are not included since they presently have variable payment criteria and a variety of evaluations are used. There is a movement toward Medicare requiring a standard outpatient assessment, such as the Continuity Assessment Record and Evaluation (CARE) item set. Medicare has added requirements for billing codes (e.g., G Codes) to indicate the severity of the client's condition and the focus of therapy, to be rated at the beginning, middle, and end of therapy. It is anticipated that further outpatient requirements will be added due to the growth of Medicare expenditures for outpatient therapy.

Medicare and Medicaid typically have stringent requirements for initial, progress, and discharge documentation. This might include the initial justification for occupational therapy as a necessary skilled service, a monthly progress report, and a discharge summary. The CMS website is one useful source of information. Also, as mentioned earlier, contacting the Medicare contractor that pays the bills would be a good place to start. A list of these contractors by state can be found on the CMS website.

	TABLE 3-1	
	Types and Focus of AOTA Official Documents	
Type of Document	**Focus of Document**	**Example**
Concept papers	Discussion of an issue or topic synthesizing different perspectives to assist the reader in understanding in response to issues, concerns, or needs.	*The Role of Occupational Therapy in Disaster Preparedness, Response and Recovery* (2011)
Guidelines	Descriptions, examples, or recommendations of procedures related to the practice of occupational therapy.	"Guidelines for Documentation of Occupational Therapy" (2013)
Position papers	Present the official stance of AOTA on substantive issues or subjects; for use within the profession or outside the profession.	*The Role of Occupational Therapy in Primary Care* (2014)
Roles papers	Provide guides to major roles common in the profession of occupational therapy.	*Guidelines for Supervision, Roles and Responsibilities During the Delivery of Occupational Therapy Services* (2014)
Specialized knowledge and skills papers	Provide detailed outline of specialized knowledge and skills needed for competent practice	"Specialized Knowledge and Skills in Mental Health Promotion, Prevention and Intervention in Occupational Therapy Practice" (2010)
Standards	Provide general descriptions of topics and define the minimum requirement for performance and quality.	*Standards of Practice for Occupational Therapy* (2010)
Statements	Describe and clarify an aspect or issue related to practice that is linked to the fundamental concepts of occupational therapy.	*Cognition, Cognitive Rehabilitation, and Occupational Performance* (2013)

Managed care organizations may require that a clinical or critical pathway be followed as a quality assurance measure in medical settings. These pathways are typically established by the facility. For example, a clinical pathway may state that an OT should see a patient who will undergo hip replacement surgery the day before his or her surgery for patient education on precautions, and then evaluate his or her ability to apply these principles after surgery. A clinical pathway for an outpatient setting may involve a protocol for patients who undergo carpal tunnel release and are covered under workers' compensation. This could include splinting, edema reduction, initiation of active movement, and follow-up ergonomic assessment of the workstation. It is essential that occupational therapy practitioners be at the table when these pathways are formulated, to ensure that our role is recognized and integrated within the care plan.

Investigating the evidence to support occupational therapy involvement with patients with various diagnoses will prepare you for convincing others that occupational therapy intervention is a key component that should be included in the clinical pathway. Collecting ongoing outcome data for patients served will contribute to the body of knowledge and likelihood of occupational therapy being seen as an essential service.

In school system practice, there may be another set of expectations to follow regarding the size of caseload, documentation, obtaining a physician prescription, and discharge guidelines. Some guidelines exist at the national and state levels, but many guidelines are formulated at the state or local district level. Each district, for example, may require different documentation of progress toward goals of the individualized education plan. One district may only require

---

TABLE 3-2

Medicare Payment Systems by Setting

	Hospital	Skilled Nursing Facility	Home Health Agency	Inpatient Rehabilitation
System Used to Determine Payment	Diagnosis-related groups (DRGs)	Resource utilization groups (RUGs)	Home health resource group (HHRG)	Case mix groups (CMGs)
Criteria for Payment	Diagnosis and outliers (exceptions resulting from long or costly stay)	Level of intensity of nursing care and rehabilitation services needed	Mix of clinical and functional indicators and therapy need, paid for a 60-day period of service	CMG determined by impairment group code and the rehab impairment category, age, comorbidities, functional independence measure motor and cognitive score
Evaluation Used	Medical diagnosis and secondary conditions	Minimum data set (MDS)	Outcomes and assessment information set (OASIS)	Inpatient rehabilitation–patient assessment instrument (IRF-PAI)
Implications for Occupational Therapy	Focus on early discharge, discharge planning, and prevention of readmission	Early assessment, deliver expected services, participate in MDS	Limited number of visits for all therapies combined, need to justify need for occupational therapy to other disciplines	Preadmission screening, work for maximal gain in the time provided, focus on functional gains, plan for discharge

---

quarterly reports on goal attainment, whereas another may require therapists to complete a narrative note or a checklist after each occupational therapy session. Some districts bill insurance companies or Medicaid for therapy services (allowable by law after the 1997 amendments), and others do not; this affects the documentation requirements for the school system practitioner. Another area of clinical practice that differs among school districts is their stance on how therapy services are to be delivered. Some districts support a consultation model, in which most of the occupational therapy services are delivered in the classroom or via consultation or training with teachers, assistants, and other staff. Other districts use a "pull-out" approach, in which the child receives therapy in a space outside of the classroom, and others may combine these approaches, depending on the needs of the child and the available space in the school. Some settings may use more group treatment, or work with the full class, and others use more individual treatment. Gathering evidence on the advantages,

disadvantages, costs, and outcomes of these different models will assist you in implementing the approach that you determine meets the needs of the constituencies you serve.

Community agencies that are not medical in nature, such as day programs for seniors or mental health vocational centers, do not typically have the stringent requirements for assessment tools, documentation, and clinical practice as described previously. However, they might have internal protocols for progress measures and outcome evaluation, which are either mandated by the Commission on Accreditation of Rehabilitation Facilities or the prerogative of the agency. In these settings, you may wish to develop guidelines, protocols, and standards for intervention if they do not exist, and you are encouraged to use the strategies suggested throughout this book to make such guides based on the most current evidence.

Finally, you are encouraged to review studies and guidelines provided by other disciplines (e.g., knowledge related to occupational therapy practice but outside the occupational therapy domain) that may help you in developing services that meet commonly accepted expectations and that fit with other disciplines' services. For example, the fields of community psychology, physical therapy (PT), special education, and nursing generate knowledge and documents of interest to, and of use by, occupational therapy practitioners.

Data, Information, and Other Forms of Evidence on Personnel

In the personnel domain, there are several sources of data that will assist with well-informed decision-making and more accurate forecasting of the need for, and availability of, new staff, as well as information about salaries. The U.S. Department of Labor, Bureau of Labor Statistics (BLS), compiles forecast information on a wide variety of fields. It projects job demand and future trends, and also reports salary trends. For example, BLS employment estimates for OTs are that jobs are projected to grow 29% from 2012 to 2022. The BLS reported that, "the need for occupational therapists is expected to increase as the large baby-boom generation ages and people remain active later in life. Occupational therapists can help senior citizens maintain their independence by recommending home modifications and strategies that make daily activities easier." It projected much faster than average growth (41% or more job growth) in OTA positions (Bureau of Labor Statistics, U.S. Department of Labor, 2014).

Every few years, AOTA completes a survey of occupational therapy practitioners. The results of the survey are available for purchase, and excerpts from the data are often available on the AOTA website or in AOTA publications such as *OT Practice*. Typical information includes annual salary, often broken down by state, region, and number of years of practice in a given work setting; hours worked per week; and degree level. For example, the 2010 report indicated that 92% of practitioners were female, more than three-quarters (85%) were employed full-time in the profession, and the median level of professional experience was 13 years (AOTA, 2010). This information could be valuable when planning staffing that utilizes part-time employees, as it shows that only 15% of those surveyed were working part-time.

Data on the supply of new graduates is important to the organizations that hire them because evaluating the supply trends may provide indications of whether there is a surplus or shortage of potential hires and how long it will take to recruit new personnel. AOTA reports data on the number of graduates in its *"Education Annual Data Report"* and reported that in the 2013–2014 year there were 108 occupational therapy graduates at the doctoral level and 5,439 at the master's level. The 5-year growth rate was reported at 23% and 38%, respectively. The projected number of OTA graduates was 4,313 and this reflected an 83% 5-year growth rate (AOTA, 2014d). This same report includes data on enrollment, as well as gender and diversity statistics. Time trend data, which compare the number of new graduates who pass the exam over time, are available from the NBCOT website (http://www.nbcot.org/), and the total number of enrolled students is available to AOTA members in the Resources for Educators section of the AOTA website (http://www.aota.org/Education-Careers/Educators.aspx). On reviewing the AOTA website, you will find that some areas and documents, such as those just cited, are limited to viewing by members only, a benefit of being a member of your professional association.

Determining if there will be a shortage or surplus of desired personnel can assist you in determining appropriate starting salaries, salary increases, the appropriateness of the use of sign-on bonuses or other recruitment incentives, and the mix of OTs and OTAs that is most desirable and most feasible to attain. Student fieldwork programs often provide a supply of potential new graduate hires, and should be seen as a recruitment strategy during phases of increased job demand or decreased supply of practitioners. Obtaining data on graduates from local universities and colleges may also assist you in planning for personnel needs, and will guide you in how aggressive you need to be in mounting a recruitment campaign.

Licensure and Certification

Understanding requirements for professional licensure and certification is critical when planning programs, especially if your programming will be provided in more than one state. Professional certification for both OTs and OTAs requires completion of an educational degree from an accredited program and passing the certification exam administered by the NBCOT. That examination provides initial certification for a period of 3 years. After that point, in order to maintain the right to use the Occupational Therapist, Registered (OTR) and Certified Occupational Therapy Assistant (COTA) designations, practitioners must complete requirements for continuing competence. Recertification must be completed every 3 years if one desires to maintain the OTR and COTA designations. A variety of activities can meet this requirement, including formal continuing education, mentorship, fieldwork student supervision, and research (National Board for Certification in Occupational Therapy, 2014). As of 2014, all 50 states, the District of Columbia, Puerto Rico, and Guam have licensure laws for the practice of occupational therapy. For OTAs, 49 states, the District of Columbia, Puerto Rico, and Guam have licensure laws. Box 3-6 defines each of these types of regulations (AOTA, 2014c).

The laws that govern occupational therapy practice vary considerably from state to state, so it is important for you to be familiar with the regulations in your state and neighboring states. Box 3-7 shows the different components that may be addressed by a licensure or practice act. If you or one of your supervisees does not follow the requirements for physician referral, supervision, documentation, signature, provisional license, or continuing competence, penalties may be invoked that range from verbal or written warning to loss of license. Not being familiar with the licensure requirements in your area is not an adequate excuse, because this is a law all occupational therapy professionals are expected to know and follow.

Imagine that you have just accepted a management position in another state. How do you find out whether the state has a practice act or licensure law, as well as what you need to do to apply? Once you begin your new position, can you hire a new graduate before he or she passes the NBCOT exam? Do you need a physician referral in order to initiate intervention? What is the minimum supervision time that OTAs are required to have? The AOTA website's licensure section has all of the answers in database format and downloadable reports (AOTA, 2014c). Table 3-3 presents a comparison of the answers to these questions from the AOTA database for two neighboring states, Mississippi and Alabama (as of August 2014; this information is subject to change). You should note how variable these components are, and recognize that they may change over

---

BOX 3-6
Types of Practice Regulations

- **Licensure:** Provides the highest level of public protection by prohibiting unlicensed individuals from practicing occupational therapy or referring to themselves as OTs or OTAs. Licensure laws reserve a certain scope of practice for those who are issued a license.
- **Mandatory certification:** Protects the public by prohibiting uncertified persons from referring to themselves as OTs or OTAs. Unlike licensure, individuals under certain circumstances can practice if they do not refer to their services as occupational therapy. Certification laws may provide for a definition of occupational therapy.
- **Mandatory registration:** Protects the public by prohibiting unregistered persons from referring to themselves as OTs or OTAs, although they can practice if they do not refer to their services as occupational therapy. Registration laws may provide for a definition of occupational therapy.
- **Trademark or title control legislation:** Prohibits individuals who have not met specific education and entry-level examination requirements from referring to themselves as OTs or OTAs, although they can practice under certain circumstances if they do not refer to their services as occupational therapy.

---

time because they are determined by legislation passed by each state.

Trend Data and Future Forecasts

In addition to uncovering evidence from all of the previously described areas, it is important to anticipate upcoming trends and changes to be prepared for the future. In fact, a keen awareness of these trends allows you to *shape* the future, because you are able to position your department in front of the pack in addressing

---

BOX 3-7

Common Components of Practice Acts

- **Scope of practice:** Defines the domain of occupational therapy, such as defining the roles of OTs and OTAs. May include specifics such as orthotics, physical agent modalities, activities of daily living intervention, and environmental modification, or may be more general in nature
- **Referral requirements:** Specify if a physician referral is necessary for evaluation or treatment.
- **Temporary license/work permit:** Defines the process for unlicensed personnel to obtain permission to work while waiting for their licenses
- **Continuing competence:** Specifies the requirements for continuing education and other means to demonstrate continuing competence
- **OTA supervision requirements:** Define what type of supervision is required for OTAs, including amount of time, frequency, and documentation requirements

---

TABLE 3-3

Comparison of Two States' Practice Act Regulations

Component of Act	Mississippi	Alabama
Referral requirement	Physician referral not necessary.	Physician, chiropractor, dentist, or optometrist referral necessary with annual confirmation of the diagnosis. Referral not required to provide services to people with educationally related needs.
Temporary license or permit	Limited permit provided until the exam scores are received; allowed to renew one time if exam is not passed.	Temporary permit until the exam scores are received; if the exam is not passed, the permit is revoked.
Continuing education requirement	OT: 20 contact hours (CHs) or 2 continuing education units (CEUs) to be accrued during the licensure period. At least 6 CHs or 0.6 CEUs must be directly related to the clinical practice of occupational therapy. OTA: 20 contact hours (CHs) or 2 continuing education units (CEUs) to be accrued during the licensure period. At least 6 CHs or 0.6 CEUs must be directly related to the clinical practice of occupational therapy.	OT: 3.0 CEUs (or 30 CHs) biennially. OTA: 2.0 CEUs (or 20 CHs) biennially.
Supervision of occupational therapy assistants	Occupational therapist must be available by phone; joint supervisory patient visit every 7 treatment days or 21 calendar days.	5% of OTA work hours per month must be spent in one-to-one supervision with an occupational therapist.

emerging needs. It is your responsibility as a manager to constantly scan the environment for information on emerging trends and ways of thinking about practice and health systems. There are numerous places to look for this information, both within and outside the field. For example, the "Presidential Address" delivered by the president of AOTA at the association's annual conference often addresses future directions of the profession, including building capacity and occupational therapy leadership (Stoffel, 2014). Other fields and disciplines often have similar forums, and because such addresses are typically published in the professional literature, they are easily accessible. Keeping abreast of AOTA Board of Directors and Representative Assembly decisions via the AOTA website is also a key strategy. Maintaining your membership in AOTA and your state association are solid strategies to receive the most recent updates. A good tool for keeping up with the latest developments in health care, financing, and legislation is using Internet services that screen news headlines for the topics you are most interested in, and then send you the relevant headlines and links to full text. The *New York Times* offers such a service at http://www.nytimes.com/. Another option is to scan an Internet site that lists headlines from health care–related articles that appear in newspapers around the country, such as the Yahoo.com full-coverage news on health care-related topics, available at http://news.yahoo.com/topics/health-care/. The Kaiser Family Foundation provides a daily health news update at http://www.kaiserhealthnews.org/. Some private resources, including health-related foundations, track changes in health-care trends over time. An example of such a foundation is the Robert Wood Johnson Foundation (http://www.rwjf.org/). Other relevant literature includes *Healthy People 2020* and subsequent versions, a compendium of desired health outcomes to be achieved by the target year. Also, literature on emerging disabilities will be relevant. This includes studies of disability prevalence and changes over time,

future projections on demographic changes and how they will impact the need for health services, and new areas on the horizon that are "hot." Reading occupational therapy literature about new program models and innovative service delivery is also recommended.

Chapter Summary

This chapter described the complex "system" of health care and other service delivery systems in which occupational therapy practitioners work. The dualistic health-care system was described, and you were introduced to basic free-market economic principles and learned how they can only be applied to the health-care market in limited ways. These concepts include supply and demand, competition, and free choice.

In Chapter 2, you were introduced to a range of types of evidence, and in this chapter you were further encouraged to consider a broad range of data, information, and other forms of evidence beyond the results of empirical investigations. You learned that strategies commonly used in research can also be used to gather these other types of evidence that are useful in planning and justifying occupational therapy programming. Evidence may be gathered on payment and the payment practices of specific sources of payment (Medicare, Medicaid, workers' compensation, out-of-pocket, and SSA), legislation, clinical practice requirements, demographics, personnel, and licensure and certification requirements. Perhaps most importantly, this chapter demonstrated a range of strategies for finding data, information, and other forms of evidence, some of which is readily accessible and some of which must be found through creativity and perseverance.

At the beginning of the chapter you were introduced to Andrea, who had accepted a new job as the sole occupational therapist in a rural health facility. Andrea used the information presented in this chapter to develop occupational therapy services at her facility.

■ Real-Life Solutions

Andrea decided to begin by learning about the larger system issues by researching payment sources and determining which of the patient populations

at her facility were covered, what sort of occupational therapy interventions were covered, the payment rates, and the requirements for referral and documentation. She consulted with AOTA, obtained resources on determining charges and payment, and obtained copies of key documents

■ **Real-Life Solutions—cont'd**

produced by the association to help guide her practice and to give credence to services as she presented them to other managers in the facility.

Despite the fact that she was initially intimidated, Andrea made contact with her Medicare contractor and obtained copies of relevant guidelines for outpatient occupational therapy under Medicare. She also began to network with her peers in her city and state, and across the country through Listservs and Internet discussion boards, to learn more about Medicare payment. Further, Andrea began to plan for a needs assessment, which would include an analysis of local demographics and illness or injury patterns, socioeconomic status, risk factors, and services currently available. She sought reference materials on developing surveys and other tools to collect information from payers and consumers.

The ADA website furnished specifics on providing accessible parking, elevators, and signage, as well as funding available for adapting the workplace for employees with disabilities. At first it seemed overwhelming that so much information was available, but soon Andrea began to feel more proficient at searching the Internet to take advantage of the many resources available, including the websites of government agencies at the national, state, county, and local levels, as well as those for private foundations.

Andrea also contacted the state regulatory agency and investigated the requirements for supervision of OTAs and recently graduated occupational therapists. She knew she would be hiring another therapy practitioner in the near future, because the evidence pointed to significant unmet needs and the potential to build a successful occupational therapy practice in a rural context. Andrea was sure that the skills she was acquiring in finding and evaluating data, information, and other forms of evidence would support her efforts.

Study Questions

1. Which of the following statements best describes the *free-market system* as it applies to our health-care system?

   a. All principles of the free-market system apply to health care in the same way as they apply to all other products.

   b. All principles of the free-market system apply to health care in the same way as they apply to all other products *except* competition, because competition is limited.

   c. All principles of the free-market system apply to health care in the same way as they apply to all other products *except* supply and demand, because supply and demand are totally under government control.

   d. All principles of the free-market system apply to health care, but in complex ways that limit consumers' free choice in various ways.

2. A state-run program that is jointly funded by states and the federal government for people who have limited income or high medical expenses where eligibility for the limited income cohort is based on the family income and size in relation to the national poverty level would best be called which of the following?

   a. Medicare
   b. Medicaid
   c. Workers' compensation
   d. Sliding scale self-pay

3. Based on data on trends in self-pay (i.e., out-of-pocket) as a payment source for complementary medicine, which of the following is most accurate?

   a. Most adults are highly unlikely to pay for complementary health care out-of-pocket and utilization is very low when there is no third-party payment.

b. Third-party payment for complementary medicine is essentially nonexistent, so almost 100% of payment for these approaches is out-of-pocket.

c. Complementary health care is an essential benefit of the ACA and therefore self-pay approaches need not be considered.

d. Adults are likely to pay for complementary approaches to health care when they have the resources, and approximately a third of self-pay payments are for complementary health care.

4. **A legislative act that provides for free and appropriate education for children with disabilities in the least restrictive environment and includes requirements for the states to develop EI programs would best be called the:**

a. Patient Protection, Education and Affordable Care Act.

b. Individuals With Disabilities Education Act.

c. Health Insurance Portability, Accountability and Education Act.

d. Rehabilitation Services Education Act.

5. **Groups of providers that provide care associated with a defined population of patients across multiple settings while being held responsible for the quality and cost of care delivered to that population would best be called:**

a. Patient-centered medical homes.

b. Post-acute care bundles.

c. Home health agencies.

d. Accountable care organizations.

6. **Which of the following is most accurate in regard to AOTA official documents such as concept papers, guidelines, or position papers?**

a. AOTA official documents represent a consensus opinion of experts, so they should influence practice and action but are not always the "final word" in decision-making.

b. AOTA official documents represent legal opinions published by AOTA on behalf of the profession and must be followed.

c. AOTA official documents are historical only in nature; they reflect past practices and not current recommendations for practice or action.

d. AOTA official documents represent a consensus opinion of experts and are often officially sanctioned and accepted by the federal government.

7. **Occupational therapy managers often need to access data, information, and other forms of evidence to guide decision-making and the development and implementation of programs. Which of the following is most accurate regarding the process of obtaining and interpreting such evidence in the current environment?**

a. Data, information, and other forms of evidence are easily accessible, easy to organize, and easy to interpret due to the abundance of resources available to the modern-day occupational therapy manager.

b. Despite the Internet and online data sources, access to relevant data, information, and other forms of evidence remains elusive; it is often difficult for occupational therapy managers to find the necessary evidence.

c. With the rise of the Internet and the development of many systems for storing and accessing data, information, and other forms of evidence, occupational therapy managers may find an overwhelming amount of evidence and may have to focus on organized and strategic approaches to gathering and interpreting the most appropriate evidence.

d. Not much has changed in the last decade; because it is often impossible to validate the sources of data, information, and other forms of online evidence, occupational therapy managers should stick to formal literature searches using electronic search engines.

8. **Which of the following is most accurate in regard to variability in licensure laws in the 50 states, the District of Columbia, Puerto Rico, and Guam?**

a. There is considerable variation in issues such as practicing without a referral, continuing education requirements, and supervision requirements for OTAs.

b. Due to the NBCOT certification examination, all licensure laws are 100% consistent across the 50 states, the District of Columbia, Puerto Rico, and Guam.

c. There is considerable variation in whether or not occupational therapists can practice without a referral, but all other elements of licensure laws are consistent across the 50 states, the District of Columbia, Puerto Rico, and Guam.

d. Most elements of licensure laws are consistent across the 50 states, but there is much variation in the territories, including the District of Columbia, Puerto Rico, and Guam.

Resources for Learning More About Health-Care Systems and Practice Contexts

Journals That Often Publish Articles Related to Health-Care Systems and Practice Contexts

Health Affairs: The Policy Journal of the Health Sphere

http://www.openclinical.org/jnl_ha.html

Health Affairs is a bimonthly, peer-reviewed journal that explores health policy issues of current concern in both domestic and international spheres.

Healthcare Financing Review

http://search.proquest.com/publication/5416

The *Healthcare Financing Review* is available through subscription from the CMS. Readers who wish to gain an improved understanding of the Medicare and Medicaid programs and the U.S. health-care system will find this a helpful resource. In addition to policy-relevant research, published articles present varied perspectives on issues including health-care policy, as well as the planning and delivery of health-care services. Articles include analyses on a broad range of health-care financing and delivery issues and promote discussion and debate from a diverse audience that includes policy makers, planners, administrators, insurers, researchers, and health-care providers. The *Review* appears quarterly, with an additional statistical supplement issue every year.

Journal of Public Health Policy

http://www.palgrave-journals.com/jphp/index.html

The *Journal of Public Health Policy* publishes scholarly articles on the epidemiological and social foundations of public health policy. Results of empirical research related to the development of public health policy as well as the implementation of such policy are included.

Health Services Research

http://www.hsr.org/hsr/abouthsr/journal.jsp

Health Services Research provides researchers, policy makers and analysts, and health-care administrators and managers with access to empirical findings as well as articles addressing policy and methodological issues. Readers interested in health-care financing, the organization or delivery of health services, or in the evaluation of health delivery outcomes will find *Health Services Research* a useful resource. The journal provides a forum for the exchange of practice-related information for individuals, health systems, and communities.

Professional Associations Concerned With Health-Care Systems and Practice Contexts

American Healthcare Association

http://www.ahcancal.org

The American Healthcare Association (AHCA) is a nonprofit association of state health organizations. Member organizations include both nonprofit and for-profit organizations representing the areas of assisted living, nursing facility, developmentally disabled, and subacute care providers. The AHCA represents the long-term care community to the general public as well as the federal and state governments and business leaders. In addition to other functions, the AHCA serves a role as an advocate for change within the long-term care field. The association provides members and the public with information, educational resources, and tools to improve the delivery of quality care.

American Public Health Association

http://www.apha.org/

The American Public Health Association (APHA) provides a forum for health researchers, health service providers, administrators, teachers, and other health workers to interact and to exchange ideas and varied perspectives. In addition, the APHA is concerned with a variety of societal and health-care system issues.

Among others, the APHA identifies issues of interest such as federal and state funding for health programs, pollution-control programs, and policies related to chronic and infectious diseases, a smoke-free society, and professional education in public health.

Website Resource List

Vocational Rehabilitation State Offices

http://askjan.org/pubsandres/res.htm

This Web page contains information about federal, state, and local resources for individuals with disabilities, service providers, and employers.

U.S. Census Bureau

http://www.census.gov

This is the main Web page of the U.S. Census Bureau website. It provides access to all possible statistical data available from every subject for which the data were collected by the U.S. Census Bureau. Statistics are arranged by themes such as the economy, employment, health, housing, population and others.

Centers for Disease Control and Prevention

- National Center for Health Statistics (http://www.cdc.gov/nchs/about.htm)
- Diseases and Conditions Section (http://www.cdc.gov/diseasesconditions/)
- Publications (http://www.cdc.gov/nchs/hus.htm)

The CDC home page has a section on diseases and conditions with an A-to-Z listing. Although the list omits some common diagnoses, such as Alzheimer disease, each listed condition has a Web page that may include a fact sheet, relevant website links, publications, and information about the prevalence of certain conditions across the United States.

The National Center for Health Statistics

http://www.cdc.gov/nchs/

The National Center for Health Statistics (NCHS) of the CDC is the United States' principal health statistics agency. The agency compiles statistical information on health-related issues. The website contains data from various national surveys on various health concerns that range from disability, nutrition, and hospice care to statistics on vital life events (births, deaths, marriages, infant mortality, etc.). The website also has links to many other government agencies, including state and local health departments and Web resources and publications, as well as software and products you can download or order.

Office of Disability Employment Policy, U.S. Department of Labor

http://www.dol.gov/odep/

The Office of Disability Employment Policy (ODEP) provides statistics on employed disabled persons, as well as the Workforce Investment Act of 1998 WIA 188 Disability Checklist. The website provides information on a wide range of issues related to disability and the workforce, including guidelines for implementation of the ADA and for return-to-work programs for workers who are injured, that is arranged in alphabetical order.

The National Organization on Disability

http://www.nod.org/

In cooperation with the Harris Poll, the National Organization on Disability (NOD) provides timely survey research data on the participation of people with disabilities in American life. The website also provides links to other disability-related surveys and studies.

Centers for Medicare and Medicaid Services

https://www.cms.gov/Research-Statistics-Data-and-Systems/Research-Statistics-Data-and-Systems.html

This Web page provides statistical data on Medicaid and Medicare, ranging from estimates of future Medicare and Medicaid spending to enrollment, spending, and claims data.

State Children's Health Insurance Program

http://www.medicaid.gov/chip/chip-program-information.html

This Web page, which can be accessed by linking from the CMS website, overviews the SCHIP program.

National Institutes of Health

http://www.nih.gov/

The National Institutes of Health website has health information for consumers, health news and events, media contacts (radio and video), grants and funding opportunities, and scientific resources (special interest groups, library catalogs, journals, research training and labs, statistical computing).

Administration for Children and Families, U.S. Department of Health and Human Services

http://www.acf.hhs.gov/reports

This Web page provides data and reports on programs and grants with the goal of improving the lives of America's most vulnerable children, families, communities, and individuals.

Administration on Aging

http://www.aoa.acl.gov/Aging_Statistics/index.aspx

This Web page provides statistical data on older adults along different dimensions, including indicators of well-being, disabilities data, and census data on aging.

Bureau of Labor Statistics, U.S. Department of Labor, and Occupational Safety and Health Administration

http://www.osha.gov/oshstats/work.html

This Web page contains Occupational Safety and Health Administration (OSHA) workplace injury and illness statistics, including data on injury and illness incidence rates; state occupational injuries, illnesses, and fatalities; and injury and illness characteristics.

American Hospital Directory

http://www.ahd.com/

The American Hospital Directory website provides online data for more than 6,000 hospitals. Its database of information is built from Medicare claims data, cost reports, and other public-use files obtained from the CMS. The data also include annual survey data from the American Hospital Association. Detailed information is available for subscribers.

General Accounting Office

http://www.gao.gov/

This website contains reports of health-care disparities among ethnic groups and by gender, SSA disability decision-making data, and the like.

Centers for Independent Living

http://www.ilusa.com/links/ilcenters.htm

This Web page contains a listing of centers for independent living, organized by state. These centers are run by people with disabilities and typically provide advocacy, peer counseling, information and referral, and community education.

Healthy People 2020

http://www.healthypeople.gov/2020/default.aspx

The *Healthy People 2020* website provides science-based, 10-year national objectives for improving the health of all Americans. For the last 3 decades, *Healthy People* has established benchmarks and monitored progress over time in order to:

- Encourage collaborations across communities and sectors.
- Empower individuals toward making informed health decisions.
- Measure the impact of prevention activities.

Office of Minority Health Resource Center

http://www.nsvrc.org/organizations/90

The Office of Minority Health Resource Center website has health information and statistics on various ethnic populations (Asian American, African American, Hispanic, Native American, etc.), health brochures and videos in various languages (covering topics such as diabetes, teen pregnancy, and hypertension), publications (*Closing the Gap*), funding resources, and a network of resource people to contact.

Reference List

ADA National Network. (2014). *Who is the ADA National Network?* Retrieved from http://www.adata.org/national-network.

American Occupational Therapy Association. (2010). *Member compensation survey*. Bethesda, MD: Author.

American Occupational Therapy Association. (2012). *AOTA fact sheet on ACOs/medical homes*. Retrieved from http://www.aota.org/Advocacy-Policy/Health-Care-Reform.aspx

American Occupational Therapy Association. (2013). *AOTA engaged in ongoing efforts to promote the role of OT in primary care*. Retrieved from http://www.aota.org/Publications-News/AOTANews/2013/Primary-Care-Promote.aspx

American Occupational Therapy Association. (2014a). Jimmo v. Sebelius: *The so-called Medicare "improvement standard" deemed illegal, skilled maintenance care now covered*. Retrieved from http://www.aota.org/Advocacy-Policy/Federal-Reg-Affairs/News/2013/Improvement-standard.aspx#sthash.8hkUKOVI.dpuf

American Occupational Therapy Association. (2014b). *Medicare regulations and guidance*. Retrieved from http://www.aota.org/Advocacy-Policy/Federal-Reg-Affairs/Pay/Medicare/Guidance.aspx

American Occupational Therapy Association. (2014c). *State OT statutes and regulations*. Retrieved from http://www.aota.org/Advocacy-Policy/State-Policy/Licensure/StateRegs.aspx

American Occupational Therapy Association. (2014d). *2013–2104 education annual data report*. Retrieved from http://www.aota.org/-/media/Corporate/Files/EducationCareers/Accredit/2013-2014-Annual-Data-Report.pdf

BB&T Program on Capitalism, Markets, and Morality. (2014). *Mixed economy*. Retrieved from http://www.uncg.edu/bae/bbt/capitalism/mixed_economy.html

Berwick, D., Nolan, T., & Whittington, J. (2008). The triple aim: Care, health and cost. *Health Affairs, 27*, 759–769.

Braveman, B., & Metzler, C. (2012). Health care reform implementation and occupational therapy. *American Journal of Occupational Therapy, 66*, 11–14.

Bureau of Labor Statistics, U.S. Department of Labor. (2014). *Occupational outlook handbook, 2014–15 edition, occupational therapists*. Retrieved from http://www.bls.gov/ooh/healthcare/occupational-therapists.htm

Centers for Medicare and Medicaid Services. (2013). *Medicare administrative contractors*. Retrieved from http://www.cms.gov/Medicare/Medicare-Contracting/Medicare-Administrative-Contractors/MedicareAdministrativeContractors.html

Centers for Medicare and Medicaid Services. (2014a). *Bundled payments for care improvement (BPCI) initiative: General information*. Retrieved from http://innovation.cms.gov/initiatives/bundled-payments/

Centers for Medicare and Medicaid Services. (2014b). *Children's Health Insurance Program*. Retrieved from http://www.medicaid.gov/CHIP/CHIP-Program-Information.html

Centers for Medicare and Medicaid Services. (2014c). *Medicare physician fee schedule*. Retrieved from http://www.cms.gov/Outreach-and-Education/Medicare-Learning-Network-MLN/MLNProducts/downloads/MedcrePhysFeeSchedfctsht.pdf

Centers for Medicare and Medicaid Services. (2014d). *Physical therapy, occupational therapy, speech language pathology services*. Retrieved from http://www.medicare.gov/coverage/pt-and-ot-and-speech-language-pathology.html

Drafke, M. W. (2002). *Working in health care: What you need to know to succeed*. Philadelphia, PA: F.A. Davis.

Fisher, G., & Cooksey, J. A. (2002). The occupational therapy workforce: Part one—context and trends. *Administrative and Management Special Interest Section Quarterly, 18*, 1–4.

Fisher, G., & Friesema, J. (2013). Health policy perspectives—Implications of the Affordable Care Act for occupational therapy practitioners providing services to Medicare recipients. *American Journal of Occupational Therapy, 67*(5), 502–506.

Fisher, G., & Keehn, M. (2007). *Workforce needs and issues in occupational and physical therapy*. Chicago, IL: UIC Midwest Center for Workforce Studies.

Frass, M., Strassl, R. P., Friehs, H., Müllner, M., Kundi, M., & Kaye, A. D. (2012). Use and acceptance of complementary and alternative medicine among the general population and medical personnel: A systematic review. *The Ochsner Journal, 12*(1), 45–56.

Hammel, J., Charlton, J., Jones, R., Kramer, J. M., & Wilson, T. (2014). Disability rights and advocacy. In B. A. B. Schell, G. Gillen, & M. A. Scaffa (Eds.), *Willard & Spackman's occupational therapy* (12th ed., Chapter 70). Philadelphia, PA: Lippincott/Williams and Wilkins.

Jacobs, K., & McCormack, G. L. (2011). *The occupational therapy manager* (5th ed.). Bethesda, MD: AOTA Press.

James, J. (2013). Health policy brief: Medicare hospital readmissions reduction program. *Health Affairs*. Retrieved from http://www.healthaffairs.org/healthpolicybriefs/brief.php?brief_id=102

Kaiser Family Foundation. (2012). *Snapshots: A comparison of the availability and cost of coverage for workers in small firms and large firms*. Retrieved from http://kff.org/private-insurance/issue-brief/snapshots-a-comparison-of-the-availability-and-cost-of-coverage-for-workers-in-small-firms-and-large-firms/

Kaiser Family Foundation. (2013). *Most uninsured Americans live in states that won't run their own Obamacare exchanges*. Retrieved from http://www.pewresearch.org/fact-tank/2013/09/19/most-uninsured-americans-live-in-states-that-wont-run-their-own-obamacare-exchanges/

Kaiser Family Foundation. (2014). *Interactive: A state-by-state look at how the uninsured fare under the ACA*. Retrieved from http://kff.org/interactive/uninsured-gap/

Lassman, D., Hartman, M., Washington, B., Andrews, K., & Catlin, A. (2014). US health spending trends by age and gender: Selected years 2002–10. *Health Affairs, 33*(5), 815–822.

Littleton, M. (2003). Cost effectiveness of a pre-work screening program for the University of Illinois at Chicago physical plant. *Work, 21,* 243–250.

Lohman, H. (2014). Payment for services in the United States. In B. A. B. Schell, G. Gillen, & M. E. Scaffa (Eds.), *Willard & Spackman's occupational therapy* (12th ed., pp. 1051–1067). Philadelphia, PA: Lippincott, Williams & Wilkins.

Mansfield, E. (1980). *Principles of microeconomics* (3rd ed.). New York, NY: W.W. Norton.

Medicaid. (2014a). 1915 (c) *Home and community based waivers.* Retrieved from http://www.medicaid.gov/Medicaid-CHIP -Program-Information/By-Topics/Waivers/Home-and -Community-Based-1915-c-Waivers.html

Medicaid. (2014b). *Money follows the person.* Retrieved from http:// www.medicaid.gov/Medicaid-CHIP-Program-Information/ By-Topics/Long-Term-Services-and-Supports/Balancing/ Money-Follows-the-Person.html

Metzler, C., Hartmann, K., & Lowenthal, L. (2012). Health policy perspectives—Defining primary care: Envisioning the roles of occupational therapy. *American Journal of Occupational Therapy, 66*(3), 266–270.

Muir, S. (2012). Occupational therapy in primary health care: We should be there. *American Journal of Occupational Therapy, 66*(5), 506–510.

National Board for Certification in Occupational Therapy. (2014). *Renewal process overview.* Retrieved from http://www.nbcot.org/ certification-renewal-process

National Center for Complementary and Alternative Medicine. (2013). *Paying for complementary health approaches.* Retrieved from http://nccam.nih.gov/health/financial

National Center for Policy Analysis. (2014). *Myths and truths about the Canadian Health System.* Retrieved from http://www.ncpa .org/sub/dpd/index.php?Article_ID=24543

National School Boards Association. (2014). *Individuals with Disabilities Education Act (IDEA): Early preparation for reauthorization.* Retrieved from https://nsba.org/sites/default/files/reports/ Issue%20Brief-Individuals%20with%20Disabilities%20 Education%20Act.pdf

Peterson, M. (2012). *OIG claims inappropriate payments to SNF's cost Medicare more than $1 billion dollars a year.* Retrieved from http:// www.healthlawyers.org/Members/PracticeGroups/PALS/ emailalerts/Pages/OIGReportClaimsInappropriatePayments toSNFsCostMedicareMoreThan$1BillionaYear.aspx

Radomski, M. V., & Trombly-Latham, C. A. (2008). *Occupational therapy for physical dysfunction* (6th ed.). Baltimore, MD: Lippincott, Williams & Wilkins.

Roberts, P. S., & Robinson, M. R. (2014). Health policy perspectives—Occupational therapy's role in preventing acute readmissions. *American Journal of Occupational Therapy, 68,* 254–259.

Sandstrom, R. W., Lohman, H., & Bramble, J. D. (2014). *Health services: Policy and systems for therapists* (3rd ed.). Upper Saddle River, NJ: Pearson Education Inc.

Stoffel, V. (2014). *Attitude, authenticity, and action: Building capacity for OT.* Presentation at the 2014 AOTA Annual Conference. Baltimore, Maryland.

U.S. Department of Education. (2012). *The IDEA 35th anniversary.* Retrieved from http://www2.ed.gov/about/offices/list/osers/ idea35/index.html

U.S. Department of Health and Human Services. (2014). *Key features of the Affordable Care Act by year.* Retrieved from http://www.hhs.gov/healthcare/facts/timeline/timeline-text .html

CHAPTER 4

Understanding and Working Within Organizations

Brent Braveman, PhD, OTR/L, FAOTA

■ Real-Life Management

Kate has been working in a large hospital system for 2 years since graduating from an occupational therapy program. The system is composed of different types of facilities, including a general hospital, a freestanding rehabilitation hospital, a skilled nursing facility, and several outpatient centers. She has followed with interest what seems to be a constant state of change in the organization. It seems that staff and services are continually changing not only within the facilities in which she has worked but also in the larger system.

Kate often hears expressions of frustration from her peers that seem to indicate that they don't understand why many of the changes are being made. Kate is interested in pursuing additional education but knows that she is not interested in a research career. She is considering enrolling in a Master of Business Administration or a Master of Health Care Administration program because she has always had an interest in how successful organizations operate and she is interested in learning more about the business side of health care. Because the curriculum in her occupational therapy program had a strong emphasis on theory, she wonders if there are theories related to how organizations are structured and managed that she'll learn about as she furthers her education. Additionally, she wonders how these theories might be helpful to her first as a clinician and later as she pursues her long-term goal of becoming an occupational therapy manager.

Critical Thinking Questions

As you read this chapter, consider the following questions:

- How can rational systems, natural systems, and open systems perspectives help you to understand the operation of an organization and how a manager may be most successful?

- What factors from an organization's external and internal environments affect organizational performance and how can understanding these factors and their influence make you a more effective manager?

- What can you do on a daily basis to observe how an organization's culture and values are demonstrated in the daily life of an employee and how can this help you be more effective as a manager?

- What are the various methods used to classify organizations by *type* and how can each method aid you in better understanding the organization's interactions with its environment?

Glossary

- **Associations:** formally named organizations composed primarily of participants who do not derive their livelihoods from the organization's activities (e.g., the members of the American Occupational Therapy Association).
- **Bureaucracy:** a typical managerial authority structure (e.g., CEO, vice president, middle managers, workers).
- **Culture:** in terms of organizations, it is widely accepted to mean a learned, shared set of basic assumptions or shared way of doing things that is based upon the underlying values and beliefs of the members of a particular society or of a group (in this context, an organization).
- **Instrumental values:** relate to the *means* for achieving ends, such as self-sufficiency or honesty.
- **Limited liability corporations (LLC):** a form of business that, unlike a sole proprietorship, is separate and distinct from the personal and business affairs of its owners.
- **Natural systems:** systems that focus on the human element that members bring, including their personal values and convictions, and recognize that personal agendas can affect the system.

- **Open systems:** systems that are capable of self-maintenance within a larger context or environment; the influence of internal and external environments is keenly recognized.
- **Organizational charts:** a management tool that visually depicts the lines of authority, organization, and reporting in an organization.
- **Partnerships:** an association of two or more persons formed to carry on a business for profit.
- **Rational systems:** systems that have specific goals, are highly organized, have tight lines of authority, and function through the implementation of rules and tight coordination of organizational units.
- **Sole proprietorships:** type of business organization that merges together the business and its affairs and the owner's personal affairs; therefore, from the standpoint of nearly all legal rights and responsibilities, the business and the owner are considered to be one and the same.
- **Terminal values:** relate to the *ends* that a person wishes to achieve, such as financial independence or a high level of self-esteem.

Introduction

Occupational therapy personnel work in a wide spectrum of organizations, including hospitals, schools, community-based organizations, and private businesses. There has been considerable theory development related to organizations, and a considerable body of research exists on various aspects of organizational development and function. Notable scholars have devoted entire careers to the study of organizations and organizational behavior. Chapter 3 provided an introduction to the health-care system and other systems in which occupational therapy managers are employed. This chapter provides an introduction to some key concepts useful in understanding the organizations that employ occupational therapy managers.

Occupational therapists (OTs) and occupational therapy assistants (OTAs) are well familiar with improving function by examining the fit between an individual and his or her environment. As an occupational therapy manager, you can more effectively direct and coordinate services and be a more effective advocate for the profession, the staff that you supervise, and consumers of occupational therapy if you improve your fit and the fit of your department with the environment of your organization. A first step is to develop an understanding of how your organization functions. To do this, you must come to recognize and understand the factors that have influenced your organization's development, its current operations, and its future. In Chapter 2, it was noted that occupational therapy managers *practice* just as clinicians do, and that becoming familiar with the data, information, and other forms of evidence available on organizations is necessary to practice effectively as a manager.

An observation made throughout this book is that, all too often, occupational therapy managers "fall" into their roles without adequate preparation and training rather than consciously choosing to pursue a career in management. Whether their roles are planned or occur by circumstance, it is also true that occupational therapy managers often remain insular, with too heavy a focus on the knowledge base of the profession, and fail to avail themselves of the considerable body of theory and evidence developed by other fields such as organizational development and behavior. You are encouraged to explore and use the full range of theory and evidence available to guide your practice as an occupational therapy manager.

In this chapter, we explore theoretical views and frameworks of the types of organizations, the relationship between organizational structure and function, the culture of organizations, and the fit between personal values and worldviews and "fit" within various types of organizations. Recent trends in theories related to organizational function and research are also presented.

A Brief History of Organizations and Organizational Theory

Organizations have played a critical role in the evolution of modern culture. The great social transformations in history have essentially been organizationally based. The expansion of the Roman Empire, the spread of Christianity, and the growth and development of capitalism and socialism were all accomplished through organizations (R. H. Hall, 1996; Shafritz, Ott, & Jang, 2011). Organizations have been present throughout history, including in early Chinese and Greek civilizations. For example, early tax collectors were "organized." Organizations assumed increased importance in regard to organized labor and developing economies in the late 1600s and the 1700s, especially as technological improvements contributed to the industrial revolution. In addition to technology, expanding trade markets and a growth in population created increased demand for goods and paved the way for new factories that brought with them the need to improve work methods and productivity. Specialization in work skills flourished during the 1800s as the concept of "division of labor" began to get a foothold and the advantages of specialization related to skill development, saved time and efficiency, and the development and utilization of specialized tools were recognized.

Frederick Winslow Taylor introduced one of the first theories of organizations, and he found an eager audience during the second part of the 19th century among factory managers and foremen. Taylor used "scientific management" to analyze work tasks and to make changes in production methods that resulted in increased productivity and a lessened need for labor. Taylor's early work on a theory of organizations has taken root in common thinking about organizational functioning. Today, theorists recognize that organizations play an even more central role in modern-day

Western civilization. Organizations have come to serve as the structure through which most critical societal needs are met. These needs include, among others, education (schools and universities), production and distribution of goods (factories and wholesale firms), health care (hospitals and community medical centers), travel (airlines, train companies, bus companies, and taxicab companies), preservation of culture (museums, art galleries, and libraries), communication (phone companies and Internet service providers), and entertainment (restaurants, movie theaters, and television and radio studios) (Scott, 2003).

R. H. Hall (1996) noted that organizing is a requisite for social change. Without organization, change cannot occur. A social cause alone, however strongly felt by its supporters, in itself is not adequate for change. However, by organizing, supporters of a cause can foster social change that may be lasting and of great importance. Changes in civil liberties, including the civil rights movement, equal opportunities for women, gay and lesbian rights, and the rights of disabled persons, have all been moved forward by groups forming organizations to garner political power and influence. Tolbert and Hall (2009, p. 2) commented that

> *Our lives are shaped by organizations, from birth to death. Although we may be vaguely aware of this fact, we often do not give much thought to just how pervasive organizational influences are. So let's think about this for a moment. Most of us were born in a hospital. The policies, rules, technologies, and other aspects of that organization affected how we came into the world, whether we got appropriate treatment for problems that could affect us throughout our lives, whether we survived. There may have been a brief respite from organizational influences in our early years, though organizations produce most children's toys, books, television shows, and movies, as well as the childcare books that parents rely on for advice. The organizational decisions made about producing these things undoubtedly, though largely imperceptibly, shaped our childhood experiences and early views of the world.*

As we continue through lives, our participation in most forms of education, employment, leisure, and worship are shaped by and often delivered through some form of an organization. In most industrialized countries, even how our deaths are handled is influenced by various organizations.

Richard Daft (2009, p. 14) identified seven things that organizations do for society. These seven things are:

1. Bring together resources to achieve desired goals and outcomes.
2. Produce goods and services efficiently.
3. Facilitate innovation.
4. Use modern manufacturing and information technologies.
5. Adapt to and influence a changing environment.
6. Create value for owners, customers, and employees.
7. Accommodate ongoing challenges of diversity, ethics, and the motivation of confrontation of employees.

Today the vast majority of persons are employed by and look to different types of organizations to provide their source of income and productivity and to meet most of their basic needs. The study of organizations has emerged only during the last century and has been promoted by various fields of study, including sociology and anthropology, and more recently within academic departments such as schools of business administration. March (1965) traced the origins of the study of organizations as an academic discipline back to the period of 1937 to 1947 in Europe. The study of organizations was further supported with the translation into English of the works of Max Weber, a German sociologist who is cited as publishing one of the first discussions of formal organizations or *bureaucracies* within modern society early in the 20th century (Weber, 1946). A much larger proliferation of literature began to be published in the 1940s and 1950s as organizations became even more central to economic and industrial development and production in the post–World War II United States.

Modern organizational theories include a systems approach, the sociotechnical approach, and the contingency or situational approach. These theories view the organization as an adaptive system that must adjust to changes in the environment in order to be successful and survive. The systems approach views the organization as a set of interrelated subsystems that rely on the individual, formal and informal organizational structures, patterns of behavior, and the physical environment (Cunliffe, 2008). The sociotechnical approach views the organization as composed of social systems located within an environment. Success for an organization under this theory relies on balancing the influence of social system factors and factors from the environment (Miner, 2007). The contingency or situational approach views the organization as composed of interrelated systems that interact with the environment. Because environments are different, successful organizations must form different relationships and structures in order to survive and thrive (Daft, 2008). Table 4-1 illustrates the development of the many organizational theories and indicates when they were developed.

Some forms of organization are relatively new. P. D. Hall (2010) noted that some charitable, organizational, and educational organizations are thousands of years old and some in the United States, such as Harvard University, were founded in colonial times. However, nonprofit organizations have only existed as a unified sector since the 1970s. Over 90% of nonprofit organizations that currently exist were created since 1950. Most nongovernmental organizations (NGOs) across the globe came into being in just the last 30 years, and they are the most rapidly growing type of organization.

Organizations as Systems

Scholars of organizational development have used three distinct perspectives to describe organizations as systems (Scott, 2003). These three perspectives view organizations as *rational*, *natural*, or *open systems*. Although the most common way of introducing how health-care organizations function is to discuss them as **"open systems,"** each perspective

TABLE 4-1
Organizational Theories and Time of Development

Year of Development and Primary Theorists	Organizational Theory
1911 Taylor	Strategic Management
1922 Weber	Bureaucracy Model
1925 Fayol	Administrative Theory
1933 Mayo	Hawthorne Studies
1965 McLelland	Achievement Theory
1966 Herzberg	Motivation–Hygiene
1968 Olsson	Management by Objectives
1969 Hersey Blanchard	Situational Leadership
1974 House Mitchell	Path–Goal
1976 Vroom	Expectancy Theory
1985 Schein	Organizational Culture
1991 Toyota	Lean
1998 Fairholm	Values-Based Leadership
1998 Scott	Rational, Natural, and Open Systems
2013 Barrick, Mount, Li	Purposeful Work Theory

adds to the overall understanding of the function of health-care organizations, and each perspective continues to be used to guide research, theory development, and the application of theory to everyday managerial action.

Descriptions of organizations as **rational systems** use language that one might expect as indicated by the term *rational*. Rationalists view organizations as having characteristics that differentiate them from other types of social groups, such as families. This view of organizations focuses on the following characteristics:

- Organizations benefit from having specific goals for their existence, and the more specific the goals, the higher functioning the organization is likely to be.
- Organizations are systems that are highly formalized, with tight lines of authority and accountability that serve to support the organization in meeting its goals.
- Organizations function through the implementation of rules and the tight coordination of organizational units.

Rationalists place high importance on the specificity of goals because goals can provide a set of criteria to guide decision-making and believe that more successful organizations have more specifically defined goals. Likewise, it is believed that the more formal the structure of an organization, the more predictable its behavior may become, leading to decreased resources being required to guide an organization. Rationalists such as Weber (1968) proposed that strictly defined structures and clearly delineated lines of authority and accountability for performance would improve organizational efficiency. Hence, an organizational leader who adopts a rationalist perspective may place high value on activities such as strategic planning and tend to favor organizational structures that are stable and formal, with clearly delineated lines of authority and accountability.

Whereas rationalists view organizations as systems constructed purposefully to pursue specific goals, **natural system** theorists view organizations primarily as collectives with characteristics similar to those of other social groups that are more important than the characteristics identified by rationalists (e.g., specificity of goals, authority, etc.). Natural system analysts focus on the "human element" that employees bring

to an organization, including their personal values and convictions as well as the fact that individual agendas of employees can impact organizational functioning. A primary theory within the natural systems perspective is that of *human relations theory* (Scott, 2003). Human relations theory is constructed on the assumptions that

- Most individuals find work and the expenditure of physical and mental effort to be as natural as play or rest.
- External control and threat of punishment are neither the only nor the most effective means for bringing about effort toward organizational objectives.
- The most significant rewards are those associated with the satisfaction of the ego and self-actualization needs.

Organizational leaders who adopt a naturalist perspective may stress activities related to the personal and professional development of personnel and favor organizational structures that are relatively more fluid and that promote individual growth.

An *open systems* perspective of organizations arises from *general systems theory*, which proposes that a change in any one part of a system causes inherent change in the total system and that living organisms maintain structure through continuous change (von Bertalanffy, 1968). An open system is a system that is capable of self-maintenance within a larger context or environment. Open systems theory has been used widely in the studies of organizations and of human behavior and is the systems perspective most commonly used to describe health-care organizations in management texts (McCormack, Jaffe, & Frey, 2003; Page, 2010).

Open systems theory points to three fundamental contradictions of organizational life (Mumford & Peterson, 1999):

- There is a constant need to balance the tendency toward stability with the need for change.
- Although they need to work together to produce a product or service, members may not agree on goals or strategies for coping with change.
- Managers must cope with meeting performance objectives and the bottom line while recognizing the unique needs of people who comprise work units.

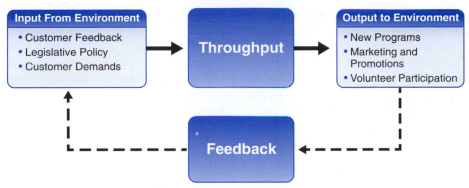

Figure ■ 4-1 An Open System.

Organizational leaders who adopt an open systems perspective may tend to focus on activities that include monitoring and assessment of internal and external organizational environments and favor a balance of formal planning and human resource development activities.

Basic to the premise of organizations as open systems are the concepts of (a) input, (b) throughput, and (c) output. Input can be thought of as the resources and influences that flow into the organization (e.g., physical resources such as money and materials or psychological and human resources in the form of energy and knowledge) that allow the organization to complete its basic functions. Throughput can be thought of as the processes that occur within an organization or the processing of input to achieve the organization's end goals. Output is simply what the organization sends back into the larger environment in terms of goods or services. Feedback is provided from the environment in which the organization functions and in return becomes an additional source of input. The key features of an open system are presented in Box 4-1, and a simple visual depiction of an open system as applied to an organization is presented in Figure 4-1.

Although an open systems perspective provides a simple way to think about the influences on and the functions of organizations, more complex frameworks are needed to help managers within an organization perform their jobs effectively. This is true because even very large and complexly structured organizations may be conceptualized as open systems. Viewing an organization as a hierarchical system adds the perspective that organizations may be structured differently in order to manage input into the system and produce the goods or services related to their missions

or the reasons they exist. Organizations have characteristics that may be examined as a first step toward understanding the day-to-day functioning of the organization. The following is a partial list of characteristics to consider:

- Organizations have boundaries that serve to define membership; these boundaries include some members of the population and exclude others.
- Organizations involve social relationships in which individuals within the organization interact with each other, as well as with persons outside of the organization.

BOX 4-1

Key Features of Open Systems as Applied to Organizations

- **Input:** Entry of resources, energy, and information into the system
- **Throughput:** Processing of input to achieve organizational goals
- **Output:** Goods or services produced by an organization and returned to the external environment
- **Feedback:** Knowledge or information returned to the organization from external sources or from internal sources interpreting the result of output
- **Environment:** Organizations exist within environments that provide input to the system and receive output from the organization

- Organizations involve a hierarchy of authority in which power to make decisions and commit resources is unequally distributed.
- Organizations involve a division of labor in which tasks are typically divided among employees based on skill, capacity, and the types of rewards associated with completion of tasks.
- Organizations exist outside the lives of their members and therefore have goals, missions, and a reason to exist on their own.

Any complex system or organization is composed of multiple subsystems. For example, a hospital may both comprise smaller subsystems such as divisions, departments, or product lines and itself operate within a larger system or "network" of health-care providers. Similarly, a school is composed of individual classrooms that function to some degree as subsystems but is located in a school district composed of individual schools that each function as distinct organizations. Within each system or subsystem, a hierarchy, or some form of levels, may be found. How these levels interact in terms of status, power, authority, and accountability may vary a great deal, but the main point to consider is that most systems in which occupational therapy personnel work are made up of smaller subsystems and are themselves typically components of larger systems. Occupational therapy managers may benefit by becoming adept at analyzing and understanding systems both within and outside of their organization. Managers who can do so, and who can recognize, respond to, and even predict the influence of environmental changes, will increase their value to the organization and the profession. In addition, a manager who develops an understanding of how organizations work can be more effective at setting questions related to managerial functions and finding relevant data, information, and other forms of evidence needed to answer these questions.

Although many veteran managers may appreciate the value of educating their staff about the influences of the greater system in which the occupational therapy department or organization functions, they are likely to also express that it can be difficult at times to convince line staff of this importance. Entry-level practitioners are often consumed by the stressors of learning a myriad of new skills, coming to terms with their professional style, understanding the dynamics of the levels of the organization in which they interact directly, and sometimes learning to integrate basic habits of daily work into their lives. Given these demands, it is reasonable to understand that placing energy into comprehending the larger political, economic, and legislative contexts in which an organization functions might not appear as a priority for the typical occupational therapy staff member. One need only consider the basic organization of a typical medical-model setting in which occupational therapy personnel work to recognize just how far removed the staff members are from the "outside world" in terms of daily work. For example, Figure 4-2 is a simple representation of the layers of an organization. In large organizations, each layer might in turn be broken into several other layers so that by the time you move from a staff OT to the level of vice president or the chief executive officer, you may have eight or more levels of reporting. By coming to understand more about how organizations function, the occupational therapy manager can help to filter information for the occupational therapy staff members and call their attention to the environmental influences that will have the most impact on employees.

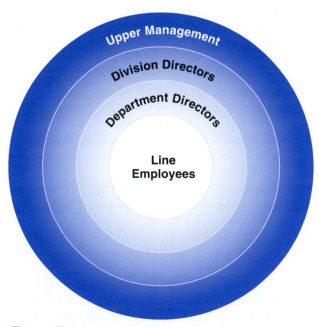

Figure ■ 4-2 The Multiple Layers of a Typical Organization.

Organizational Environments

Occupational therapy personnel are well aware of the importance of the interaction and fit between an individual and his or her environment as it relates to the individual's capacity for satisfactory occupational performance. Likewise, organizations operate within environments, and the organization's capacity to meet environmental demands and anticipate and prepare for future demands impacts the organization's performance capacity. In today's world, the organizations in which occupational therapy personnel work may interact not only in local environments, but sometimes on a state, national, or even global basis. It is useful as an occupational therapy manager for you to understand the environments in which your organization operates and the forces and pressures to which the organization must respond. For example, after the Patient Protection and Affordable Care Act became law in 2010 the environment in which most occupational therapy practitioners practice in the United States changed, and the law is affecting various organizations in different ways (Braveman & Metzler, 2012). It is likely that the influence of the law will continue to evolve over at least the next decade.

Managers can have great influence on those whom they supervise. Managers can be mentors, inspiring others to work beyond their own expectations for performance and helping those they supervise to make a positive contribution to the organization and their community. However, managers can also add to a subordinate's sense of dissatisfaction, frustration, and lowered productivity. Working to actively monitor and understand the organization's internal environment can help to have a positive influence on subordinates' job satisfaction and performance.

External Environments

R. H. Hall (1996) made the interesting and important observation that, with regard to the influence of external environmental factors on health-care organizations, environmental factors have both *theoretical* and *practical* outcomes for these types of organizations. This holds true today; in other words, we cannot rely on theory or evidence alone to help us understand the decisions that a health-care organization may make. For example, although hospitals may increase services or invest monies in updated facilities based upon patient needs, this may not be the only or even the primary environmental influence to which they are responding. Hospitals and other health-care or public service organizations also need to compete in a competitive, market-driven environment. In Chapter 3 you were introduced to the concept of supply and demand. Based upon this economic theory alone, we might expect that an organization would make the rational decision to not invest monies in inpatient hospital beds if the market in which it operates were already saturated. However, in the year 2000, Cook County in Illinois began construction on a new 464-bed hospital in Chicago despite the fact that, during that same year, the average occupancy rate for Illinois hospitals was only 58.5% and it was estimated that, in the city of Chicago and its suburbs, there might be as many as 10,000 more inpatient hospital beds than required (Illinois Hospital Association, 2003). The practical outcome of remaining competitive in the market by improving the physical facilities outweighed the theoretical outcome of contributing to an already saturated marketplace.

A number of specific arenas within the external environment should be of concern to occupational therapy managers. These include:

- The *legislative arena* at a state and national level where new laws influence access to services, reimbursement, and the scope of care that can legally be provided.
- The *economic arena*, as the availability of resources and the local, state, and national economy influence organizational plans for the future.
- The *technology arena*, because finding and managing information becomes more sophisticated and complex and new products and services are constantly introduced.
- The *demographic arena*, as the age, socioeconomic status, racial mix, and other characteristics of local and national populations change.
- The *sociocultural arena*, where societal values and beliefs about what is acceptable and expected are constantly shifting.

Organizations survive and sometimes thrive in turbulent environments by responding to change at multiple levels. The issues or problems of external adaptation and survival specify the coping cycle that any system must be able to maintain in relation to its changing environment (Schein, 1992). Edgar Schein, a noted organizational psychologist and a professor of management at the Massachusetts Institute of Technology Sloan School of Management, described five stages of a cycle of adaptation for an organization, which are outlined in Box 4-2. When reviewing the stages suggested by Schein, it is of interest to note that the most commonly identified functions of management (i.e., planning, organizing and staffing, directing, and controlling) are easily recognizable within them.

Typically an organization's mission (a statement of why the organization exists) remains fairly stable and can be thought of as a rudder that guides the organization in the direction envisioned by its founders. Highly successful organizations maintain a sense of focus but are flexible in serving multiple functions and meeting the needs of numerous constituent groups. For example, the major initiatives pursued, products produced, and services provided by a community or health-care agency typically reflect the organization's core mission, but the interests and desires of key personnel or customer groups may also be reflected in programming and service offerings that come and go over time. The extent to which large amounts of the organization's financial and human resources are

not diverted from the core mission to these "side projects" is one measure of the success of organizational leadership in making the organization's mission "real." Organizational missions are not impervious to challenge, however, especially when the survival of the organization itself comes into question. Few organizations ever willingly state, "Our mission has been achieved, so we are disbanding," or "It is clear in the marketplace that our competitors are better equipped to serve the public than we are, so we are closing up shop in the best interests of the public." In today's society, one commonly recognized function of an organization is to provide a living wage for those it employs, and reaching this goal can at times seem to take precedence over goals related to the very reason an organization was created in the first place.

It might seem that, if an organization's mission were kept front and center in the minds of personnel through the actions of leadership, then establishing goals to match the mission would be an easy task. However, doing so is more complicated than you might imagine. Establishing a common understanding of mission does not automatically translate to having a shared understanding of how that mission is best served or the strategies that should be pursued. It is through the management functions of strategic and operational planning (discussed in Chapters 6 and 9) that a concrete and articulated set of specific goals with specific time frames is developed. Planning is an ongoing process that must include consistent monitoring of the external environment to cue the organization to when it must adapt strategies and pursue contingent actions.

Organizations cannot reach their goals unless there is a clear and articulated consensus on the specific means and methods by which they intend to do so. Moving from long-range planning focused on the goals of the year or next few years to day-to-day planning for tomorrow and next week requires vigilant attention on the part of all levels of leadership and management. Managers must decide how to best *organize* resources to accomplish work tasks and must assure that the right combination of skills and talents are assembled for the work to be done. Schein (1992), a major organizational development theorist, made the interesting observation that deciding how things will be done often also inadvertently assigns ownership of who will do what in many ways. He noted that various amounts of status, access to rewards, and certain privileges inevitably accompany the assigned roles, and the

---

BOX 4-2

The Stages of Organizational Adaptation to External Change

1. **Mission clarification:** Obtaining and maintaining a shared and functional understanding of the organization's core mission, functions, and products
2. **Goal setting:** Developing consensus on goals that match the stated organizational mission
3. **Means to goal obtainment:** Developing consensus on the means and methods to reach stated goals
4. **Measurement:** Establishing clear criteria to use to measure how well the organization is doing to meet stated goals
5. **Correction:** Developing consensus on appropriate remediation or strategies to take if goals are not being met

means by which things get done in the external environment become "property" in the internal environment. Such a sense of ownership can both facilitate the work of an organization if personnel are appropriately involved in making decisions, and inhibit work if changes to processes are perceived as threats or as a means of lowering one's status in the workplace.

Preestablished criteria or indicators of performance allow an organization to monitor whether it is meeting its goals and to identify when contingent action must be taken to get it back on course. Such *operational definitions*, if properly applied, remove any doubt regarding expectations for middle managers, who are often responsible for direct supervision of those who do the primary work of the organization. These operational definitions also allow managers to take swift action when it becomes apparent that a unit is not on target. Applying such criteria is often described as the *control* function of management. Again, such steps may seem as if they would be relatively simple, but often agreeing on performance "targets" as well as the process for measuring performance against a target can be difficult. Common criteria for performance that are encountered by occupational therapy personnel and managers include volume or productivity targets. Agreeing on performance criteria, such as the number of billable hours per day per OT or OTA to be provided, may be difficult enough, but coming to consensus on how to factor the many situations OTs and OTAs encounter into such criteria becomes very difficult indeed. Information, including some of the most basic financial information, can be analyzed and interpreted in a variety of ways. Assuring not only that operational definitions are in place but also that there is discussion about the underlying rationale for criteria can help maintain consensus.

Finally, when things are not going according to plan and it appears that goals are not being met, organizations must make decisions about what strategies are to be assumed. Alternatively, sometimes organizations exceed expectations for performance; managing unexpected success and taking full advantage of such situations are also forms of contingent actions.

Internal Environments: Organizational Culture

The term **culture** is widely accepted to mean a learned, shared set of basic assumptions or shared way of doing things that is based upon the underlying values and beliefs of the members of a particular society or of a group. Shared values serve to impact the actions of the members of an organization in several ways. Shared values:

- Help turn commonplace, routine work into valued activities.
- Create a connection between the mission of the organization and society's values.
- Provide a source of competitive advantage to the organization.

Individual values are developed through interactions between a person and the environment and culture in which he or she resides. As we might expect, because the experiences of individuals vary even within the same cultural context, different persons develop different values. Values are typically thought to be resistant to simple influences and to persist over time because they develop over periods of many years as we interact with the world. A commonly recognized method of classifying values was developed by psychologist Milton Rokeach, who identified two classes of values: **instrumental values** and **terminal values** (Rokeach, 1973). Instrumental values relate to the *means* for achieving ends, such as self-sufficiency or honesty. Terminal values relate to the *ends* that a person wishes to achieve, such as financial independence or a high level of self-esteem. It has been hypothesized that, as workers age, a shift occurs so that terminal values are less influential and instrumental values exert more influence on worker actions. If this is true, understanding the difference in how these values can be supported in the workplace can be useful for the occupational therapy manager.

The relationship between organizational values and individual values has important implications for the workplace. As one might expect, it is generally believed that having a high level of *congruence* between the values of an organization and those of individual employees facilitates improved organizational performance. When values do not match, or are *incongruent*, it is typically expected that the level of conflict may be higher and that organizational performance may be lower. The connection between value congruence and organizational performance has an implication for managers. If it is true that individual values are resilient to simple influences and not easily changed, it may be easier for managers to select employees who have values that match and support those of the organization than to try to instill a set of values within employees after they are hired. Although fully assessing the values of potential employees may be beyond the scope of time and resources available to most managers while recruiting employees, a manager can effectively communicate recognized organizational and department values by:

- Sharing copies of mission and vision statements for the organization and department during the recruitment process
- Including current staff in the interview process and encouraging candidates to ask questions of staff regarding shared values and common practices and what it "feels like" to work for the organization, as well as providing examples of group norms that represent shared values
- Sharing explicit statements of personal values as a manager and making expectations clear by giving examples of how he or she hopes that values are translated into action and behavior by staff

One useful aspect of organizational culture is that it implies structural stability in a group. This stability means that there are elements of an organization or group that can be *observed*. Moreover, these elements are often just below the level of consciousness of most organizational members. An astute manager can use these observations to his or her advantage when joining an organization or attempting to create change. As noted by Schein (1992), "If the concept of culture is to have any utility, it should draw our attention to those things that are the product of our human need for stability, consistency, and meaning." Schein identified 10 phenomena associated with organizational culture that may be overtly observed. These phenomena and common examples of each are listed in Box 4-3.

We must understand that we are not born into a culture, but rather are born into a society that teaches us its culture. Similarly, as we enter a new organization, we may come to understand the underlying or shared values and beliefs as we become exposed to the way things are done within the organization. The notion of organizational or "corporate" culture is pervasive in the management literature and has been widely investigated. In their influential book, *In Search of Excellence*, Peters and Waterman (1982) stressed the contribution that the development of specific organi-

zational cultures made to what they defined as "best-run" organizations. They noted that:

The dominance and coherence of culture proved to be an essential quality of the excellent companies. Moreover, the stronger the culture and the more it was directed toward the marketplace, the less need there was for policy manuals, organization charts, or detailed procedures and rules. In these companies people way down the line know what they are supposed to do in situations because the handful of guiding values is crystal clear.

Uhl-Bien, Schermerhorn, and Olson (2013) identified three levels of analysis for understanding organizational culture, as shown in Figure 4-3:

First level: observable culture, or "the way we do things around here," including the unique stories, ceremonies, and corporate rituals that make up the history of the organization
Second level: shared values that link organizational members together and provide a motivation for organizational behavior
Third level: common assumptions or taken-for-granted truths that collections of corporate members share as a result of their joint experience

These levels are shown in an inverted triangle to indicate that common assumptions are at the most basic layer and may be limited in number but not tacitly expressed. An example might be the assumption that all persons deserve the same level of care regardless of the ability to pay. Shared values are based on these assumptions and are reflected in the day-to-day behavior of organization members. These values may be more easily identified and sometimes are specifically indicated. For example, an organization might include the values of respect, quality, customer service, and efficient care in the annual performance appraisal of employees. The observable culture is most easily recognized in employee behaviors and is at the surface. Not all employee behavior is consistent with an organization's values or underlying assumptions. However, in highly effective organizations many employees will demonstrate the organization's values and underlying assumptions in their daily work, and this will be visible. For example, the assumption that all persons deserve the same level of care and the value of respect can be demonstrated by the nurse, physician, occupational

BOX 4-3

Observable Phenomena Related to Organizational Culture

1. *Behavioral regularities*, including the language used and the customs, traditions, and rituals that evolve, such as expectations to attend department functions, including holiday parties or company picnics.
2. *Group norms*, or implicit standards and values, such as a norm of offering to cover each other's patients during vacations.
3. *Espoused values*, or publicly announced principles and values, such as customer service.
4. *Formal philosophy*, or the broad policies and ideological principles that guide a group's actions toward employees, customers, and other key stakeholders, such as rewarding seniority among employees or providing special privileges to loyal customers.
5. *Rules of the game*, or the unspoken rules for getting along that are often described as "the way we do things around here," such as staying late in the office to finish paperwork and submit it on time.
6. *Organizational climate*, or the feeling that is conveyed in a group by the way members interact with each other, customers, and other outsiders, such as staff routinely asking "May I

help you?" when they see someone who appears to be lost in the building.
7. *Embedded skills*, or the special competencies that group members display in accomplishing certain tasks, such as communicating with parents who do not speak English about their children's therapies.
8. *Habits of thinking, mental models, or linguistic paradigms*, or the cognitive frameworks that guide the perceptions, thought, and language used by the members of a group, such as commonly used conceptual practice models.
9. *Shared meanings*, or the emergent understandings that are created by group members as they interact with each other, such as meanings associated with eating lunch together, or in regard to common events, such as having all referrals assigned to an evaluating therapist in a timely manner.
10. *Root metaphors*, or the ideas, feelings, and images groups develop to characterize themselves that become embedded in the physical spaces and material artifacts of the group, such as group photos, awards given to the department, or souvenirs on display from group outings.

Adapted from Schein, E. H. (1992). Organizational culture and leadership. New York, NY: Jossey-Bass.

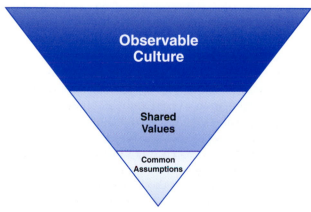

Figure ■ 4-3
Three Levels of Analysis in Studying Organizational Culture.

therapy practitioner, and other employees when they take the time to use common words rather than medical jargon so that a patient with a lower level of education might understand and remain in control of medical decision-making.

These levels of analysis can be used by a new or veteran manager who wishes to understand more about the values, beliefs, and shared assumptions of the organization's members. Listening to the stories told about the organization, sharing observations about common practices with other managers, listening to other managers' interpretations, and carefully noting the feedback and reaction you receive both in times that you are succeeding and when you are struggling are strategies that you can use to gain insights into your organization's culture.

Organizational cultures will present both opportunities and challenges to you as a new manager as you enter an organization and must interpret the explicit and implicit messages that you receive about the way that things are to be done. Through shared experiences, veteran organizational members will likely have developed ways of accomplishing day-to-day work that tacitly incorporate strategies to meet challenges previously encountered and overcome. It is likely that members will have also developed strategies that tacitly manage the expectations, demands, and work styles of other units within the organization. Unconscious ways of working such as those just described may not only provide key insights into the underlying values and assumptions of an organization's members, but they may also serve to improve the effectiveness and efficiency of work groups. Unfortunately, systems, processes, and procedures sometimes outlive their usefulness, and you may find that it seems that members of an organization complete tasks in an almost ritualistic fashion without being quite sure why. The tendency to challenge such behavior as ineffective, wasteful, or unneeded is understandable, but you must remember that, in doing so, you may be perceived as challenging not just the way things are done but also the underlying values that drove members to assume the action in the first place.

All organizations have some things in common, most notably that each organization exists for a particular reason (e.g., the organizational mission) and that each makes particular contributions to society by its output or products. Recognizing the commonalities among organizations is helpful in understanding how they function; however, it is also useful to recognize the differences between organizations. The next section of the chapter briefly overviews some typologies for making distinctions between organizations. Practitioners who wish to start their own businesses or assume leadership roles in nonprofit agencies will need more detailed information on the structure of those types of organizations.

Types of Organizations

Relatively large numbers of systems for classifying organizations, or *typologies*, have been presented in the organizational development literature. However, R. H. Hall (1996) made the point that any single typology may or may not be useful depending on the needs of the reader. Taking a cue from Hall, the following is not intended as a specific system of classification but is actually a mix of typologies that focuses on making the distinctions that are most helpful for the occupational therapy manager to understand the types of organizations in which occupational therapy personnel most often work.

Bureaucracies and Associations

Jaques (1998) made a distinction between a bureaucracy, or a typical managerial authority structure, and an association. This distinction is helpful in understanding the relationship between the types of organizations in which most occupational therapy personnel are employed and the voluntary organization that represents OTs and OTAs, the American Occupational Therapy Association (AOTA), or similar associations that represent other health disciplines or professionals. Although the term **bureaucracy** has generally come to hold a negative connotation, indicating an organization that is inefficient and overly structured, in organizational development literature it simply indicates the type of authority structure found in most businesses where employees are paid for the work they produce and is not meant to hold either a negative or a positive connotation. **Associations** are formally named organizations composed primarily of participants who do not derive their livelihoods from the organization's activities. When speaking of AOTA, it is important to distinguish whether you mean the OTs and OTAs who pay to be members of the association in order to have their professional interests represented, the paid staff members who work for the bureaucracy (the authority structure), or both. The distinction between bureaucracies and associations has become less clear in modern times as associations have assumed more responsibility for activities such as continuing education, marketing, and product development, yet it is still helpful at times to recognize the unique combination of paid and volunteer leadership in professional associations and how it influences decision-making.

For example, in AOTA, the executive director is a paid employee (often *not* educated in occupational therapy) who is hired by the Board of Directors. The Board of Directors is composed of mostly OTs or OTAs elected to the Board by members of the association in voluntary elections. The executive director leads a group of paid employees composed of occupational therapy personnel and non–occupational therapy personnel hired for their expertise in marketing, sales, program development, information management, or other skill sets required to carry out the work of the association and meet the varied needs of the membership. There is also a very large volunteer leadership structure comprising members who are elected or appointed, or who volunteer to assume various roles, led by the president of AOTA, who is elected for a 3-year term. One important part of most associations is a policy-making group that is typically composed of elected members who represent various segments of the association. For example, AOTA's Representative Assembly (RA) is composed of representatives elected from the 50 states and territories (e.g., Puerto Rico) and persons who fill other key volunteer leadership positions. The RA sets policy for the association, such as strategic directions, the cost of membership dues, and the membership structure, and charges association bodies with projects to meet the needs of the membership and to promote occupational therapy. Other professional associations have similar policy-making and decision-making groups.

For-Profit and Nonprofit Organizations

A simple but sometimes important way of distinguishing between organizations is whether they are *for-profit* or *nonprofit* organizations. To the outsider, at first glance it might be difficult to distinguish between for-profit and nonprofit organizations that have similar missions and produce similar products and services. For example, there are both for-profit and nonprofit hospitals and skilled nursing facilities that provide similar services to similar populations and that are structured in almost identical ways. Simply by examining their organizational charts, or even the mission statements, you might not be able to distinguish the for-profit from the nonprofit organization. Further, if you were to speak to managers from each type of organization, you might hear very similar descriptions of what their responsibilities and concerns entail. Both are likely to report being responsible for the traditional management functions (e.g., planning, organizing and staffing, directing, and controlling) and facing the same pressures of operating with limited resources to produce a quality product with high levels of productivity. Moreover, managers in nonprofit organizations may be as concerned—if not more concerned—than managers in for-profit organizations with helping to create a positive "bottom line," or assuring that the organization makes money in any given year. In fact, nonprofit organizations must make a profit in order to be able to maintain and improve physical facilities, buy new equipment, and pay for the same expenses faced by for-profit organizations, such as advertising and marketing. So, if for-profit and nonprofit organizations can have so much in common, you are likely asking, "How are they different?"

There are many financial and legal differences, such as whether the organizations are taxed on their profits or must pay taxes on goods that they purchase, how the organizations are legally structured, and who is legally responsible for debt and contractual obligations entered into by the organization. In addition, a primary difference is that the for-profit organization exists to make money for a group of investors and the nonprofit exists solely to meet its mission and reinvests all profits into the organization. Another difference may be represented in the decisions the organizations make about the nature of the programming they provide and how flexible they are willing to be in accepting various forms of payment for services. Managers in for-profit organizations are likely to feel more pressure to examine the impact that service design and delivery will have on reimbursement and to maximize services that are highly reimbursed while avoiding, when possible, services that are not reimbursed. It must be noted, however, that even many for-profit organizations provide some level of "indigent" or uncompensated care.

The for-profit sector of the profession not only includes large health-care organizations but also includes the private practitioner and business entrepreneurs who may provide traditional occupational therapy services or other services such as the manufacture and sale of assistive and adaptive equipment. Owning and operating your own business can be rewarding both financially and professionally, but is also very challenging, and requires the development of business and marketing skills in addition to a devotion to hard work and to making the business successful. Resources for the private practitioner or business entrepreneur can be found through AOTA, the Small Business Association, and other associations, including associations dedicated to helping women or people of color to succeed as small business owners. The next section of this chapter provides a brief description of the most common types of private businesses and the advantages and disadvantages of each type.

Common Types of Private Business Organizations

Sole Proprietorships

The majority of small businesses start out as sole proprietorships (Small Business Administration, 2013). **Sole proprietorships** merge together the business and its affairs and the owner's personal affairs; therefore, from the standpoint of nearly all legal rights and responsibilities, the business and the owner are considered to be one and the same. In sole proprietorships, the owner directs business activities and may hire employees; however, this does not alter the legal nature of the business. The owner of a sole proprietorship has legal ownership of all assets of a business but also assume responsibility for all debt. If credit is used in the operation of the business, it is important to maintain separate financial records for business and personal finances. Interest payments on personal debt are not a deductible expense for federal and state income tax purposes; however, interest payments on business borrowing are fully deductible.

Advantages of sole proprietorships are:

- They are the easiest and least expensive form of business ownership to organize.
- They can be established, bought, sold, or terminated very quickly.
- They do not require public notification to start, terminate, or be modified beyond routine permits and licenses.
- The size and structure can change, and others (family, etc.) can be involved according to the proprietor's wishes.
- Complex business planning or organizational arrangements (bylaws, organizational charter, etc.) are not required by law.

Disadvantages of sole proprietorships are:

- Both personal and business assets are at risk unless they are protected in a trust or some other protective mechanism.
- Mixing business and personal finances can make it more difficult to measure the financial success of the business.
- The business ends with the death of the proprietor, and a new business must be formed if others wish to continue the business.
- In family sole proprietorships, each generation must purchase or inherit the business assets, paying any applicable taxes and costs, upon death of the sole proprietor.
- The availability of credit and ability to respond to opportunities may be restricted because of limited resources.
- Conflicts or disagreements within the family can stagnate the business and delay needed decision-making.

Partnerships

A **partnership** is an association of two or more persons formed to carry on a business for profit. All partnerships should be based on a written partnership agreement that lays out in advance how decisions are to be made in the case of disagreement and how funds and property are to be handled upon dissolution of the partnership. With few exceptions, a partnership is not an income-tax-paying entity because profits from the partnership flow directly to the partners' personal tax returns. Unless arrangements are made to continue the partnership beyond death or withdrawal of a partner in the partnership agreement, the partnership is dissolved in such situations.

Advantages of partnerships are:

- They are relatively easy to establish because the partners may combine resources.
- The partners may capitalize on their skills and interests by specializing in certain aspects of management or operations.
- There may be a greater capacity for obtaining credit by partners than what either partner might obtain on his or her own.
- The necessary record-keeping and income tax filing requirements are only slightly more complicated than for individuals.
- They provide opportunities for family members or friends to work together in starting or operating a business.

Disadvantages of partnerships are:

- The personal assets of all partners are put at risk.
- Business is disrupted upon the death or withdrawal of a single partner.
- Alienation of a partner with minority interests can occur if partners with majority interests vote together and block the interests of the minority.
- They must be carefully planned to allow succession to a new generation or the next generation, and tax laws related to inheritance apply.
- They can lead to fragmented leadership if the division of management responsibility among the partners results in no one having an overall understanding of the financial standing of the partnership.
- They may be difficult to end without undue financial loss or interpersonal conflict with the other partners.
- They can lose productivity and profitability if conflicts or disagreements among the partners immobilize business decision-making.

Limited Liability Corporation

The **limited liability corporation (LLC)** is a form of business that, unlike a sole proprietorship, is separate and distinct from the personal and business affairs of its owners. The LLC, a newer form of *hybrid* business that is now permissible in most states (Small Business Administration, 2013), is designed to provide the limited liability features of a corporation and the tax efficiencies and operational flexibility of a partnership. One or more persons may organize an LLC by preparing and filing copies of articles of organization with the designated state agency. The name, the purpose for which the LLC is organized, its principal place of business, the resources to be invested in it, and the identity and addresses of managers must be stated in the articles. Upon issuance of a certificate of organization by the designated state agency, the LLC can begin business activities.

An LLC may be dissolved when (a) the identified life span specified in the articles of organization expires, (b) the members unanimously agree in writing that it should be dissolved, (c) any other dissolution cause specified in the articles of organization occurs, or (d) it is dissolved by a court. Operating procedures are also articulated in the articles of organization.

With the exception of liabilities for unpaid taxes, members and managers of an LLC are not liable for LLC debt or liabilities.

Advantages of LLCs are:

- They provide the owners with a flexible and adaptable form of business organization that provides liability protection comparable to the protection provided by incorporation.
- They can be established at moderate cost in a relatively short time.
- All members, one or more members, or a nonmember individual or business entity may manage an LLC.
- The interests of the owners can be transferred to others upon approval of the LLC members as articulated in the articles of organization.

Disadvantages of LLCs are:

- They can be more difficult to establish than sole proprietorships or partnerships and require legal assistance and public notification.
- Conflict can arise among members because it may be more difficult to correctly anticipate ownership and management issues.
- Corporations are monitored by federal, state, and some local agencies and so may require more paperwork to comply with regulations.
- Incorporation may result in higher overall taxes.

S Corporations

An *S corporation* is a corporation that is taxed under Subchapter S of the Internal Revenue Code and receives Internal Revenue Service (IRS) approval of its request for Subchapter S status. Eligibility for S corporation tax status is based on compliance with IRS regulations regarding the number and characteristics of stockholders, type of stock issued, and other characteristics specified in the regulations. Because it is a separate legal entity, the corporation finances and records are established and maintained completely separate and distinct from the finances and records of the stockholders. One or more officers of the corporation are authorized to conduct business on behalf of the corporation. If the corporation is new and has a limited credit record, personal guarantees by one or more officers or stockholders may be required to obtain the necessary credit to conduct business, which then may create personal liability for those individuals.

Advantages of S corporations are:

- The liability of stockholders is limited to their investment in the corporation and their personal assets are protected.
- These corporations can raise additional funds through the sale of stock.
- They can continue operating despite the death of one or more stockholders.
- They accommodate multiple owners but provide for decision-making mechanisms that base influence on percentage of ownership.
- They allow for change of ownership through sale or gift without disturbing business operations.
- They may benefit from communication between stockholders, legal counsel, and other groups to maximize management knowledge.

Disadvantages of S corporations are:

- Personal guarantees from officers or stockholders may be required if the corporation has limited credit.
- Conflict can erupt if a small but powerful group of stockholders join together and limit decision-making.
- Minority stockholders may be limited from being able to recover the value of their investment in the corporation.
- Stock ownership can become fragmented among many persons who are not active in or knowledgeable about the business through gift or sale to others.
- The corporate shield of limited liability may be lost in some instances when corporate formalities are not followed, and shareholders can become personally liable in rare instances.

C Corporations

A *C corporation* is a corporation that is taxed under Subchapter C of the Internal Revenue Code and receives IRS approval of its request for Subchapter C status. As a legal entity, the C corporation is separate and distinct from the owners of the corporation (stockholders). The C corporation must pay taxes on its taxable income before making dividend distributions to stockholders. It is allowed to issue more than one type of stock and can have any number of stockholders. One or more officers or employees of the corporation are authorized to conduct business on behalf of the corporation. As with an S corporation, if the corporation is new or has a limited credit record, a lender may require personal guarantees by one or more officers or stockholders before approving a credit application from the corporation. If personal guarantees are given, the signer(s) usually have unlimited liability for the corporation's debts. Some legal costs are incurred in setting up a C corporation, and the formation and continued operation of a corporation is required and is accomplished through filings with the designated state office.

Advantages of C corporations are:

- The perpetual life of the corporation makes possible its continuation, as well as the relatively undisturbed continued operation of the business, despite the incapacity or death of one or more stockholders.
- Fractional ownership interests are easily accommodated in the initial offering of stock.
- The purchase, sale, and gifting of stock make possible changes in ownership without disturbing the corporation's ability to conduct business.
- The required separation of finances and records for the corporation reduces the risk of unrecognized equity liquidations.
- To the extent the corporate shield is maintained and other investments and savings of the stockholders are not at risk, the personal life of stockholders is simplified.
- The annual meetings of stockholders and consultations with legal counsel can provide a stimulus for improved communication with the stockholder group (usually a family group) and can provide more comprehensive guidance for management.
- Life insurance up to $50,000 per person, health insurance, housing costs, and other benefits for employees (including stockholder–employees) can be tax-deductible expenses for the corporation.

Disadvantages of C corporations are:

- They must pay income tax on their net income before distribution of dividends to stockholders, and the dividends are taxable to the stockholders, resulting in double taxation of corporation income distributed to stockholders.

- Personal guarantees from corporate officers may be required if credit is limited, resulting in loss of the corporate shield to limit liability.
- Conflict among a small group of stockholders may stagnate decision-making.
- Stock ownership can become fragmented among many persons who are not active in or knowledgeable about the business through gift or sale to others.
- Corporation-paid benefits for stockholder–employees may become costly and exceed the business's ability to pay.

For more in-depth information on starting a business and on the advantages and disadvantages of various forms of structuring private practices or entrepreneurial ventures, you are encouraged to review the resources at the end of the chapter, particularly those provided by the U.S. Small Business Administration (http://www.sba.gov/). Your local Chamber of Commerce may also provide a network of peers and learning opportunities for persons interested in starting and managing their own business.

Organizations by Societal Sector

A common sense way that organizations have been classified is according to their societal "sector," such as medical, educational, or community-based. Although R. H. Hall (1996) pointed out that this manner of classifying organizations is limited because there are dimensions of organizations that can overlap in unpredictable ways (e.g., many universities operate hospitals), this classification is functional and commonly used to describe the settings in which OTs and OTAs work. For example, it is common to refer to occupational therapy practitioners who work in the "school system," and much has been written about the increased number of occupational therapy practitioners who have returned to practice in the "community." Classifying organizations in this manner is useful because, for the occupational therapy manager and practitioner, it typically has significant implications for the type of services provided.

Hospitals and other medical-model settings are still a popular area of practice for occupational therapy across the full age span of patients and the entire continuum of care from acute trauma to skilled nursing facilities. These settings are often referred to as "medical-model" settings because the focus of much of the intervention is on remediation of an underlying physical impairment in order to restore health and function. It should not be assumed, however, that practicing in a medical setting prevents the delivery of holistic care, the provision of occupation-based practice, or the use of strategies to lessen disability by adapting the environment. Effective managers in medical-model settings must develop a working knowledge of a wide range of reimbursement policies because these can have dramatic effects on the services provided, patterns of staffing, and organizational structure. For example, the 1997 Balanced Budget Act drastically decreased the amount of covered services in skilled nursing facilities and imposed caps on Medicare reimbursement for outpatients. Outpatient caps to Medicare payment and other changes to reimbursement introduced as part of the Patient Protection and Affordable Care Act (2010) continue to provide challenges to practice today.

A large percentage of OTs and OTAs work in school systems and provide services under the Individuals With Disabilities Education Act (IDEA), which was discussed in Chapter 3. As with hospitals, choosing to practice in a type of organization such as a school system typically has implications for the nature of practice. Often, services in a school are provided through consultative models by collaborating with a student's teacher and adapting the environment to promote learning while providing limited individual service. Occupational therapy managers who work in the school system often supervise therapists over a large geographic area, therapists in a number of different schools, or therapists from other disciplines, including physical therapy (PT) and speech–language pathology (SLP).

Occupational therapists and occupational therapy assistants work in a wide range of community-based organizations, including those providing early intervention, work rehabilitation, mental health, and adult day programs (Scaffa & Reitz, 2013). Although it is common to refer to "community-based organizations" as a single type of organization, the diversity within these organizations must be recognized. Community-based organizations can be small organizations focused on the delivery of a single type of service to a very specific population, or they can be large and serve a range of needs experienced by the community they serve. The range of roles assumed by occupational therapy managers in community-based organizations must be recognized. Whereas it is common for the role of the OT or OTA in a medical-model setting such as a hospital to be more narrowly defined because of the presence of numerous other disciplines, occupational therapy practitioners in community-based organizations often assume a wider variety of duties. In addition to managing and providing traditional occupational therapy services, they may assume responsibility for supervision of volunteers, case management of clients, or organizing and running special events.

Regardless of type, organizations can be structured in various ways. Understanding the relationship between organizational structure and performance is important and can help the occupational therapy manager more effectively navigate the flow of daily challenges. The next section of this chapter provides a brief overview of concepts related to organizational structure.

Organizational Structure

Organizations can be structured in a wide variety of manners, from simple to extraordinarily complex. Depending on the size and age of an organization, it may have undergone a number of restructurings intended to improve efficiency and effectiveness, often undertaken to reduce costs. These restructurings may have been planned and executed in a logical manner, or they may have happened organically as the organization grew, added new services, or had to respond to environmental influences. A good place to start to understand an organization's structure is the **organizational chart,** a management tool that visually depicts the following aspects of an organization (Nosse & Friberg, 2010):

- Major functions, usually by department
- Relationships of functions or departments
- Channels of supervision
- Lines of authority and of communication
- Positions by job title within departments or units

It is important to remember a number of things when considering an organizational chart. First, the organizational chart typically is a static picture of an organization. It may be out-of-date, may not reflect current vacancies or temporary employees such as consultants, and may not accurately reflect staffing that changes based on volume or work demand. Second, organizational charts usually represent only formal chains of command and authority and do not indicate informal communication systems between departments or units, or power and informal authority that may evolve as members remain in an organization for extended periods of time.

Examining the organizational charts of many large organizations may provide evidence to support that systems are not only "open" but often quite organic in how they grow and structure themselves over time. The architect Louis Sullivan noted, "form follows function." Of course, Sullivan was referring to the physical structures of organizations, but his idea has often been used to explain how the organization of personnel and resources follow the function completed by an organization. Unfortunately, it sometimes happens that organizational forms remain as artifacts that no longer serve the purpose for which they were developed—and may even contribute to dysfunction in the organization.

According to R. H. Hall (1996), organizational structures serve three basic functions (Box 4-4). First, structures are intended to produce organizational outputs and to achieve organizational goals. Second, structures are designed to minimize or at least regulate the influence of individual variations on the organization. Structures are imposed to ensure that individuals conform to the requirements of the organization and

---

BOX 4-4

The Three Purposes of Organizational Structure

1. Structures produce outputs to achieve organizational goals.
2. Structures minimize or regulate the influence of individuals on the organization.
3. Structures are the settings in which power is exercised, decisions are made, and activities are carried out.

not vice versa. Third, structures are the settings in which power is exercised, in which decisions are made, and in which the organization's activities are carried out. These three purposes are important to remember because changes in structure may also change how the organization achieves its goals and may unintentionally increase or decrease the formal power and authority of individuals.

Although few large organizations perfectly fit the profile of any "named" organizational form or structure, there are a few basic structures commonly found in health-care organizations that are useful for a new manager or practitioner to understand. These structures include the *dual pyramid* form of organizing, *product line* or *service line management* organizations, and *hybrid* or *matrix* organizations. The term *dual pyramid* has been used to describe the common structure found in many medical-model settings, such as acute and general hospitals. The symbol of a pyramid has been used to represent a typical organization of personnel, with upper management at the top of the pyramid and line staff at the bottom (Figure 4-4).

In the *dual pyramid* form of organizing, the traditional relationship between medical staff and administration results in the pyramid structure shown in

Figure 4-5 being duplicated. One pyramid represents the structure of professional staff organized in departments, including top management (with the chief executive officer at the top of the pyramid); allied health professionals such as occupational therapy, physical therapy, and social work in the middle; and all support services, such as engineering, housekeeping, and human resources personnel, as line employees. A second pyramid mimics that structure but

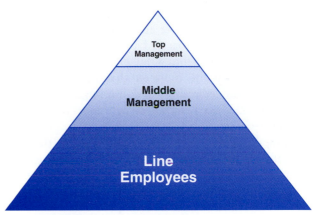

Figure ■ 4-4   The Pyramid Form of Organizing.

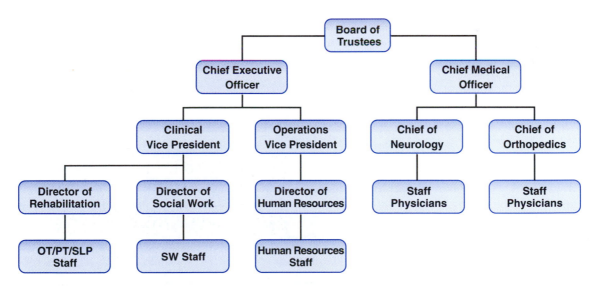

Note: Due to size constraints some departments are not shown. For example, there might be line units with directors (i.e., marketing, finance, etc.) and there may be other medical departments, each with their own chief (i.e., oncology, pediatrics, surgery, etc.). There might be other departments reporting to the Clinical Vice President as well, such as nursing or case management.

Figure ■ 4-5
A Sample Dual Pyramid Form of Organizing. (CEO, chief executive officer; CMO, chief medical officer; OT, occupational therapy; PT, physical therapy; SLP, speech–language pathology; SW, social work)

represents the organization of the medical staff, with the chief medical officer at the top of the pyramid, department heads as middle management, and staff physicians as line employees. The major role of the medical staff organization is to recommend to the hospital board of directors the appointment of physicians to the medical staff (Sultz & Young, 1997). Medical staff also provides oversight and peer review of the quality of medical care in the hospital.

Both pyramids report to the ultimate authority, which is typically a board of trustees or board of directors. However, there are two distinct chains of command; this results in authority and accountability systems being separated depending on function within the organization. The "bricks" of the pyramid are based upon the function that individuals complete or upon education and training. An example of a typical dual pyramid structure is provided in Figure 4-5.

An alternative form of organizing to the dual pyramid is the *product line* or *service line management* form of organizing. In a product line management organization, personnel are organized according to the service or product that they provide rather than according to the specific function that they complete or according to departments based upon education or training. A board of directors maintains ultimate authority, and the chief executive officer and chief medical officer often still maintain parallel but distinct responsibilities and authority. An example of the orga-

nizational chart for an organization with a product line management form of organizing is provided in Figure 4-6.

A *matrix* or *hybrid* organization is one that combines elements of organizing by department, as found in a dual pyramid form of organizing, with the functional approach found in the product line management form of organizing. Combining the key elements of the dual pyramid and product line management forms provides increased flexibility. In matrix organizations, there is typically a more fluid organizational chart, including the use of project management teams and strategies in which subject matter and technical experts are borrowed from departments or functional units to lead key projects on a temporary basis. Project teams may form for periods of weeks to months to guide the implementation of a new organizational system and disband when their work is done. This results in a constant shifting of the organizational chart.

Each of the methods of organizing has advantages and disadvantages, and understanding how they influence the function of your organization can help you capitalize on the benefits and compensate for the limitations within your system. Health-care organizations formed in a dual pyramid structure rely on departmentalization according to discipline or professional education and training to provide for strong supervision of staff and oversight of clinical performance. As such, communication within a professional discipline is

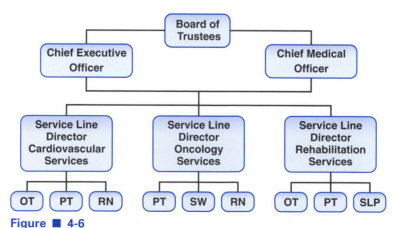

Figure ■ 4-6

A Sample Product Line Management Form of Organizing. (CEO, chief executive officer; CMO, chief medical officer; OT, occupational therapy; PT, physical therapy; RN, nursing; SLP, speech–language pathology; SW, social work)

facilitated and the daily work of a unit may be completed more efficiently. For example, planning staffing levels or coverage for staff members who might be absent becomes easier in this type of organization. Continuous quality improvement (CQI) of processes and outcome measurement of single types of interventions are also easier to measure in a dual pyramid organization, typically because of the presence of a department manager or supervisor from each discipline who has direct access to staff and data related to routine processes and interventions. For the same reason, it may be easier for discipline-specific managers to work with staff from their own discipline to plan for professional development and continuing education. There are also disadvantages to the dual pyramid

form of organizing. Communication across disciplines may be more complicated and pose potential hazards for developing and managing new programs. Problem-solving and process improvement in existing programming may be cumbersome because staff members may feel it necessary to communicate up through the chains of command. The advantages and disadvantages of both the dual pyramid and the product line management form of organizing are summarized in Table 4-2.

Regardless of the form that an organization takes, another important concept to recognize related to organization form and function is the difference between what have been termed *line functions* and what have been termed *staff functions*. Line units or

---

TABLE 4-2

Advantages and Disadvantages of Common Forms of Organizing

	Dual Pyramid	Product Line Management
Communication	Communication within a discipline is facilitated.	Communication between disciplines becomes harder.
Planning	Planning for activities such as professional development and clinical supervision is facilitated but program planning becomes harder.	Program planning and planning for interprofessional activities such as program evaluation is facilitated but functions within disciplines become harder.
Budgeting	Tracking and planning for finances related to single-discipline costs is facilitated but that for interprofessional activities (e.g., cost per unit of care) is harder.	Tracking and planning for finances related to programmatic costs is facilitated (e.g., cost per unit of care) but that for discipline-specific activities is harder.
Staffing	Some needs, such as providing coverage for leaves or vacancies, may be easier, but the need to communicate with other managers increases. Recruitment activities are facilitated.	Staffing activities influenced by other disciplines, such as scheduling programmatic elements, may be facilitated, but coverage for leaves or vacancies becomes more difficult. Recruitment of staff may be more difficult or you may need to rely upon managers from other disciplines for assistance.
CQI, Program Evaluation, and Outcomes	Improving discipline-specific processes is easier, as is measuring single-discipline outcomes and indicators of program evaluation, but interprofessional programs require extra effort.	Improving interdisciplinary or program processes is easier, as is measuring program outcomes and indicators of program evaluation, but discipline-specific elements require extra effort.
Professional Development	Development of discipline-specific skills related to assessment and intervention may be facilitated by the ease of access to disciplinary specialists.	Development of interprofessional skills related to the needs of a population or program development or implementation may be facilitated.

employees conduct the major business that is directly related to the primary outputs of the organization. For example, in a typical hospital, physicians, nurses, and therapists complete line functions. Staff functions or employees assist the line units by providing specialized services and bring specialized supportive knowledge such as human resource management, accounting, or information technology. Staff functions are critical to the operations of an organization, and a new occupational therapy manager would benefit from establishing and maintaining relationships with contacts in other departments, including areas such as human resources, planning and marketing, information technology, engineering, and accounting.

Trends in Organizational Development, Behavior, and Function

In recent decades, many organizations that employ occupational therapy practitioners have faced considerable change as a result of new legislation, turbulent economic times, increased competition in the marketplace, and myriad other factors. An example would include responding to decreased reimbursement under the Balanced Budget Act of 1997, which resulted in large numbers of providers of rehabilitation to skilled nursing facilities "downsizing" by laying off occupational therapy and physical therapy personnel. Other examples include the impact of decreased levels of reimbursement under managed care and the effects of the September 11, 2001, terrorist attack on the economy and charitable giving to nonprofit organizations, including those that employ occupational therapy practitioners. The Patient Protection and Affordable Care Act (2010) will provide both opportunities and challenges as new care structures and payment mechanisms, such as accountable care organizations (ACOs) and bundled payments, are explored in trials and evolve over the coming decade. At the same time, OTs and OTAs have had an increasing influence in community-based practice and in the area of work disability in industry, and new opportunities have presented themselves in these types of organizations. As organizations struggle to keep pace with their changing environments, a number of trends have emerged. Three of these trends are briefly reviewed in this section.

Continuous Quality Improvement

Most health-care organizations, such as hospitals, have had formal systems to evaluate and improve quality for many years. In the last 2 decades, however, there has been a shift from what was referred to as *quality assurance* to *CQI*. Chapter 13 explores CQI in depth, including the history of CQI and the common concepts, strategies, tools, and techniques used for "process improvement," so only a brief explanation is provided here. The primary change that has resulted in moving from quality assurance to CQI has been a shift from focusing on gathering data on stable processes to *control* or *assure* quality to a focus on customer satisfaction by improving the efficiency and effectiveness of the common or *critical processes* completed in the course of everyday work. This shift has included both a change in management philosophy, including increased involvement of employees in decision-making about how to best meet the needs of customers, and a change in the strategies for examining the flow of work. The principles behind CQI (commonly known as *total quality management* in industry) find their origins in the 1940s and 1950s in efforts to rebuild the post–World War II economy in Japan. Since that time, these principles have been effectively implemented in a wide range of industries in the United States, including the automobile, hotel, and manufacturing industries, and most recently have been widely implemented in health-care settings.

Operations Improvement and Process Reengineering

A second trend in organizations, particularly in medical-model health-care settings such as hospitals, has been a focus on cost savings through *operations improvement* and *process reengineering*. Operations improvement should not be confused with CQI; they are not the same thing, but neither are they mutually exclusive. Many hospitals have undertaken both CQI and operations improvement efforts at the same time. In CQI, the relationship between costs and customer satisfaction is such that, by focusing on customers' needs, you also improve efficiency and effectiveness and hence reduce costs. In operations improvement approaches, you are likely to reexamine work processes and change or "reengineer" how things are done, although the primary focus is on reducing costs. In addition to an examination of work processes, operations improvement includes an examination of staffing and ways of doing business, such as purchasing practices focused on eliminating unnecessary costs.

A key difference between CQI and an operation's improvement initiative is *who* is involved and *how* they are involved. In CQI, an outside consultant or consulting firm may very often be involved in the initial orientation and training of staff. After training of organizational leadership is complete, the consultants turn over all responsibility for the CQI effort to the organization, and it becomes the organizational leadership's responsibility to plan for ongoing training of staff. A focus of CQI is involving staff at all levels (e.g., all key stakeholders in the process) in process improvement. As a result, staff members may feel positively about their involvement in making decisions and creating change within the organization.

Consultants are also a typical part of operations improvement initiatives, as is training of organization leadership and department managers. However, in operations improvement initiatives the focus is definitely on cutting costs from the budget, whereas less attention may be paid to involving all levels of staff in the process. Still, these initiatives may often include a brainstorming or idea generation phase in which employees are invited to submit ideas. Naturally, both CQI and operations improvement efforts will be heavily influenced by the values of organizational leadership, and may be experienced as positive or negative processes by managers and staff depending on how the initiatives are rolled out. It is important to understand, however, that operations improvement initiatives do not target the management philosophy of organizational leadership, as does CQI. Rather, the central target is cost cutting. The fees of operations improvement consulting firms and their reputations may be heavily dependent upon their success in cutting costs from a budget in a relatively short period of time. Some of the most common strategies used in operations improvement efforts include

- Combining departments to eliminate duplications of effort in both management and support positions, such as receptionists and secretarial support
- Leveraging tasks to the most appropriately trained but lowest-paid staff members, resulting

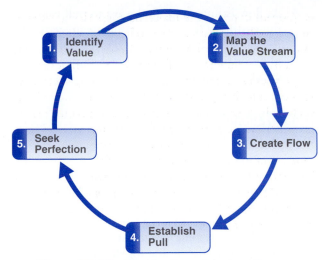

Figure ■ 4-7 The Five Steps of the Lean Process.

in decreased use of professional staff and increased use of assistants and support staff
- Purchasing strategies such as buying all office supplies from the same supplier so that larger volumes are purchased at one time and discounts can be negotiated
- Process reengineering and automation of processes to eliminate rework and delays and to eliminate or decrease the number of work hours devoted to routine processes

There are other approaches that combine CQI principles and methods focusing on efficiency that have gained attention in the last 2 decades. One, for example, is "lean." Lean principles simply seek to create more value for the customer by minimizing waste (Lean Enterprise Institute, 2013).

The five steps used to implement the lean techniques are listed next and are shown in Figure 4-7:

1. Define value from the standpoint of the end customer for each service or product you deliver.
2. Identify all the steps in the value stream for each service or product and eliminate steps that do not create value.
3. Tighten the sequence of the value-creating steps so that delivery of the product to your customer is efficient and smooth.

4. As flow is improved, find ways to pull value for the customer from the next upstream activity.

5. Repeat steps 1 to 4 and continue it until a state of perfection is reached in which perfect value is created with no waste.

Organizational Learning and Learning Organizations

Organizational learning and *learning organizations* are concepts that have appeared in the organizational development and organizational behavior literature over the last 3 decades and have been met with mixed reaction. Whereas some organizational development theorists have had high praise for the concepts, others have dismissed these ideas as fads.

Argyris (1977), who is also a major theorist in organizational development, defined organizational learning as the process of "detection and correction of errors." Organizations detect and correct errors, or "learn," through individual employees who function as agents of change and learning for the organization. Argyris (1999, p. 157) stated, "Organizations learn by individuals acting as agents for them. The individuals' learning activities, in turn, are facilitated or inhibited by an ecological system of factors that may be called an organizational learning system." When a person or an organization learns by processing information and experiences, the range of potential behaviors of the employee or organization is changed. Although the process of learning can be extremely complicated, the types of learning that occur with organizations have been described simply as learning related to (Haines, 2002)

- New knowledge, or the understanding of concepts, facts, and opinions
- New attitudes, or the willingness and motivation to act
- New skills, or the ability to demonstrate or perform an action or function

What Is a Learning Organization?

According to Ortenblad (2013), the term *learning organization* was introduced in academic works as far back as the 1970s; however, it gained considerably more attention with the publication of the very famous book *The Fifth Discipline: The Art and Practice of the Learning*

Organization (Senge, 1990). In this book, Senge defined the learning organization as the organization in which "you cannot *not* learn because learning is so insinuated into the fabric of life." He described a learning organization as an organization in which "a group of people [are] continually enhancing their capacity to create what they want to create." McGill, Slocum, and Lei (1992) defined the learning organization as "a company that can respond to new information by altering the very 'programming' by which information is processed and evaluated." Simply stated, a learning organization is one in which the organization strives to have everyone working at his or her best, and to recognize how this happens and to consciously facilitate that state. A key concept related to the learning organization is that of *generative* or *double-loop* learning.

Single-Loop (Adaptive) Learning Versus Double-Loop (Generative) Learning

Much of the traditional view of organizations is based on *adaptive learning*, or what some refer to as "single-loop learning." Adaptive learning or single-loop learning focuses on solving problems in the present without examining the appropriateness of current learning behaviors. Adaptive organizations focus on incremental improvements, often based upon the past track record of success. Essentially, they don't question the fundamental assumptions underlying the existing ways of doing work. Senge (1990) noted that increasing adaptiveness is only the first stage; companies need to focus on generative learning or "double-loop learning" (Argyris, 1977). *Double-loop learning* emphasizes continuous experimentation and feedback in an ongoing examination of the very way organizations go about defining and solving problems (Bakacsi, 2010). In Senge's (1990) view, generative learning is about creating—it requires systemic thinking, shared vision, personal mastery, team learning, and creative tension between the vision and the current reality. Generative learning, unlike adaptive learning, requires new ways of looking at the world.

To become most adaptable through the use of generative or double-loop learning and to survive in fast-changing and unpredictable environments, organizations need to learn to incorporate experimentation as a way of daily life. Learning organizations must become comfortable with frequent change in structures, processes, domains, goals, and the like, even in the face of apparently optimal adaptation (Hedberg,

Nystrom, & Starbuck, 1976; Starbuck, 1983). The consequences of an ongoing state of experimentation are that organizations learn about a variety of design features and remain flexible.

What Is the Managers' Role in the Learning Organization?

Senge (1990) suggested that the leaders of learning organizations must adopt the role of designer and teacher. He argued that leaders can build a shared vision and challenge the status quo by suggesting alternative mental models to those that have traditionally driven managerial action. In other words, leaders are responsible for learning.

The key ingredient of the learning organization is in *how* organizations process their managerial experiences. In learning organizations, managers *learn* from their experiences rather than being *bound* by their past experiences. In generative learning organizations, the ability of an organization or manager is not measured by *what* it knows (that is the product of learning), but rather by *how* it learns—the process of learning. Management practices encourage, recognize, and reward openness, systemic thinking, creativity, a sense of efficacy, and empathy.

Evidence on Learning Organizations

There is a growing body of literature on the concept of learning organizations; their success in innovation; the relationships between organizational learning, innovation, and performance; the attributes thought to foster their development; and descriptions of the implementation of discrete strategies (Jiménez-Jiménez & Sanz-Valle, 2011). Early research conducted consisted of qualitative, descriptive studies, typically performed in a case study format (Gardiner, 1999; B. P. Hall, 2001; Kasl, Marsick, & Dechant, 1997). These studies described the characteristics of managers that were thought to empower employees to learn, as well as the limitations of existing perspectives. Argote and Miron-Spektor (2011, p. 1123) noted that, "Because organizational learning occurs over time, studying organizational learning requires time-series or longitudinal data." This has limited the large-scale publication of strong empirical data on learning organizations.

The evidence to support the concept of learning organizations is becoming more convincing to support managerial action as the general findings are consistent with better developed perspectives on learning, employee development, and mentoring, and so may warrant a review by an occupational therapy manager interested in employee learning. A sample of evidence on learning organizations is summarized in Table 4-3.

As was asserted in Chapter 1, many of the topics overviewed in this introduction to organizations would lend themselves to the development of questions to be answered through the identification and evaluation of evidence. The literature presented in Table 4-3 is just one example of such evidence.

Chapter Summary

Organizations play a critical role in the functioning of modern life in industrialized nations. Some types of organizations—whether public or private, profit or nonprofit—employ most occupational therapy personnel. By becoming familiar with the range of scholarship, theory, and evidence related to the development and functioning of organizations, occupational therapy managers can become more effective as managers and as advocates for those they represent. Although healthcare and community-based organizations are perhaps most commonly described as "open systems," the three perspectives on organizational functioning described in this chapter (rational, natural, and open) each contribute something valuable to our understanding of the internal and external environments in which we operate. Learning to assess how the culture and values of an organization are demonstrated in the everyday behaviors of its employees is a critical skill for the occupational therapy manager that can aid him or her to have increased influence. As more OTs and OTAs develop and manage private businesses, it is necessary for these entrepreneurs to become aware of resources to guide them in choosing the most appropriate business structure. Finally, three trends in organizational development and behavior (CQI, operations improvement, and learning organizations) were overviewed. Other aspects of organizational functioning are discussed in later chapters, but you are encouraged to remain open to the new knowledge that is constantly being generated by a variety of fields that will guide you as you work within various types of organizations.

TABLE 4-3

Summary of Selected Evidence on Learning Organizations

Author	Study Type	N (Sample Size)	Level of Evidence	Results
Campbell, T. T, & Armstrong, S. J. (2013)	Longitudinal testing using causal cognitive mapping	4 organizations	Fair	Organizational learning can increase shared managerial understandings that may lead to organizational benefits derived from higher degrees of unified action. However, the study also revealed potentially dysfunctional aspects of organizational learning such as cohesive managerial mental models inhibiting learning and organizational learning can be slower than individual learning.
Rouzbahani, Khazai, Farah, & Nasr (2013)	Descriptive survey methodology	210 employees	Fair	There is a significant relationship between the seven dimensions of learning organizations and organizational readiness for change.
Mojab & Gorman (2003)	Literature review using Marxist–feminist analysis	Not stated	Poor	Authors suggest based on their review that learning organizations have limited capabilities to support democratic, grass-roots, and gender-conscious organizations and do little to promote the economic interests of women.
Lahteenmaki, Toivonen, & Mattila (2001)	Literature review	Not stated	Poor	Identifies proposed gaps in organizational learning research, including a lack of empirical validation of concepts, continued focus on individual learning rather than social structure, and the continued proliferation of new models rather than efforts to validate currently proposed models.
B. P. Hall (2001)	Case study	1 shipping company	Poor	Values exploration and values mentoring of organizational leaders increases leadership decision-making capability and the consciousness of the system as a whole, which are critical factors in developing the organization as a learning environment.

■ Real-Life Solutions

Kate wondered about theories related to how organizations are structured and how those theories might help her as an occupational therapy clinician and manager. Kate decided to enroll in a master's program in business administration, and she took an introductory course in organizational behavior. She quickly discovered that scholars had been studying how organizations develop and function for decades and that, indeed, there was a range of theories on organizations that she would learn. She also began to see how these theories might be applied within organizations. She considered continuing her education with a postprofessional clinical doctorate (OTD) to gain advanced skills and knowledge specific to occupational therapy leadership and management.

She noted that different organizations within the hospital system where she was employed were structured differently. She had previously worked in the system's acute care facility, which was organized in a dual pyramid structure, but now worked in the rehabilitation hospital, which was organized in a product line management structure. In her class, they discussed that all structures had advantages and disadvantages, and she could see now that that was true. She appreciated how easy it seemed to be, in a product line management structure, to solve interprofessional problems, but worried whether the new OTs and OTAs, who reported to a physical therapist, were getting the clinical supervision they needed.

Kate was most excited about how she was able to apply what she was learning about organizational culture and values to her current job, and could see how knowledge from other fields such as organizational behavior could be helpful in her future as an occupational therapy manager. She had only recently moved to the head injury team and had been confused at first at all of the seemingly "unwritten" rules that all the other staff members seemed to know about. She began to enjoy the idea that, by observing the actions of the other members of her team and how the team members responded to each other, she could not only learn "how things are done" but also gain important insights into the underlying values that were shared among the team members but were not explicitly articulated.

Finally, Kate was impressed with the range of research that she was being exposed to and began to formulate questions about the strength of some of the evidence related to these questions. Although she felt a little overwhelmed at the prospect of all that she could learn to help her succeed as a manager, she also knew that the same evidence-based skills that helped her answer clinical questions could guide her in finding possible answers to questions about organizations and any other aspect of being an occupational therapy manager.

Study Questions

1. A shared set of basic assumptions or shared way of doing things that is based upon the underlying values and beliefs of the members of a particular society or of a group might best be called a(n):

   a. Organizational vision.
   b. Strategic plan.
   c. Code of ethics.
   d. Organizational culture.

2. Rebecca works part-time for AOTA as an associate in the Practice Department. When she functions in this paid work role, it is most appropriate to say she is working within a structure most accurately described as a(n):

   a. Association.
   b. Bureaucracy.
   c. Trade bureau.
   d. Professional hierarchy.

3. **A type of system that is capable of self-maintenance within a larger context or environment, and in which the influence of internal and external environments are keenly recognized, is best called a(n):**

   a. Rational systems organization.
   b. Natural systems organization.
   c. Open systems organization.
   d. Market economy systems organization.

4. **Two types of values related to the means to achieve the ends, as well as the ends a person wishes to achieve, are commonly referred to as:**

   a. Instrumental values and terminal values.
   b. Personal values and cultural values.
   c. Organizational values and societal values.
   d. Formative values and summative values.

5. **An organizational chart is a management tool that:**

   a. Shows the location of an organization in a larger system such as a city or county.
   b. Visually depicts the lines of authority, organization, and reporting in an organization.
   c. Defines the sources of revenue and expenses and how these affect the tax status of an organization.
   d. Helps leaders determine the impact of an organization's culture to guide leaders in choosing the most effective leadership styles.

6. **Which of the following is not a commonly cited purpose of organizational structures discussed in Chapter 4?**

   a. Structures produce outputs to achieve organizational goals.
   b. Structures minimize or regulate the influence of individuals on the organization.
   c. Structures are the settings in which power is exercised, decisions are made, and activities are carried out.
   d. Structures dictate administrative policies and procedures that guide organizational decision-making.

7. **A commonly recognized form of organizing in hospital systems where a managerial hierarchy is duplicated for physicians and nonphysicians would best be called:**

   a. Dual pyramid.
   b. Medical-model.
   c. Mirror model.
   d. Traditional administrative model.

8. **The primary characteristic of double-loop (generative) learning would best be described as which of the following?**

   a. It emphasizes concrete problem-solving and application of solutions in the here and now.
   b. It emphasizes continuous experimentation and feedback in an ongoing examination of the very way organizations go about defining and solving problems.
   c. It is most applicable for slow-paced environments where there is little change.
   d. It focuses on learning from the past and applying that learning to the present.

Resources for Learning More About Organizations

Journals Related to Organizations

Journal of Organizational Behavior

http://onlinelibrary.wiley.com/journal/10.1002/(ISSN)1099-1379

The *Journal of Organizational Behavior* reviews international and multidisciplinary, as well as qualitative and quantitative, research. Published articles address both research and theory on a wide range of topics related to occupational organizational behavior. Topics noted for inclusion in the journal include motivation, work performance, equal opportunities at work, job design, career processes, occupational stress, quality of work life, job satisfaction, personnel selection, training, organizational change, research methodology in occupational or organizational behavior, employment, job analysis, behavioral aspects of industrial relations, managerial behavior, organizational structure and climate, leadership, and power.

Journal of Occupational and Organizational Psychology

http://www.wiley.com/WileyCDA/WileyTitle/productCd-JOOP.html

The *Journal of Occupational and Organizational Psychology* publishes empirical research as well as papers addressing theory and emerging issues with the goal of improving readers' understanding of people and organizations. The journal publishes articles that address a variety of contexts and areas of knowledge. Published articles relate to contexts and domains including industrial, organizational, engineering, vocational, and personnel psychology, as well as behavioral aspects of industrial relations, ergonomics, human factors, and industrial sociology.

Journal of Organizational Excellence

Global Business and Organizational Excellence

http://onlinelibrary.wiley.com/journal/10.1002/(ISSN)1932-2062

Global Business and Organizational Excellence (GBOE) presents applied research and first-hand case studies of best practices of people in organizations, including common management and organizational behavior techniques as well as knowledge that help people lead their organizations to excel.

Professional Organizations and Associations Concerned With the Study of Organizations

The Academy of Management

http://www.aomonline.org/

The Academy of Management's central mission is to enhance the profession of management by advancing the scholarship of management and enriching the professional development of its members. The academy is also committed to shaping the future of management research and education. The Academy of Management is a leading professional association for scholars dedicated to creating and disseminating knowledge about management and organizations. Founded in 1936 by two professors, the Academy of Management is the oldest and largest scholarly management association in the world. Today, the academy is the professional home for over 14,000 members from 90 nations.

The American Society for Training and Development

http://www.astd.org/astd/

Founded in 1944, the American Society for Training and Development (ASTD) is the world's premier professional association and leading resource on workplace learning and performance issues. The ASTD provides information, research, analysis, and practical information derived from its own research; the knowledge and experience of its members; its conferences, expositions, seminars, and publications; and the coalitions and partnerships it has built through research and policy work. The ASTD's membership includes more than 70,000 people working in the field of workplace performance in 100 countries worldwide. Its leadership and members work in more than 15,000 multinational corporations, small and medium-sized businesses, government agencies, colleges, and universities.

The Society for Organizational Learning

http://www.solonline.org/

The Society for Organizational Learning (SoL) is an intentional learning community composed of organizations, individuals, and local SoL communities around the world. SoL was created to connect corporations and organizations, researchers, and consultants to generate knowledge about and capacity for fundamental innovation and change by engaging in collaborative action inquiry projects. While bringing together "specialists," the society's goal is more than simple collaboration. The purpose of the SoL is to discover (research), integrate (capacity development), and implement (practice) theories and practices of organizational learning for the interdependent development of people and their institutions and communities, such that they continue to increase their capacity to collectively realize their highest aspirations and productively resolve their differences. With this intention, organizations are truly worthy of the commitment of their employees and communities.

U.S. Small Business Administration

http://www.sba.gov/

The mission of the Small Business Administration (SBA) is to maintain and strengthen the nation's economy by aiding, counseling, assisting, and protecting the interests of small businesses and by helping families and businesses recover from national disasters. The SBA provides resources on starting, financing, and managing small businesses, including the basics of developing business plans, applying for loans, and resolving tax issues.

Reference List

Argote, L., & Miron-Spektor, E. (2011). Organizational learning: From experience to knowledge. *Organization Science*, *22*(5), 1123–1137.

Argyris, C. (1977). Double-loop learning in organizations. *Harvard Business Review*, *55*, 115–134.

Argyris, C. (1999). *On organizational learning* (2nd ed.). Oxford, UK: Blackwell Business.

Bakacsi, G. (2010). Managing crisis: Single-loop or double-loop learning. *Strategic Management*, *15*(3), 3–9.

Braveman, B., & Metzler, C. A. (2012). Health care reform implementation and occupational therapy. *American Journal of Occupational Therapy*, *66*(1), 11–14.

Campbell, T. T., & Armstrong, S. J. (2013). A longitudinal study of organisational learning. *The Learning Organization*, *20*(3), 240–258.

Cunliffe, A. L. (2008). *Organization theory*. London, UK: Sage Publications.

Daft, R. L. (2008). *Management* (8th ed.). Mason, OH: South-Western Cengage Learning.

Daft, R. L. (2009). *Organization theory and design* (10th ed.). Mason, OH: South-Western Cengage Learning.

Gardiner, P. (1999). Soaring to new heights with learning oriented companies. *Journal of Workplace Learning*, *11*, 255–277.

Haines, S. (2002). *What is learning and the learning organization?* San Diego, CA: Center for Strategic Management.

Hall, B. P. (2001). Values development and learning organizations. *Journal of Knowledge Management*, *5*, 19–26.

Hall, P. D. (2010). Historical perspectives on nonprofit organizations in the United States. In D. O. Renz (Ed.), *The Jossey-Bass handbook of nonprofit leadership and management* (3rd ed., pp. 3–31) Somerset, NJ: Jossey-Bass.

Hall, R. H. (1996). *Organizations: Structures, processes and outcomes* (6th ed.). Englewood Cliffs, NJ: Prentice Hall.

Hedberg, B. L., Nystrom, P. C., & Starbuck, W. H. (1976). Camping on seesaws: Prescriptions for a self-designing organization. *Administrative Science Quarterly*, *21*, 41–65.

Illinois Hospital Association. (2003). Homepage. *Illinois Hospital Association*. Retrieved from http://www.ihatoday.org

Jaques, E. (1998). *Requisite organization*. Arlington, VA: Cason Hall.

Jiménez-Jiménez, D., & Sanz-Valle, R. (2011). Innovation, organizational learning, and performance. *Journal of Business Research*, *64*(4), 408–417.

Kasl, E., Marsick, V. J., & Dechant, K. (1997). A research-based model of team learning. *Journal of Applied Behavioral Science*, *33*, 227–246.

Lahteenmaki, S., Toivonen, J., & Mattila, M. (2001). Critical aspects of organizational learning research and proposals for its measurement. *British Academy of Management*, *12*, 113–129.

Lean Enterprise Institute. (2013). *Principles of lean*. Retrieved from www.lean.org/whatslean/Principles.cfm

March, J. G. (1965). *Handbook of organizations*. Chicago, IL: Rand McNally.

McCormack, G. L., Jaffe, E. G., & Frey, W. F. (2003). New organizational perspectives. In G. L. McCormack (Ed.), *The occupational therapy manager* (4th ed., pp. 85–126). Bethesda, MD: AOTA Press.

McGill, M. E., Slocum, J. W., & Lei, D. (1992). Management practices in learning organizations. *Organizational Dynamics*, *21*, 5–17.

Miner, J. B. (2007). *Organization behavior 4: From theory to practice*. Armonk, NY: M. E. Sharpe, Inc.

Mojab, S., & Gorman, R. (2003). Women and consciousness in the "learning organization": Emancipation or exploration. *Adult Education Quarterly*, *53*, 228–241.

Mumford, M. D., & Peterson, N. G. (1999). The O*NET content model: Structural considerations in describing jobs. In N. G. Peterson, M. D. Munford, W. C. Borman, P. R. Jeanneret, & E. A. Fleishman (Eds.), *An occupational information system for the 21st century: The development of O*NET* (pp. 21–30). Washington, DC: American Psychological Association.

Nosse, L. J. & Friberg, D. G. (2010). *Managerial and supervisory principles for physical therapists* (3rd ed.). Philadelphia, PA: Lippincott Williams & Wilkins.

Ortenblad, A. (2013). *Handbook of research on the learning organization: Adaptation and context*. Cheltenham, UK: Edward Elgar Publishing Limited.

Page, C. G. (2010). *Management in physical therapy practices*. Philadelphia, PA: F.A. Davis.

Peters, T. J., & Waterman, R. H. (1982). *In search of excellence*. New York, NY: Harper & Row.

Rokeach, M. (1973). *The nature of human values*. New York, NY: Free Press.

Rouzbahani, M. T., Khazai, M., Farah, E. N., & Nasr, S. M. (2013). The relationship between learning organizations and organizational readiness for change according to seven dimensions of learning organizations. *Journal of Basic and Applied Scientific Research*, *3*(5), 631–636.

Scaffa, M. E., & Reitz, S. M. (2013). *Occupational therapy in community-based practice settings* (2nd ed.). Philadelphia, PA: F.A. Davis.

Schein, E. H. (1992). *Organizational culture and leadership*. New York, NY: Jossey-Bass.

Scott, W. R. (2003). *Organizations: Rational, natural and open systems* (5th ed.). Englewood Cliffs, NJ: Prentice Hall.

Senge, P. (1990). *The fifth discipline: The art and practice of the learning organization*. New York, NY: Doubleday.

Shafritz, J. M., Ott, S. J. & Jang, Y. S. (2011). *Classics of organizational theory* (7th ed.). Belmont, CA: Wadsworth.

Small Business Administration. (2013). *Choosing your business structure*. Retrieved from http://www.sba.gov/category/navigation

-structure/starting-managing-business/starting-business/choose-your-business-stru

Starbuck, W. H. (1983). Organizations as action generators. *American Sociological Review, 48,* 91–102.

Sultz, H. A., & Young, K. M. (1997). *Health care USA.* Gaithersburg, MD: Aspen.

Tolbert, P. S., & Hall, R. H. (2009). *Organizations: Structures, processes and outcomes* (10th ed.). Englewood Cliffs, NJ: Prentice Hall.

Uhl-Bien, M., Schermerhorn, J. R., & Osborn, R. N. (2013). *Organizational behavior* (13th ed.). New York, NY: John Wiley & Sons.

von Bertalanffy, L. (1968). *General systems theory: Foundations, development, and application.* New York, NY: Braziller.

Weber, M. (1946). *From Max Weber: Essays in sociology* (Transl. ed.). New York, NY: Oxford University Press.

Weber, M. (1968). *Economy and society: An interpretive sociology.* New York, NY: Bedminister Press.

CHAPTER 5

Communicating Effectively in Complex Environments

Brent Braveman, PhD, OTR/L, FAOTA

■ Real-Life Management

Charlotte, a level II fieldwork student, is completing her fieldwork in a large mental health setting that provides services ranging from an inpatient unit to a variety of day treatment options. She has always wanted to work in psychosocial practice and has typically excelled academically. She entered her fieldwork expecting that she would excel there as well, but she has encountered some difficulties. Much to Charlotte's surprise, she has received constructive criticism from a number of the occupational therapy staff on her style of interpersonal communication with staff and with clients. What is most concerning to Charlotte is that the feedback she has received seems to indicate that there is often a mismatch between what she hopes to communicate and how her message is being received.

Charlotte's clinical fieldwork educator has been very supportive and has suggested to Charlotte that she take advantage of a fieldwork assignment to develop and present an in-service education session for unit staff by exploring strategies for improving the effectiveness of interpersonal communication. Charlotte begins by visiting the library to find some resources on communication theory and strategies for improving her verbal, nonverbal, and written interpersonal communication.

Critical Thinking Questions

As you read this chapter, consider the following questions:

- Which of the many theories of communication related to interpersonal communication, communication to the public and groups, communication in the mass media, and intercultural communication are most relevant to you as an occupational therapy practitioner and manager?

Continued

Critical Thinking Questions—cont'd

- What resources would help you improve your written communication and verbal and non-verbal aspects of vocal communication with individuals and groups?
- How can planning your communication and paying conscious attention to aspects of communication that are often unconscious, such as rate of speech, facial expressions, or body

orientation, help you become a more effective communicator?
- What are the many different forms of communication used by an occupational therapy manager, such as conversations, presentations, memos, business letters, business plans, and grant proposals?

Glossary

- **Cybernetics:** a theory of communication focused on the study of regulation and control in systems.
- **Dramatism:** a theory of communication focused on the study of the use of metaphor in communication.
- **Narratives:** stories; in communication studies, the examination of stories as a method to

communicate information is common, including research in occupational therapy.
- **Paralinguistics:** nonverbal aspects of communication, such as tone of voice, pitch, volume, and so on.
- **Proxemics:** a theory of communication that is focused on the impact and use of space, distance, and territory.

Introduction

The topic of communication has become exponentially broader in scope and depth in the last few decades. Communication theory and research have moved far beyond focusing on the transmission and receipt of an idea between people in the same room. In little more than 2 decades, we moved from needing to mail information to a collaborator and wait for a period of several days for it to arrive to being able to have a document arrive in moments as an "e-mail attachment" or have live "online chats" with someone on the other side of the country or world. Effective communication has become a major challenge for organizations and is a central competency for the effective occupational therapy manager.

The range of communication theories that might be useful to the occupational therapy manager is summarized in this chapter. Strategies for increasing the effectiveness of communication in person and in various written and electronic formats also are presented.

A Short History of Communication Theory

Communication as a subject of inquiry is as old as civilization itself. We know that it was a major area of interest to the ancient Greeks and Romans. In the 5th century B.C., Plato and Aristotle developed the first recorded communications theories in the West. Others, such as Cicero, Seneca, Quintilan, and Longinus, followed them (Trenholm, 1991). The ancient Greeks focused their communication theories on persuasive argument and public communication.

Modern rhetoric refers to the body of communication study that occurred roughly between 1600 and 1900 A.D. The primary work during this time reversed earlier "prescriptive" approaches to communication. Modern rhetoric raised questions about how humans come to know, be, believe, and act. In addition, it focused on aspects of delivery, including verbal and nonverbal behaviors, that a speaker could use to embellish his or her presentation. Scholarship and study related to communication during this time was both theoretical and practical (Cisneros, McCauliff, & Beasely, 2009).

During the 19th century, the primary focus of investigation was on how speakers transmitted ideas to a listener. A major change during the 19th century was the application of the scientific method to investigation of communication theory, including the use of experimental studies focusing on finer aspects of communication and the manipulation of specific variables such as the context, timing, or aspects of delivery. This focus continued during the 20th century, with the application of behavioral methods added to the study of communication. The goal of communication theory became specifying the invariant laws and describing the functional relationship between different variables that could affect the delivery or interpretation of communication. In addition, as technology has rapidly progressed over the last 2 decades, the influence of modes of transmission has been introduced to the study of communication theory.

Communication theory and research has expanded to become a discrete discipline; organizations have formed around the study of communication, and multiple journals have been developed where communication scholars publish their research (Littlejohn & Foss, 2010). Park and Pooley (2008) noted that the discipline of communications research is relatively "youthful"; primary development began since the mid-1950s and lagged behind the development of other social science disciplines. Modern-day topics of communications research include cognition and emotion, conflict, health communication, communications technology, persuasion and social influence, and political communication (University of Texas at Austin, 2013).

Theories of Communication

Communication as a field of study is well developed and there are a large number of theories intended to explain various aspects of communication. The full range and scope of communication theories is far beyond what can be covered in this book. For example, Griffin (2011) introduces over 50 separate communication theories in his introductory text *A First Look at Communication Theory!* Theories have been developed related to interpersonal communication, communication to the public and groups, communication in the mass media, and intercultural communication. Grouping theories according to the area of communication that they seek to explain is one helpful way of organizing communication theories. Another method of classifying communication theories is according to seven traditions in the field of communication theory, as outlined in Box 5-1.

Within each of these traditions, numerous theories have been developed; to add to the complexity of understanding communication theory, some theories also cross more than one tradition. In addition to the theories, multiple models of communication have been developed to explain the application of the theory in everyday communication. As is explained in Chapter 15, a theory provides an explanation of how or why a particular phenomenon occurs and how that phenomenon might be influenced, whereas a model helps to generate theory and the methods that are used to apply that theory.

Trying to address all theories of communication is simply beyond the scope of one chapter, and probably beyond the need of the typical occupational therapy manager. However, as is the case with all the topics in this book, the occupational therapy manager can benefit from exploring theories, models, and evidence to improve his or her effectiveness in communication. At this point, it would be useful to comment on the *context* of communication. As managers, we communicate in varied contexts, ranging from a conversation with an individual staff member we supervise, another manager, or our boss, to communicating with large groups of people, such as when we run a staff meeting, present an in-service education program, or communicate with a continuous quality improvement team. More and more often we communicate with managerial peers from multiple disciplines from other organizations to benchmark data and share ideas. Just as we may be able to choose more than one appropriate occupational therapy conceptual practice model to guide intervention, multiple communication theories can be applied to each of these contexts of communication. Recognizing the commonalities of these situations helps to make this process less confusing.

BOX 5-1

Seven Traditions in the Field of Communication Theory

1. The *sociopsychological tradition* uses the scientific method to discover communication "truths" and cause-and-effect relationships through careful systematic observation.
2. The *cybernetic tradition* views communication as information processing where communication is the link connecting the separate parts of any system, such as a computer system, a family system, an organizational system, or a media system.
3. The *rhetorical tradition*, grounded in Greco–Roman history, examines communication as an "artful address" and focuses on effective verbal communication of ideas.
4. The *semiotic tradition* views communication as the process of sharing meaning through signs (a sign is anything that can stand for something else).
5. The *sociocultural tradition* views communication as the creation and enactment of social reality based on the premise that, as people talk, they produce and reproduce culture.
6. The *critical tradition* views communication as a reflective challenge of unjust discourse arising from the Marxist tradition of critiquing society, including the use of communication to control power, the role of mass media in dulling sensitivity to repression, and blind reliance on the scientific method and uncritical acceptance of empirical findings.
7. The *phenomenological tradition* views communication as the experience of self and others through dialogue, or an analysis of everyday life from the standpoint of the person who is living it through the communication process.

Common problems faced by all communicators regardless of the context of communication can be identified. In other words, all communicators have these problems in common no matter what the situation and what form of communication they are using to convey their message (Trenholm, 1991; Trenholm & Jensen, 2011). Five common problems are identified next and applied to the example of a director of occupational therapy who needs to communicate regarding initiation of a rotation system for therapy staff in a large hospital.

1. *Communicator acceptability*, or identifying the characteristics of the audience, how members of the audience might respond, and what the likely rewards or punishments for communication might be. An example would be giving a presentation to a large group of nursing directors about the rotation system you wish to implement and identifying their level of knowledge about your department, their concerns, possible responses, and the positive and negative outcomes that might occur in order to plan your communication.
2. *Signification*, or choosing the appropriate verbal and nonverbal means to create meaningful messages, accurately interpreting the signs from the communication partner or audience, and making the greatest impact on the listener. An example would be deciding when to use e-mail to communicate versus scheduling meetings or face-to-face communication and accurately reading the response from key customers.
3. *Social coordination and relational definition*, or defining the rules to be followed throughout the interaction and coming to understand how you are expected to act within the context of a specific communication. An example would be understanding when higher-ups in your division and in nursing should be included on communication and when you should ask for feedback versus informing others about decisions.
4. *Achieving communicative outcomes*, or discovering how you can construct a message in order to most effectively achieve the goal for your intended communication. An example would be deciding what information to include in a general announcement about the planned rotation system in order to build support and allay concerns among physicians, nurses, and other key customers.
5. *Evolution and change*, or the fact that communication occurs over time and with the context;

therefore, goals for communicating and the demands on the communicators can change within the context of a communication. An example would be identifying the information that needs to be included in each message and the time between messages as the rotation system is implemented and adjusted based on customer feedback.

Much of our daily communication happens quickly and naturally. We could not possibly stop and examine the context of *every* communication before it happens. However, just as we sometimes stop and use our clinical reasoning skills and processes to examine interventions that are new to us, that are complicated for some reason, or that aren't going "just right," we can also use communication theory to examine new, complex, or problematic communications to more effectively solve common problems in communication.

The next sections of this chapter provide a brief overview of several communication theories that are most directly related to management. These theories were chosen because of the particular contributions they can make to help the occupational therapy manager understand communication in the workplace. It may be notable that there is no theory presented specific to *mass communication*, or communication to the broad public, in this chapter. Although some have identified theories specific to mass communication, others have argued that organizing communication according to a "level" or context of communication reinforces the tendency to think of these communications as a type that are different from other "levels" of communication (Littlejohn & Foss, 2010). Because occupational therapy managers have fewer needs to organize mass communication and often do so without the assistance of a public relations department, I have chosen to follow the suggestion that mass communication is simply a type of communication to which you can apply appropriate communication theories. Therefore, the theories chosen for review are:

- *Cybernetics and information theory*, because of their relationship to the area of *health informatics*, including written communication in the form of e-mail or documentation
- *Dramatism and narrative*, because of their focus on the analysis of discourse through examination

of metaphors and stories, and their applicability to understanding how clinical and interpersonal stories play out in the workplace
- *Proxemics and expectancy violation theory*, because of their contribution to aiding us in seeing how nonverbal communication, space, and distance impact relationships and understanding

Each of these theories is briefly reviewed, and then the remainder of the chapter focuses on the pragmatic strategies for communicating more effectively in the workplace.

Cybernetics and Information Theory

Cybernetics is the study of regulation and control in systems (Handy & Kurtz, 1964; Krippendorf, 2009). The term *cybernetics* is a translation of the Greek word for "steersman" or "governor," and describes the way feedback makes information processing possible in our heads and on our computers (Griffin, 2000). Cybernetics deals with the ways a system gauges its effect based on both positive and negative feedback and makes the necessary adjustments to maintain effective functioning. Cybernetics may be viewed as a way of thinking that emphasizes circular reasoning and challenges the idea that one thing causes another in a linear fashion. It has been applied not only to engineering and mathematics but also to states, armies, families, and individual human beings.

One of the most common and relevant theories in the tradition of cybernetics is *information theory*, as developed by Shannon and Weaver (1949). Figure 5-1 shows Shannon and Weaver's model as applied to a conversation between a supervisor and an employee.

Shannon, a Bell Telephone Company research scientist, developed a mathematical theory of signal transmission while seeking to improve the transmission of information over telephone lines with minimal distortion. His focus was on the technical aspects of communication, with little concern for the message. It might be difficult at first to see the relevance of such a "hands-off" approach for the occupational therapy manager; however, it becomes more apparent when you consider the rapid move toward electronic documentation of intervention in settings where occupational therapists (OTs) and occupational therapy assistants (OTAs) are employed, including hospitals,

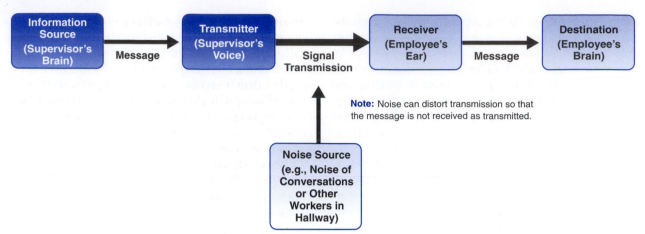

Figure ■ 5-1 Shannon and Weaver's Model of Communication Applied to a Conversation Between a Supervisor and an Employee.

school systems, and even community-based settings. When moving from paper-based communication to electronic communication, we are certainly concerned with *what* is communicated; however, at first we must be concerned with *how* information is communicated. Shannon's theory views information as a *reduction of uncertainty* that increases the use and reliability of communication. An example of this concept might be waking up in the morning to go to work in a New England town in January. When you first wake up, you are never completely sure of how your commute to work will be influenced by the weather; you are *uncertain*. However, by watching the weather report before you go to bed or upon getting up, you receive information through communication that reduces your uncertainty. You learn either that it is going to be a brisk but sunny day with an easy drive to work, or that snow is on the way and you should plan plenty of extra time.

In interpersonal communication, the speaker's brain is the *information source*, the vocal system is the *transmitter*, and the air medium is the *channel*. The listener's ear is the *receiver*, and the listener's brain the *destination*. The final element in the model, *noise*, is any disturbance in the channel that distorts or otherwise interferes with the signal. Whether the message is coded in regular language, electronic signals, or some other code, the problem of transmission is the same: to reconstruct the message accurately at the destination (Littlejohn & Foss, 2010). Applied to our example of electronic documentation, the communication problem becomes building a system (of drop-down menus, checks, documentation flowsheets, narrative text, etc.) that allows the practitioner (the source) to transmit information to be accurately received by other staff (the destination).

Information theory has been influential in a number of ways, particularly in communication technology and engineering, which have become so much more relevant in health care in the last decade. Shannon and Weaver's model is commonly cited as a method of introducing the basic elements of communication. It has been criticized, however, for its simplicity and limited application to communication areas beyond electronic means.

Dramatism and Narrative

Dramatism and **narrative** are two closely associated theories that both deal with stories. Stories are one of the most important ways people use symbols to create meaning and to communicate that meaning to others.

Dramatism was developed by Kenneth Burke and focuses on the use of metaphor in communication. Burke believed that "Verbal symbols are meaningful acts from which motives can be derived" (Griffin, 2000). Further, Burke held the conviction that "Action requires symbolicity and that language use must be understood as a form of *symbolic action* in which both actor and object and events are defined, interpreted, and acquire meaning" (Meister & Japp, 1999). Burke saw the use of metaphor and persuasion as the communicator's attempt to get an audience to believe his or her view of reality to be true.

Key to persuasion in dramatism is the concept of *identification*, or the common ground that exists between a speaker and his or her audience. The more similarity in the physical characteristics, talents, occupation, background, personality, beliefs, and values between a speaker and an audience, the greater the identification of the audience with the speaker. Of course, these characteristics may be weighted such that two persons who have similar physical characteristics and occupation but come from very different backgrounds, personalities, and beliefs may not identify with each other as much as two persons who look very different and have different occupations but share similar beliefs, values, and personality. An implication of identification for the communicator is that, to some extent, he or she can attempt to alter his or her presentation to increase identification by the audience and therefore increase his or her level of persuasion. For example, when presenting an in-service education program to a group of occupational therapy practitioners, a speaker can share personal and professional information that demonstrates to the listeners how the presenter is like the audience.

The most comprehensive narrative theory in the communication field is that of Walter Fisher. Fisher believed that human rationality in all its forms is based essentially on narrative, and, as such, communication in all its forms can be understood as narrative. Fisher defined *narration* as "symbolic actions—words and/or deeds—that have sequence and meaning for those who live, create, or interpret them" (Fisher, 1989). Griffin (2000) offered an expanded definition:

Narration is communication rooted in time and space. It covers every aspect of our lives and the lives of others in regard to character, motive, and action. The term also refers to every verbal or nonverbal bid for a person to believe or act in a certain way. Even when a message seems abstract—is devoid of imagery—it is narration because it is embedded in the speaker's ongoing story that has a beginning, middle, and end, and it invites listeners to interpret its meaning and assess its value for their own life.

Fisher saw narrative as a rational approach to communication. He summarized this view on the rationality of narrative to highlight his perspective that narrative can include a broad range of types of reasoning and rationality. He stated, "In narrative, no form of discourse is privileged over others because its form is predominantly argumentative. No matter how strictly a case is argued—scientifically, philosophically, or legally—it will always be a story, an interpretation of some aspect of the world that is historically and culturally grounded and shaped by human personality" (Fisher, 1987).

Fisher offered what he referred to as a *narrative paradigm* built on five assumptions. The narrative paradigm represents a shift from the more traditional *rational-world paradigm*, which purports that people are rational beings who make decisions on the basis of arguments and who see the world as a set of logical puzzles that we can solve through rational analysis. The five assumptions of the narrative paradigm are presented in Box 5-2 (Fisher, 1987).

Two key concepts related to Fisher's narrative paradigm are those of *coherence* and *fidelity*. Narrative coherence is how probable the story appears to the listener. Stories are more likely to be perceived as probable by a listener when the listener believes that he or she has been told all of the most important details of a story and that key information has not been omitted. Listeners must also believe that the story they are told is the most likely explanation and that an alternative story is not more plausible. Narrative fidelity is the extent to which a story "rings true" with a

---

BOX 5-2

The Five Assumptions of Fisher's Narrative Paradigm

1. People are essentially storytellers.
2. We make decisions on the basis of good reasons.
3. History, biography, culture, and character determine what we consider good reasons.
4. Narrative rationality is determined by the coherence and fidelity of our stories.
5. The world is a set of stories from which we choose, and thus constantly re-create, our lives.

listener's experiences. Narratives have strong fidelity when they provide sound logic for our actions.

Concepts related to narrative have become increasingly visible in the social and health sciences, and particularly in the field of occupational therapy, over the last several decades (Boydell, Goering, & Morrell-Bellai, 2000; Braveman, Helfrich, Kielhofner, & Albrecht, 2003; Bury, 2001; Helfrich & Kielhofner, 1994; Helfrich, Kielhofner, & Mattingly, 1994; Lee, 2001; Lieblich, Tuval-Mashiach, & Zibler, 1998; Lindström, Sjöström, & Lindberg, 2013; Mattingly, 2007; Nochi, 2001; Robinson, 1990). The use of narrative interviews and narrative analysis of life stories or accounts of disability experiences has been validated as an approach to understanding the experiences both of individuals and of groups of individuals who share a common illness or disability (Fredriksson & Erikson, 2001; Helfrich & Kielhofner, 1994; Mattingly, 2007; Robinson, 1990). Crepeau and Cohn (2014) describe a "narrative turn" that occurred in occupational therapy after medical anthropologist Cheryl Mattingly directed an ethnographic study of OTs and OTAs in a large teaching hospital as part of a study on clinical reasoning funded by the American Occupational Therapy Association (AOTA) and the American Occupational Therapy Foundation (AOTF). Mattingly's work was pivotal in bringing narrative and storytelling to the forefront of the awareness of occupational therapy scholars and practitioners. More recently, Kielhofner et al (2004) documented that the "slope" of a narrative (e.g., did things generally get better, worse, or stay about the same) might have value in predicting outcomes within a vocational rehabilitation program for people with acquired immunodeficiency syndrome (AIDS).

Narratives are important because they describe what happened, define outcomes, or present the stages of a social process. The process of integrating past, present, and future selves involves the construction of personal narratives (Ingvar, Joakim, & Ingegerd, 2000; Kielhofner et al, 2002; Mattingly, 1998). Narrative thought stresses that humans create meaning about what they encounter in everyday life by plotting or framing experiences within narrative structures (Bruner, 1986; Gergen & Gergen, 1983; Jonsson, Josephsson, & Kielhofner, 2000; Polkinghorne, 1988). Narratives create a "symbolic bridge between a person's past, present and future; they can mediate multiple—apparently disparate—elements into a heterogeneous synthesis anchored in human experience" (Ricoeur, 1991).

It may be argued that individuals not only use narratives to understand their everyday lives but also use narratives as a guide to create a particular future (Jonsson et al, 2000; Kielhofner, Borell, Burke, Helfrich, & Nygård, 1995; Mattingly, 1998). Narratives are a way of creating meaning as life unfolds and as new circumstances present themselves. As noted by Kielhofner et al (2002), "What we do continues our stories, sometimes by accepting what we perceive as inevitable, sometimes in response to a set of external events, and sometimes by aiming to create a particular outcome." Thus, narratives are created and refined in response to experiences, or as challenges are encountered as individuals seek to meet goals they set as a way of creating an outcome. Bury (2001) stated, "Not only do narratives help sustain and create the fabric of everyday life, they feature prominently in the repair and restoring of meaning when they are threatened."

It must be noted that, because a narrative is told or retold at a particular point in time, a narrative always reflects the temporal, physical, social, and emotional context of the narrator. The process of narrating experience is always set within a historical and temporal frame that the teller brings to the story (Sanchia & Street, 2001). Thus, narratives by their very nature are susceptible to change. As noted by Ricoeur (1984), "through the recreation of a narrative, new meaning can evolve in the creative imitation of the person's experienced world." This has led to some caution regarding the value and limitations of the use of narratives in the research process, because narratives are always told within a specific context and can change when told in a different context (Sanchia & Street, 2001), because it is questioned whether some information is stored by individuals within narratives or perhaps as problems without solutions (Kluwin, McAngus, & Feldman, 2001), and because narratives can be told as an effort to convince a listener who was not present that events occurred in a particular way (Riessman, 1990).

Proxemics and Expectancy Violations Theory

Proxemics is a term that was originally coined by Edward T. Hall, who was an anthropologist at the Illinois Institute of Technology, to refer to the study of people's use of space as an elaboration of culture (Hall, 1966). There are three fundamental areas related to proxemics: space, distance, and territory.

Three types of *space* have been identified by Hall: fixed-feature, semifixed-feature, and informal space. *Fixed-feature* space is one of the ways in which people organize activities. Houses, buildings, cities, rooms, and the like are organized spatially. Objects and activities are related to these spatial arrangements, and if objects or activities are moved, people react. *Semifixed-feature* space is of primary importance in interpersonal communication, because it can be used in many different ways to convey meaning. Hall mentioned two types of semifixed-feature space: "socio-petal" spaces are those that bring people together and stimulate involvement, whereas "socio-fugal" spaces keep people apart and promote withdrawal. Socio-fugal space transmits connotative meanings such as "large," "cold," and "impersonal," whereas socio-petal arrangements usually connote the opposite. *Informal space* is significant because it includes the distances people unconsciously maintain when they interact. According to Hall, "informal spatial patterns have distinct bounds and such deep, if unvoiced, significance that they form an essential part of culture. To misunderstand this significance may invite disaster." The three types of space identified in proxemics are summarized in Box 5-3.

A classic description of the types of *distance* (commonly referred to as personal space) for various types of interpersonal communications was first presented by Hall in 1966 and continues to be used today. The categories of distance identified by Hall—public,

BOX 5-4

Proxemics: Four Categories of Distance

1. *Public space* ranges from 12 to 25 feet and is the distance maintained between the audience and a speaker, such as a presenter at a conference.
2. *Social space* ranges from 4 to 10 feet and is used for communication among business associates, as well as to separate strangers using public areas, such as beaches and bus stops.
3. *Personal space* ranges from 2 to 4 feet and is used among friends and family members, as well as to separate people waiting in lines, such as at automated teller machines.
4. *Intimate space* ranges out to 1 foot and involves a high probability of touching. We reserve it for whispering and embracing.

social, personal, and intimate space—and their definitions are presented in Box 5-4 (Hall, 1966).

Personal comfort with distance during interpersonal communication varies from culture to culture, and understanding this is extraordinarily important for health-care providers (Dreachslin, Gilbert, & Malone, 2013). When Americans interact with people from other cultures, they need to be aware of how the other parties view space. Low-contact cultures (North American, Northern European, Asian) favor the social distance for interaction and little, if any, physical contact. High-contact cultures (Mediterranean, Arab, Latin) prefer the intimate and personal distances and much contact between people. Misunderstandings can occur when these two groups interact and either invade or avoid space and contact. Violations can also occur between people of the same culture. Differences in personality can lead to different interpretations of personal space and touching. Remaining aware of cultural and personal preferences for distance and attending to others' styles and reactions can increase your effectiveness in communicating in the workplace.

Finally, the concept of *territory* has important implications for interpersonal communication. It refers to any area controlled and defended by an individual or group of individuals, with emphasis on

BOX 5-3

Three Types of Space

1. *Fixed-feature space* is used to organize houses, cities, and spaces where people expect the organization to remain the same and will react if changes are made.
2. *Semifixed-feature space* includes socio-petal spaces that facilitate involvement and socio-fugal spaces that promote separation.
3. *Informal space* includes the distances people unconsciously maintain when they interact.

possession of physical space. There are *public territories*, or places anybody can enter, such as a reception area; *home territories* into which entrance is restricted to members, such as an office for one or more managers or staff members; *interaction territories*, or areas where people meet informally, such as a cafeteria; and *body territories*, or the space we use ourselves. Understanding the "rules" about entering various territories can help prevent you from unintentionally violating another person's or group's assumption about the use of a territory. In addition, as a manager you'll want to consider the impact that the verbal and nonverbal signals you send about your office and accessibility as territory have on the culture of your department. Many managers claim to have an "open door" policy but give a clear nonverbal signal that interrupting their work without an appointment is not a welcome intrusion.

Expectancy violations theory (EVT) is a theory of *personal space and nonverbal communication* that falls within the sociopsychological tradition of communication theory and is closely aligned with proxemics. Judee Burgoon defined *personal space* as the "invisible, variable volume of space surrounding an individual that defines that individual's preferred distance from others" (Burgoon, 1978). EVT sees communication as the exchange of information that is high in relational content and on occasion can be used to violate the expectations of another, which will be perceived either positively or negatively depending on the liking between the two people. Violation of our expectations produces arousal, which heightens the salience of cognitions about the communicator and his or her communication behavior. Arousal mediates the violation of the expectation and the subsequent communication behavior. When a violation has been perceived and arousal is triggered, the recipient evaluates the violation and the violator. Violations initiated by highly attractive sources may be evaluated positively, whereas those initiated by unattractive sources may be evaluated negatively (Dainton & Zelley, 2011).

The tenets of Burgoon's theory do contradict Hall's notion that people have expectations about how close others should come, but offer the counterpoint that there are times when it is best to break the rules. Burgoon believed that at times violating social norms and personal expectations is a superior strategy to conformity. In addition to proximity, EVT applies the same theoretical propositions to facial expressions, eye contact, touch, and body lean. For example, although

BOX 5-5
Propositions of Expectancy Violation Theory

1. As communicators, we develop expectations about the verbal and nonverbal communication of others.
2. Violations of communication expectations are arousing and cause a shift in our attention to the communicator, our relationship with the communicator, and the characteristics of the violation and meaning we attach to it.
3. Communicator reward valence (i.e., the strength of the reward), or the reactions we give or receive to violations, moderate the interpretation of ambiguous communicative behaviors.
4. Communicator reward valence moderates how we evaluate communicative behaviors.
5. Violation valences (i.e., the degree of the violation) are a function of
   a. The evaluation of the enacted behavior
   b. The direction of the discrepancy between the expected and enacted behavior toward a more favorable or unfavorably valued position
   c. The magnitude of the discrepancy such that enacted behaviors that are more favorably evaluated than expected behaviors constitute positive violations; enacted behaviors that are less favorably evaluated than expected behaviors are negative violations
6. Positive violations produce more favorable outcomes and negative violations produce more unfavorable outcomes relative to expectancy confirmation.

putting one's arm around the shoulders of a coworker might normally violate the expectations of employees in a particular setting, an employee who likes the "offender" might view the violation as positive if it is clear that it is meant to show appreciation for a special achievement. The propositions of EVT are further summarized in Box 5-5 (Burgoon, Stern, & Dillman, 1995).

Pragmatic Strategies for Improving Communication

Communicating effectively to individuals and groups in either verbal or written format is an important skill for any manager. Understanding communication theory helps you design what will be said to most effectively transmit your message to the receiver or listener. Unfortunately, things that we do consciously and unconsciously during the process of communicating can make it less likely that our message is going to be heard and interpreted as intended. Some of the most common problems that can limit your effectiveness when communicating, as well as strategies for making your verbal and written communication more effective, are presented next.

Simple Suggestions for Effective Conversations

Some of the most important communications you will have on a daily basis are the one-to-one conversations you have with staff, other managers, or members of the public, including consumers of occupational therapy. Particularly when you are busy, it is important to focus on strategies that you can use to assure your listeners that you are interested in what they have to say, so they leave your conversation sensing that you feel they are important and that you heard what they needed to say. Six simple strategies to help you be more effective in conversations with others in the workplace are listed in Box 5-6.

Paralinguistics and Nonverbal Communication

You are most likely already familiar with the experience of receiving communication in which *what* is said does not have as much impact as *how* it is said. *How* communication is conveyed may include verbal aspects, such as tone or volume, that do not relate to the content or words (e.g., **paralinguistics**), and nonverbal aspects, including facial expressions and body movements. There are many easily accessible overviews and lists of strategies for improving effectiveness in nonverbal behaviors, such as those provided by Ritts

---

BOX 5-6

Six Strategies for Effective Conversations

1. *Ask open-ended questions* to elicit informative answers to learn new information and to avoid giving the impression that you have already made decisions.
2. *Ask focused questions* that aren't too broad to limit extraneous information and help guide listeners to the type of information that will help them best make their point or advocate for their position.
3. *Ask for additional details*, examples, and the speaker's thoughts and impressions to show genuine interest and to indicate that you are open to the speaker's message.
4. *Paraphrase*, or restate what you heard, remembering that the real purpose of paraphrasing is not to clarify what the other person actually meant, but to show what it meant to you.
5. *Check perceptions of your impressions of another person's feelings* by describing them, being careful to avoid any expression of approval or disapproval. Objectively state what you believe the other person seems to be feeling.
6. *Describe behavior without making accusations or generalizations* about motives, attitudes, or personality traits.

---

and Stein (2014). Paralinguistics include the following facets of verbal communication:

- *Tone*, which generally indicates the overall quality of a person's voice. Tone is often referenced to give context to the manner in which voice contributes to communication, such as indicating that a person spoke in a "conversational" or a "nervous" tone of voice.
- *Pitch*, which refers technically to the frequency of the sound waves produced and heard by the listener's ear, but generally is referenced as higher or lower, and is typically thought to communicate the speaker's emotional state and level of excitement. Raising the pitch of your voice may communicate increased emotion.

- *Rhythm*, or the pattern of speech, indicated by the extent of variation in tone and volume. Varying the rhythm of your communication can help to hold the interest of your audience and, along with other aspects of vocal communication, can intentionally or unintentionally communicate your level of arousal or the nature of your emotion.
- *Volume*, or the loudness or softness of voice, can not only communicate emotion (by increasing voice volume) but also can increase interest on the part of the listener (by lowering voice volume to "pull" the listener into the message). Lowering your voice volume to a whisper during a presentation can sometimes be more effective than speaking more loudly in gaining attention.
- *Inflection* is sometimes used to reference changes in pitch or tone. In linguistics, it specifically represents the change in the shape of a word, generally by adding an affix, such as a prefix or suffix, to the root word. By doing this, a change of meaning or relationship to some other word or group of words can be indicated. Inflectional operations ground the semantic content of a root word according to place, time, and participant reference, without substantially affecting the basic semantic content of the root. They often specify when an event or situation took place (e.g., pre- or post-); who or what were the participants (e.g., non-); and sometimes where, how, or whether an event or situation really took place (e.g., -like). By means of inflection, we can creatively communicate information by inferring meaning beyond the static meaning of our words, thereby increasing listener attention.

All of us develop styles of speaking over our lives, yet we may not be aware of the impact of the various facets of our speech. In addition, the novice speaker may be more likely to be influenced by the context of communication such that the emotions of nervousness, anger, frustration, or a deep intellectual commitment may be evident in how he or she communicates via paralinguistics. Videotaping or audiotaping yourself during a presentation is a helpful way to become more familiar with your communication style so you can identify behaviors you wish to change, including those paralinguistic elements just described. Ultimately, becoming more confident in communicating

with others in the work setting is achieved through practice and conscious focus on skill development. Practicing verbal communications, especially to a group, may be fostered by looking for opportunities to make presentations in low-risk situations, such as presenting part of a lunchtime in-service, copresenting at small conferences, or even making very short presentations such as public toasts or an acknowledgment of thanks.

It is worth noting that paralinguistics are heavily influenced by culture, and, as the workplace continues to become more diverse, recognizing cultural variations in communication becomes more important. Stephan Dahl (2001) pointed out that differences in the volume, speed, and other aspects of paralinguistics are interpreted differently in different cultures. He noted, for example, "The notion that Americans are talking too loud is often interpreted in Europe as aggressive behavior or can be seen as a sign of uncultivated behavior. Likewise, the British manner of speaking quietly might be understood as secretive by Americans." Similarly, the speed of talking is different in various cultural settings. For example, Finnish is spoken relatively slowly in comparison to other European languages. This slowness of speaking has often resulted in the Finnish being regarded as somewhat "slow" and lax. Further importance is given to the amount of silence that is perceived as appropriate during a conversation. A Japanese proverb says, "Those who know do not speak—those who speak do not know." This purposeful use of silence by individuals from Oriental cultures must come as a slap in the face to Americans, for whom even a short silence is seen as embarrassing, and hence is filled up with often random speech, something often perceived as hypermanic by persons from other cultures. Similarly, there is an avoidance of silence in Arabic countries, where word games are played and thoughts repeated to avoid silence (Dahl, 2001).

Some major areas of nonverbal communication to consider are discussed in the following sections.

Eye Contact

Maintaining eye contact helps to regulate the flow of communication by signaling interest in others and can increase a speaker's credibility. When you speak, your eyes involve your listeners in your presentation; the easiest way to break a communication bond between you and the listeners is failing to look at them. By looking at your listeners, you communicate that you are sincere and are interested in them, and that you care that they hear what you have to say. Eye contact can also help you to overcome nervousness by making a connection with listeners who do care about your message.

Laskowski (2002) presented a series of tips on using your eyes effectively during presentations and communications with others:

- Know your material well so that you don't have to devote your mental energy to the task of remembering the sequence of ideas and words.
- Establish a personal bond with listeners by selecting one person and talking to him or her personally. Maintain eye contact with that person long enough to establish a visual bond (about 5 to 10 seconds). This is usually the equivalent of a sentence or a thought. Then shift your gaze to another person.
- Monitor visual feedback. While you are talking, your listeners are responding with their own nonverbal messages. Use your eyes to actively seek out this valuable feedback.

Facial Expressions

Expressions are a key part of effective communication. Facial expressions such as smiling can be powerful cues that transmit friendliness and openness to communication, but they might also communicate impatience, frustration, disagreement, or disappointment. It is important to be aware of your facial expressions and use them consciously so that your expressions match the context and tone of your intended communication. Nervous speakers may make unconscious expressions such as frowning. Frowning may occur when a speaker attempts to deliver a memorized speech or when the speaker is feeling frustrated because listeners do not understand what he or she is attempting to communicate. There are no rules governing the use of specific expressions.

Gestures

Gestures, including head nods or arm movements, can animate a presentation and capture the attention of

listeners, make the material more interesting, and facilitate learning. Like unconscious facial expressions, however, unintended gestures can be distracting and make it harder for the listener to receive your message. When you make a verbal mistake (either saying the wrong thing or using inappropriate tone or volume), it is easier to correct it because you may hear it yourself. It may be harder to discontinue distracting gestures of which you are not aware. If you are going to be giving public presentations frequently, or if giving a presentation is a particularly nerve-wracking experience for you, you might consider the previously suggested strategy for improvement of videotaping yourself giving a presentation. At first you may be very aware of the camera, but after a while you are likely to drift into your normal style of presentation, and on playback of the tape you will be able to see both effective and ineffective strategies and behaviors that you commonly use.

Some of the most common behaviors of inexperienced or nervous speakers include:

- Gripping or leaning on the lectern or podium
- Finger tapping
- Lip biting or licking
- Playing with coins in your pocket or with jewelry, such as a necklace or a watch
- Frowning when nervous or frustrated that listeners don't seem to understand
- Adjusting hair or clothing
- Head wagging or nodding and beginning to react to a question or comment from a listener before he or she is finished speaking

Posture and Body Orientation

Posture and body orientation communicate numerous messages by the way you walk, talk, stand, and sit. Standing erect, but not rigid, and leaning slightly forward communicates to listeners that you are approachable, receptive, and friendly. If you are involved in a one-to-one conversation, maintaining an "open" posture with both feet on the floor, arms resting comfortably in your lap or on the arms of the chair (not crossed on your chest) with no objects between you and the person with whom you are speaking, such as a desk, can indicate your attention to the conversation. Often conversations begin without the speakers realizing the importance of the discussion, and your posture and body orientation can inadvertently communicate that you are not invested in the conversation. For example, if you continue to face a computer workstation and keep your fingers on the keyboard when someone enters your office to ask a question, you may communicate that you do not wish to take the time to fully attend to the conversation. By consciously using posture and body orientation, such as by turning to face the person to whom you are speaking and leaning forward, or standing up and coming out from behind a desk, you can indicate that you are truly invested in the discussion.

During presentations, varying your body orientation can help maintain the attention of an audience as long as it is used judiciously. Moving away from a podium or lectern and walking toward the audience can effectively communicate interest and increase the sense of the audience's participation in the presentation. Naturally, moving too much or pacing nervously can detract attention from your message. During formal presentations, you may also be limited by factors beyond your control, such as the size of the room, the placement of audiovisual controls or screens, or limited ability to move around the room because of acoustics or the need to use a microphone.

Effective Presentations

Public speaking can be intimidating for many people, but being able to give an effective presentation is a critical management skill. Speaking confidently to a group can establish instant authority and credibility. Like many skills in life, learning to give effective presentations is simply a matter of knowledge, planning, and practice. A wide variety of available resources are easily accessible on the Internet and at your local bookstore to help guide the development and preparation of a presentation. Some basic strategies for giving an effective presentation are summarized next.

When planning a presentation, it is helpful to think about the *purpose* of your communication. Most presentations fall into one of three purposes: efforts to inform, explain, or persuade. These three types of presentations are briefly summarized in Box 5-7. Simple strategies for more successful development of content for presentations are provided in Box 5-8. The strategies in Box 5-8 apply regardless of the purpose of your presentation, although thinking about these types of presentations separately when planning your

> ### BOX 5-7
> #### Three Common Purposes for Presentations
>
> 1. Presentations to *inform* provide your audience with information. Your goal is that the audience leaves with information they did not have when they arrived.
> 2. Presentations to *explain* help your audience become more familiar with new information they have received. Your goal is that the audience better understands the process or procedure that is your topic.
> 3. Presentations to *persuade* are designed to convince your audience to think differently about an issue. Your goal for this type of presentation is to change the audience's beliefs and sometimes to get them to take action.

content helps you to be more on target with the goal of your communication. Table 5-1 also provides strategies for success in the three types of presentations.

A good place to start when you are planning an important presentation is by thinking about your audience. Conducting an *audience analysis* is simply a process of doing the best you can to get to know your audience so that you can tailor your presentation to the occasion. A common mistake is to try to use a "one size fits all" approach and use the same presentation materials, style, and format for very different groups and situations. I recently gave a presentation to a group of OTs and OTAs to introduce them to evidence-based practice. Before the presentation, a colleague shared a PowerPoint presentation that she had previously prepared. Happy to save time, I removed the slides that did not apply to my presentation and printed the handouts for use with my talk. As I moved through the presentation, however, I became aware of more and more instances in which the language on the slides was not a perfect fit for that day's audience. I kept having to refer to bulleted points by saying, "That should say. . . ." The presentation was not only more confusing for the audience, but it also lessened my credibility with the group. With just a little more work, I could have customized the

BOX 5-8

Strategies for Developing Successful Presentation Content

- **Focus your take-home message:** Write one to three simple messages you want to deliver and organize your presentation around these messages.
- **Brainstorm, then focus:** Balance creativity with focusing on your topic. Begin by quickly writing the things that come to mind about your topic in any order, but stop when you need to pause for more than a moment. Now organize your list into groups and put them in logical order. Finally, ask yourself what is missing and where it belongs in your outline.
- **Develop a strong and convincing introduction and conclusion:** Catch the attention of your audience right from the beginning. Writing your conclusion first will actually help you stay focused on where you are going and what you need to say to get you there.
- **Highlight three to five key points:** A common mistake is to plan too much for one presentation, especially when you care very much about what you have to say. Deciding on three to five key points will help you distinguish between what *could* be said and what *must* be said. Develop supporting evidence or information for each key point, writing first in bulleted points to help you

keep your message *simple and focused*. Include statistics, facts, or stories where appropriate.
- **Write and rewrite:** Write a section of your remarks and then come back to them later. Often presenters speak from notes or in an unscripted fashion using a slide show as their notes. This can make presentations seem more conversational and less formal, but the speaker must be comfortable and familiar with the topic and the slides. Other times, even for an expert speaker, a completely scripted presentation may be more appropriate. Still, a scripted presentation does not have to be boring or even sound like it is being read. If you put your presentation on paper or on note cards, be sure to number them so that, if you drop them or get lost while presenting, you can easily find your place.
- **Practice, practice, practice:** You've heard the adage "Practice makes perfect." Perfection may be a lot to hope for, but practice certainly can improve the quality of a presentation. Read your presentation or review your notes frequently. For formal presentations that must fit a time frame closely, be sure to read your remarks out loud. You may find that, when speaking aloud, your pace slows or quickens.

presentation, given full credit to my colleague, and been more effective in meeting the needs of my audience. Some simple questions to ask yourself to *analyze* your audience are listed in Box 5-9.

Effective Written Communication

In addition to communicating verbally, managers often use various modes of written communication, including memos, business letters, e-mail, business plans, and grant proposals. Confidence in business writing, as in verbal communications, comes with practice, but can be greatly improved by conscious attention to practicing and learning specific skills.

Writing effectively in the workplace can be very different than other sorts of writing because communicating ideas objectively and succinctly is highly valued. Well-written documents clarify issues, guide coworkers' thinking, and help to build agreement on courses of action.

The foundation of effective business writing is clear thinking. Grammar and style matter, but critical thinking is even more important (Alpha Books, 2002). Critical thinking starts by carefully thinking through what *could* be communicated and what *should* be communicated to help achieve your objective. Much like with a verbal presentation, identifying the purpose of written communication (e.g., to inform, to explain, or to persuade) is a good first step that will guide your decision-making about what to put in and what to leave out of

---

TABLE 5-1

Strategies for Successful Presentations

Types of Presentations	Success Strategies

• **Presentations to inform**
• **Presentations to explain**
	• Tell them what you will tell them, tell them what you want them to know, then tell them what you told them.
	  • *"Today I'm going to introduce you to four key principles of continuous quality improvement."*
	  • *"The first key principle of CQI is. . . ."*
	  • *"To summarize, today you were introduced to the four key principles of CQI, which were. . . ."*
	• Relate new information to something they already know.
	  • *"You are already familiar with. . . ."*
	• Begin with simple concepts and move to complex concepts.
	  • *"The most basic CQI principle is customer service; later we'll talk briefly about more complicated strategies for meeting customer needs."*

• **Presentations to persuade**	• Start by establishing agreement with something you have to say, or establishing a common view with which there can be no dispute.
	  • *"Can we all agree that we want to be effective as occupational therapists?"*
	• Get them in a "yes" mode (ask several questions in a row related to your point of view to which the audience will respond "Yes!")
	  • *"Do you want to improve your services?"*
	  • *"Do you care about your clients?"*
	  • *"Do you want to be more effective in meeting client needs?"*
	• Number your reasons for your point of view.
	  • *"There are four reasons you should attend the Continuous Quality Improvement Leadership Course. The first is. . . ."*
	• Close the deal by asking for agreement.
	  • *"So, can I plan on each of you attending the CQI Leadership Course?"*
	• What will it take to convince them? Ask for a firm commitment before they leave the presentation.
	  • *"How do I convince you to sign up for the CQI Leadership Course today?"*

BOX 5-9

Analyzing Your Audience

• How many people will be in the audience, and how does this affect your plan for use of audiovisual equipment, handouts, or discussion questions and exercises?

• What are the background, gender, age, careers, and interests of the audience members? Can you include references in your presentation to each major demographic group to customize your presentation?

• What do you think the audience already knows about your topic? How can you make ties to what is already familiar to them as a way of introducing new topics?

• How much more will they want to know? Are you able to tell them everything they need to know in one presentation, or do you need to plan for "unfinished business"?

• Why are the members of the audience attending? Are they there voluntarily or because their boss told them to attend?

• Will there be other speakers? If so, can you coordinate your presentations ahead of time to minimize duplication and reinforce key issues?

• How much time have you been given for your presentation, including questions and answers? Can you meet the audience's expectations in the time you have been allotted, or do you need to start by reframing their expectations?

any document. Regardless of the form of writing, you should be able to clearly state the purpose of your writing in a single sentence before you begin. The "Seven *C*'s of Effective Business Writing" are commonly identified factors to consider when writing for business, These factors are (1) consideration (the "your" or "we" approach instead of "I"), (2) conciseness, (3) correctness (accuracy), (4) courtesy, (5) clarity, (6) completeness, (7) and concreteness (Notes Desk, 2013).

Resources for specific forms of writing (e.g., memos, letters, e-mails, business plans, and grant proposals) abound and can easily be located at your local bookstore or on the Internet. The following sections briefly overview key strategies for increasing effectiveness in each form of writing. You are encouraged to find and use some of the many resources specific to the format of writing you are using.

The Business Memo

Memos are appropriately used for communication internal to your organization. They typically confirm conversations, request actions, inform others of problems, or update others on events or progress. Memos are not appropriate for communicating to outside parties and have limited use in establishing policy. They should not be used as a substitute for initial conversations or for dealing with issues that can be settled with a short telephone conversation, especially if the situation evokes strong emotions. You should never write a memo in anger; it is better to wait until the next day, when you can decide whether the communication is necessary and if a memo is the most appropriate form of communication; by doing so, you can compose the memo in a calm manner. Some additional tips for writing memos are included in Box 5-10.

Business Letters

As opposed to memos, which are written to an audience internal to your organization, a business letter is written to communicate to an outside audience. Business letters must be taken very seriously because you will most likely be considered a representative of your organization. Many of the strategies for writing an effective memo also apply to writing an effective business letter (e.g., the Seven *C*'s of Business Writing). As

---

BOX 5-10

Tips for Writing Effective Memos

- Keep paragraphs short and to the point. Be concise, yet try to be complete.
- Paragraphs should be in block form with no indentation and may be organized according the following framework:
  - Introduction: a few sentences that state the reason for the communication
  - Background: one or two paragraphs describing the context for the request or recommendation included in the memo
  - Recommendation or request: a concise statement of what you desire to have happen
  - Rationale: two to three paragraphs proving the reasoning for your recommendation
  - Conclusion: a brief statement restating your position
- Accent or highlight major points by using underlining, bullets, or bold type, but use these approaches sparingly.
- Use short headings to separate major topics in your memo to keep things organized, provide structure, and make for smooth reading.
- The title (RE: . . .) to your memo should reflect its contents and should be no more than a few words long.
- Make sure your distribution list is relevant. Send your memo or e-mail only to those who are directly concerned with the issues contained or raised in your message.
- Be considerate of the recipients' time and don't use memos or e-mails as a way to reinforce or defend your position, or to indirectly put down other people in your firm.
- Proofread carefully for errors before distributing.

---

with a memo, you should be able to answer these questions clearly before you begin to write:

- Why are you writing?
- Whom are you writing to?
- What information do you want to convey, or what do you want to ask the receiving party to do?
- Why should the receiving party care or agree?

Business letters typically include three major sections: the opening, the body, and the closing. The opening paragraph should introduce your reason for writing, stated in clear, concise, and candid language. The reader should easily be able to understand why you are writing and what you are going to ask or convey by the time he or she has finished reading your opening. Your opening will make an impression on your reader that will set the context as he or she reads the remainder of your communication. You may ask yourself, "What do I want the reader to be feeling or thinking when he or she finishes reading this first paragraph?" and then examine your opening to see if it is likely to have the desired impact on your reader.

In the body of your letter, you will concisely state and explain what you want or what information you are writing to share. It is important to have reasonable expectations for a business letter. If you expect that your reader will need additional information or the opportunity for a face-to-face meeting to discuss your topic or ask questions, then the body of your letter should set the stage for the next step in the process. For example, consider a fieldwork coordinator at a university who wishes to establish a relationship with a new practice setting in order to place fieldwork students there. The ultimate goal is to get the manager of the setting to agree to take several students each year. Including all the information that might be necessary to convince the manager to make an affirmative decision in a single letter would not be an effective strategy. A face-to-face meeting is a more effective strategy; thus, the goal of the business letter would more appropriately be to ask the manager to agree to a meeting to discuss taking fieldwork students.

It is critically important that you pay close attention to the tone of your letter and that you neither write in a style that is overly "familiar" if you do not have an established relationship with the reader, or in a style that is aggressive or demanding. If you are uncertain about how a letter might be received, asking a colleague to read the letter for you and respond to its tone is always a good idea. In addition, business letters should seldom exceed one to three pages. If necessary, additional documents can be included with the business letter that provide supporting documentation or reference material. These documents can be cited in the body of your business letter or listed at the end of your letter as appendices or enclosures.

The closing or final paragraph of your letter needs to accomplish two goals. The first of these goals is to provide a concise summary of the letter's purpose in no more than a sentence or two. This may seem like a daunting task, especially if the subject matter of your letter is of considerable importance. The most common mistake, however, is trying to "overshoot" or accomplish too much in one letter. The second goal of the closing is to request a specific action and suggest a time frame for action, if appropriate. This action might be to adopt a point of view based on information provided in the letter, or it might be a task that you want the reader to agree to complete. If asking for a task to be completed, it is important to also include a time frame in which you would like the reader to act.

E-Mail

The use of e-mail has virtually exploded over the last decade. There is no doubt that it has become an extraordinary convenience that has impacted the business environment in many positive ways and has fostered communication, especially in terms of speed and ease. However, there are dangers inherent in this form of communication both in terms of what is communicated inadvertently and in terms of some negative impacts of e-mail on work productivity. E-mail is simply a communication tool that must be used wisely to remain an advantage rather than a disadvantage.

Electronic communication is different from traditional written communication in a number of fundamental ways. E-mail tends to be more conversational because messages can be exchanged very quickly. In other forms of written communication, such as the memo or business letter, you must make everything clear because your reader may not have a chance to ask clarifying questions. With e-mail, the reader can ask questions immediately, and this tends to make e-mail seem more as if you are having a conversation. Therefore, it is easy to forget key differences between a face-to-face conversation and e-mail. In e-mail, your reader won't have access to the nonverbal and paralinguistic cues described earlier that communicate emotion and help the receiver of communication interpret meaning. Therefore, meaning can easily be misconstrued. For example, efforts to be humorous that might be effective if the reader could see you smiling or hear you chuckling as you write the message might be perceived as sarcastic or rude.

Some aspects of paralinguistics can be incorporated into e-mail messages; however, these can sometimes indicate unintended meaning. For example, TYPING IN ALL CAPITAL LETTERS may be understood as the e-mail equivalent of increasing the volume of your voice; this may effectively indicate a word you wish to stress but can also be interpreted as shouting. The term *emoticons* has developed to indicate the use of symbols or punctuation to indicate emotion. For example, one particular combination of symbols—written as "<G>"—may be used to indicate that you are "grinning" or saying something in jest. The word *netiquette* has been coined to describe rules of e-mail behavior that have found common acceptance. You should keep in mind that the content of messages could be guided by the same rules for effective written communication as other forms (again, the Seven *C*'s of Business Writing) but that strategies for adding context or emotional cues need to be considered separately. There are many easily accessible guides to netiquette and strategies for communicating emotion or other aspects of vocal speech, such as a *pause equivalent*, that can be found by conducting a simple Internet search or in books on business writing found in your local bookstore. Box 5-11 includes a short list of how to avoid the most common mistakes in the use of e-mail. Remember, once you hit the Send button, you lose complete control over where your message goes and who will see what you write.

Business Plans and Program Proposals

Writing a business plan or a proposal for a new program is an example of a specific and complex writing task faced by some occupational therapy managers. A business plan is a detailed document that describes the need and the costs and benefits of a new program or service. The written document itself actually summarizes a complicated process of collecting and analyzing a range of data, which may occur over many months. Full-scale business plans for the initiation of a new business enterprise may be many pages in length, whereas shorter program proposals are sometimes requested by administrators to justify the need for more discrete services, such as expanding services to an existing population. These shorter proposals still may be difficult to write, especially if you are not provided with a lot of guidance as to how the proposal should be structured and what should be included.

Writing a business plan for the first time is not a venture that should be undertaken without preparation and assistance. The development of effective business plans requires both skilled business writing and strong organizational, financial, and data-analysis skills. Outlines for business proposals can commonly be found through organizations such as the Small Business Administration (http://www.sba.gov/), and these outlines can also be used to help you organize shorter program proposals. A sample outline showing the common elements of a business plan is included in Box 5-12 to highlight the complexity of what is typically included in such a plan (Small Business Administration, 2014).

BOX 5-11

Ways to Avoid Common Mistakes in E-Mail Use

- Never write and send e-mail when you are angry.
- Do not attach unnecessary files.
- Do not overuse the High Priority option.
- Don't reference earlier messages without including part of the "message thread."
- Read the e-mail before you send it.
- Do not overuse Reply to All.
- Be careful with abbreviations and emoticons.
- Do not copy a message or attachment without permission.
- Do not use e-mail to discuss confidential information.
- Don't send or forward e-mails containing libelous, defamatory, offensive, racist, or obscene remarks.
- Use the c: field (copying others on an email) sparingly.
- Adhere to Health Information Portability and Accountability Act of 1996 (HIPPA) and organizational security guidelines on protected health information.

Grants

Another form of business writing in which the occupational therapy manager might participate is grant writing. Although grants as a form of funding may

---

BOX 5-12

Sample Elements of a Business Plan

Executive Summary
- Short (2- to 3-page) summary of what will be presented
- Sets the context for the program you are trying to "sell"
- Appears first in the document but must be written after all other sections of the document are prepared

Market Analysis
- Describes your target market, including
  - Demographics of consumers
  - Characteristics of payers and the payer mix
- Your market niche

Demographic Analysis
- Age, gender, nationality, educational level, and so on, of consumers
- Diagnostic criteria or statistics representing challenges to activity and participation

Competitive Analysis
- Do you have competitors?
- What are their relative strengths and weaknesses?
- How do consumers view your competition?

Referral Analysis
- Do you have established referral mechanisms?
- Are there potential referral sources not yet tapped?

Financial Plan
- Projections for 3 to 5 years (often called a Pro Forma)
- Analysis of revenue, expenses, and discounts or bad debt

Marketing Plan
- Needs assessment summary
- Consumers and payers to be targeted
- Strategies for promotion
- Year-by-year plan to support growth

Operational Plan
- Organizational chart
- Description of key personnel
- Description of fit of systems such as billing and documentation with existing organizational systems

Program Evaluation
- Plan for program evaluation and documentation of outcomes

---

most often be associated with research, some grants support the development and implementation of new programs. Such grants may pay for the development or evaluation of model programs, to prove the effectiveness of an intervention, to assist with capacity building of an organization, to provide a service, or to cover start-up costs of new programming, including equipment and sometimes staff for a limited period of time. These types of grants are often sought by community-based organizations. Grants may be available through city, state, or federal government sources or through a wide range of nonprofit foundations. A short, nonexhaustive list of various types of grants that are available is provided in Box 5-13.

Like business plans, grant writing should not be entered into without some preparation, because this will increase your likelihood of success. The response

BOX 5-13

Common Types of Grants

- Research (including investigator awards)
- Program or demonstration
- Training (including postdoctoral awards)
- Operating
- Technical assistance
- Publication
- Infrastructure
- Technology development

to a *request for proposals* (RFP) issued by a funding source can sometimes be very competitive. You may initially have to submit a letter of intent in which you are asked to summarize your request for funds, including the need for the program, the intervention, a brief description of how the funds will be used, and anticipated outcomes, in as little as two to four pages. Once again, using a guide such as the Seven *C's* of Business Writing to review your work can be helpful.

Identifying Funding Sources

Finding the right match for a funding source is an important first step in grant writing. Writing grants can be extraordinarily time consuming, and you do not want to invest days or weeks of work to write a strong proposal only to hear from the funding source that it does not match the source's priorities. Key to finding the right match is having a clear understanding of your interests and what you want to accomplish. Completing the first steps of program development and marketing, including a demographic and market analysis, will provide you with some of the information you will likely need to include in your proposal (see Chapters 14 and 15).

A helpful strategy for finding potential funding sources is to develop a network of others who are interested in the same types of programming. Although sometimes they may be your competitors in submitting a response to an RFP and might not be willing to share much information about strategy, you will be surprised how often your peers in occupational therapy and other professions will be willing to direct you to opportunities. One of the best ways to promote such behavior is by doing that yourself. As you develop a network, watch for those occasions when you find an RFP that does not exactly fit your needs or for which the timing may be wrong for you but that might be a match for someone in your network, and forward the information to him or her. Soon you will likely notice that others are doing the same for you.

Other key strategies include conducting an Internet search for foundations that relate to your interests and putting yourself on lists to receive e-mail notifications of RFPs. A number of websites include search engines that list funding sources. Websites useful for searching for federal grants (e.g., http://www.grants .gov/) include links to allow you to receive e-mail notifications of new grant opportunities as they are announced. Another important source of announcements for government grants is the *Federal Register*. All federal announcements of grants are published in the *Federal Register*, and a search engine for announcements can be found on the Federal Grant Opportunities website (www.fedgrants.gov/). An excellent resource for finding opportunities with private foundations is The Foundation Center (http://fdncenter.org/).

Once you find opportunities for funding, you need to determine which ones are good matches. A helpful tool is to create and use a "matching worksheet" to evaluate the fit between what you want to do and what the funding source is willing to pay for. The sample matching worksheet in Table 5-2 is for a program for children from birth to 5 years of age with a physical disability to expose them to play and social interests, for which you desire funding for equipment. Although not a perfect match on all criteria (listed along the left side of the table), funding source 1 is a better match than the other funding sources even though none of the funding sources is a strong match related to leisure or funding of equipment.

In the matching process, you need to consider the following factors:

- Do you match the eligibility criteria as stated by the funding source?
- Are there types of expenses listed as funding exclusions (e.g., indirect costs, food, etc.)?
- Can you meet the deadline for responding to the RFP?
- How quickly will reviews be conducted and a funding decision made?
- What are the typical funding amounts and is the potential payoff worth your investment of time in writing the proposal?
- What percentage of proposals is commonly funded?

Writing the Grant Proposal

When preparing your submission, you must be sure to read the rules carefully and highlight the key points. It is important to pay special attention to rules about the allowable number of pages, type size, margins, and any defined sections or budget exclusions. Funding sources typically take these rules very seriously and will often not even review a proposal that does not fit the criteria. You can imagine that it would be very demoralizing to

TABLE 5-2			
Sample Funding Matching* Worksheet for a Program to Introduce Children From Birth to 5 to Play and Social Options			
	Funding Source 1	**Funding Source 2**	**Funding Source 3**
Develop a Direct Service Program	5	5	3
For Children Birth to 5	5	5	5
Who Have a Physical Disability	5	3	3
To Expose Them to Play and Social Options	3	3	3
Need Funding for Equipment	3	3	3

*1 = weak match; 5 = strong match.

spend days, weeks, or even months writing a proposal only to have it rejected because your narrative was a half-page too long or you used too small a type size!

You need to plan your writing strategy—develop a timeline, obtain necessary support, divide the labor, and pull in experts (e.g., evaluators, statisticians). You should consider if writing alone is a wise strategy for you. Sometimes grant proposals are strengthened greatly by including other organizations as collaborators. Even though the grant dollars may have to be split between organizations, your proposal may be perceived as having a greater impact if funded. A local university is the best place to start to obtain help with complicated proposals. There you can find mentors and critics who can help along the way by reviewing your work and giving you suggestions to strengthen your proposal, but you should be sure to ask for their assistance with plenty of notice.

When writing, it is helpful to use the headings of your proposal sections to format your work and to keep track of requirements and rules for formatting your submission. Formatting your proposal, using any criteria provided by the funding source that will be evaluating submissions, is a great way to keep your writing organized and clear. You must do your research and make sure you "know your stuff." It is not uncommon for your first submission to be rejected; however, you will often be invited to submit your proposal again after incorporating reviewer feedback. It is important to remember that experts in your area of interest are often serving as reviewers, and you do not want to

damage your credibility in the future by making factual mistakes or assertions that are poorly supported because you have not adequately prepared yourself to write a sophisticated proposal.

Your statements of purpose and outcomes should be clear, and your argument should be logical and well supported by current and appropriate references. The proposal is your "sales pitch" to a funding source, and you want them to buy your argument. In addition to describing the purpose and outcomes, there are other common components of grant proposals. These components are listed in Box 5-14.

Some errors commonly made in writing grant proposals that you will want to avoid include:

- Lack of definitions for key concepts or terms that may be unfamiliar to the reviewers
- Too much jargon (words or abbreviations familiar to those in your setting but not to others)
- Inconsistencies in language across proposal (this can commonly happen if you have multiple people working on a proposal)
- Logic leaps that assume that the reviewers are familiar with your topic
- Errors in spelling and grammar
- Failure to address all points in the RFP
- Lack of current and comprehensive references
- Promising more than is possible in the time frame you have to implement your proposal or for the funds you are requesting
- Underbudgeting or overbudgeting

BOX 5-14

Common Components of Grant Proposals

- **Statement of need:** Why is your proposal important?
- **Objectives:** What will you accomplish if funded?
- **Literature review:** What prior work has been done in this area, including research or other program implementations, to support the need for you to carry out your proposed work?
- **Proposal narrative:** This portion of the proposal includes procedures, expected outcomes, and how you will measure outcomes. This is the main body of your proposal that ties together the other pieces.
- **Management plan:** This is a listing of project goals and objectives, including time frames and accountability for major project tasks.
- **Evaluation:** How will you know that your project is being implemented as planned (formative evaluation), and how will you measure its outcomes and success (summative evaluation)?
- **Budget:** This is a year-by-year breakdown of expenses, often presented in table format,

including personnel, overhead (indirect cost recover, or ICR), and supplies and equipment.
- **Budget narrative:** This is a 1- to 3-page written explanation justifying your budget proposal.
- **Institutional resources:** Will your organization match funds and donate time or supplies, and does it have adequate space to allow you to achieve your objectives?
- **Team qualifications:** Do you have personnel, including a project director (principal investigator), who have the skills and experience to warrant the amount of funds you are requesting?
- **Dissemination plan:** Will you share what you learn or the outcomes of your program with others, and, if so, how will you do that?
- **Appendices:** These are documents referenced in your narrative, including letters of support from collaborators. (Sometimes you can shorten your narrative to the required length by putting some items in an appendix.)

Other mistakes are commonly made in the process of submitting proposals to funding sources that can result in proposals being rejected. For example, you need to know who in your organization has to sign the proposal. If there is any research element to the proposal, or if you will be collecting protected health information as defined by HIPAA, you must meet all of the requirements listed for involving an Investigational Review Board or managing the protected health information (U.S. Department of Health and Human Services, 2013). You must be very careful to note and understand correctly the due date for the proposal. Some due dates reference the "received by" date, meaning your proposal must be received by the funding source by that date, whereas others reference the "postmarked by" date, meaning that your proposal must be postmarked by the due date. It is becoming more common for proposals to be submitted electronically, and in this case be sure to note carefully if the submission deadline includes a time zone (i.e. 5:00 PM EST). If possible, you should plan to submit your

proposal a few days early so that, if you hit an unexpected roadblock, you will have a few days to recover and still meet your deadline. Rushing at the last minute is often why writers make some of the common errors described previously.

You must be careful to submit the correct number of copies of the proposal; often the RFP states that an original (with all original signatures) and a specified number of copies must be submitted. If submitting electronically pay close attention to directions for e-signing or initialing. A cover letter citing what is included with your submission is recommended, and you should check your submission against the cover letter and the original RFP criteria as you are preparing to mail, ship or submit it. In addition, you should follow directions as to how to present your proposal (e.g., some RFPs state specifically *not* to use binders and to only use clips).

Grant proposals are typically reviewed by a panel of experts, or by a *peer-review panel* in the case of many federal RFPs. As noted earlier, many first submissions are not funded, but you should not be overly discouraged if this happens to you. Many funding sources report funding rates of fewer than 10% of the submitted proposals. If your proposal is rejected, it may be possible to resubmit it at another time. Some funding sources only accept proposals in response to published RFPs, but others have open calls for proposals at designated times of the year. When resubmitting your proposal, you should review your feedback carefully and make revisions to address the comments. A detailed explanation of how you addressed the reviewer comments can be included in your cover letter to the agency or explained within the proposal.

Writing a successfully funded grant proposal is a very rewarding experience and can even be fun. You should approach the process as a contest and continually strategize about what you can do to make your submission stronger. Once you are funded, you are responsible to deliver the product as proposed—you have essentially established a contract with the funding source. Included in that contract is the fact that you may be committing yourself to employment at a site for a specified period of time. Many grants cannot be "ported," or moved to another organization, even in the same community, and some funding sources may stop funding if key personnel cited in the proposal leave the organization and there is doubt whether those remaining are qualified or able to finish the project. In addition, a part of the understood contract is that you are typically not free to significantly alter your program (objectives, procedures, budget) without permission from the funding source. Additional resources for helping you with the process of finding funding sources and preparing effective grant proposals are included at the end of the chapter.

Communicating in Virtual Meetings and Social Media

Over the last decade there has been an explosion in the use of social media websites and the use of electronic mechanisms for communication. As a result, conducting meetings using these forms of media has become commonplace. These communication formats and tools allow occupational therapy managers an ever-widening opportunity to communicate. Using these tools effectively requires the development of a unique set of communication skills and new challenges that come with use of the medium.

Common Virtual Work Tools

The various types of online and wireless communication and the virtual work tools available to us continue to evolve, and it appears inevitable that electronic and wireless communication tools will continue to become more commonplace. Braveman (2013) summarized some of the common types of virtual communication's work tools, which are presented in Table 5-3.

Advantages and Cautions

There are great advantages in terms of time, cost, and efficiency in the use of virtual communication, but there are also cautions that should be considered. For example, it is not uncommon for virtual written communication to quickly become informal; this increases the likelihood that misunderstandings may occur. It is all too easy to unintentionally insult others and it is critical to remain aware that once you post information in an electronic format you lose control of the information, who will read it, and who they will share it with. Because these sites can blur the lines of personal and professional communication, you should use them with caution.

Skills and Strategies for Running Effective Virtual Meetings

As a leader or as a participant, it is important to understand that there are stated or *explicit* rules, as well as unstated (tacit) or *implicit* rules. Implicit rules are often related to the culture of the group or organization in which the meeting is occurring. Group cultures include the values and beliefs of a group that drive shared understandings about rites, rituals, and behaviors. Because these beliefs are frequently unwritten, it can be easy to violate them. Before running your first virtual meeting, it is wise to consider the following:

1. Who will be attending?
2. Do you know all of the participants?

TABLE 5-3	
Common Types of Virtual Communication Work Tools	
Listservs and Bulletin Boards	Allow for creation and management of electronic distribution lists and the ability to communicate with multiple people at the same time. Discussions are often by topic, allowing participants to participate in focused virtual discussions.
Virtual Live Meetings	Use Web conferencing software or websites to hold virtual meetings over the Internet. Participants can deliver a presentation, collaborate and edit documents, or hold a typical business meeting while physically being in different locations. There is often a cost for this type of service and the features vary from product to product.
Social Media Sites	Social media sites such as Facebook® or the recently introduced OTConnections© allow participants to share information ranging from blogs to photos, or to update others about their current activities. OTConnections© (which is owned and operated by AOTA) can be used to conduct asynchronous meetings. Asynchronous means that messages are posted at the convenience of the poster and other participants are not necessarily at their computers viewing the same information at the same time.
Podcasts	Podcasts are audio files available for download so that you may listen to them at your convenience. Podcasts are useful to communicate with workers on various shifts or people in different time zones. Newer forms of podcasting allow for the integration of images with the audio file, which can enrich the learning environment.

3. Do you have an established relationship with the participants, or will this be your first opportunity to make an impression?
4. Think about your first posts and interactions as an opportunity to create your own personal *brand image*.

Braveman (2013) identified a few common suggestions for running effective face-to-face meetings that can also be used in virtual meetings:

- Distribute an agenda in advance of the start of the meeting with discussion items listed and include a time frame for each item.
- Clearly state the start and end time of the meeting and do not deviate from these time frames without the agreement of group members.
- Establish ground rules to guide meeting behavior such as being logged on and "in" the meeting before the stated start time and having all phones on "mute" so that the meeting is not disturbed by background noise.
- Decide how members will indicate that they wish to ask a question or comment. Are you using a system (in synchronous meetings) that allows someone to virtually *raise his or her hand*?
- Decide how you will decide. How will decisions be made? Do you have time to work for

consensus, or will you allow decision-making by voting? If you will be voting, will members state their vote publicly, and so on?
- Consider starting the meeting with an icebreaker if members are new to each other. This can vary from simple introductions to sharing more in-depth information about each person's background and experience.

Preparing Group Members to Effectively Handle Virtual Meeting Agendas and Business

Preparing members for participation in a virtual meeting or for conducting business in an ongoing manner online can require a great deal of time and can be more complex than one might expect. However, the more prepared and the better informed the participants are, the more likely they will be to actively contribute to your group's work. Helping to prepare group members for virtual work goes beyond setting ground rules, an agenda, and shared expectations. It is also important to prepare members technically. You must make sure that participants have the necessary hardware, software, and access to be online at the right times. Some participants may need technical assistance to download the software needed for some online meeting formats. Reliable Internet access may be an issue for some participants, whereas use of the software or program may be an issue for others. Younger workers may have grown up using platforms like Facebook or OTConnections©; however, there are many people in today's workforce who are less technologically savvy and may require additional coaching to find the meeting, know how to post, and know how to manage multiple discussions that are occurring at the same time. Braveman (2013) also shared strategies for helping to prepare your participants for a virtual meeting:

1. Send directions for joining the meeting several times in advance. If using a Web-conferencing system that requires downloading software, strongly encourage participants to do that ahead of the meeting.
2. Offer a training session that demonstrates the Web-conferencing program or social media site to be used. Send screen shots if possible to make directions clearer.
3. Establish a practice site. If you will be running multiple discussion threads, set up at least two mock discussions and have participants practice posting.
4. Ask that all participants be "at" the meeting (i.e., sign on and call in) 15 minutes before your first meeting.
5. For large groups, have several volunteers who will be willing to work one-to-one with participants who have trouble. The volunteers can call the participants who are struggling and walk them through any procedure he or she is struggling with.

Ending the Virtual Meeting

Bringing a virtual meeting to a close has much in common with the process of ending a face-to-face meeting. First, assure that everyone is in agreement that the planned business has been concluded. Second, give participants an opportunity to identify business that they would like to have added to the next meeting agenda. Third, consider the "thank you" or other messages you may want to share before adjourning the meeting. Thank those who made special contributions and "first-timers" for attending, and acknowledge any participant who may be leaving the group. Finally, be sure that everyone is clear about the next steps and when the next meeting will occur if you will be having one.

SBAR Communication in Medical Settings

Clear and effective communication is important in all settings in which occupational therapy practitioners work, but can be especially critical for its impact on others in medical settings such as hospitals. The SBAR communication technique is an approach to standardized communication that provides a logical sequence of communicating key medical information (Massachusetts Department of Higher Education, 2007). SBAR stands for situation, background, assessment, and recommendation. For example:

- Situation includes the reason you are calling or contacting another provider, what is currently happening, and a short explanation.
- Background includes specific and critical historical information related to the current situation, including how it happened and any circumstances that caused the situation, that the other provider must know to take appropriate action.
- Assessment includes an evaluation or definition of the current problem that must be addressed.
- Recommendation includes suggestions of what should be done to address and resolve the problem or the action you are recommending to the other practitioner.

SBAR communication can be employed in critical situations, such as when contacting a physician to communicate concern over a patient's deteriorating status, or it can be employed in more common situations, such as end-of-shift "handoffs" from one practitioner to another.

Chapter Summary

This chapter introduced you to the wide range of theories that have been developed to explain communication, including theories of interpersonal communication, communication to the public and groups, communication through mass media, and intercultural communication. You learned that the many theories of communication are sometimes organized according to seven "traditions" of communication research, and you were provided with an introduction to a number of theories that are useful for the occupational therapy manager, including *cybernetics* and information theory, *dramatism* and narrative, and proxemics and expectancy violation theory.

In addition, this chapter provided you with a basic introduction to common problems in verbal and written communication and to some strategies for improving the effectiveness of your communication during conversations, in presentations, and in various forms of business writing. Although there are strategies specific to each form of communication, paying close attention to what is said or written (content), how it is said or written (delivery), and the context of the communication can help you prepare so that there is a greater likelihood that your listener or audience receives the same message that you intend to send.

Occupational therapy managers spend much of their time involved in interpersonal communication, and developing skills through conscious effort and practice is a valuable investment of time. Luckily, many resources are available to guide you in your practice. Some of those resources are listed at the end of this chapter, but many more can be found by conducting an Internet search or visiting your local library or bookstore.

■ Real-Life Solutions

At the beginning of the chapter, you were introduced to Charlotte, a fieldwork student who had received some feedback indicating that she needed to improve her communication skills. Charlotte agreed to prepare an in-service education program for the staff members of the unit to which she was assigned on strategies for effective interpersonal communication.

Charlotte began to prepare for her in-service for the unit staff by visiting the local university library. She was pleased to find that there was a large selection of books on communication that addressed both communication theory and "hands-on" strategies for improving various types of communication. She had difficulty understanding how some of the theories might be helpful at first, but found a number of introductory communication textbooks that organized theories using a variety of frameworks. By investigating these frameworks, she began to see that some communication theories were more easily applied to communication in the work environment than others, and that, just like occupational therapy theory, no single theory seemed to provide everything she would need for every type of communication or context.

As Charlotte read about some of the theories, she could easily see how they might be utilized to guide her communication. She was surprised to find narrative theory as a theory of communication because she had read a number of research studies in occupational therapy that used narrative approaches to explore interactions with clients. She also found that she and some of the unit staff members discussed issues related to proxemics and violation expectancy theory without realizing there was a theory that addressed issues of personal space.

In addition to including an overview of several of the most relevant theories of communication, Charlotte decided to provide staff with some handouts that listed specific strategies for improving communication during conversations, in presentations, and in written communication. She found strategies and information on paralinguistics and nonverbal communication especially helpful because much of the feedback she had received about her own style involved mismatches between the content of her communication and how it was conveyed. She chose to include resources from university communication department websites, from commercial websites, and from government websites (she also included information on evaluating websites!).

Finally, Charlotte was proud to be able to pass on valuable information on business writing and grant writing to her supervisor, who had recently suggested at a staff meeting that the occupational therapy staff should investigate possible alternative sources of funding to expand elements of their programming for the most at-risk populations.

Study Questions

1. **Which of the following are examples of common challenges faced by communicators regardless of the mode of communication?**

   a. *Communicator acceptability*, or identifying the characteristics of the audience, how they might respond, and what the likely rewards or punishments for communication might be

   b. *Signification*, or choosing the appropriate verbal and nonverbal means to create meaningful messages, accurately interpreting the signs from the communication partner or audience, and making the greatest impact on the listener

   c. *Achieving communicative outcomes*, or discovering how you can construct a message in order to most effectively achieve the goal for your intended communication

   d. All of the above

2. **A key element of Shannon and Weaver's *information theory* related to improving the reliability and use of information is:**

   a. Reduction of uncertainty.

   b. Visual mapping.

   c. Information coding.

   d. None of the above.

3. **A theory of communication often used in occupational therapy that helps us examine interpersonal communication through the use of stories and storytelling is best named:**

   a. Proxemics.

   b. Dramatism.

   c. Cybernetics.

   d. Narrative.

4. **Paralinguistics is best described as:**

   a. Aspects of communication not related to content or words, such as tone, pitch, inflection, or volume.

   b. The study of cultural influence on how words originate and their meaning.

   c. Aspects of communication that relate to expectations established between the person speaking and the person listening and what happens when these expectations are violated.

   d. The study of the influence of space on interpersonal communication.

5. **Which of the following is true in regard to expectancy violations theory?**

   a. EVT supports the notion by Hall that there is a most desirable personal space that remains constant across cultures.

   b. A violation of expectations can be perceived as either positive or negative.

   c. Violations in expectations are always undesirable because they lower attention and make it less likely that your message will be heard.

   d. All of the above are true.

6. **A common type of business document that outlines the needs, costs, and benefits of a new program in order to justify obtaining new resources would best be called a:**

   a. Grant request for proposals.

   b. Market analysis.

   c. Business plan.

   d. SWOT plan.

7. **Which of the following is most accurate regarding communication in virtual meetings and social media?**

   a. Use of virtual meetings and social media is uncommon and not recommended for effective communication in occupational therapy practice.

   b. The strategies for virtual meetings are essentially the same as in face-to-face meetings.

   c. These meetings are preferred because the implicit and explicit rules for participation are more commonly understood.

   d. There can be significant advantages in terms of time, cost, and efficiency, but you must be careful of some of the inherent problems with using these communication venues.

8. **The four elements of SBAR communication are:**

   a. Situation, background, assessment, resolution.

   b. Symptoms, background, assessment, recommendation.

   c. Situation, background, assessment, recommendation.

   d. Symptoms, background, appraisal, resolution.

Resources for Learning More About Communication

Journals Related to Communication

Communication Theory

http://onlinelibrary.wiley.com/journal/10.1111/(ISSN)1468-2885

Communication Theory publishes original quantitative and qualitative research related to the theoretical development of communication from varied disciplines, such as communication studies, sociology, psychology, political science, cultural and gender studies, philosophy, linguistics, and literature.

Writer's Digest

http://www.writersdigest.com

Writer's Digest, a popular magazine for writers, provides a wide range of informational, instructional, and inspirational offerings for writers. Examples of such offerings include a variety of books, magazines, special interest publications, educational courses, conferences, websites, and more.

Associations Concerned With Communication

The American Communication Association

http://www.americancomm.org/

The American Communication Association (ACA) is a not-for-profit organization, a virtual professional association with actual presence in the world of scholars and practitioners alike. The ACA was created to promote academic and professional research, criticism, teaching, practical use, and exchange of principles and theories of human communication. The ACA embraces researchers, teachers, businesspersons, and specialists located in North, Central, and South America and in the Caribbean.

Resources for Learning More About Writing Grant Proposals

The Foundation Center

http://www.fdncenter.org/

The Foundation Center's mission is to support and improve philanthropy by promoting public understanding of the field and helping grant seekers succeed. The center collects, organizes, and communicates information on U.S. philanthropy, conducts and facilitates research on trends in the field, provides education and training on the grant-seeking process, and ensures public access to information and services through its website, print and electronic publications, five library or learning centers, and a national network of cooperating collections.

The Catalog of Federal Domestic Assistance

https://www.cfda.gov

The online Catalog of Federal Domestic Assistance provides access to a database of all federal programs available to state and local governments (including the District of Columbia); federally recognized Indian tribal governments; territories (and possessions) of the United States; domestic public, quasi-public, and private profit and nonprofit organizations and institutions; specialized groups; and individuals. After you find the program you want, contact the office that administers the program and find out how to apply.

The Grantsmanship Center

http://www.tgci.com

The Grantsmanship Center (TGCI) was founded in 1972 to offer training and low-cost publications and other resources to nonprofit organizations and government agencies. The TGCI conducts annual workshops in grantsmanship and proposal writing. The *Grantsmanship Center Magazine*, published by the TGCI, is mailed to the staff of 200,000 nonprofit and government agencies in the United States and 58 other countries. TGCI's *Winning Grant Proposals Online* collects the best of funded federal grant proposals annually and makes them available on CD-ROM. The TCGI proposal-writing guide, *Program Planning and Proposal Writing* (PP&PW), is a widely read resource for both new and experienced grant seekers.

Reference List

Alpha Books. (2002). Business writing. In J. Chisolm (Ed.), *Every manager's desk reference* (pp. 826–920). Indianapolis, IN: Pearson Education.

Boydell, K. M., Goering, P., & Morrell-Bellai, T. L. (2000). Narratives of identity: Re-presentation of self in people who are homeless. *Qualitative Health Research, 10*(1), 26–38.

Braveman, B. (2013). Conducting online meetings: A new form of communication. In R. V. Whitney & C. A. Davis (Eds.), *A writer's toolkit for occupational therapy and health professionals* (pp. 259–276). Bethesda, MD: AOTA Press.

Braveman, B., Helfrich, C., Kielhofner, G., & Albrecht, G. (2003). The narratives of 12 men living with AIDS. *Journal of Occupational Rehabilitation, 13*, 143–147.

Brunner, J. (1986). *Actual minds, possible words.* Cambridge, MA: Harvard University Press.

Burgoon, J. K. (1978). A communication model of personal space violations: Explication and initial test. *Human Communication Research, 4*, 130–146.

Burgoon, J. K., Stern, L. A., & Dillman, L. (1995). *Interpersonal adaptation: Dyadic interaction patterns.* New York, NY: Cambridge University Press.

Bury, M. (2001). Illness narratives: Fact or fiction? *Social Health and Illness, 23*, 263–285.

Cisneros, J. D., McCauliff, K. L., & Beasley, V. B. (2009). The rhetorical perspective, doing, being, shaping and seeing. In D. W. Stacks & M. B. Salwen (Eds.), *An integrated approach to communication theory and research* (pp. 232–244). New York, NY: Routledge.

Crepeau, E. B., & Cohn, E. S. (2014). Narrative as a key to understanding. In B. A. Boyt Schell, G. Gillen, & M. E. Scaffa (Eds.), *Willard & Spackman's occupational therapy* (12th ed., pp. 96–102). Philadelphia, PA: Wolters Kluwer-Lippincott Williams and Wilkins.

Dahl, S. (2001). Communications and culture transformation. *Stephweb.com.* Retrieved from http://www.stephweb.com/capstone/

Dainton, M., & Zelley, E. D. (2011). *Applying communication theory for professional life* (2nd ed.). Thousand Oaks, CA: Sage Publications, Inc.

Dreachslin, J. L., Gilbert, M. J., & Malone, B. (2013). *Diversity and cultural competence in health care.* San Francisco, CA: Jossey-Bass.

Fisher, W. R. (1987). *Human communication as narration: Toward a philosophy of reason, value, and action.* Columbia, SC: University of South Carolina Press.

Fisher, W. R. (1989). Clarifying the narrative paradigm. *Communication Monographs, 56*, 55–58.

Fredriksson, L., & Erikson, K. (2001). The hidden disability dilemma for the preservation of self. *Journal of Occupational Science, 2*(1), 13–21.

Gergen, M. M., & Gergen, K. J. (1983). Narrative of the self. In T. R. Sarbin & K. E. Scheibe (Eds.), *Studies in social identity* (pp. 254–272). New York, NY: Prager.

Griffin, E. (2000). *A first look at communication theory* (4th ed.). New York, NY: McGraw-Hill.

Griffin, E. (2011). *A first look at communication theory* (5th ed.). New York, NY: McGraw-Hill.

Hall, E. T. (1966). *The hidden dimension.* New York, NY: Anchor Books.

Handy, R., & Kurtz, P. (1964). A current appraisal of the behavioral sciences: Communication theory. *American Behavioral Scientist, 7*, 99–104.

Helfrich, C., & Kielhofner, G. (1994). Volitional narratives and the meaning of therapy. *American Journal of Occupational Therapy, 48*, 318–326.

Helfrich, C., Kielhofner, G., & Mattingly, C. (1994). Volition as narrative: An understanding of motivation in chronic illness. *American Journal of Occupational Therapy, 42*, 311–317.

Ingvar, F., Joakim, O., & Ingegerd, B. (2000). On the use of narratives in nursing research. *Journal of Advanced Nursing, 32*, 695–703.

Jonsson, H., Josephsson, S., & Kielhofner, G. (2000). Evolving narratives in the course of retirement: A longitudinal study. *American Journal of Occupational Therapy, 54*, 463–470.

Kielhofner, G., Borell, L., Burke, J., Helfrich, C., & Nygård, L. (1995). Volition subsystem. In G. Kielhofner (Ed.), *A model of human occupation: Theory and application* (2nd ed., pp. 39–62). Baltimore, MD: Williams & Wilkins.

Kielhofner, G., Borell, L., Freidheim, L., Goldstein, K., Helfrich, C., Jonsson, H., . . . Nygard, L. (2002). Crafting occupational life. In G. Kielhofner (Ed.), *Model of human occupation: Theory and application* (3rd ed., pp. 124–144). Baltimore, MD: Williams & Wilkins.

Kielhofner, G., Braveman, B., Finlayson, M., Paul-Ward, A., Goldbaum, L., & Goldstein, K. (2004). Outcomes of a vocational program for people with AIDS. *American Journal of Occupational Therapy, 51*, 64–72.

Kluwin, T. N., McAngus, A., & Feldman, D. M. (2001). The limits of narratives in understanding teacher thinking. *American Annals of Deafness, 146*, 420–428.

Krippendorf, K. (2009). *On communicating: Otherness, meaning and information.* New York, NY: Routledge.

Laskowski, L. (2002). *Five effective ways to make your body speak.* Retrieved from http://www.ljlseminars.com/bodyspeaks.htm

Lee, C. S. (2001). The use of narrative in understanding how cancer affects development: The stories of one cancer survivor. *Journal of Health Psychology, 6*, 283–293.

Lieblich, A., Tuval-Mashiach, R., & Zibler, T. (1998). *Narrative research.* Thousand Oaks, CA: Sage.

Lindström, M., Sjöström, S., & Lindberg, M. (2013). Stories of rediscovering agency home-based occupational therapy for people with severe psychiatric disability. *Qualitative Health Research, 1049732313482047.*

Littlejohn, S., & Foss, K. A. (2010). *Theories of human communication* (10th ed.). Long Grove, IL: Waveland Press.

Massachusetts Department of Higher Education. (2007). *Communication and documentation.* Retrieved from http://www.mass.edu/mcncps/orientation/m1Documentation.asp

Mattingly, C. (1998). *Healing dramas and clinical plots: The narrative structure of experience.* Cambridge, UK: Cambridge University Press.

Mattingly, C. (2007). Acted narratives: From storytelling to inquiry. Mapping a methodology. In J. C. Clandinin (Ed.), *Handbook of narrative inquiry* (pp. 405–425). Thousand Oaks, CA: Sage Publications.

Meister, M., & Japp, P. M. (1999). Analyzing narratives of expertise: Toward the development of a burkeian pentadic scheme. *Sociology Quarterly, 40*, 587–613.

Nochi, M. (2001). Reconstructing self-narratives in coping with traumatic brain injury. *Social Science and Medicine, 51*, 1795–1804.

Notes Desk. (2013). *The seven C's of effective business communication.* Retrieved from http://www.notesdesk.com/notes/

business-communications/the-seven-cs-of-effective-business-communication/.

Park, D. W., & Pooley, J. (2008). *The history of media and communication research*. New York, NY: Peter Lang Publishing.

Polkinghorne, D. E. (1988). *Narrative knowing and the human sciences*. Albany, NY: State University of New York Press.

Ricoeur, P. (1984). *Time and narrative*. Chicago, IL: The University of Chicago Press.

Ricoeur, P. (1991). *From text to action: Essays in hermeneutics, II*. Evanston, IL: Northwestern University Press.

Riessman, C. K. (1990). Strategic uses of narrative in the presentation of self and illness: A research note. *Social Science and Medicine, 30*, 1195–1200.

Ritts, V., & Stein, J. R. (2014). *Six ways to improve your nonverbal communications*. Retrieved from TLSIG website: http://www.tlsig.cba.neu.edu/tip-5-fall-2011/

Robinson, I. (1990). Personal narratives, social careers, and medical courses: Analysing life trajectories in autobiographies of people with multiple sclerosis. *Social Science and Medicine, 30*, 173–186.

Sanchia, A., & Street, A. (2001). From individual to group: Use of narratives in a participatory research process. *Journal of Advanced Nursing, 33*, 791–797.

Shannon, C. E., & Weaver. W. (1949). *The mathematical theory of communication*. Urbana, IL: University of Illinois Press.

Small Business Administration. (2014). *Create your business plan*. Retrieved from http://www.sba.gov/category/navigation-structure/starting-managing-business/starting-business/how-write-business-plan

Trenholm, S. (1991). *Human communication theory* (2nd ed.). Englewood Cliffs, NJ: Prentice Hall.

Trenholm, S., & Jensen, A. (2011). *Interpersonal communication* (7th ed.). New York, NY: Oxford University Press.

University of Texas at Austin. (2013). *Department of Communication Studies*. Retrieved from http://commstudies.utexas.edu/research

U.S. Department of Health and Human Services. (2013). *Sample business associate agreement provisions*. Retrieved from http://www.hhs.gov/ocr/hipaa/contractprov.html#2

Roles and Functions of Managers: Planning, Organizing and Staffing, Directing, and Controlling

Brent Braveman, PhD, OTR/L, FAOTA

■ **Real-Life Management**

Marty was recently hired as director of occupational therapy services for a small occupational therapy department in a community hospital. He is excited about this new opportunity and confident in his leadership skills. However, Marty has only been practicing as an occupational therapist (OT) for a few years. He thinks that he began to develop solid skills as a supervisor in his last position through experiences supervising fieldwork students and several occupational therapy assistants (OTAs). In addition, he had some prior experience supervising staff in an earlier career as a director of marketing for a community-based agency. However, he is concerned that he may be getting himself in over his head. Marty has always been a self-directed learner

and is confident that, if he can identify the new tasks that he will have to perform, he can seek out information and resources to help him in his new job. As a place to start, he begins to conduct information interviews with other occupational therapy managers in his local area to identify the most common roles and functions that they perform in their daily work. To help make his interviews more effective, he develops the following questions:

1. What are the most common functions that you serve for your organization in your role as a manager?

2. What are some of the specific skills I will need to learn to run and manage my department?

3. What do I need to learn to help the employees that I supervise grow and develop as occupational therapy professionals?

Critical Thinking Questions

As you read this chapter, consider the following questions:

- What do the four commonly identified functions of managers (e.g., planning, organizing and staffing, directing, and controlling) have to do with the day-to-day functioning of an occupational therapy department?

- How can you categorize the management tasks, including recruitment, hiring, discipline, and financial and information management, into one of the four management functions?

- What are some of the variety of activities commonly completed by occupational therapy managers that require the development of a wide range of skill sets not learned in your entry-level education?

- What are some of the ways that managers interact with other professionals in organizations to complete complex tasks such as financial planning, recruiting and retaining staff, or planning new clinical spaces and facilities?

Glossary

- **Controlling:** the process of establishing performance standards and measuring, evaluating, and correcting performance.
- **Directing:** the process of providing guidance and leadership so that the work performed is goal oriented.
- **Organizing:** the process of designing workable units, determining lines of authority and communication, and developing and managing patterns of coordination.
- **Planning:** the process of deciding what to do by setting performance objectives and identifying the activities needed to accomplish these activities.
- **Requisite managerial authority:** the level of control and discretion that a manager must have

to be fairly held responsible for the outcomes of work groups, including the authority to hire and fire employees and determine rewards.
- **Skill mix:** the appropriate ratio of OTs, OTAs, and service extenders or aides needed to provide care that is effective but also cost efficient.
- **Staffing:** the process of assuring that the right person is completing the right tasks within predetermined work units and that these persons have the necessary skills to do the job.
- **Strategic planning:** the process of determining the long-term goals of an organization, developing concrete measures of success and achievement, and formulating the strategies and general action plans needed to accomplish these goals.

Introduction

Chapter 1 introduced the topic of leadership, and reviewed the primary theories related to leadership as well as evidence supporting each theory. The relationship between leadership and management was

discussed and the four functions of a manager (i.e., planning, organizing and staffing, directing, and controlling) were briefly introduced. Chapters 6 and 7 provide an overview of what managers and supervisors "do" as well as a sample of theories and evidence that can be used to guide the work of a manager or supervisor. Chapter 6 explores key areas of each of the managerial functions in more depth, whereas Chapter 7 focuses specifically on the roles and functions of managers as supervisors. As you read these two chapters, you should keep in mind that the roles and functions of managers and supervisors are closely related. Later, in Chapter 17, some of the key concepts presented in these two chapters are applied to promoting evidence-based and occupation-based practice within a *community of practice*.

Managers by their very nature supervise the work of others; however, in many of the settings in which occupational therapy practitioners are employed, it is not always true that those asked to assume supervisory responsibilities have full managerial control. An important difference that distinguishes a manager from a supervisor is that of **requisite managerial authority**. Elliot Jaques (1998) defined requisite managerial authority as the level of control and discretion that a manager must have to be fairly held responsible for the outcomes of work groups. Requisite managerial authority includes the authority to hire and fire employees, an authority that many supervisors do not possess.

Managers are usually concerned with solving problems with long-range implications and planning for the future of work units, such as departments or an entire organization. Mary Parker Follet, an early organizational theorist, said that, "Management is the art of getting things done through other people" (Daft & Marcic, 2011). Although this may be what managers often do, it is through the process of supervision that managers interact with employees who "get things done." Peter Drucker (1974) encouraged us to define management and supervision by emphasizing the contribution that managers and supervisors make to organizations and not the amount of responsibility and control they have. By doing so, we place the emphasis for the manager and supervisor on the goals of management and supervision rather than on the subordinate; this prevents the manager or supervisor from becoming primarily a controller rather than a leader.

When considering management and supervision, it is important to recognize that, although there are overlaps between the two functions, the focus of top management in most organizations is certainly different from that of first-line supervisors. The focus of top management and first-line supervision for common management functions vary but are clearly

---

BOX 6-1

Commonly Identified Functions of Management

- **Planning:** The process of deciding what to do by setting performance objectives and identifying the activities needed to accomplish these activities
- **Organizing and staffing:** Designing workable units, determining lines of authority and communication, and developing and managing patterns of coordination
- **Directing:** Providing guidance and leadership so that the work performed is goal oriented
- **Controlling:** Establishing performance standards and measuring, evaluating, and correcting performance

---

related. These functions (i.e., planning, organizing and staffing, directing, and controlling) are briefly defined in Box 6-1, and the focus of managers versus supervisors is compared in Table 6-1. These common management functions will help set the stage for understanding the manager's roles and functions and are explored in more depth in subsequent sections of this chapter.

Planning

Planning is the process of establishing short-term and long-term goals, measurable objectives, and action plans related to the organization's mission. Goals are usually distinguished from objectives in terms of the scope of the accomplishment.

Objectives are measurable steps that are taken to reach a goal that is a major accomplishment related to the organization's or system's output. In addition to establishing goals and objectives, planning includes determining the needs for the human resources, materials, supplies, facilities, and equipment required to meet goals and objectives. Sometimes the words *goals* and *objectives* can be reversed; the objective is the

TABLE 6-1

Functions of Management: Comparison of Focus of Top Management Versus First-Line Supervisors

Function	Focus of Top Management	Focus of First-Line Supervisors
Planning Forecasting Budgeting Establishing objectives Scheduling Developing policies	• Long range • Growth • Capital procurement • Service mix • Initiating • Overall financial	• Short range • Day-to-day • Week-to-week • Converting "what" to "how to" • Activities lists • Scheduling tasks and facilities
Organizing Designing the organization Establishing work relationships Workflow Delegating	• Overall structure • Establishing lines of responsibility and authority • Determining line and staff relationships	• Coordination of people, equipment, and supplies to accomplish results • More concerned with relationships between things and specific activities than with overall structure
Staffing Recruiting Hiring Promotion Training Development	• Developing personnel policies • Providing total training system to support • Negotiating union contracts	• Hiring good staff • Training and developing workers • Assessing staff needs
Directing Motivating Leading	• Modeling good behavior • Developing and promoting a positive overall approach to leadership • Providing a good image in the community	• Leading in such a way as to create a positive climate in which workers operate with optimum efficiency and professionalism
Controlling Establishing standards Measuring, evaluating, and correcting performance	• Monitoring total organizational results • Setting standards and goals	• Tracking work in progress • Appraising work and results • Correcting performance

longer-term outcome and the goals are the measurable steps taken to reach an objective. Don't let the interchange of these terms confuse you, as the main ideas and approaches remain the same. Writing the policies and procedures that guide the use of materials, supplies, facilities, and equipment, as well as guide staff in daily activities, is also commonly considered a component of planning, as is the financial planning involved in developing and managing a department budget. Some simple

guidelines for effective planning are included in Box 6-2.

Operational Planning Versus Strategic Planning

Managers are responsible for planning for the day-to-day activities within a department and organization

---

BOX 6-2

Guidelines for Effective Planning

- Make plans specific and measurable, avoiding vague indicators or terminology.
- Be neither too idealistic nor too practical and limited.
- Avoid underplanning by recognizing potential roadblocks and developing contingency plans, as well as overplanning by not being too rigid or detailed to allow flexibility.
- Communicate plans consistently and concisely to those above and below you in the organization and ensure two-way communication.
- Assign clear responsibilities for completing plan activities and monitoring progress on goals and objectives.
- Troubleshoot plans before their implementation.

---

but are also responsible for longer-term planning. This longer-term planning, commonly referred to as **strategic planning,** is the process of determining the long-term goals of an organization, developing concrete measures of success and achievement, and formulating the strategies and general action plans to accomplish these goals. Over the last several decades, strategic planning has come in and out of favor as organizations have struggled to keep up with the almost frenetic changes in technology and the economy. And yet, operating in an environment fraught with change may be when long-term planning, especially the processes of *mission review* and of *visioning*, becomes most important. Strategic planning, including mission and vision statements, is discussed briefly in this chapter and more fully in Chapter 9.

Given the demands for high productivity in most of today's workplaces, it is sometimes difficult to convince managers and staff members to take time from their busy schedules to think creatively about the future. A precursor to beginning or revising a strategic plan should be to spend some time reviewing—and perhaps revising—a department's mission and vision

statements. A mission statement is a setting forth of an organization's or department's purpose, including definition, products, and services. A vision statement expresses the aspirational and inspirational messages about what a department or organization would like to become as it seeks to fulfill its mission.

Mission Statements

Mission statements are typically established by an organization's founders and usually remain fairly stable over time, although, as discussed in Chapter 4, they can sometimes become diluted or lose focus as organizations age and come to serve not only the purpose for which they were created, but also the practical purpose of providing a source of income for their employees. Although most organizations have established mission statements, many individual departments do not. The process of writing a departmental mission statement can help to refocus and re-energize staff members by helping them better understand the role they serve within an organization and the beliefs and values they hold in common. These beliefs and values are what hold them together as a "community of practice." The concept of a community of practice is explored in more depth in Chapter 17.

Mission statements often communicate the answer to four questions that provide an organization's internal and external publics with an understanding of the organization's role in society:

1. Why does the organization exist?
2. What function does the organization perform?
3. For whom does the organization perform this function or who are the primary beneficiaries?
4. How does the organization go about filling this function?

There is a wide variety in the length and style of mission statements for different organizations. Some mission statements can be as short as a single sentence and may only imply the answer to some of the questions listed here, whereas others can be relatively lengthy and provide additional information. Regardless, a mission statement should be used often as a management tool to guide planning and to direct resources. Time and other resources are not limitless, and choosing to invest them in one direction means they cannot be invested in another. By asking the question, "Is this central to our mission?" you can use your mission statement as a tool in carry out the daily functions as a manager.

Vision Statements

Elaine Hom (2013) described the nature and importance of vision statements to organizations. She stated, "Aspirational in nature, vision statements lay out the most important primary goals for a company. Not to be confused with business plans vision statements generally don't outline a plan to achieve those goals. But by outlining the key objectives for a company, they enable the company's employees to develop business strategies to achieve said goals." Visioning can be a fun, creative, and motivating process that communicates the valuable role that employees can play in helping a department or organization to survive and thrive. At the same time, it is important for the person leading employees in a visioning exercise to set clear and appropriate boundaries for the exercise so employees do not become frustrated or waste time. An effective vision statement reflects a vision or dream of a future state that is both sufficiently clear and powerful to arouse and sustain the actions necessary for that dream to become a reality. However, it could be said that a vision that is not based in reality is a *mirage*. Sample portions of vision statements are listed in Box 6-3. The process of developing a vision statement may take a number of meetings during a number of weeks or even months if done in a thoughtful manner. Additional strategies for engaging staff in the process of visioning are included in Chapter 9.

BOX 6-3

Sample Portions of Vision Statements

- To become the health-care provider and employer of choice in the city of Boston
- To be a global leader in innovation in providing high-quality, cost-effective service
- To become a national model for provision of creative and highly effective fieldwork education

---

Once a vision for your department is clear, a plan of action to bring that vision about is necessary. Strategic planning is the process of developing a plan to achieve a vision. As the pace of information exchange and technological development has increased, the very definition of "long term" has changed. At one point in time it was not unusual for organizations to have strategic plans spanning up to 10 years. However, given the current pace of change, it is difficult for many organizations to look a decade into the future; many strategic plans today cover periods of 3 to 5 years.

Whether short term or strategic, the management function of planning can be complicated and should not be underestimated by the new manager. As noted, strategic planning is discussed in more detail in Chapter 9; however, a full discussion of strategic planning is beyond the scope of this book. Additional resources for further investigation are provided at the end of this chapter, and readers and new managers are encouraged to seek assistance and mentorship when first involved in formal planning activities.

Policies and Procedures

Writing the policies and procedures that guide supervisors and staff members in their daily work and in the use of materials, supplies, facilities, and equipment is a specific aspect of planning that typically rests with a department manager. Policies are statements of values that are consistent with the mission and frame the reasons for boundaries governing the services provided. Policies set the broader principles and parameters for making day-to-day decisions about operations. Most organizations have a standard format that is followed to guide managers in deciding what to include in a specific policy and procedure and in knowing which policies should be included in general in a department's policies and procedures manual. For business owners or new managers who do not find existing resources within their organizations, numerous resources are available for purchase that can be found by conducting an Internet search. These products include preformatted tables of contents and policy and procedure forms that can be customized to your department or business. Networking with other managers or business owners can help you in the process of choosing a product appropriate to your practice setting and customizing your policies and procedures

---

BOX 6-4

Basic Components of a Policy and Procedure

- **Policy statement:** A brief statement of the guiding principle to be communicated
- **Purpose statement:** A brief statement outlining the reason for inclusion of the policy and procedure
- **Scope:** Lists the employee groups to which the policy and procedure apply (e.g., all occupational therapy department staff members)
- **Materials:** Any materials needed to carry out the procedures outlined
- **Procedures:** Statements outlining the specific actions to be taken by the identified employee groups and criteria for determining adherence to the policy
- **References:** Any related policies and procedures that should also be reviewed
- **Approvals:** Names the persons responsible for oversight of the policy and procedure (e.g., all occupational therapy team leaders)
- **Implementation date and review date:** Lists the date of the last review and update of the policy and procedure (typically policies and procedures are reviewed on an annual basis)

---

manual to your setting. The basic components of a policy and procedure are included in Box 6-4 and a sample policy and procedure is included in Box 6-5.

Like mission statements, policies and procedures are most useful if they are highly visible to both management and staff. Policies and procedures should be frequently reviewed and updated as needed, and copies should be easily accessible to staff. Effective managers must not only be able to identify a policy and procedure but also be able to clearly articulate its necessity and underlying logic. In organizations such as hospitals that undergo an accreditation process by accreditors such as the Joint Commission, the organization is typically held accountable for following its own policies and procedures; therefore, keeping them up-to-date is critical. Policies and procedures can relate to processes as commonplace as requesting time off to complex processes related to surgical operations,

infection control, patient sedation, or how a "do not resuscitate" order is signed and recorded.

Financial Planning

One of the most important functions of many managers is the development and oversight of a department budget. Budgeting is both a planning and a controlling function. Financial planning and management is discussed in more depth in Chapter 11, but is discussed briefly here so that its connection to the management function of planning is clear.

Budgets are typically planned for a fiscal year. A fiscal year is a period consisting of one budget cycle that coincides with a calendar year (January 1 to December 31) or to another cyclical calendar (e.g., many organizations operate on a fiscal year that runs from July 1 to June 30). Developing and managing a budget is a complex process, and occupational therapy practitioners who have the goal of becoming a manager or director of an occupational therapy department are encouraged to attend a course on financial planning and management. Graduate education such as a master's in business administration (MBA) or master's in health administration (MHA), or an advanced degree in occupational therapy such as a clinical doctorate (OTD) may also be beneficial. Planning and managing a budget that can easily include millions of dollars of revenue and expenses in larger departments requires a working knowledge of a wide variety of information and systems, including:

- Health-care systems, including city, county, state, and national systems
- Payment and reimbursement structures such as Medicare, Medicaid, workers' compensation, private insurance, and grant and foundation support
- Human resources systems and costs, including salary and benefit administration, training and educational costs and systems, and recruitment and retention structures
- Equipment and materials purchasing and management, including medical supplies such as splinting or assistive and adaptive equipment and office and other supportive supplies
- Facilities management and improvement systems, including cleaning and maintenance of physical plant structures

BOX 6-5

Sample Policy and Procedure: Infection Control for Trial Wheelchair Cushions

Policy and Procedure: Trial Wheelchair Cushions and Infection Control

Purpose

The purpose of this policy is to minimize the risk of transmitting infections from trial wheelchair cushions from patient to patient, among treatment areas, or between patient equipment and staff.

Policy Statement

Infection control measures are particularly important when dealing with equipment that is utilized by several patients over time. Most of the special seat cushions are primarily used with those patients who have special needs because of tissue pressure problems, decubitus ulcers, pain, or positioning difficulties. Any of these patients may have infectious disease, draining wounds, or incontinence. The transmission of infection is a risk because various patients will be utilizing these items. The Department of Occupational Therapy is committed to infection control; therefore, the following procedure is to be carefully administered.

Scope of the Policy

Licensed occupational therapists (OTs), licensed occupational therapy assistants (OTAs), and occupational therapy aides

Materials

1. Institutionally approved sanitizer

Procedure

Each cushion will be checked out to the specific patient following the checkout procedure in occupational therapy.

1. All foam-based cushions must have an incontinent cushion cover on them before distribution to a patient.
2. All seat cushions will be picked up by 4:30 p.m. daily and returned to the department by an occupational therapy aide (unless preapproval is obtained by a supervisor for a specific sitting protocol).
3. Occupational therapy staff must wear gloves when handling a used cushion.
4. After the patient has completed the use of the cushion, it will be necessary for the cushion to be returned to the Occupational Therapy Department in a closed plastic bag to prevent the spread of infection during transport.
5. Once the cushion is picked up, it will be labeled as dirty and placed in the soiled utility room until appropriately cleaned by a staff member.
6. Cushions will be wiped down with the appropriate disinfectant cloth to disinfect thoroughly.
7. Roho cushions: Thoroughly wipe all of the cushion's air cells and the spaces between. Use the edge of a basin to spread the air cells for good access to the base. Cushions should have excess water taken off with a towel but will need to air dry completely.
8. Foam-based cushions: In the case of a foam-based cushion that is soiled and not able to be cleaned, a supervisor must be contacted to make a decision about discarding the cushion.
9. Cushion covers will be washed in the washing machine, dried, and placed back on the appropriate cushion.
10. All cleaned cushions will be stored in the designated location.

References

Institutional Infection Control Disinfection & Sterilization Policy (Institutional Policy # IC 412).

BOX 6-5

Sample Policy and Procedure: Infection Control for Trial Wheelchair Cushions—cont'd

APPROVALS

_____   ___/___/___

Director   Date

_____   ___/___/___

Steward   Date

Implementation Date: 08/08/2015

Review/Revision Date: 07/08/2015

Budgeting is often categorized as a planning function because it is necessary to plan or budget both your projected revenues and expenses, which can be surprisingly complicated for new programs. Occupational therapy managers who assume responsibility for existing services may rely on historical data to help them with the process of projecting work volume, revenue, and expenses. However, when planning a new program, you may have to gather data and information from outside sources and peers.

Facility Planning

Planning for new facilities and space can be daunting for occupational therapy managers if they are poorly prepared for the task. Although the accreditation standards for occupational therapy educational programs include a standard related to maintaining and organizing treatment areas, equipment, and supply inventories, few programs include detailed content related to planning and designing treatment areas. A full discussion of the process is beyond the scope of this chapter; however, it is important that you know that resources are available if needed, and that finding yourself in the position of having to guide development of an occupational therapy clinic is not unimaginable. Twice in my career as an occupational therapy department director, I have found myself responsible for planning new spaces. In both instances, it was because the

TABLE 6-2

Overview of the Stages and Steps for Planning Facilities

Stage	Step
Predesign	1. Planning team selection for those involved in facility planning 2. Preplanning
Design development	3. Detailed planning 4. Final planning 5. Keeping track of the project
Construction	6. Construction and equipment procurement
Preoperations	7. Final checkout
Occupancy and startup	8. Occupancy 9. Revisions and critique

hospitals in which I worked were building new outpatient centers and chose to move rehabilitation services into a new facility. In addition, some practitioners choose to open private practices or businesses that require planning for space and materials. Nine steps in the process of designing and planning a therapy facility are outlined in Table 6-2. You are encouraged to consult this and additional resources on planning facilities for additional information. In addition, you might consider these simple steps to better prepare you:

- Visit other facilities to get ideas for planning and look at the space used by multiple disciplines.
- Ask other managers in your facility and at others what they like best about their space and, more importantly, what mistake were made in its design.
- Have staff brainstorm a "wish list" for use of space.
- Put a blank sheet of paper on the wall in each room and have staff members make notations of problems or suggestions for new space as they think of them.

Organizing and Staffing

Organizing is the process of designing workable units, determining lines of authority and communication, and developing and managing patterns of coordination. Organizing involves creating the most effective grouping of activities together with the necessary guidelines and coordinating systems so that the organization's goals can be achieved as efficiently as possible. If carried out properly, organizing will provide clear identification of

- Who is responsible for work tasks and outputs of critical work processes
- Who has the authority to make decisions
- The functional separation of work activities
- The expected levels of performance for individuals and groups

Organizing as a management function is discussed in depth in Chapter 4, but is reviewed briefly here as well. Organizing is more often associated with mid-level or upper management than first-line supervisors. However, all levels of managers and supervisors are involved in overseeing and supporting organizational structures on a daily basis. First-line supervisors often can provide valuable input into the effectiveness of or problems with existing organizational forms. The basic steps of organizing are listed in Box 6-6.

BOX 6-6

Basic Steps of Organizing

1. Recognize organizational goals and objectives.
2. Review the internal and external organizational environments.
3. Determine the organizational and departmental structures needed to reach the goal.
4. Determine the authority of relationships, and develop organizational charts and job descriptions.

Staffing is the process of assuring that the right person is completing the right tasks within predetermined work units and that these persons have the necessary skills to do the job. Staffing ensures that the organization will have sufficient quantity and quality of personnel to achieve its mission and goals. This ongoing process accounts for recruiting, hiring, training, firing, and replacing personnel as necessary. The primary activities associated with staffing are described in Box 6-7 (Lyles & Joiner, 1986).

Human Resources Planning

Developing a staffing plan includes identifying the number, type, and qualifications of staff needed to meet the needs of a department and its customers. Staffing plans must account for the expected work volume, including fluctuations for various days of the week or seasons, and the length of time spent with each client, including the full range of billable and nonbillable services (an example of a service that is often not billable to a third-party payer or to the client is a team conference). Defining the **skill mix**, or the appropriate ratio of OTs, OTAs, and service extenders or aides needed to provide care that is effective but also cost efficient, is also part of developing a staffing plan. Finally, staffing plans must consider the skills of staff members within an employee classification. For example, in a hospital setting in which policies state that occupational therapy practitioners provide services in a neonatal intensive care unit on a

Primary Activities Associated With Staffing

- **Human resources planning:** Collaborating with management and supervisors at all levels of the organization to forecast the organization's short-term and long-term personnel needs based on the organizational mission, leadership vision, and strategic plans
- **Recruitment:** Seeking out and attracting adequate numbers of qualified personnel to meet the organizational needs on an ongoing basis, including contingencies such as resignations and leaves of absence
- **Hiring:** Selecting the appropriate personnel for vacant positions and associated activities such as benefits counseling, background, and reference checks
- **Orientation:** Introducing the new employee to organizational policies, procedures, values, personnel, and environments
- **Training and development:** Meeting the short- and long-term education and professional development needs of employees at all levels of the organization
- **Separation:** Terminating the employment of personnel because of resignation, inadequate job performance, or a decrease in organizational resources; disciplinary activities may preclude separation as necessary

7-day-a-week basis, the staffing plan must accommodate the need for an occupational therapy practitioner who has demonstrated age-specific competencies to be available each and every day. Another example would be a hospital that has an OT on call 24 hours a day to see patients in the emergency center. These OTs must have demonstrated the competency to respond to these patients, must be paid for their on-call hours, and may require compensatory time off if they are called in to work. Factors such as this can make scheduling staff and assuring appropriate staffing levels are available a complicated management task.

Recruitment and Hiring

Recruiting new employees can be fun and rewarding, but it may also be a difficult, confusing, and sometimes frustrating responsibility. It is one of the most important functions that managers perform, however, and must be approached with the utmost care and attention. Recruitment of an employee includes identification of the type of employee needed based on an established staffing plan, advertising for candidates, and screening and interviewing candidates to identify a candidate who is a good match for the vacant position.

Typically the process of identifying the type of employee needed begins by reviewing the position's job description. Often you may hire someone with skills similar to those of the last person who held the now-vacant position; however, it is important to recognize that, over time, the nature of a department's work can change with shifts in referral sources such as changes in physicians or midlevel providers or the addition or deletion of programs. Because a wide variation may exist in the salaries of an OT, an OTA, and an occupational therapy aide, comparing the work to be done against current job descriptions can help to assure that you are hiring the right type of employee and making the most effective use of resources. For example, if an experienced OT leaves an organization, his or her $88,000 salary might cover the salary of both an OTA and an occupational therapy aide. However, in making the decision to hire an OTA or occupational therapy aide, you would need to be sure that you still have a sufficient number of OTs to complete the evaluation and intervention planning tasks that are not appropriate for an OTA or occupational therapy aide. You should also consider whether the employee you are hiring needs to have prior experience or if you might be able to hire a new graduate or a practitioner with less experience. At times you may need to take advantage of the increased independence and lowered supervision needs of an experienced practitoner, whereas at other times the enthusiasm and fresh outlook that many new graduates bring, along with lower salary expectations, may justify the increased costs for training and supervision necessary for new graduates.

Advertising includes writing and placing an ad or announcement in a newspaper, professional magazine, or journal; placing an ad on a website or Listserv; or working with a professional recruiter. The best way to decide what to put in your ad is to spend time reviewing ads placed by other organizations both within and outside of health care. Advertising can be very expensive (more than $1,200 for a small ad in a single edition of some professional magazines), so you need to be sure that your advertising contains all of the necessary information to attract the sort of candidates you hope to reach while being concise and attractive or "eye catching" to the reader. The American Occupational Therapy Association (AOTA) (http://www.aota.org/) has both a professional magazine (*OT Practice*) and an Internet-based service ("OTJobLink") that sell space for employment advertisements. *Advance for Occupational Therapy Practitioners*, a private publication, is also a popular medium for advertising for new employees (http://www.advanceforot.com/). The advantage of the services just mentioned is that they allow you to recruit on a regional or national basis. This allows you to reach a broader net of potential candidates, but it also means that you may have to consider negotiating expenses for interviews or for relocation if you hire someone who is not local. Advertising in local papers, posting on a state occupational therapy association Listserv or website, or buying mailing labels (also available from AOTA and some state occupational therapy associations) allows you to narrow your recruitment to a smaller geographic area, but limits your potential candidates.

A newer development and approach to staff recruitment is the use of social media. Many organizations maintain a presence on sites such as Facebook and develop networks through sites such as LinkedIn. The advantage of these strategies is that they can be low cost and may allow almost immediate access and communication with potential candidates. The disadvantages include the staff time it takes to keep these sites and networks up-to-date. Obtaining a substantial following may require frequent, regular, and interesting posts and monitoring the sites on a daily basis to watch for feedback, questions from followers, or spam or inappropriate posts. It is very common, for example, to hear about a famous person or an organization posting a "tweet" only to remove it later because it had an unintended controversial consequence. A problem is that once something is posted, it is almost impossible to make it completely go away once users take and save screen shots or forward your message to others. The use of social media should not be taken lightly and it has become commonplace for organizations to have social media policies to manage issues like recruitment, as well as protect consumer privacy.

A different alternative for recruiting is using a professional health-care recruiter who will identify potential candidates for you and help to arrange interviews. In some ways, this saves you time and may save the expense of advertising; however, professional recruiters or "headhunters" can charge high fees if they successfully place a candidate in your organization. Often there is no fee charged unless you hire a candidate referred by the recruiter; however, if successful, the recruiter may charge a fee equal to a large portion of the employee's annual salary, so it can be an expensive method of recruitment. A disadvantage is that some potential employees are reticent to use recruiters, and you will only reach the candidate pool with which the recruiter has contact. In addition, you may waste valuable time if the recruiter is unsuccessful and end up spending money on advertising anyway. In times when there are shortages of available OTs and OTAs, you may have to consider using recruitment alternatives such as health-care recruiters or "sign-on bonuses" that you would not otherwise use. Developing and maintaining a peer network will allow you to keep up with trends in recruitment practices as they change and allow you to remain competitive.

Screening employees involves reviewing applicants' basic qualifications and experience to determine if they meet the preestablished criteria for hiring. This process is done so that you only offer interviews to candidates who might be a match for your work setting. Preestablished criteria may include factors such as whether candidates are licensed or eligible for licensure in your state, if they have the level and type of experience matching your needs, if there are large gaps in their employment history that cannot be explained, or if they can demonstrate specialized competencies related to a patient population or program (e.g., sensory integration certification). In addition, you may screen candidates out of the interview process because of poorly written cover letters or résumés, which indicate a lack of professionalism. Using preestablished criteria is important and particularly helpful when you receive a large number of résumés. When this happens, an intermediate step between screening résumés and conducting face-to-face interviews can be conducting telephone or videoconference interviews.

Videoconferencing methods can include fee-based services such as copy shops or other businesses with rental conference services available. The use of programs like "Skype" or "Face Time" through a personal computer, computer tablet, or phone may also provide a way to conduct a screening interview with more intimacy than just speaking over the phone. Interviewing is essentially a process of finding the best match between potential employees and both the open position *and* the culture of your department and organization.

An effective method of interviewing that helps to match an employee to both the job and the culture of the department and organization is attribute-based interviewing. In this approach, the desired employee's attributes are identified and described in writing, and then open-ended questions are developed that allow the interviewer to get a sense of how closely the potential employee matches the desired attributes. Examples of desirable attributes in a new occupational therapy team leader, as well as sample open-ended questions, are provided in Table 6-3. It is also important to consider who will be involved in an interview process and the extent to which those persons will be involved in selecting a preferred candidate. There may be value in including subordinates, peers both from within the occupational therapy department and from other departments, or other key supervisory and managerial personnel in the interviews.

It is also critical that managers are aware of the questions that cannot be legally asked in an interview. Asking questions about a candidate's age, his or her marital status, if he or she has children or plans to have children, or if he or she has any impairments or a disability is illegal because these questions could indicate an intent to discriminate. The U.S. Equal Employment Opportunity Commission makes it clear that it is illegal to discriminate in employment practices because of race, color, religion, sex (including pregnancy), national origin, age (40 or older), disability or genetic information (U.S. Equal Employment Opportunity Commission, 2014). Typically, human resources will provide guidance to new managers who do not have experience; however, it is easy to inadvertently offend a candidate by asking a prohibited question while attempting casual conversation to make a candidate feel more comfortable. You must remain aware that real discrimination in hiring practices occurs!

Hiring a new employee includes checking references and negotiating salary, benefits (including relocation expenses), and the date the employee will begin work. A full history of previous employment, including the start and end dates, the title of the position held by the candidate, the reason for leaving the job, and the names of supervisors, should be obtained. All previous employers should be contacted to verify that the information is correct. You should be aware that, because of fear of liability in litigation, some employers will only verify factual information and may not comment on the employee's skills or performance. Only after references are checked should a formal written offer be extended. Two copies of an offer letter, stating the rate of compensation, benefits, and starting date, along with a job description, should be mailed to the candidate. The candidate should then sign both copies, indicating acceptance of the position, and return one to you and keep the other for himself or herself.

TABLE 6-3

Sample Employee Attributes and Open-Ended Interview Questions

Employee Attribute	Open-Ended Question
Direct style of conflict management	Tell me about a time that you had to give someone you supervised some difficult feedback and how you went about doing it.
Committed to maintaining a role in patient care	If you could design your perfect job, what would be the mix of supervisory duties and patient care responsibilities?
Creative problem-solver	Tell me about a time that you faced a complex problem and how you led your team in the process of solving it.

Orientation

McNamara (2003) provided a helpful list of suggestions for orienting an employee to a new position in a manner that both provides information and makes the new employee feel welcome in his or her new organization. Some of these suggestions include:

- Send a letter of welcome before the employee begins, providing him or her with a contact number if he or she has questions.
- Meet with the employee the first day, even if just for a few moments, before he or she reports to the human resources department, if required to do so.
- Give the employee a tour of the facilities, including basics such as the location of lockers and bathrooms, kitchen and telephone use, and the location of the cafeteria, if one is present.
- Provide a schedule for the first few days.
- Provide an orientation checklist to assure that nothing is missed.
- Assign a fellow employee as a buddy to answer questions and to have lunch with the new employee on the first day. Join them for lunch if possible.
- Meet with the employee at the end of the first day.
- Meet on at least a weekly basis for the first few weeks.

Before orientation begins, you should start a departmental personnel file in which you keep copies of important documents such as the signed letter of offer and job description; a copy of the employee's license, if applicable; and a checklist of all activities completed during orientation.

Bacal (2003) noted that there are two related kinds of orientation. The first, "overview orientation," deals with the basic information an employee will need to understand the broader system he or she works in; this is often conducted by the human resources department. Overview orientation includes helping employees understand:

- The system in which the organization functions in general (e.g., schools, community, medical model)
- Important policies and general procedures (non–job specific)
- Information about compensation and benefits
- Safety and accident prevention issues
- Employee and union issues (rights, responsibilities)
- Physical facilities

The second type of orientation, "job-specific orientation," is the process used to help employees understand:

- The function of the organization, and how the employee fits in
- Job responsibilities, expectations, and duties of the employee
- Policies, procedures, rules, and regulations
- Layout of the workplace

An important part of the orientation process for occupational therapy personnel is the assessment of competencies. Competencies are specific statements of an individual's ability to perform a specific skill or activity in a particular situation. Assessment of competencies is discussed in more depth in Chapter 12. Although some competencies should be assessed on an annual basis, especially in organizations subject to accreditation by bodies such as the Joint Commission, others may only be assessed at the time of initial orientation. For example, an employee's understanding of procedures related to electrical or fire safety or to blood-borne pathogens should be assessed on an annual basis. Other competencies, such as the ability to safely transfer a patient or to fabricate a common splint, might only be assessed as part of the orientation process.

Training, Education, and Development

McNamara (2003) identified a variety of reasons for organizations to provide for the training and development of employees. These reasons include:

- When a performance appraisal indicates performance improvement is needed
- To "benchmark" the status of improvement so far in a performance improvement effort
- As part of an overall professional development program
- As part of succession planning to help an employee be eligible for a planned change in role in the organization
- To train about a specific topic to meet customer service or other needs of the department or organization

Schein (1992) differentiated the functions of training, education, and development. The differences in these functions relate to the focus of the learning activity and when it will be applied in an employee's professional development. Briefly, these functions can be described as follows:

- *Training activities* are related to improving an employee's capacity to perform his or her current job, such as learning a new treatment technique related to a patient population that he or she currently treats.
- *Education activities* are related to improving an employee's capacity for a specific but future job, such as a staff therapist taking an introductory course on supervising others.
- *Development activities* are related to overall capacities that may be used in any job, such as time management or communication skills.

The manager of a department is typically responsible for integrating information from multiple systems to identify and meet the training, education, and development needs of staff. These systems include employee performance appraisals, competency assessment systems, strategic plans, program evaluation results, and staffing plans, among others. Meeting the training, education, and development needs of staff is accomplished through a variety of strategies, including department in-service education, sending staff members to outside continuing education programs, and individual supervision.

Discipline and Separation

Managers (along with supervisors) are responsible for overseeing performance and providing feedback and guidance to employees to correct inappropriate behavior (such as tardiness to the workplace), as well as to improve the quality and quantity of performance if it does not meet minimal standards. Feedback for minor concerns or feedback focused on helping employees develop as persons and professionals is routinely delivered as part of an ongoing performance appraisal system. Performance appraisal systems are discussed in more detail in Chapter 7.

When a manager must provide feedback on unacceptable or substandard performance, he or she must utilize a formal disciplinary process. Such a process typically consists of several steps. The specific action to be taken depends on the seriousness of the behavior or problem being addressed, whether the employee has received feedback before, and the length of time since the employee last exhibited the behavior. The steps of a sample disciplinary process applied to the problem of a tardy employee are provided in Box 6-8.

Although often difficult for the manager or supervisor, disciplinary procedures are beneficial and necessary for the safety and well-being of those the organization serves, as well as the organization's health and survival. In the long run, these procedures are also in the best interest of the employee who experiences difficulty meeting the performance or behavioral expectations of his or her job.

Although the word *discipline* likely conjures up negative thoughts, the first steps of an effective disciplinary procedure focus on providing the employee (or fieldwork student) with the information and skills to bring his or her behavior and performance into compliance with organizational expectations. Progressive disciplinary systems provide multiple opportunities for the employee to correct deficiencies by providing progressively more stern feedback and increasingly severe consequences. Such systems should also provide multiple opportunities for the manager to offer assistance and to ask the employee what the manager or organization could do to help the employee overcome the difficulty he or she is experiencing. Most often, employees are able to correct the problem behavior or bring performance up to standards, and it is not necessary to continue the process to the employee's termination.

Terminating an employee is undoubtedly one of the most difficult things a manager must do. Although it will not eliminate the discomfort, you should know that no manager should act alone when terminating an employee. In large organizations, someone from personnel or human resources should always be involved, and in private businesses where the manager is also the owner, legal counsel, another business owner, or a supervisor should be involved in the process to provide guidance and support to the manager and to be a witness to the actions taken.

It should be stressed that there is considerable room for sound managerial judgment in the process just presented. Like any staged model, you may skip steps if behavior warrants, or, with the passing of time, steps may be repeated. An employee with a solid

---

BOX 6-8

A Sample Disciplinary Process Applied to Tardiness to Work

- **Step 1—Remind or reinstruct:** On a first instance of unexcused tardiness, the behavior is brought to the employee's attention and he or she is reminded of the importance of being on time, the problems that being late causes, and that it is always necessary to call in to a supervisor if he or she is going to be late.
- **Step 2—Verbal warning:** On a second instance of unexcused tardiness within a short period of time in relation to the first, the behavior, problems associated with the behavior, the policy or expectation, and that this is the second (or more) instance of the unacceptable behavior is brought to the employee's attention.

    A second reminder of the necessary behavior is provided and the possible ramifications of continued unacceptable behavior are pointed out. A dated notation is placed in the employee's personnel file.
- **Step 3—Written warning:** On a third instance of unexcused tardiness within a short period of time in relation to the second, the actions in Step 2 are repeated. This time the employee should be invited to a formal meeting to discuss the behavior, the resulting problems, and what the manager might do to assist the employee to prevent the behavior from continuing, and to problem-solve with the employee. A referral to an employee assistance program (EAP) is made.* The seriousness of the situation and the possible

implications for the employee are stressed, and again a dated notation is placed in the employee's personnel file. The human resources department may need to be consulted or informed at this point.
- **Step 4—Suspension:** On the next instance of unexcused tardiness within a short period of time in relation to prior instances, and after consulting with human resources, the employee is suspended from work without pay for a period of time (1 day to 1 week, depending on the seriousness of the behavior). Offers of assistance to help prevent the behavior are made, a second referral to an EAP is made, the fact that the employee may be headed for termination is stressed, and all facts and conversations are documented in the personnel file.
- **Step 5—Termination:** On the next instance of unexcused tardiness within a short period of time of returning from suspension, the employee will be terminated. Immediately upon noticing the behavior, the human resources department is contacted and a plan is developed. The employee's manager and a representative from human resources meet with the employee, review briefly the cause for termination, and stay with the employee until he or she gathers personal belongings and leaves the building. All facts and conversations are carefully documented in the personnel file.

Many large organizations have employee assistance programs (EAPs) that aid employees with a range of personal problems that might affect performance, including stress management, substance abuse, and a range of other issues. Such services are typically provided in a confidential manner to the employee and are often free of charge.

---

performance history who is tardy 1 day after not having been tardy for a year most likely deserves to be reminded of the importance of being on time and likely does not warrant a verbal warning. Of course, behaviors such as theft, patient abuse, or serious ethics violations may warrant moving directly to termination on the first instance of the behavior. Other than for very serious infractions, you should only move to terminating an employee if you have:

- Given the employee a clear indication of what you originally expected from him or her via a written job description previously provided to him or her.
- Supplied clearly written personnel policies that specify conditions and directions about firing employees, and the employee initialed a copy of the policy handbook to verify that he or she had read the policies.

- Warned the employee in successive and dated memos that clearly described the continuance of the problem behavior over a specified time despite your specific and recorded offers of assistance and any training.
- Clearly observed the employee still having the performance problem. (You should note that, if the employee is being fired within a probationary period specified in your personnel policies, you might not have to meet all of these conditions.)

Directing

Directing can be defined as the process of providing guidance and oversight so that the work performed is goal oriented and focused on achieving desired departmental and organizational outcomes. The manager uses his or her leadership, motivational, and supervisory skills to teach, coach, and motivate workers. Management activities that might be grouped under the function of directing include mentoring or coaching, in addition to elements of traditional performance planning and supervision. Typically a department manager is responsible for the creation of an overall staff development plan or program, including support of continuing education and professional development in the department budget, allowing for release time for staff to attend professional development activities. Supervisory approaches and strategies, including appraisal of performance and the creation of individual professional development plans, is the focus of Chapter 7, so the remainder of this section of the chapter focuses on mentoring.

Mentoring

Mentoring is a process in which a more experienced professional enters into a formal relationship with a typically younger, less experienced professional focused on guiding the professional development of the younger professional. Mentoring relationships are different and can be much more significant than the typical relationship between a supervisor and supervisee. Mentors (the more experienced professional) and "mentees" (the less experienced professional) may work at the same organization and may also have a supervisor–subordinate relationship, but this is not necessarily the case. There is wide variation in what mentoring means to different persons, and Haggard, Dougherty, Turban, and Wilbanks (2011) identified over 40 separate definitions in their review of 117 articles published between 1980 and 2011. They did, however, note that "many scholars share the general view that a mentor is a more senior person who provides various kinds of personal and career assistance to a less senior or experienced person (the 'protégé' or 'mentee')" (p. 286).

Naturally occurring mentoring relationships can be intense for both parties, with the mentor feeling a sense of responsibility for the mentee's development and the mentee feeling a sense of responsibility to meet the mentor's expectations. Becoming involved in a mentoring relationship requires a commitment of time and effort by both parties. The mentor invests time in meeting with the mentee, looking for opportunities that will promote growth, listening to and meeting with the mentee to discuss concerns and plans for the future, and providing praise for accomplishments. The mentee also invests time in meetings, in communicating regularly with the mentor, in following up on suggestions for activities made by the mentor, and in making himself or herself available by displaying a willingness to learn.

Mentoring relationships sometimes happen naturally when two professionals meet in the course of their work lives, recognize their affinity for each other, and begin to commit to a professional relationship that is sustained over time. Mentoring relationships typically include four stages: birth, engagement, sustainment, and transition. These stages are defined in Box 6-9 (Robertson & Savio, 2003).

As an OT, I have been fortunate enough to find not one, but two mentors. As I have progressed in my career I also have had the opportunity to mentor others in both formal ongoing relationships and less formal or briefer experiences. I met my first mentor as a level II fieldwork student in the Continuing Education Division of AOTA. My fieldwork educator was an experienced occupational therapy practitioner, Susan Robertson, who immediately became a professional inspiration and role model for me. Our relationship flourished during my fieldwork experience and continues over 30 years later. During my first decade of practice, Susan served as my mentor. My experience is presented in Box 6-10 as a case example of mentoring.

BOX 6-9

The Four Stages of a Mentoring Relationship

1. **Birth of the relationship:** The mentor and mentee meet and negotiate expectations for satisfying expectations of each other within the relationship. Each member of the mentoring relationship gains a clear understanding of what he or she will contribute.
2. **Engagement:** Short-term goals and actions to achieve these goals are identified. Engagement is task-focused and this shared focus helps to strengthen the relationship as each partner in the mentoring process focuses on achievement of the mentee's long-term goals.
3. **Sustainment:** This occurs through continued focus on activities to achieve the mentee's goals but is characteristically marked by honest, mutually respectful, and positive interactions. Both the mentor and the mentee continually evaluate both process and outcomes and provide feedback on what is working and what is not and must be corrected. It is through this feedback that energy to maintain the relationship and the positive aspects of the relationship are reinforced.
4. **Transition:** This is the final stage that occurs when the mentee's goals have been attained or the time commitment of each partner in the process is fulfilled. Successful transition is marked by the development of a new but different relationship that is not solely focused on the developmental needs or goals of the mentee.

Although the mentoring described so far has been in regard to naturally occurring mentoring relationships, formal mentoring programs in which professionals are paired with each other by the program or employing organization have also been developed. Mentoring in general has been connected in the human resources literature with positive organizational outcomes, including increased job satisfaction, higher pay, and more promotions for protégés (Allen,

Eby, O'Brien, & Lentz, 2008; Eby, Allen, Evans, Ng, & DuBois, 2008; Underhill, 2006).

Orchestrated mentoring experiences are typically shorter in duration than naturally occurring relationships; are often less intense, with predetermined meeting frequency and prescribed activities; and may be limited because the mentors fear the perception of favoritism because the relationship may be very public (Blake-Beard, 2001).

The theme of this book is using evidence to guide the management of occupational therapy services. Almost every function of management can be guided by theory and some form of evidence. Presenting the evidence on *every* topic discussed in this text would not be helpful; however, occasional illustrations of the strategies presented in Chapter 2 would be of use. Therefore, the evidence related to orchestrated mentoring will be used as an example. Let's assume that you have become aware of the benefits of mentoring and wonder if it would be a good use of your organization's resources to develop a mentoring program for new managers. Your question then would be

What does the evidence presented in the literature suggest about the effectiveness of formal mentoring programs compared to naturally occurring mentoring relationships?

When searching the literature on mentoring, limiting your search to empirical studies, you would find that there are only a handful of empirical studies that have compared the effectiveness of formal programs to naturally occurring mentoring relationships. Each of these studies found that naturally occurring or "informal" mentoring relationships resulted in greater outcomes for the mentees in terms of career development than did participation in a formal mentoring program. Two of the three studies reported that informal mentees perceived higher levels of psychosocial support. That evidence is summarized in Table 6-4.

Controlling

Controlling is the process of measuring performance against expectations and taking action to eliminate obstacles to achieving organizational goals. One primary method of controlling everyday functions is

BOX 6-10

A Case Example of Professional Mentoring

I began my first day of my level II fieldwork experience at the AOTA Division of Continuing Education by meeting with my fieldwork educator, Susan Robertson. Susan's unbridled enthusiasm for educating others was immediately evident. During my fieldwork, I benefited from the opportunities that Susan orchestrated for me, including involvement in a wide range of projects and interaction with leaders in the profession. Some of the specific actions that Susan took were:

- To assign me strategically to projects that fit my goals and strengths but that challenged me to grow
- To introduce me to key leaders at meetings
- To call the attention of others to the contributions I made to association projects
- To challenge me to set development goals for myself

As I continued my fieldwork, I began to feel a sense of responsibility to do well on all assignments not only to meet my own performance expectations but to also make Susan proud of me.

After I completed my fieldwork, Susan and I agreed to keep in touch and did so. Over the next few years, I kept Susan informed of my professional activities. Susan followed my career with great interest, not only providing me with praise for accomplishments, but also challenging me to think ahead to my next job and to constantly think strategically about the activities with which I became involved. At Susan's urging, I became involved in state occupational therapy association activities and pursued volunteer leadership experiences that helped me with skill development. Despite being uncomfortable at first, I made presentations at local and national conferences with Susan's support, and these experiences proved valuable to me later in my career when I had to make presentations to other groups. I also furthered my education by obtaining a master's degree.

As my mentoring relationship with Susan matured, the nature of the interactions we had changed and Susan began to share more about how she was working on developing her own career; however, she continued to challenge me to grow. Even as I accumulated years of professional experience and became the director of an occupational therapy department, Susan and I maintained regular contact. For example, each year at the AOTA annual conference, we would have dinner and, after catching up on what was going on in our personal lives, Susan would inevitably shift the conversation to discussing my career and what I should be doing next.

Eventually I reached a point in my career at which I began to primarily seek mentoring from a new boss as I accepted a job in academics and changed the focus of my career. Rather than expressing loss or even jealousy, Susan expressed sincere joy and respect for my accomplishments. Although my maturation as a professional led to the end of our formal mentoring relationship, Susan and I remain close colleagues and friends to this day. This mentoring relationship was effective because of the actions that both Susan and I took to support the relationship.

As a mentor, Susan

- Fostered self-reflection
- Instructed and motivated me to achieve new goals and develop new skills
- Supported my critical thinking and clinical reasoning
- Facilitated problem-solving and decision-making as I progressed through the first decade of my career
- Encouraged the application of learning to new situations and challenges

As a mentee, I

- Actively reflected on the advice and observations shared by Susan
- Sought self-motivating learning opportunities to build on the suggestions and guidance provided by my mentor
- Engaged in critical thinking, clinical reasoning, and reflective self-examination
- Collaborated actively with Susan to solve problems and make key career decisions
- Related learning to the professional goals that Susan and I identified

TABLE 6-4

Summary of Selected Evidence on Formal Mentoring Programs

Author	Study Type	N (Sample Size)	Level of Evidence	Results
Ingersoll & Strong (2011)	Critical review	15 studies	Strong	Provided empirical support for the claim that support and assistance for beginning teachers have a positive impact on three sets of outcomes: teacher commitment and retention, teacher classroom instructional practices, and student achievement.
Ragins & Cotton (1999)	Quantitative analysis of survey	510 informal mentees, 104 formal mentees	Good	Informal mentees rated their mentors as more effective and received higher salaries than mentees with formal mentors. Informal mentees also reported higher levels of psychosocial support.
Hurley & Fagenson-Eland (1996)	Qualitative interview and survey	16 informal, 30 formal mentees	Good	No difference between groups in the level of career development or role modeling reported, but informal mentees did report higher levels of psychosocial benefit.
Chao, Walz, & Gardner (1992)	Quantitative analysis of survey	212 informal, 53 formal mentees	Good	Informal mentees reported greater career support and higher salaries than peers in informal relationships, but no support for a hypothesis that informal mentors provide greater levels of psychosocial support.

through the use of control mechanisms or control indicators. A control mechanism or control indicator is a "check" or measure that is in place to constantly monitor the output or product of a system. When the check indicates that performance falls below a previously established limit, it means there is an unacceptable variation in the system or a problem to be addressed. Control mechanisms can be related either to *outcomes*, or the desired targets for a process, or to *processes* themselves, or controls intended to specify the manner in which tasks will be completed through the use of policies, procedures, and rules.

Common examples of control mechanisms that might be used by an occupational therapy manager include taking the temperature in a refrigerator that stores patient food each day so action can be taken if the temperature is not sufficiently cool, noting the length of time it takes to respond to a referral after it is received by the occupational therapy department so action can be taken when the time exceeds a predetermined period of time, or checking the cords on all electrical equipment once monthly so action can be taken if a cord is frayed or damaged. Monitoring the productivity level of OTs and OTAs by counting the number of units of care that they provide or enter into a computerized billing system to identify when productivity levels drop below minimum standards would also be an example of controlling as a managerial function.

The process of controlling includes three phases: (1) establishing standards, (2) measuring performance, and (3) correcting deviations (Box 6-11). There are various types of controls (sometimes also referred to as standards) that can be used depending upon the process or mechanism that is being monitored. Controls can relate to physical characteristics of a product or to quantity, quality, or cost. The most common types of controls and brief definitions of each are listed in Box 6-12.

Regardless of the type of control, in order to be effective, the control must be structured so you become aware of the problem in a timely and efficient manner and you receive adequate information to take

---

BOX 6-11

Controlling: A Three-Phase Process

- **Establishing standards:** Determining the specific indicators or quantifiable measures of acceptable work
- **Measuring performance:** Comparing outputs of processes to established standards
- **Correcting deviations:** Taking action to improve outputs of processes that do not meet established standards

---

BOX 6-12

Types of Controls

- **Physical:** Standards related to tangible elements of a product or outcome of a process, such as smoothness, texture, or size
- **Quantity:** Amounts or counts that provide a measure of conformance and efficiency, such as the number of units of care provided or hours billed
- **Quality:** Quantitative measures of quality, such as outcome measures or patient or customer satisfaction
- **Cost:** The cost of a process, such as the cost per unit of service provided, or the cost of materials associated with a process, such as fabricating a splint

---

BOX 6-13

Characteristics of Adequate Control Mechanisms

- **Timeliness:** The control signifies a problem in a timely manner so corrective action can be taken before serious harm or loss of resources is experienced.
- **Economy:** The control is conducted in a routine manner that does not require significant human or financial costs or resources.
- **Comprehensiveness:** The control measures a sufficient variety and extent of available data so problems are caught and are not inadvertently overlooked.
- **Specificity and appropriateness:** The control is specific to the process being measured so false alarms do not consume time or effort.
- **Objectivity:** The control is easily understood by all personnel and there is no question as to when measures fall below or above preestablished standards.
- **Responsibility:** Responsibility for monitoring the control on an ongoing basis is clear to all personnel so measures are checked regularly according to a predetermined schedule.

---

appropriate action. The characteristics of adequate control mechanisms are listed in Box 6-13.

Information Management

With improved technology, the amount of data and information that managers receive on a daily basis can be overwhelming. The ability to transmit large amounts of information to a person in another department or across the world in seconds through e-mail, to access millions of Internet sites or search multiple databases for current evidence, or to have statistics and data automatically collected and reported from documentation or billing systems has clear advantages. However, time can also be wasted sorting through meaningless data. On any single day, an occupational therapy manager may receive reports related to budget, staff productivity, rates of client visits, client charges, equipment usage, continuous quality improvement efforts, and clinical outcomes. It has been said that *information* is *data* that have been organized so they are useful and can be easily interpreted.

So, if the possibility exists of excess data and information overload, what are the most common types of data and information to which you must attend? Luckily, in many larger organizations, some data are

TABLE 6-5		
Common Types and Sources of Data and Information and Possible Uses		
Type of Data	**Source**	**Use**
Demographics (age, sex, educational level, etc.)	• Admissions records • Public data sets	• Program planning • Program evaluation
Revenue (payer source, rates, discounts)	• Accounting • Budget reports	• Budgeting • Program planning
Expense (accounts payable)	• Financial reports • Purchasing records	• Budgeting • Program planning and evaluation
Payroll (salary, benefits, leave usage)	• Accounting • Budget reports	• Staffing plans • Recruitment and retention
Productivity (visits, staff activity)	• Automated charge systems • Department billing records or productivity tracking sheets	• Staffing plans • Performance appraisal • Recruitment
Personnel (licensure, competencies, professional development, performance)	• Human resources • Departmental personnel files • Professional association data sets	• Accreditation visits • Staffing plan development • Professional development plans
Clinical (diagnosis, intervention, outcomes)	• Medical records • Outcome databases	• Continuous quality improvement • Program evaluation
Legal (contracts, leases)	• Legal or grants and contracts department	• Facility planning

organized into useful information for you and often delivered to you automatically in the form of paper or electronic reports. With increasingly sophisticated and automated systems, data and information at the departmental level may also be available in this manner. At other times you may need to collect data yourself, such as when you are in the process of developing new programming for a target population for which your organization does not have an existing data collection mechanism. A simple question to ask yourself before you begin data collection is "What do I want to know and what will this data help me learn in order to improve the performance of my department?" If you cannot identify the specific use for the data before collecting it, you should reexamine whether it is worth the resources to collect the data in the first place. Turning *data* into *information* requires that you know what question you are seeking to answer before you begin to collect the data. Table 6-5 lists common types and sources of data, information, and other forms of

evidence used by managers and a sample of how these can be utilized.

Chapter Summary

This chapter reviewed the commonly identified functions of a manager (planning, organizing and staffing, directing, and controlling) and provided an introduction to some of the key activities associated with each of those functions. It was noted that managers are most often also supervisors, but then many occupational therapy supervisors do not have requisite managerial authority. Hopefully you have begun to get a flavor for the diversity that characterizes what managers "do." Moreover, you have likely begun to appreciate why it is that any introductory text on management typically presents a wide range of topics at a basic level. It is also likely that this chapter left you with many unanswered questions about becoming an occupational therapy manager. Some of those questions will be answered in the remaining chapters. However, for those questions that remain, you should have confidence that, if you master the basic skills of evidence-based practice, you will be able to seek out and identify the most current information to guide your decision-making in choosing an effective answer.

At the beginning of this chapter, you were introduced to Marty, who had just accepted a position as the director of occupational therapy. Although he had some experience as an occupational therapy supervisor, he was unsure of what he needed to learn and so conducted a number of information interviews.

■ Real-Life Solutions

Marty completed a number of information interviews with other local occupational therapy department directors before beginning his new job. Although he was somewhat overwhelmed at the wide range of tasks that these managers completed, he was comforted to hear from most of his interviewees that he should begin by reviewing an introductory text on management. He was surprised to hear repeatedly that he could organize his learning needs and objectives according to the commonly identified management functions of planning, organizing and staffing, directing, and controlling.

Marty began to see that, like the practice of occupational therapy, management is guided by both theories and models that help you to conceptualize how to begin to address a set of responsibilities and by specific skill sets that help you perform discrete management tasks. Similarly, he began to understand that the principles of evidence-based practice could be applied to any type of occupational therapy practice, including management. When Marty considered the different activities that his peers had mentioned (strategic planning, policies and procedures, budgeting, planning facilities, recruitment of staff, discipline, and mentoring), he began to appreciate more how what he had learned about the functioning of health-care systems, organizations, and leadership would help him in his new job. He also took solace in how often the directors that he interviewed encouraged him to rely on the expertise of other professionals in his new organization, including those in human resources, finance, continuous quality improvement, information management, and facilities management.

Marty was probably most surprised by how much the directors felt they still had to learn, and the extent to which they noted that they relied on a peer network to find the answers and solutions to their everyday questions and problems. Based on recommendations from his information interviews, Marty decided that he would be wise to do the following to help assure his success in his new role as an occupational therapy manager:

1. Join the special interest sections (SISs) in administration and management offered by both his state occupational therapy association and AOTA.
2. Develop and maintain contact with the network of peer managers he created while conducting his information interviews.
3. Seek to establish a relationship with a professional mentor.
4. Immediately establish contacts in the departments responsible for key staff functions, including human resources, finance and accounting, continuous quality improvement, and facilities management.
5. Explore learning opportunities offered by his organization, his state occupational therapy association, AOTA, and a local university, as well as those in the community, to develop skills for completing key management functions such as interviewing and budgeting skills.
6. Continue to read and search the literature from diverse disciplines and journals, including business administration, organizational development, human resources, and psychology, to remain aware of current developments in research and evidence related to his job as an occupational therapy manager.

Study Questions

1. Deciding which staff are most appropriate to work on a specific patient care unit and assigning them work tasks would best be described as which of the following key functions of a manager?

   a. Planning
   b. Controlling
   c. Organizing and staffing
   d. Directing

2. Determining the costs for staff salaries and benefits, equipment, and other operational expenses, as well as the amount of revenue anticipated, would best be described as which of the following functions of a manager?

   a. Planning
   b. Controlling
   c. Organizing and staffing
   d. Directing

3. A management tool that describes why your department or organization exists and its key functions would best be called a:

   a. Vision statement.
   b. Strategic plan.
   c. Policy and procedure.
   d. Mission statement.

4. An aspirational description of the future state of an organization that identifies the organization's primary goals would best be called a:

   a. Vision statement.
   b. Strategic plan.
   c. Policy and procedure.
   d. Mission statement.

5. Which of the following was described as a function of the manager?

   a. Recruiting and retaining staff
   b. Developing and implementing policies and procedures
   c. Establishing performance standards and measuring, evaluating, and correcting performance
   d. All of the above

6. A description of the appropriate ratio of OTs, OTAs, and service extenders or aides needed to provide care that is effective but also cost efficient would best be called a:

   a. Staffing plan.
   b. Skill mix.
   c. Case mix ratio.
   d. Staffing index.

7. Which of the following is not true of mentoring programs based on the discussion and evidence presented in this chapter?

   a. Both naturally occurring and formally structured mentoring experiences can be beneficial to newer employees.
   b. Mentoring relationships often transition and "end" when goals are met, the mentee has gained skills and experience, and he or she is ready to establish a new relationship with his or her mentor as an equal colleague.
   c. The advantage of mentoring as an approach to staff development is that there is a standard definition of the concept that is widely accepted and utilized.
   d. Orchestrated mentoring relationships are often less intense and often last for a shorter period of time than naturally occurring mentoring relationships.

8. Which of the following is not one of the identified phases of controlling?

   a. Establishing standards
   b. Negotiating goals
   c. Measuring performance
   d. Correcting deviations

Resources for Learning More About the Roles and Functions of Managers

Journals That Often Address Management and Management Issues

Management Science

http://pubsonline.informs.org/journal/mnsc

Management Science is a scholarly journal that scientifically addresses the problems, interests, and concerns of organizational decision-makers. Through publication of relevant theory and innovative applications, the journal serves the needs of both academicians and practitioners.

Journal of Management Development

http://www.emeraldinsight.com/journals
.htm?issn=0262-1711

The *Journal of Management Development* covers a broad range of topics in its field, including competence-based management development, developing leadership skills, developing women for management, global management, the new technology of management development, team building, organizational development and change, and performance appraisal.

Journal of Management Studies

http://onlinelibrary.wiley.com/journal/10.1111/
(ISSN)1467-6486

The *Journal of Management Studies* provides in-depth coverage of organizational problems and organization theory, reports on the latest developments in strategic management and planning, presents cross-cultural comparisons of organizational effectiveness, and includes concise reviews of the latest publications in management studies as well as lively debate on topical and important issues in management.

Associations That Are Concerned With Management and Management Issues

The American Occupational Therapy Association

http://www.aota.org/

The stated mission of AOTA advances the quality, availability, use, and support of occupational therapy through standard setting, advocacy, education, and research on behalf of its members and the public. AOTA provides its members with a variety of resources related to the supervision of occupational therapy personnel, including a number of papers that provide guidelines for the occupational therapy supervisor;

access to special interest sections (SISs) that provide Listservs and quarterly newsletters, including the administration and management SIS; and continuing education options.

American Management Association

http://www.amanet.org/index.htm

The American Management Association (AMA) states that its mission is to provide managers and their organizations worldwide with the knowledge, skills, and tools they need to improve business performance, adapt to a changing workplace, and prosper in a complex and competitive business world. The AMA serves as a forum for the exchange of the latest information, ideas, and insights on management practices and business trends. The AMA disseminates content and information to a worldwide audience through multiple distribution channels and its strategic partners by offering seminars, conferences, current issues forums and briefings, books and publications, research, and online self-study courses, which cover such topics as supervisory skills.

Miscellaneous Resources Related to Management

The National Mentoring Partnership

http://www.mentoring.org/index.adp

MENTOR/National Mentoring Partnership is an advocate for the expansion of mentoring and a resource for mentors and mentoring initiatives nationwide. For more than a decade, MENTOR/National Mentoring Partnership has been leading the effort to connect America's young people with caring adult mentors. MENTOR was created in 1990 by financiers and philanthropists Geoff Boisi and Ray Chambers. The website includes downloadable resources on mentoring, a list of research on the effectiveness of mentoring, and resources for developing mentoring programs.

Reference List

Allen, T. D., Eby, L. T., O'Brien, K. E., & Lentz, E. (2008). The state of mentoring research: A qualitative review of current research methods and future research implications. *Journal of Vocational Behavior*, 72, 269–283.

Bacal, R. (2003). *A quick guide to employee orientation.* Retrieved from the Work911 Workplace Supersite website: http://www.work911.com/articles/orient.htm

Blake-Beard, S. D. (2001). Taking a hard look at formal mentoring programs: A consideration of potential challenges facing women. *Journal of Management Development*, 20, 331–345.

Chao, G. T., Walz, P. M., & Gardner, P. D. (1992). Formal and informal mentorships: A comparison on mentoring functions and contrast with non-mentored counterparts. *Personnel Psychology*, 45, 619–636.

Daft, R. L., & Marcic, D. (2011). *Understanding management principles.* Manson, OH: Cengage Learning.

Drucker, P. (1974). *Management: Tasks, responsibilities and practices.* New York, NY: Harper & Row.

Eby, L. T., Allen, T. D., Evans, S. C., Ng, T., & DuBois, D. (2008). Does mentoring matter? A multidisciplinary meta-analysis comparing mentored and non-mentored individuals. *Journal of Vocational Behavior*, 72, 254–267.

Haggard, D. L., Dougherty, T. W., Turban, D. B., & Wilbanks, J. E. (2011). Who is a mentor? A review of evolving definitions and implications for research. *Journal of Management*, 37(1), 280–304.

Hom, E. J. (2013, February 1). What is a vision statement? *Business News Daily.* Retrieved from http://www.businessnewsdaily.com/3882-vision-statement.html

Hurley, A. E., & Fagenson-Eland, E. A. (1996). Challenges in cross-gender mentoring relationships: Psychological intimacy, myths, rumors, innuendoes, and sexual harassment. *Leadership and Organizational Development Journal*, 17, 42–49.

Ingersoll, R. M., & Strong, M. (2011). The impact of induction and mentoring programs for beginning teachers: A critical review of the research. *Review of Educational Research*, 81(2), 201–233.

Jaques, E. (1998). *Requisite organization.* Arlington, VA: Cason Hall.

Lyles, R. I., & Joiner, C. (1986). *Supervision in health care organizations.* New York, NY: John Wiley & Sons.

McNamara, C. (2003). *Basics: Definitions (and misperceptions) about management.* Retrieved from http://158.132.155.107/posh97/private/management-general/definition.pdf

Ragins, B. R., & Cotton, J. L. (1999). Mentor functions and outcomes: A comparison of men and women in formal and informal mentoring relationships. *Journal of Applied Psychology*, 84, 529–550.

Robertson, S. C., & Savio, M. C. (2003, November 17). Mentoring as professional development. *American Occupational Therapy Association OT Practice Online.* Retrieved from http://www.aota.org/-/media/Corporate/Files/Secure/Publications/OTP/1999-2003/2003/11-17-2003.PDF/

Schein, E. H. (1992). *Organizational culture and leadership.* New York, NY: Jossey-Bass.

Underhill, C. M. (2006). The effectiveness of mentoring programs in corporate settings: A meta-analytic review of the literature. *Journal of Vocational Behavior*, 68, 292–307.

U.S. Equal Employment Opportunity Commission. (2014). *Prohibited employment policies/practices.* Retrieved from http://www.eeoc.gov/laws/practices/

CHAPTER 7

Roles and Functions of Supervisors

Brenda Koverman, MBA, MS, OTR/L
Brent Braveman, PhD, OTR/L, FAOTA

■ Real-Life Management

Chris has worked as an occupational therapist in a hospital for 6 years. During this time, she was promoted to senior occupational therapist and acts as a resource for other occupational therapy practitioners, including occupational therapists (OTs), occupational therapy assistants (OTAs), and students. Other staff members often ask for her opinion on alternative treatment interventions and she sometimes will observe a treatment session with a coworker to give advice. She also has supervised multiple fieldwork students and has found great satisfaction in these experiences. She has co-led a lab with the academic faculty at the university located on campus.

Recently, a supervisory position has become available and Chris is considering applying for the position. Chris previously passed up opportunities to be promoted into a position with more formal supervisory responsibilities because she has always been nervous about having to be someone's "boss." She thinks that she would enjoy a job where she would spend more of her time coaching and mentoring others and contributing to their professional development, but is not as sure about having to give constructive criticism, especially to her current peers. Chris also is not sure about "moving up the ladder" and becoming a department director. She feels certain that her passions rest in working with clients, as well as in helping others become better occupational therapy practitioners.

Chris wonders too if she can assume the role of supervisor without also taking on responsibilities such as budgeting and personnel management that seem to be such a source of frustration and conflict for her own boss. She wonders if there is a difference between being a manager and a supervisor and, if so, what those differences might be. Chris decides to speak to Craig, the occupational therapy manager, to find out what responsibilities would be included in a supervisory job.

Critical Thinking Questions

As you read this chapter, consider the following questions:

- What are ways that OTs and OTAs become involved in the supervision of other OTs, OTAs, fieldwork students, and volunteers without accepting full managerial responsibilities?

- What do the terms *formal authority* and *power* mean and what do they have to do with each other and being an occupational therapy supervisor?

- Where can you find models and resources to guide the supervision of others within the human resources and the occupational therapy literature?

- What types of theories of motivation exist that are helpful in guiding supervision strategies as well as strategies for rewards and recognition of others?

- What are the characteristics of a formal performance appraisal system that are likely to make it most effective?

Glossary

- **Formal authority:** (also legitimate power) the right to issue orders or direct action by virtue of one's formal position.
- **Personal power:** power that is separate from the formal authority associated with an organizational position; it is power that comes from knowledge, personal attractiveness, or demonstration of effort.
- **Power:** the ability to force compliance to one's wishes through coercion despite resistance.
- **Service competency:** defined as the process of teaching, training, and evaluating through which

the OT determines that the OTA or other occupational therapy personnel performs tasks in the same way that the OT would and achieves the same outcome.
- **Span of control:** defined as the number of immediate subordinates who report to any one supervisor.
- **Supervision:** the control and direction of the work of one or more employees in a manner that promotes improved performance and a higher-quality outcome.

Introduction

Chapter 1 introduced leadership as an overarching theme relevant to both management and supervision. Both managers and supervisors are in positions to provide leadership to others regardless of the level of formal power or authority that they hold within an organization. The major theories of leadership were introduced, as was evidence related to the effectiveness of adopting leader behaviors based on each theory. Chapter 6 reviewed the major management functions (planning, organizing and staffing, directing, and controlling) and noted that, although most managers are supervisors, many supervisors do not have what is referred to as *requisite managerial authority*. Chapter 7 focuses on the supervisor's role and functions in more depth and summarize the common duties of the occupational therapy supervisor. Theory related to the motivation of employees is introduced and selected evidence related to a number of key issues of concern to the supervisor is presented.

Supervision

After reading Chapter 6, you might be asking yourself, "If managers are responsible for the planning, organizing and staffing, directing, and controlling functions in an organization, what do supervisors do?" In the previous chapter, it was noted that there are many areas of overlap between the management and supervision functions in organizations, but that not all supervisors have requisite managerial authority. Many OTs and OTAs supervise others relatively early in their careers (and without formal training) as they accept fieldwork students, collaborate with and supervise OTAs and rehabilitation aides or technicians, or utilize volunteers.

Management was previously defined as:

The process of guiding an organization by planning for future work obligations, organizing employees into functional units, directing employees in the process of completing daily work tasks, and controlling processes and systems to assure adequate quality of work output.

Supervision is the aspect of management that relates to directing employees in their daily work tasks and seeks to assure that their performance meets established standards and supports the organization's goals and objectives. Therefore, supervision is defined as:

The control and direction of the work of one or more employees in a manner that promotes improved performance and a higher-quality outcome.

Supervisors typically are responsible for the progress and productivity of those employees who directly report to them within an organization. Supervision often includes conducting basic management tasks (decision-making, problem-solving, planning, delegation, and meeting management), organizing teams, noticing the need for and designing new job roles in the group, training new employees, managing employee performance (setting goals, observing and giving feedback, addressing performance issues, etc.), and ensuring conformance to personnel policies and other internal regulations. At times, supervisors may have the ability to hire and fire employees or give input to this process, although this is a responsibility often reserved for managers. In order to maintain requisite managerial authority and to be fairly held ultimately responsible for the outcomes of work groups, you *should* have authority to hire and fire employees and have full direction over the employees for whose work outcomes you will be held responsible. However, it is common in health care, school systems, and community settings for occupational therapy practitioners to be responsible for supervising others without being responsible for the full range of managerial functions.

The Roles and Functions of Supervisors

Although there are variations in the exact job responsibilities of supervisors from one setting to another, there are also typical functions that most supervisors serve. Some of the most common duties of supervisors include:

1. Determine daily priorities for workers.
2. Schedule workers.
3. Coordinate the efforts of others.
4. Observe and evaluate employees' performance.
5. Give accurate and honest performance-based feedback.
6. Coach and train employees.
7. Handle administrative duties and relevant paperwork.
8. Communicate clearly about policies, procedures, and processes.
9. Address problems and conflicts in a timely manner.
10. Look for ways to improve the efficiency and effectiveness of work processes.

These duties can be grouped conceptually into three main supervisory functions: (1) management, (2) education, and (3) support (Hawkins & Shohet, 2006; Nicklin, 1995). The management function of supervisors includes those duties related to monitoring and evaluating the work of others. The education function of supervisors includes those duties related to the development and evaluation of competencies of staff. The support function of supervisors includes duties related to professional development, including promotion of self-awareness and emotional growth.

Supervisors carry out managerial, educational, and support functions within an organizational environment (see Chapter 3), and their jobs and their level of influence on others are heavily influenced by structures within that environment. Two important supervisory concepts influenced by the organization's internal structure that are important to understand when examining the supervisor's role and influence are *span of control* and *power or authority*. These concepts are discussed next.

Span of Control

One structural decision that must be made by management that has a direct impact on the day-to-day life of supervisors is determining the span of control for each supervisor. **Span of control** is defined as the number of immediate subordinates who report to any one supervisor. For occupational therapy supervisors, this can range from just a few employees to large groups of 30 or more practitioners. They may be located in a single site or may be spread across different locations. If a supervisor's span of control is too large, he or she may be ineffective because of the inability to adequately attend to the needs of individual employees and to monitor the quality of employees' work on a close enough basis.

However, if a supervisor's span of control is too small, there may be unnecessary labor costs to the organization and time may be wasted as a result of unnecessary layering of the organization and duplication of tasks. Determining the most effective span of control relies on a number of factors related to the organization's size, structure, and history. The most commonly identified factors influencing span of control are identified in Box 7-1.

BOX 7-1

Factors Affecting Span of Control

- **Type of work:** Routine and repetitious work on the part of employees supports a larger span of control, whereas complex or unpredictable work tends to limit span of control.
- **Degree of training:** The presence of highly trained staff supports a larger span of control, whereas less trained staff tend to require more supervision and limit span of control.
- **Organizational stability:** Stable organizations with little change and staff turnover support a larger span of control, whereas constant change and high turnover tend to limit span of control.
- **Geographic location:** The location of staff to be supervised in one or in easily accessed locations supports a large span of control, whereas supervising staff dispersed in various or hard-to-access areas limits span of control.
- **Flow of work:** Regular and even flow of work in a predictable manner supports a larger span of control, whereas work that flows unevenly or

in an unpredictable manner may limit span of control.
- **Supervisor's qualifications:** The presence of more qualified and experienced supervisors supports a larger span of control, whereas less qualified or inexperienced supervisors limit span of control.
- **Availability of staff specialists:** The availability of specialists to provide consultation in specific areas (e.g., someone who is a specialist in assistive technology) supports a larger span of control, whereas reliance on only formal supervisors limits span of control.
- **Value system of organization:** Organizations that most highly value minimizing salary expenses paid for supervision, very high productivity, and profit may support a larger span of control, whereas organizations that mostly value close supervision of new staff and less stringent productivity may limit span of control.

Power and Formal Authority

Although different supervisors may use varied supervision styles, all supervisors rely on others to respond to requests or orders to do what they are asked or told to do. Supervisors rely on power or formal authority to achieve compliance by those that they supervise to achieve daily goals. Scholars of organizational development and functioning frequently distinguish between the concepts of **power** (the ability to force compliance to one's wishes through coercion despite resistance) and formal authority (the right to issue orders or direct action by virtue of one's formal position). **Formal authority** has also been termed *legitimate power* (Liebler, Levine, & Rothman, 2011).

Although power is often associated with positions of authority, it must be recognized that power within organizations comes in many forms. For example, labor unions may hold great power to coerce management to act in ways against its wishes through threats of labor strikes. Even individual employees may hold power over managers or supervisors regardless of rank if they have a great deal of influence among other employees or have some characteristic that brings them power. A common example in occupational therapy may be the power that a practitioner with specialized skills, such as a certified hand therapist, may hold when it is evident that an employee would be difficult to replace if he or she were to leave the organization.

Formal authority typically is associated with specific positions or ranks within organizations. Liebler et al (2011) identified several sources of formal authority studied by theorists in the fields of social psychology, management, and political science. These sources are (1) acceptance of or consent to authority, (2) formal organizational patterns, (3) cultural expectations, (4) technical competence and expertise, and (5) characteristics of authority holders. The key concepts associated with each of these potential sources of authority are summarized in Table 7-1.

Whetten and Cameron (2011) named the type of power that is separate from the formal authority associated with an organizational position **personal power.** Although a manager or supervisor uses position power to exert influence over those at lower levels in the organization, he or she typically has little or no formal authority to influence persons at higher levels of the organization. In order to influence one's supervisor or organizational leaders, one must rely upon personal power. As a result, anything that a manager or supervisor can do to increase his or her personal power will help in the important types of negotiations that they complete on behalf of their departments (e.g., negotiating operating and capital equipment budgets or gaining resources to provide training for staff). Personal power may be enhanced through increasing one's knowledge or expertise, by improving one's personal attractiveness, through demonstration of effort, and through legitimacy.

Whetten and Cameron (2011) also provided four general suggestions for enhancing one's position power. It is easy to imagine that a cynical person might view these strategies as underhanded or false flattery. This might be an accurate characterization for those who only occasionally utilize these strategies and demonstrate limited follow-through. However, those managers and supervisors who use these strategies consistently and with the sincere intent to combine personal success with a contribution to organizational success are likely to find themselves more valuable and central to an organization's functioning. The suggested strategies for increasing position power are outlined in Box 7-2.

As a supervisor, you need to feel comfortable with increasing your personal and professional power in order to become more effective and influence others. Translating power into influence is a way to get your department objectives met in the overall organizational hierarchy. In doing this, you will better position your area within the overall organizational structure. This can lead to program development and ultimately greater employee and patient satisfaction.

Becoming an Effective Supervisor

Supervisors can have dramatic influence on the quality of daily work life, job satisfaction, and retention of employees. Being effective as a supervisor goes beyond being respected, appreciated, or well liked by employees, however, because the supervisor has responsibilities to both employees and the organization. Although many large organizations provide ongoing training for supervisors and managers, smaller organizations may not have the resources to conduct training, and relatively few OTs receive formal training before becoming a fieldwork educator or beginning to supervise an OTA. So what does it mean to be *effective* as a

TABLE 7-1

Key Concepts Related to Identified Sources of Formal Authority

Acceptance of or Consent to Authority	• Authority involves acceptance of a superior's decision by a subordinate. • Subordinates often accept orders without conscious questioning. • Subordinates seek to act in a manner that is acceptable to the superior even when there has been no explicit order. • Subordinates are part of a psychological contract that includes acceptance of authority in return for appropriate rewards for compliance.
Formal Organizational Patterns	• The rights and duties of members of organizations are consistent with the rules accepted as rational in society in general. • Jurisdictions of authority are reasonably fixed. • Authority rests with a position independent of the individual who fills that position.
Cultural Expectations	• Individuals in a society are culturally induced to accept authority. • Acceptable use of authority is predefined by social structures such as laws or organizational policies. • Acceptance of authority is learned through normal socialization.
Technical Competence or Expertise	• Technical competence carries inherent limited authority to control specified activities. • Authority may vary and move from person to person and is influenced by the demands of the situation in addition to recognized positions.
Characteristics of Authority Holders	• Authority rests in individuals. • The talents and traits of an individual may become the source of authority. • Characteristics that influence authority may relate both to the individual and to the interaction between the individual and the position he or she holds within an organization.

BOX 7-2

Four Strategies for Increasing Personal Power

1. Increase your centrality in the organization by looking for opportunities to include new functions central to the flow of work in your job. Volunteer for committees where you can build networks with other department leaders.
2. Increase the personal discretion and flexibility of your position by replacing routine activities with involvement in new projects in the early stages of decision-making.
3. Increase the visibility of your job performance by developing and nurturing relationships with organizational leadership. Volunteer to make presentations from task groups, offer suggestions and examples when a presenter asks for input from a large group, or volunteer to become a trainer.
4. Increase the relevance of your job tasks to the organization by finding ways to develop programs that align with the organization's top priorities.

supervisor, and how do you gain these skills? Commonly identified characteristics of effective supervisors are listed in Box 7-3.

One key to becoming an effective supervisor is to clearly understand what is expected of you. A good place to start is to review your job description with *your* manager. These duties should be outlined when you interview for the position. These duties can also be reviewed periodically to ensure similar job performance expectations with you and your manager. Before meeting with your supervisor, highlight the formal supervisory functions listed in your job description so that you and your manager can review them to be sure that performance expectations for these functions are clear and reasonable. In addition, try to identify any unwritten expectations of supervisors by observing others with the same or similar positions and discussing these responsibilities with them. For example, it might be a common expectation that supervisors regularly check in with supervisors from other disciplines to assess their satisfaction or to volunteer for committees outside of the department. A detailed list of responsibilities may help in starting the conversation with your supervisor. Another helpful strategy is to consider the various *customers* you serve. All employees (and employee groups) have multiple customers within an organization. An internal customer is anyone who uses or relies on the work of another in order to do his or her job. For supervisors, two key customers are the subordinates who report to them and the supervisor to whom they report. Strategies for identifying the requirements of customers are covered in more depth in Chapter 13, but a simple strategy for the

supervisor is to ask his or her subordinates and his or her boss: "What is most important to you?" Although you might assume that the answers to this question would be easy to identify, sometimes the most valued requirements of customers are not among the formal duties listed in job descriptions.

Another key strategy to becoming an effective supervisor is conducting a self-assessment. Self-assessment is a reflective process of identifying the demands and responsibilities of your position and the needs of your customers and objectively comparing them to your ability to satisfy them through your skills and personal characteristics. Self-assessments can be completed in a number of ways. It is recommended that all practitioners, whether clinicians, educators, researchers, or managers, have a professional development plan that is updated on a regular basis.

The first step in developing such a plan is self-assessment. Formal assessment methods such as the Professional Development Tool, available from the American Occupational Therapy Association (AOTA) to its members, provide a structured approach to self-assessment, including the use of peer reviews, assessment of customer satisfaction, and the development of written learning objectives to guide professional growth (Case-Smith, 2003). Maintaining membership in AOTA and your state occupational therapy association is one of the best strategies for finding resources to become a more effective occupational therapy supervisor.

Another method of self-assessment is completing a self-assessment matrix. Matrices such as the one for Chris from our introductory case scenario (Table 7-2) are a simple way of planning for any aspect of professional growth. The horizontal axis includes the three commonly identified domains of learning, which are *knowledge*, *skills*, and *attitudes*. The vertical axis includes supervisory duties related to the management, education, and support functions of the supervisor found in your job description. Each cell of the matrix includes a goal, professional activity, or area of growth for the coming year. Completing a self-assessment matrix can be part of the process of planning for participation in your annual performance appraisal. The matrix can be shared with your supervisor so that he or she will be aware of your goals and be able to help you achieve them.

Another approach to self-assessment is to apply an adapted strategic planning process to planning for your professional growth. Such an adaptation is

TABLE 7-2

Chris's Sample Supervisory Self-Assessment Matrix

	Knowledge	Skills	Attitude
Management	I need to know more about how formal job descriptions are used in the process of giving feedback to those I supervise, so I will attend a workshop on writing job descriptions at the AOTA Annual Conference and Exposition. I plan to co-lead my first few performance evaluations with my manager so he can give me feedback on my ability to evaluate others.	I am familiar with the rules for providing effective feedback, but I need to practice giving feedback and maintaining body language and facial expressions that communicate confidence and don't contradict what I am saying verbally. I can evaluate my feedback skills with past level II students. I plan to ask other supervisors to observe me over the coming 2 months and give me feedback on my presentation.	I need to become more comfortable with the concept that giving feedback to staff members as a supervisor is a positive activity that contributes to their growth and to improved quality of service to our clients. By becoming more involved in the planning of the overall staff development program, I may become more comfortable with my role in providing feedback as a supervisor.
Education	I need increased familiarity with the competencies for the OTA to identify appropriate tasks and activities for delegation in the hospital setting. I also require additional information on the various ways to assess competencies. AOTA has a number of resources on assessment of competencies.	I am interested in improving my presentation skills so that I am more comfortable providing in-service education to staff. I will investigate presenting or co-presenting at our state occupational therapy association conference as an opportunity to plan and deliver an educational presentation. I also plan to present to internal hospital professionals.	I need to value more the influence that supervisors can have on the professional development and competency of staff and realize that this can be a means to employee and client satisfaction. By developing enhanced skills, I hope to feel more satisfied with my role in competency assessment and skill development of staff.
Support	I am going to complete an evidence-based review on theories of employee motivation in order to increase my understanding of factors that contribute to employee satisfaction and dissatisfaction.	I plan to attend a course offered by the human resources department on conflict resolution to increase my mediation skills so that I can be more effective and perceived as more supportive in helping staff resolve conflicts with other staff, parents, and teachers.	I tend to want to solve problems for employees immediately, when sometimes they just want someone to empathize with them. I need to put more value on taking time to listen to employees and help them solve their own problems so that they feel more emotionally supported. I realize that employee performance issues impact the whole team and ultimately client services.

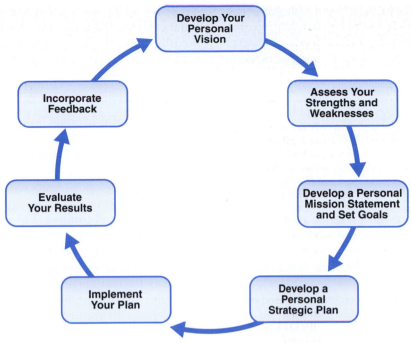

Figure ■ 7-1 Application of Strategic Planning to Development as a Supervisor.

suggested by Harvey and Struzziero (2000). The steps involved in this approach (Figure 7-1) include:

1. Developing a vision for your personal growth
2. Conducting an internal assessment of strengths and weaknesses and an external assessment of opportunities and threats (e.g., SWOT analysis)
3. Defining a personal mission and establishing goals for growth to enable you to achieve your mission
4. Developing a strategic plan, including measurable goals and objectives
5. Developing an action plan, including specific actions you will take and target dates for completing these actions related to each objective
6. Implementing your personal strategic plan
7. Conducting a formative evaluation (was the plan implemented as intended?) and a summative evaluation (were results what you expected?)
8. Feeding the evaluation results back into your personal strategic plan to begin the process again and to plan for additional growth

Certainly a large part of becoming an effective supervisor is coming to understand the needs of those you supervise and learning strategies to promote their growth, performance, and motivation. Throughout this book, you are encouraged to recognize the wide range of related knowledge (i.e., knowledge developed by other fields or disciplines not included in the occupational therapy paradigm) that can be used by the occupational therapy manager or supervisor to guide his or her daily work. In the following sections of this chapter, knowledge and evidence related to models of supervising others and to theories of motivating others are summarized.

Models of Supervision

Much of the supervision provided by occupational therapy supervisors is intended to guide OTs and OTAs in intervening with patients and clients. The fields of psychology, education, and social work have produced much of the research data that has been completed on developing models of supervision specifically related to the supervision of therapy practitioners. These models are generally split into four categories: (1) psychotherapy-based models, (2) developmental models, (3) social role models, and (4) eclectic or integrationist models. Each of these models is briefly explained.

Psychotherapy-Based Models

Therapy practitioners of any discipline work from an implicit theory of human nature that reflects how the practitioner views reality. Psychotherapy-based models of supervision tend to make the same assumptions about the nature of what constitutes an effective supervisor–trainee relationship as they do about what constitutes an effective therapist–client relationship.

The *person-centered supervision model* is based on the client-centered psychotherapy approach of Carl Rogers and tends to transfer client–therapist theory to the supervisee–supervisor relationship. Therefore, the emphasis is on the relationship between the supervisor and supervisee rather than the process of supervision. The most important aspects of supervision are the modeling of the necessary and sufficient conditions of empathy, genuineness, and unconditional positive regard (Kadushin, 2002). In this model, the supervisor establishes a welcoming and collaborative environment where the supervisee feels comfortable to bring up concerns.

The *cognitive-behavioral model* of supervision applies learning theory to supervision and generally comprises the following five elements: (1) establishing a trusting relationship, (2) skill analysis and assessment, (3) setting goals, (4) construction and implementation of strategies to accomplish goals, and (5) follow-up evaluation. This model of supervision assumes that being an effective occupational therapy practitioner is primarily a function of skills, with the purpose of supervision being to teach appropriate practitioner behaviors. A professional role is thought to consist of identifiable tasks requiring specific skills, and the supervisor assists the professional in developing skills that can be applied and refined (Patterson, 1986). The supervisor will help the supervisee learn how his or her cognitions affect his or her skills and how to change these cognitions to improve outcomes (Haynes, Corey, & Moulton, 2003).

The *feminist model* of supervision affirms the feminist theory that the individual's experiences are reflective of society's institutionalized attitudes and values (Smith, 2009). The supervisor–supervisee relationship strives to be egalitarian to the extent possible, with the supervisor maintaining focus on the supervisee's empowerment.

Developmental Models

Developmental approaches to supervision became popular in the 1990s. A main concept underlying developmental models of supervision is the notion that we each are continually growing, in fits and starts, in growth spurts and patterns. The object is to maximize and identify growth needed for the future at any given time (Leddick, 2004). Under a developmental model, it is assumed that close supervision is needed for a new occupational therapy practitioner but, as the practitioner gains experience, his or her need for supervision is lessened and the relationship with the supervisor changes also.

Stoltenberg and McNeil (2010) described a developmental model with three levels of supervisees: beginning, intermediate, and advanced. More recently, a fourth level was added that is an integration of the first three levels. Within each level, the authors noted a trend to begin in a rigid, shallow, imitative way and move toward more competence, self-assurance, and self-reliance at each level. In the final level (3i), the supervisees move fluidly through various aspects of the first three levels. Particular attention is paid to (a) self- and other awareness, (b) motivation, and (c) autonomy. For example, typical development in beginning supervisees would find them relatively dependent on the supervisor to diagnose clients and establish plans for therapy. Intermediate supervisees would depend on supervisors for an understanding of difficult clients, but *may* resent suggestions about the types of clients they have treated before. Resistance, avoidance, or conflict is typical of this stage, because supervisee self-concept is easily threatened. Advanced supervisees function independently, seek consultation when appropriate, and feel responsible for their correct and incorrect decisions.

Social Role Models

The basic tenet of the social role models is that as the needs of the supervisee change, the role of the supervisor should change to better meet those needs. For example, at times the supervisor may need to assume more of a role as a teacher and at other times may need to assume the role of counselor or consultant. Under this mode the style of the supervisor is determined by his or her theoretical orientation and the focus of supervision is determined according to the role the supervisor is assuming at any given time (Patterson, 1986). The Situational Leadership Theory discussed in Chapter 1 provides clear guidelines for how to alter supervision based on the needs of a particular employee at a particular time in a given situation.

Eclectic or Integrationist Models

Eclectic or integrationist models blend a number of different supervision theories (i.e., a social role model as well as a developmental approach). The main components of these models include a customized approach, needs assessment, and consideration of the supervisee's developmental level and cognitive style, as well as an assessment and evaluation of the supervisee's skills.

The *discrimination model* combines an attention to three supervisory roles with three areas of focus. Supervisors might take on a role of teacher when they directly lecture, instruct, and inform the supervisee. Supervisors may act as counselors when they assist supervisees in noticing their own "blind spots" or the manner in which they are unconsciously "hooked" by a client's issue. When supervisors relate as colleagues when discussing specific therapeutic cases, they might act in a consultant role. Each of the three roles is task-specific for the purpose of identifying issues in supervision (Bernard & Goodyear, 2014). The discrimination model also highlights three areas of focus for skill building: process, conceptualization, and personalization. Process issues examine how communication is conveyed. For example, is the supervisee reflecting the client's emotions and concerns in how he or she responds, or did the supervisee reframe the situation for the client? Conceptualization issues include how well supervisees can explain their application of a specific theory to a particular case—how well they see the big picture—as well as what reasons supervisees may have for what to do next. Personalization issues pertain to issues related to therapeutic use of the self in therapy to establish an effective interpersonal relationship.

Management Approaches to Supervision

In addition to the models of supervision just described, there are four management approaches supervisors can take to handle operational situations that are commonly identified in the management literature: (1) the *systematic management approach*, (2) the *human relations approach*, (3) the *quantitative approach*, and (4) the *contingency (or situational) approach*. The systematic management approach (also known as the traditional, classic, or scientific approach) relies on measurement and analysis of various tasks and activities that take place in the work environment. This approach to supervision has a greater reliance on established organizational policies and procedures and on prescribed relationships in formal work groups. In the human relations approach, it is assumed that a manager or supervisor who understands people's behaviors will be able to get his or her employees to cooperate and accomplish an organization's goals. This approach to supervision has a greater reliance on participatory techniques and upon individuals and groups to solve operational problems. The next type of approach is the quantitative approach, or systems theory of management, which relies on the use of numbers and statistics, as well as the sciences. This approach to supervision has a greater reliance on staff-directed or automatic programs to prescribe operating procedures. The fourth and last approach is the contingency (or situational) approach, which is where a manager's decision and action depend on the particular situation at hand. This approach requires a greater need for sensitivity to deal with different situations, as well as skills and flexibility to apply all the different management approaches. These four approaches are summarized in Table 7-3.

It is important to determine your approach to supervision. In this way, you can use these approaches or methods to handle new or difficult problems. For instance, if you want to implement a new program with staff, you can use many ways to achieve this goal. When using the human relations approach, you would allow the staff to participate in the way the program would be implemented. When using the systematic approach, you would prescribe specific steps to meet the new program objective. Your approach should depend on the successful implementation of past programs and the cultural approach to change within your work group. You also need to tailor your approach to the demands and knowledge

TABLE 7-3			
Four Commonly Identified Management Approaches to Supervision			
Systematic	**Human Relations**	**Qualitative**	**Contingency**
Relies on measurement and analysis of tasks	Relies on participatory techniques	Relies on numbers, statistics, and the scientific approach	Relies on the manager's judgment to choose the right approach
Uses policies, procedures, and formal relationships in work groups	Uses informal group relations to solve problems	Uses self-directed and automated programs such as statistical analysis software	Uses any of the strategies from any approach

level of your direct reports and your direct boss. If your supervisees do not understand how statistics relate to client care, you may need to use another approach.

Occupational Therapy Perspectives on Supervision

The supervision models presented in the previous section of the chapter were developed by disciplines other than occupational therapy. Limited theoretical work has been completed specifically related to the supervision of occupational therapy personnel. However, discipline-specific information and resources are available to the occupational therapy supervisor. The focus of these resources tends to be more on the supervisory relationships, responsibilities, and recommended levels of supervision for various categories of occupational therapy personnel (e.g., OTs, OTAs, and occupational therapy aides).

For example, AOTA provides its members with a document entitled "Guidelines for Supervision, Roles, and Responsibilities During the Delivery of Occupational Therapy Services" (AOTA, 2014). This document suggests that the amount of supervision required by an occupational therapy practitioner depends upon a "mutual understanding between the supervisor and supervisee about each other's competence, experience, education, and credentials." The frequency and method of supervision may vary according to the complexity of the clinical situation, the type of practice setting, regulatory requirements, and the number and diversity of clients. These supervision guidelines

follow a developmental approach to supervision as was described earlier in this chapter.

The American Physical Therapy Association (2012) provides similar definitions of supervision to guide the level of supervision of physical therapy personnel. It must be noted that the requirements stated in a state licensure law for supervision always supersede any recommendations for supervision made by a professional association. Such licensure laws may change over time, and it is the responsibility of the occupational therapy manager or supervisor to remain aware of requirements for supervision, especially when they may have an impact on staffing or productivity expectations, because it is unlikely that higher level non-occupational therapy managers will be familiar with the licensure laws for individual disciplines.

In addition to the amount of supervision required, a distinction is often made in the *type* of activity to be supervised. One common strategy is to distinguish between supervision of *client-related* and *non–client-related tasks*. This distinction is especially important in regard to the supervision of occupational therapy aides. Client-related tasks include all elements of intervention when the patient or client is present and there is contact between the occupational therapy personnel and the client.

Non–client-related tasks include clerical tasks and preparation of the environment or work area when there is no direct contact with the patient or client. The following conditions should be present when a client-related task is assigned to an occupational therapy aide (AOTA, 2014):

- The anticipated outcome of the intervention is predictable.

- The situation will not require judgment or adaptation by the aide.
- The client has demonstrated some competency to complete the task before and the task process is routine.

A final helpful concept found specifically in the occupational therapy literature related to supervision is that of **service competency** (Sladyk & Ryan, 2005). Service competency is defined as the process of teaching, training, and evaluating through which the OT determines that the OTA performs tasks in the same way that the OT would and achieves the same outcome. Although service competency is usually defined in regard to the supervision of an OTA by an OT, it is a useful concept in the supervision of OTs and occupational therapy fieldwork students as well. Establishing service competency between two practitioners simply means that, if both persons perform a particular task, they will achieve the same outcome. The process of completing competency checks on a new employee is essentially the process of establishing service competency. Service competency may be established or verified in a number of ways, including:

- Observation of a supervisee by a supervisor, comparing performance against a predetermined checklist
- Having two practitioners complete a task independently (i.e., take range of motion measurements) and comparing results
- Use of videotapes or "master cases" in which both practitioners review the tape or case and compare their analyses of problems, goals, or results
- Use of written tests or checklists of performance.

It is important to be honest with your strengths and weakness and determine what type of supervision model works best for you and your setting. Some organizations are beginning to develop management competencies. These are similar to clinical competencies and may include areas such as budgeting, employee relations, and organizational goal achievement. In addition to models of supervision, there are a number of theories that seek to explain the levels of motivation and satisfaction of employees and the impact that these have on employee retention. These theories are reviewed in the next section of this chapter.

Theories of Motivation, Employee Satisfaction, and Retention of Employees

Organizations invest huge sums of money and time in orienting, training, and developing the skills of personnel. Losing a well-trained and productive employee can have numerous negative consequences for an organization, including:

- Increased workload and dissatisfaction among the employees who remain
- Lost revenue as a result of lowered production and billing
- Customer dissatisfaction resulting from difficulties meeting customer expectations because of short staffing
- Lost business and referrals resulting from lowered customer satisfaction
- Potential of encouraging other employees to leave the organization

Loss of an employee, or employee "turnover," is not uncommon in the health-care industry or in community-based organizations. Estimates of the cost of replacing an employee have ranged from 25% to 150% of the employee's annual salary, including hiring and recruiting costs, training costs, lost productivity during the first 6 months of employment, and use of temporary employees during transitions (Bliss, 2013; Keller, 2012). Particularly in the fields of occupational therapy, physical therapy, and nursing, where jobs are often plentiful, changing jobs several times in the first decade of practice is not uncommon. However, although supervisors and managers can do little to lessen turnover driven by personal factors such as the desire to move geographically or enter a new area of practice, you can influence an employee's decision to stay with your organization by understanding theories related to employee motivation and satisfaction.

Motivation

Motivation can be thought of as the level of arousal, direction, and persistence of behavior related to a goal. The simple idea that people have needs continues to be the best explanation for what activates behavior. Satisfaction can be thought of as a consequence of performance in the workplace that is influenced by the types of rewards that individuals receive (both intrinsic and extrinsic rewards) and their connection to performance (Lawler, 1994).

Employee engagement is a more recent concept that builds on employee satisfaction. Employees engaged in their work are more likely to be motivated, to remain committed to their employer, and to stay focused on achieving business goals and driving the organization's future (Vorhauser-Smith, 2013).

Edward E. Lawler III (1994), professor of management and organization and founding director of the Center for Effective Organizations at the University of Southern California, stated that any theory of motivation must answer three questions:

1. What activates behavior?
2. What directs behavior?
3. What reactions do individuals have to the outcomes that result from their behavior?

Theories of motivation in the workplace can be organized into two basic types: (1) content or need-based theories, which stress the analysis of human needs, and (2) process theories, which focus on the thought processes of employees that influence behavior. Not all theories that have been utilized to explain employee motivation and satisfaction address all three of Lawler's questions. The most contemporary of each of these types of theories and the evidence related to their application to the workplace are briefly reviewed next.

Content Theories

Content theories describe the needs, motives, and goals of people, and these theories help us to understand how objects or outcomes become goals for people. Such theories specify why people value some outcomes and identify the factors that influence the values that people assign to their goals. Employees' goal-directed behavior is used to satisfy a need. For example, an employee who volunteers for a task force group may be satisfying a need for companionship. Content theories are useful for managers because they help them understand what people will and will not value as work rewards or as need satisfiers. Essentially, content theories suggest that managers must:

- Understand that different employees have different needs in terms of what they need and desire from work.
- Identify how an organization can meet the varying needs of employees.
- Create ways that different employees can meet individual needs and simultaneously contribute to the organization.

Maslow's Hierarchy of Needs

One content theory with which you are most likely familiar is Abraham Maslow's theory of human motivation (Maslow, 1970). The theory is based on a simple premise: Human beings have needs that are hierarchically ranked (Bauer & Erdogan, 2009). Maslow's hierarchy has been utilized as a framework for considering how factors in the work environment might influence the motivation and satisfaction of employees, and hence the likelihood that they will stay with their employer. Applications of Maslow's theory to work settings emphasize the meaning and significance of human work and focus on the fact that humans are motivated to obtain both intrinsic and extrinsic outcomes. As such, this theory addresses the second two of Lawler's questions (What directs behavior, and what reactions do individuals have to the outcomes that result from their behavior?) but does not provide a clear answer to the question as to why needs originate.

According to Maslow, the behavior of an individual related to meeting basic needs or satisfying primary drives decreases as these needs are satisfied. Basic needs and drives may be viewed as a hierarchy in which higher-order needs cannot be pursued unless lower-order or more basic needs are already satisfied. The categories of needs in the hierarchy are not completely exclusive, however. In other words, one category of needs does not need to be fully met before an individual may turn his or her attention to other needs higher in the hierarchy. Rather, as one level of need becomes gratified, another begins to emerge.

In regard to motivation, Maslow argued that, unlike motivation based on primary drives, motivation based on growth needs does not decrease as the needs become satisfied. To the contrary, Maslow stated that as people experience growth and self-actualization, they simply want more. Obtaining growth creates a desire for more growth, whereas

BOX 7-4

Maslow's Hierarchy of Needs

- **Physiological needs:** Basic human needs to sustain life itself, such as food, clothing, and shelter, that must be satisfied before a person can focus on other needs or before the pursuit of other needs provides a source of motivation for action
- **Safety needs:** The need to be free from danger and to seek self-preservation for today and the future
- **Social or affiliation needs:** The need to belong and to be accepted by social groups and persons of importance to the individual
- **Esteem needs:** The need to develop positive self-esteem and to gain recognition and acceptance from others
- **Self-actualization needs:** The need to maximize one's potential, whatever that might be

obtaining food decreases one's desire for food (Lawler, 1994). Still, the stages may be used as a general framework through which to view the progression of needs. Maslow identified five categories of needs that, in order from lowest to highest, are (1) *physiological* needs, (2) *safety* needs, (3) social or *affiliation* needs, (4) *esteem* needs, and (5) *self-actualization* needs. These categories of needs are explained further in Box 7-4.

Most persons in Western society are able to meet their most basic needs. Granted, we are all familiar with the plight of the homeless or those who must live in extreme poverty; however, most of those with whom we will interact in the workplace as employees will have found a way to meet these most basic needs. For those individuals, other needs become more central; however, we must understand that, in a turbulent economy, all workers may feel threatened even at the most basic levels when workplaces experience layoffs or downsizing. Unfortunately, it seems that layoffs and downsizing have become commonplace in most organizations. It is up to the supervisor to build a level of trust with employees so that they feel realistically secure about employment.

When a worker feels that his or her job is safe and that he or she will be able to maintain food and shelter not only for today but also in the future, affiliation needs will begin to surface. Employees will seek mechanisms by which they feel they are accepted as members of the work group and gain a sense of belonging, and will strive to develop meaningful relationships with their peers. Once affiliation needs are met, employees will seek more than just being a member of a group and will hope to gain a sense of satisfaction that is based in self-confidence and the recognition and respect that is gained from others in the workplace. Most employees seek opportunities that provide them with mechanisms to feel useful and competent in their work. In addition, most workers seek opportunities to gain recognition from their supervisors and peers as well as to be rewarded for their efforts. All of these opportunities help to meet the esteem needs of workers. Finally, once esteem needs begin to be satisfied, employees may seek to become the best at what they do within their work life, or to seek self-actualization. This can mean different things for different workers. For some, it may mean taking on a leadership role within the organization or developing advanced or specialized skills. For others, it may mean becoming involved in other venues within the work environment, such as task forces or committees, through extra volunteer efforts. The employee who is ready for self-actualization is likely to be the employee who stands out in terms of performance and extra effort.

Early research provided strong evidence related to Maslow's hierarchy to establish that unless existence needs are satisfied, none of the higher-order needs will come into play. There is also evidence that unless security needs are satisfied, people will not be concerned with higher order needs. There is little evidence to support the view that a hierarchy exists above the security level. Thus, functionally using a hierarchy that attempts to do anything beyond grouping the most basic needs together (e.g., existence and security) and grouping all higher-order needs together cannot be supported by evidence (Lawler, 1994). Also, there is little support that once a need is satisfied, it will no longer serve as a motivator and that only one need is dominant at a time (Bauer & Erdogan, 2009). Although management would benefit from addressing both security and higher-order needs, different employees may experience different higher-order needs, with one focusing on autonomy and another focusing more on esteem.

Herzberg's Hygiene or Motivation Theory

Frederick Herzberg's hygiene or motivation theory, developed out of work originally conducted with 200 Pittsburgh engineers and accountants, has become one of the most replicated studies in the field of workplace psychology. According to this theory, employee satisfaction and dissatisfaction at work nearly always arise from different factors, and are not simply opposing reactions to the same factors. Satisfaction and dissatisfaction are not opposite ends of a single continuum, but instead are two separate constructs. An important implication of this theory is that employees can be both very satisfied and very dissatisfied at the same time. If this is true, managers and supervisors must recognize that different factors contribute to employee satisfaction than to dissatisfaction. In other words, employees will not automatically be satisfied if there is an absence of dissatisfiers, nor will employees be automatically satisfied with the presence of satisfiers.

The hygiene or motivation theory states that the primary drive for persons to work is for their own self-satisfaction and contentment, because work or the engagement in healthy occupations contributes to individuals' happiness and satisfaction. Applied to the workplace, this theory identifies two sets of factors related to human needs: *hygiene factors* and *motivation factors*. Hygiene factors are defined as factors that are part of the context in which the job is performed, whereas motivation factors are factors that are intrinsic to the job (Bauer & Erdogan, 2009). Examples from these two sets of factors are listed in Table 7-4.

Because hygiene factors and motivation factors are separate constructs, managers and supervisors need to attend to both types of factors to maximize employees' satisfaction with the workplace and to minimize dissatisfaction. It is also important to recognize that the strength of factors may vary and that employees may value different factors to different extents. For example, whereas one employee may place primary importance on salary and be willing to accept the presence of some dissatisfiers if his or her salary is sufficiently high, another employee might highly value recognition from superiors and work that is interesting and satisfying and be willing to accept a lower salary. Hygiene factors and motivating factors cannot be used in an exact formula to assure employee satisfaction, but can be used as a guide to examine the status of the workplace and to guide managers and supervisors to assess the workplace and make changes that are likely to appeal to a range of employees' values and needs.

Evidence related to this "two-factor" theory is mixed, with some evidence showing support and some providing reasons to question the theory, but neither body of evidence is sufficiently strong to validate or completely reject the theory. Lawler (1994) noted that even proponents of the theory have accepted that some factors may cause both satisfaction and dissatisfaction, and the thought that satisfaction and dissatisfaction are indeed separate constructs has been questioned. He pointed out, however, that simply because some factors can influence both satisfaction and dissatisfaction, this does not mean that they are not on separate continua. Rather, the fact

---

TABLE 7-4

Hygiene and Motivation Factors

Hygiene Factors	Motivation Factors
• Rewards (financial) that are perceived to correlate with performance and the current marketplace • Safe, pleasant, and comfortable working environments • Pleasant and supportive interpersonal relationships with peers and supervisors • Competent and supportive supervision and management • Job security	• Recognition from peers and supervisors for positive contributions to the workplace • Opportunities for promotion and advancement within a career track • Levels of authority, decision-making, and responsibility that match one's responsibilities • Work that is satisfactory and matches the psychological contract entered into with the employer • Personal growth and development

TABLE 7-5
Work Preferences of Persons High in Need for Achievement, Affiliation, or Power

Individual Needs	Work Preferences	Example
High need for achievement	Prefers to work alone and accept responsibility, desires challenging targets and goals, and desires specific feedback on performance	Private practitioner who opens her own business providing work injury prevention services with the opportunity to earn based on how successfully she sells her products
High need for affiliation	Prefers to work with others; values team activities and opportunities to communicate and collaborate with others	Senior therapist in a rehabilitation hospital who accepts a role as coordinator of continuing education and collaborates with team supervisors to plan for the professional development of staff
High need for power	Prefers to take charge of work tasks and influence others; seeks attention and recognition for playing a central role	A department director who assumes responsibility for supervision of therapy practitioners and volunteers for high-profile task groups within the organization

that a single factor may influence both may simply highlight the importance of that factor in a given environment.

McClelland's Acquired Needs Theory

According to the acquired needs theory, three types of human needs are acquired over time as a result of life experiences. These needs result in motivation that is driven by how needs are associated with individual work preferences. The three types of needs are:

1. Need for *achievement,* or the desire to do something better or more efficiently and to master more and more complex tasks.
2. Need for *affiliation,* or the desire to establish and maintain friendly and warm relations with others in the environment.
3. Need for *power,* or the desire to control others, to influence their behavior, or to be responsible for others.

The acquired needs theory is most useful when each need is matched with a set of work preferences specific to a work environment, because the preferences may look very different in various settings, such as a school system, a medical-model setting or hospital, a private business, or a community-based organization. Creating an explicit process of examining the various needs of employees within a setting and including employees in generating statements of work preferences and examples of work forms that meet their needs is a concrete way that this theory can be applied.

There is limited evidence to date to support this theory, but some research has generated interesting questions about the role of culture in influencing the balance of needs in terms of achievement, affiliation, and power. Table 7-5 relates each of these needs to individual work preferences and provides examples of each.

Process Theories

Although content theories emphasize what employees need in regard to motivation, they do not address how employees become motivated or why they choose one action over another in the workplace. Process theories place higher emphasis than content theories on "how" to motivate employees.

Vroom's Expectancy Theory

Victor Vroom developed the expectancy theory of motivation, which postulates that motivation depends on individuals' expectations about their ability to perform assigned work tasks and receive desired rewards. In simple terms, outcomes have value if they lead to other valued outcomes (Vroom, 1964). The theory does not address the question of what causes people to value particular outcomes nor what other outcomes are likely to be valued.

The three main constructs of this theory are *valence*, *expectancy*, and *instrumentality*. Valence is the importance placed upon a specific reward by an employee, recognizing that not all employees equally value the same rewards and experiences. Expectancy is the belief by an employee that his or her efforts are linked to performance or that, if he or she develops increased skills or makes extra efforts, this will result in improved performance. Instrumentality is the belief that the quality of performance within a workplace is related to the rewards that are given in return. For example, consider an occupational therapy practitioner working as a salesperson for a company that sells assistive and adaptive equipment. The practitioner's expectancy is the belief that more sales calls will result in higher sales (performance). The practitioner's instrumentality is that higher sales (performance) will result in higher commissions (rewards). Finally, the practitioner's valence is the importance attached to the commissions (rewards). These three factors result in motivation. If any one of these factors doesn't exist, then motivation vanishes. If the salesperson does not believe greater effort leads to performance, then there is no motivation. Similarly, if commissions don't increase with sales, then instrumentality disappears. If commissions are not important to the salesperson, he or she will likely not extend effort even if he or she has high expectancy and instrumentality.

Vroom's motivation theory is often illustrated by the following equation:

Motivation =

$$\text{Expectancy} \times \text{Instrumentality} \times \text{Valence}$$

This equation indicates that motivation is determined in a multiplicative relationship, so expected levels of motivation should be very low if any one of these variables is very low; conversely, to expect that motivation will be very high, one must expect that all three variables are very high. For example, suppose a manager wonders whether a cash bonus program would have any effect on productivity levels. He or she might anticipate that if an employee feels any of the following conditions exist, there is low likelihood that motivation will be positively affected:

- The employee feels he or she cannot meet the performance targets to qualify.
- The person is not confident that a high productivity level will truly be recognized and result in bonuses being distributed.
- The person does not value the reward of a cash bonus.

The implication of this theory for managers and supervisors is that they must focus on increasing all three variables as they relate to employees by fostering employees' sense of competency, drawing concrete relationships between desired work behaviors and the outcomes of those behaviors, and customizing rewards to match individual employee desires to the extent possible.

The evidence relating to expectancy theory has been generally supportive, although research to more specifically articulate aspects of the theory, such as the suggested multiplicative effect, has not been presented (Salancik & Pfeffer, 2003). A generally supported aspect of the theory that is of particular interest to managers and supervisors is that the rewards linked to improving performance can vary from employee to employee and from culture to culture. As a result, managers must consider how they may vary rewards for the performance of employees within organizational structures that sometimes prescribe how rewards are provided in very structured manners.

Equity Theory

John Adams developed the equity theory of motivation, which postulates that motivation depends on individuals' perception of fairness in their interactions (Bauer & Erdogan, 2009). Employees compare their inputs and outcomes to those of others during daily work routines. The comparison person is referred to as the referent. There is a tension created with these perceived inequities, and the employee will make adjustments to reduce these inequalities. For example, an employee works after hours to develop several new protocols for an emerging patient population (input), but does not receive additional pay or recognition (output). This situation is then perceived as being unfair to the employee. It must be noted that the inequality is a subjective process. The supervisor could view this as fair as the employee could be a senior occupational therapist and this is part to the inherent job description.

TABLE 7-6
Examples of Employee Reactions to Perceived Inequities

Reactions to Inequity	Example
Distort perceptions	Changing one's thinking to believe that the referent actually is more skilled than previously thought
Increase referent's inputs	Encouraging the referent to work harder
Reduce own input	Deliberately putting forth less effort at work; reducing the quality of one's work
Increase own outcomes	Negotiating a raise for oneself or using unethical ways of increasing rewards such as stealing from the company
Change referent	Comparing oneself to someone who is worse off
Leave the situation	Quitting one's job
Seek legal action	Suing the company or filing a complaint if the unfairness in question is under legal protection

Employees react differently to these perceived inequities. Table 7-6 illustrates these responses (Bauer & Erdogan, 2009).

As a supervisor, you need to be aware of the perceptions of your employees relating to issues of inequality. Of note, the concepts of equal and fair are not the same. Equal refers to treating everyone exactly alike, whereas fair means treating in a way that does not favor some over others. For example, all occupational therapy practitioners in a department may not work weekends depending on their primary work area (e.g., the outpatient clinics do not have patients scheduled on weekends, whereas acute medicine does). It is up to the supervisor and manager to justify the reasoning behind their decisions.

Employee Retention

Retaining valuable employees is of critical importance to organizations, and the impact of rewards and recognition on employee retention is well documented in the literature. Determining monetary rewards in the form of salary increases may be reserved as a function of the manager, but both managers and supervisors can provide praise and recognition to employees in various forms.

Rewards and Recognition

Most organizations (88%) have some type of recognition programs, according to World at Work (2013). The types of recognition programs include length of service, acknowledgement of above-and-beyond performance, and peer-to-peer recognition. One more recent recognition type of program that is emerging consists of programs that motivate specific behaviors. An example of this is a wellness program. Many organizations are offering employees options to improve their health or prevent illnesses. These can include smoking cessation education programs or reduction in health insurance premiums if the employee decreases body mass index (BMI). At this time, debate continues regarding the effectiveness of these programs and if they actually change behavior or decrease organizations' health-care costs.

One reward program that is fairly easy to implement and has good results is the peer-to-peer recognition program. This usually involves a peer recognizing a fellow employee for a simple act in the workplace. This recognition can cross disciplines and is a great way to demonstrate noticing an employee's good work. The employee usually receives some type of small monetary reward (e.g., movie tickets) and a button or certificate. There can also be more substantial peer recognition programs including employee of the month or team of the year.

TABLE 7-7	
Examples of Intrinsic and Extrinsic Rewards	
Intrinsic Rewards	**Extrinsic Rewards**
• Gratification for making a contribution to the public good	• Increased salary and merit raises tied to performance
• Positive self-regard that comes with developing new skills	• Public recognition such as words of praise and thanks
• Enjoyment when spending time in pursuits of interest	• Promotions and increased power and authority
• Feelings of achievement when successfully completing assigned work and overcoming obstacles	• Safety and security that comes with other benefits such as health and retirement benefits

Many managers and supervisors pay insufficient attention to providing their subordinates with rewards and recognition outside of the formal performance appraisal meeting that typically occurs once a year. There have been a number of theories related to motivation and retention of employees in organizations. Most theories address two types of rewards that are thought to influence employee motivation: (1) *intrinsic rewards*, which are rewards received as a direct result of a person's actions, and (2) *extrinsic rewards*, which are rewards given by another person, often a manager or supervisor. Typical examples of each of these types of rewards are presented in Table 7-7.

Ensuring that intrinsic rewards become available to employees can be particularly challenging for the manager or supervisor. To facilitate adequate intrinsic rewards, you must balance the organization's needs and ensure that work is completed in an effective and efficient manner while designing work processes and environments with the flexibility to provide for different employees' individual needs and desires. Planning and specifying job tasks, as well as work settings in which they are accomplished, in a way that is motivational for employees is referred to as *job design*. Job design includes four strategies managers can use to provide adequate intrinsic rewards for employees while also facilitating employee satisfaction and organizational productivity:

1. Job *simplification*, or standardization of work procedures, and using employees in clearly defined and specialized tasks.
2. Job *enlargement*, which includes strategies to increase the breadth of a job by adding to the variety of tasks performed by a worker.
3. Job *rotation*, or increasing the variety of tasks completed by periodically shifting workers between jobs and different tasks.
4. Job *enrichment*, which is the practice of building motivating factors into job content by expanding job content and adding work functions typically performed by higher-level employees, such as planning or supervision functions.

When providing extrinsic rewards, careful consideration of the impact that a particular reward may have is warranted. You must also consider if the reward may have consequences that are not anticipated. Unfortunately, managers and supervisors may sometimes assume that employees would appreciate and enjoy the same types of rewards and recognitions that they might, and inadvertently provide a reward that is in fact experienced as punishing or unpleasant. For example, although you might assume that any employee would appreciate being taken out to lunch or dinner, having to stay late in the evening in order to free up the time during the day to attend a lunch or spending hours outside of work with the boss on a usually free evening might *not* be perceived as a reward. Providing an employee with a gift certificate so that he or she might enjoy a meal with a family member or friend might be more rewarding. Similarly, you might assume that recognizing an employee in a public manner, such as presenting him or her with a certificate or plaque as a "thank-you" in front of a large gathering of his or her peers, would be a welcome event. However, for the employee who is fearful of appearing in front of large groups of people, this "reward" might be experienced as punishing or embarrassing. Another unexpected negative impact of providing rewards and recognitions is that often success is a team effort, and providing a reward or recognition to an individual may unintentionally send a message to other employees that their efforts are not appreciated. An employee who volunteers to take on a special project or join a task group, such as a continuous quality improvement team, may only be able to do so because the employee's peers cover part of his or her workload. Careful consideration of when to reward or recognize an individual and when to reward an entire department or team for achievements will help to avoid sending unwanted messages. Remember, not all extrinsic rewards need to be tied to large monetary events. A department newsletter is one way to recognize others. Factors to consider in regard to rewards and recognitions are included in Box 7-5.

Several factors influence the success of these programs. Managers and supervisors need to have training or knowledge that these programs exist and inform new hires of these programs to increase their use. Senior management also needs to buy into these programs and see them as an investment rather than as an expense.

BOX 7-5

Factors to Consider in Selecting Rewards and Recognitions

- Investigate and consider whether to reward or recognize an individual or a team or department.
- Don't assume that all persons equally value the same types of rewards and recognition.
- Associate the reward or recognition with specific accomplishments rather than general performance.
- Individualize rewards and recognition whenever possible, such as writing individual thank-you notes or choosing rewards related to an employee's personal interests.
- Consider recognition that demonstrates your personal awareness of the employee's contribution to the organization.
- Provide reward and recognition in a timely manner close to the time of achievement.

Retention of Employees

Retention of valued employees is a major concern for occupational therapy managers and supervisors. As noted earlier, there can be tremendous costs associated with employee turnover, including recruitment expenses, lost revenue, and the need to train a new employee. Traditionally, retention of employees was primarily a human resources function, but responsibility for staff recruitment and retention has shifted over the last few decades to be a responsibility of line managers because organizations have trimmed staff functions such as their human resources departments to save costs. In addition, the knowledge of the disciplinary manager and supervisor about what contributes to satisfaction and dissatisfaction for employees has become highly valued. Although studies on employee retention from various disciplines (e.g., occupational therapy, physical therapy, nursing) reveal that similar factors influence retention regardless of discipline, designing effective strategies to improve retention is easier with discipline-specific input. The most effective way to address recruitment and retention concerns is for the occupational therapy manager to develop a collaborative working relationship with the organization's human resources professionals. It is also important to identify the reasons that employees continue their employment and the reasons that employees leave.

Although it is common for new practitioners to stay in their first jobs for a relatively short time (1 to 3 years) and for some employee turnover to be related to uncontrollable factors such as moving because of a spouse's relocation or choosing to be a stay-at-home parent, there are some factors that contribute to turnover that can be influenced. Nosse, Friberg, and Kovacek (2009) identified factors related to employee turnover and actions that could be taken by managers to limit the impact of these factors. Sample factors included (1) poorly defined responsibilities, (2) work that does not utilize employee skills, (3) limited growth opportunities, (4) lack of recognition for performance, and (5) pay inequities. In examining causes of turnover, the actions that managers can take are often easy to identify given the problem. For example, staff dissatisfaction caused by poorly defined responsibilities can be addressed by clearly outlining duties in job descriptions and in day-to-day direction. Perceptions that work does not utilize an employee's skills can be addressed in the performance

TABLE 7-8
Summary of Selected Evidence on Employee Retention

Author	Study Type	N (Sample Size)	Level of Evidence	Results
Vornholt, Uitdewilligen, & Nijhuis (2013)	Literature review	48 articles	Good	The acceptance of employees with disabilities is influenced by three main variable groups: characteristics of coworkers, of the persons with disabilities, and of the employers or organizations.
Scanlan, Still, Stewart, & Croaker (2010)	Survey of mental health occupational therapists	38	Good	Examines factors that attract employees to positions, as well as those that impact retention.
Zangaro & Soeken (2007)	Meta-analysis	31	Strong	Job satisfaction was most strongly correlated with job stress, nurse–physician collaboration, and autonomy.
Gowda (1997)	Survey of case managers	218	Good	Active coping, salary, role stress, and opportunity for promotion correlated with burnout and job dissatisfaction.
Irvine & Evans (1995)	Meta-analysis	23	Strong	Work content and work environment had a stronger relationship with job satisfaction than economic or individual difference variables in nursing job satisfaction.
Will (1995)	Survey of paramedics	299	Good	Satisfaction with work and coworkers contributed more than pay or promotion to job satisfaction and retention.
Smith, Schiller, Grant, & Sachs (1995)	Survey of OT managers	320	Good	The top retention strategies used were fostering interpersonal staff relationships, employee appraisals, and continuing education, although more than 70% used 17 similar strategies.

appraisal cycle by development of collaborative goals to focus on the application of skills. Not all turnover factors are within the manager's control. For example, the salary and benefits may be set by the organization, but by recognizing and listing potential turnover factors in your setting, you can identify strategies to directly address them. A sample of selected evidence related to the retention of employees is provided in Table 7-8.

Box 7-6 lists the most common factors shown to contribute to employee retention in the occupational therapy, physical therapy, and nursing literature. Although some strategies are beyond the simple control of the occupational therapy manager or supervisor because they require the commitment of organizational resources, there are strategies that can be implemented in the course of your daily work. These strategies are listed in Box 7-7.

Employee engagement, a recently used term correlated with employee retention, incorporates past concepts of employee satisfaction and adds the concepts of organizational commitment and job involvement. Many organizations are using surveys to measure employee satisfaction or engagement. Supervisors and managers must use the information gathered on the surveys objectively and incorporate necessary changes into their departments. Engagement scores have been shown to correlate with higher financial performance,

---

BOX 7-6

Factors Shown to Contribute to Employee Retention

- Potential for promotion
- Autonomy in decision-making
- Positive staff relationships
- Health benefits
- Flexible schedule
- Adequate supervision and feedback

- Vacation and holiday leave
- Part-time options
- Job security
- Competitive salary
- Educational reimbursement
- Continuing education

BOX 7-7

Everyday Strategies for Retaining Employees

1. Ask employees "What do you think?" on a regular basis.
2. Provide verbal praise and say "Thank you" for a job well done.
3. Follow up on expressions of concern or dissatisfaction from employees even if you are not sure you can solve the problem.
4. Use ad hoc work groups and committees to solve departmental problems and ask for volunteers.
5. Look for ways to increase flexibility, such as offering to let employees leave early or come in late when work volume is temporarily low.
6. Don't always try to immediately "fix" an employee's problem; sometimes he or she just wants you to listen and understand his or her daily frustrations.

---

lower employee turnover, and higher productivity (MacLeod & Clarke, 2008).

Performance Appraisal

"If performance evaluations were a drug, they would not receive F.D.A. approval, they have so many side effects, and so often fail" (Sutton, 2013). Although there is some partial truth to this statement and the process of performance appraisal can be unnerving for both the employee and the unseasoned supervisor, this does not have to be the case. If the supervisor has effectively shared information with employees on a routine basis throughout the performance cycle, the appraisal meeting itself need not be confrontational or unnecessarily unpleasant. However, this assumes that there has been ongoing communication, and unfortunately this is often not the case. All too often, supervisors only provide casual feedback to employees unless there is a serious problem. This practice results in two types of problems. First, it can result in missed opportunities for professional growth for employees. Second, it can result in the employees feeling as if the feedback is coming as a surprise. If an employee feels surprised in a performance appraisal meeting, even if the appraisal is going better than he or she expected, it can only mean that the supervisor has not done an adequate job in providing supervision.

An effective performance appraisal process is cyclical and can be thought of as occurring in four stages: (1) assessment, (2) performance planning, (3) intermittent review, and (4) accomplishment review. Each of these stages is reviewed in more detail in this section.

Stage I: Assessment

Assessment occurs at the beginning of a performance cycle, which is typically a 12-month period in most organizations. Assessment is most effective when it is a collaborative process between the employee and his or her immediate supervisor and includes a self-assessment by the employee. A comprehensive self-assessment includes a review of the current job description for any area for which the employee feels he or she could use additional guidance as well as identification of areas for personal and professional growth. Self-assessment can assist with the identification of goals related to training (learning needs for the current job), education (learning needs for future professional opportunities), and development (general learning needs and skills that can apply to any employment situation). The supervisor should guide the self-assessment process so that it also includes identification of any organizationally determined *key result areas*. Key result areas may relate to standard sections of job descriptions or to organizational values such as "customer service," "continuous quality improvement," or "cost-effectiveness." Although assessment of performance is typically included in the human resources policies and procedures of most organizations, structured tools to guide assessment for employees are not always provided. Use of structured tools such as AOTA's Professional Development Tool or a self-assessment matrix similar to that shown in Table 7-2 adapted to a specific job description can make the self-assessment process easier and contribute to the identification of realistic goals. Assessment also includes examination and integration of feedback from one's supervisor on performance for the previous performance period.

Stage II: Performance Planning

Performance planning is the process of identifying mutually agreed-upon goals related to programmatic needs and individual desires for growth. It also includes identification of the actions that will be taken by both the employee and his or her supervisor to facilitate the employee reaching established goals. Occupational therapists and occupational therapy assistants are well familiar with the process of setting goals because it is a key part of the occupational therapy process. Setting goals as part of a performance planning process is not so different. Just as when setting goals for a client, when an employee and his or her supervisor collaborate on goals for a performance period, it is important that the goals be (a) specific, (b) measurable, (c) attainable, (d) relevant, and (e) time bound (SMART goals). Goals should be specific in that each should clearly indicate what is and is not to be covered by the goal. Goals should be measurable so that it is possible for both the employee and his or her supervisor to know exactly when the goal has been achieved. Goals should be

attainable during the performance period and within the employee's capacities to develop. In addition, goals should be relevant to the specific employee's job responsibilities and to the work he or she is assigned. Finally, goals should be time bound in that a specific and reasonable time frame for their achievement is identified within the performance period. Employees may have long-term goals that extend over several performance periods, but these should be broken down into short-term goals that can be achieved within a single performance period. This is important because, in most organizations, raises in salary (e.g., merit increases) are typically based upon achievements in one 12-month period.

In addition to establishing specific, measurable, attainable, relevant, and time-bound goals, action plans should be developed that clearly identify the steps that will be taken by the employee to reach his or her goals, as well as those actions that the supervisor will take to support the employee in goal attainment. In many organizations, the goals and action plans may typically be documented in writing and signed by both the employee and the supervisor to indicate that they have collaborated on the development of the performance plan.

Stage III: Intermittent Review

During this stage, the supervisor evaluates the performance of employees both in their standard assigned duties and on their progress toward achieving their development goals. One of the most basic and most commonly overlooked principles of the performance appraisal process is that feedback should be *frequent and ongoing*. It is very easy to get caught up in the many responsibilities that most supervisors have in today's organizations, and it can be difficult to sequester the time to prepare and deliver feedback to employees in a timely and constructive manner. It can also be difficult at times to give negative feedback to an employee. Keeping simple rules of feedback in the forefront of one's attention can help a supervisor stay on track with providing intermittent review in an effective manner. A few of these rules for providing feedback are provided in Box 7-8.

Many organizations now have online performance evaluation systems that allow and remind the employee to document progress toward goals and achievements accomplished throughout the year. This is an easy way

Simple Rule for Making Feedback Constructive

Give Feedback in a Timely Manner

- *Timely:* "This morning your response to Sharon seemed abrupt, and that concerned me."
- *Untimely:* "Sometimes your responses to coworkers are abrupt when they ask for help."

Make Feedback Objective and Descriptive Rather Than Subjective and Judgmental

- *Descriptive:* "This morning you seemed intent on people understanding your point of view."
- *Judgmental:* "You were so stubborn in the meeting this morning."

Make Feedback Specific Rather Than General

- *Specific:* "I'm concerned that you were late for the last two meetings."
- *General:* "It bothers me that you're never on time."

Deal Only with Things That the Employee Can Change: The Behavior Instead of the Characteristics

- *Behavior:* "If you spoke a little more slowly, your patients may not feel so overwhelmed."
- *Characteristics:* "Your voice is so high and squeaky."

Consider Your Motives When Giving or Receiving Feedback

- *Constructive motives:* "If I share this with Dave, he'll be a better clinician."
- *Destructive motives:* "Dave's such a hotshot, I'll bring him down a notch."

to document employee performance throughout the performance cycle.

Once an action plan is established and the performance period begins, it is important that some planning for contingencies occurs as the employee goes about trying to achieve his or her goals. Although it is important to hold employees accountable for diligently working on their development plans, it is also important that, as managers or supervisors, we hold ourselves accountable for providing adequate support to the employee. We must recognize when circumstances within the organization interfere with the employee's ability to reach his or her goals. A common example might be when vacancies occur in staffing or budgets are reduced and the supervisor is unable to follow through on commitments to send an employee to a continuing education course. In the case of this or other contingent events that interfere with a performance action plan, alternative actions can be identified, but only if the employee and supervisor are meeting on a regular basis.

Stage IV: Accomplishment Review

The fourth stage in the performance appraisal cycle includes the process of providing feedback to the employee to objectively note the extent to which he or she met or exceeded expectations for the essential job functions and other assigned duties, and the extent to which he or she achieved the goals developed at the beginning of the performance cycle. If intermittent reviews have been conducted and the employee has been provided both regular praise and suggestions for improving performance throughout the year, the accomplishment review should be essentially a time to summarize earlier discussions and begin planning for the next appraisal cycle. Whether positive or negative, employees should never be surprised during this step of the performance appraisal process. If employees enter an accomplishment review and feedback does not match what they expect to hear, the manager or supervisor should reexamine how he or she is providing feedback to the employee.

With the exception of new employees, stage IV and stage I are typically completed together. After providing feedback on the past year, it is time to return to the process of reviewing a current self-assessment and establishing goals for the next performance appraisal period.

Maintaining a perception by employees that an appraisal by a supervisor is not heavily influenced by bias and subjectivity can be difficult. One strategy to increase the perceived fairness and objectivity of performance appraisals is by including multiple sources, including peers and managers or supervisors from other departments who are familiar with the performance of the employee being evaluated. Peer reviews often have a high level of worker acceptance and involvement; they tend to be stable, task relevant, and accurate. By helping peers to understand each other's work and by airing grievances in a nonthreatening manner, peer reviews may also help people to get along better. For the organization, this means higher performance.

These reviews are often referred to as a "360-degree" performance appraisal or a multisource appraisal. This system can be used for subordinates and managers and helps to assess several work behaviors including clinical skills and team skills. This means that there is an assessment driver in the system to demand a minimum performance in terms of interpersonal behaviors, which would not be there in the absence of the multisource feedback (MSF) (Wood, Hassell, Whitehouse, Bullock, & Wall, 2006).

According to Wood et al (2006), there are 10 tips in the development of an MSF system:

1. Develop a positive culture. This helps motivate change.
2. Be clear about the purpose. It must be owned by all and used to correctly identify high and low performers.
3. Clearly express any desired behaviors. Opportunity exists to make known desired behaviors.
4. Keep the number of items to be scored to a few. Large numbers of items do not add discrimination.
5. Keep the scale simple and fit for purpose.
6. Use 6 to 10 raters. This helps to solidify good results.
7. Compare results with self-assessment. A large discrepancy between the two can represent a lack of insight.
8. Train those who give feedback. Skilled feedback needs to be backed up by educational training.
9. Involve those being assessed. Involvement in development of the system likely enhances quality and maximizes its potential.
10. Incorporate development. This will help standardize understanding across raters and assessors.

For the employees, this means a better place to work and less frustration; it may also help employees to concentrate less on politics or working around other people, and to spend more time on their work (or to put in less overtime) (Toolpack Consulting LLC, 2002). A team of evaluators may be assembled to increase the accuracy and completeness of the picture of performance assembled by management (Ewen, 1994). The advantages of such an approach may include the following:

- Feedback on a wider variety of work behaviors may be gathered, including cooperation, planning, delegation, and teamwork.
- Direct reports from multiple sources may be more reliable than supervisory judgments alone; this can add insight into employees' perceptions of their skills and abilities.
- There is less chance that feedback will be perceived as discriminatory if peers are involved in providing the feedback, and especially if the employee influences which peers provide feedback.
- Multirater evaluations may do better to empower employees to assume responsibility for their own career development.
- The employee helps to identify those who are involved in the appraisal process, and this increases the perception of fairness.
- The process motivates behavior change as a result of process credibility, accuracy, and validity.
- The process can also make organizational values explicit, such as teamwork and excellent clinical skills.

Challenges and limitations to implementing a multisource performance appraisal system include the following:

- There may be perceived threats to the traditional role and authority of the manager and supervisor.
- Feedback on the same skill or behavior may vary from source to source and must be integrated into a single report.
- Feedback from peers may focus on personal characteristics or behaviors not related directly to work performance.

- Staff members may require training in the process of providing objective feedback.
- The process requires additional time and effort to collect information and integrate the information collected.
- Feedback may be lower if the rater is vying for the same promotion.
- There must be an organizational culture change to accept this process, including a culture of communication, trust, and senior management support.

Chapter Summary

This chapter reviewed the supervisor's major roles and functions. The concepts of power and formal authority were differentiated and strategies for increasing both personal and position power were provided. Several strategies for conducting a self-assessment in order to develop a plan for becoming a more effective supervisor were covered in this chapter, and you were encouraged to take full advantage of the many resources available that were provided both within and outside the profession of occupational therapy. This chapter provided just a sample of the many theories and models that might guide you as a supervisor, and you are reminded that the evidence on these models and theories continues to be developed. Finally, the chapter provided an overview of the processes of performance appraisal and of providing rewards and recognition to employees. Together, Chapters 6 and 7 have provided a solid introduction to the primary roles and functions of the manager and supervisor.

At the beginning of this chapter, you were introduced to Chris, who was interested in learning more about the roles and functions of a supervisor. She was interested in some aspects of becoming a supervisor but wondered if she could assume supervisory responsibilities without also assuming managerial tasks such as budgeting. Chris decided to consult with Craig, the director of the occupational therapy department, to find out what responsibilities might be included in the job of senior therapist.

■ Real-Life Solutions

After a conversation with Craig, Chris felt much more comfortable with the idea that there are opportunities to become involved in the supervision of others without also accepting all the typical duties of a manager. Chris learned that not having "requisite managerial authority" can sometimes be a complicating factor because you do not have control over who reports to you. At the same time, she became excited about the extent of resources available to help her develop as a supervisor.

Craig shared with Chris that the hospital offered professional development courses related to supervision for employees with supervisory roles and that potential supervisors could attend with their supervisor's support. He also shared that he had discovered a wealth of information on topics such as conducting performance appraisals, motivating and retaining employees, and providing rewards and recognition in the human resources literature while working on papers for a master's degree in human resource development that he was pursuing. In addition, he told Chris that whenever he encountered a new challenge and was unsure of how to proceed, he turned to his network of peers locally and nationally who were available to him through his participation in state and national occupational therapy associations.

Craig encouraged Chris to become a member of both the state association and AOTA, as he had done, and to begin networking with peers. Finally, he offered to support Chris by guiding her through the completion of a self-assessment in order to form a professional development plan that included goals related to becoming a supervisor. By the end of their conversation, Chris was ready to agree to formally interviewing for the position of supervisor.

Study Questions

1. **Power that is obtained because of knowledge, personal attractiveness, or demonstration of effort is best defined as:**

   a. Legitimate authority.
   b. Organizational influence.
   c. Personal power.
   d. Individualized control.

2. **The term *span of control* is best defined as:**

   a. The number of immediate subordinates who report to any one supervisor.
   b. The range of influence that any supervisor or manager has in an organization.
   c. The extent to which you have requisite authority over employees in a department.
   d. How broadly or narrowly your reports are distributed over a geographic area.

3. **A model of supervision in which supervisory skills are modified as the person serving as supervisor moves from a beginner toward an advanced practitioner would best be called:**

   a. Integrationist models.
   b. Developmental models.
   c. Motivational models.
   d. Psychotherapy-based models.

4. **Which of the following is not one of the management approaches to supervision presented in this chapter?**

   a. Systematic management approach
   b. Achievement approach
   c. Human relations approach
   d. Contingency (or situational) approach

5. **Which of the following regarding supervision of others by occupational therapy practitioners is not true?**

   a. State licensure laws supersede organizational policies or official documents of AOTA.
   b. Establishing service competency is an important step in determining the amount and type of supervision that is appropriate.
   c. Occupational therapy practitioners may only formally supervise others in client-related tasks and job functions.

   d. The amount and type of supervision provided may vary according to the complexity of the clinical situation, the type of practice setting, regulatory requirements, and the number and diversity of clients.

6. **Service competency is best defined as:**

   a. Assuring that the OTA performs tasks in the same way that the OT would and achieves the same outcome.
   b. A designation that employee orientation has been successfully completed.
   c. A category of feedback typically provided during the review step of a performance appraisal cycle.
   d. None of the above.

7. **Commonly recognized formal steps in a performance appraisal system include which of the following?**

   a. Intermittent review
   b. Assessment
   c. Performance planning
   d. All of the above

8. **A theory of motivation that identifies factors related to employee satisfaction and employee dissatisfaction along different continua is best named:**

   a. Maslow's hierarchy of needs.
   b. Content or process theory.
   c. Vroom's expectancy theory.
   d. Herzberg's hygiene theory.

Resources for Learning More About Supervision

Journals That Often Address Supervision

The Healthcare Manager

http://journals.lww.com/healthcaremanagerjournal/pages/default.aspx

The Healthcare Manager provides practical, applied management information for managers in institutional health-care settings. This quarterly journal, written for health-care professionals in a managerial or supervisory role, focuses on strengthening management and supervisory skills.

Supervision Magazine

http://www.supervisionmagazine.com

This journal, published by the National Research Bureau, features articles aimed at helping to guide and develop skills, attitudes, and abilities of managers and supervisors. Full-text articles are available online through many university libraries.

Management Decision

http://www.emeraldinsight.com/loi/md

Management Decision, published by Emerald Group Publishing, features articles and commentary on practical applications of theories applied to real situations in organizations for business managers, consultants, teachers, and students concerned with general management, policy, and strategy. Full-text articles are available online through many university libraries.

Management Today

http://managementtoday-magazine.com

Management Today, published in London by Haymarket Business Publications, features articles, research, commentary, profiles, training, and book reviews on all aspects of business management. Full-text articles are available online through many university libraries.

Associations That Are Concerned With Supervision

American Management Association

http://www.amanet.org/index.htm

The American Management Association (AMA) promotes the goals of individuals and organizations through a comprehensive range of solutions, including business seminars, blended learning, Webcasts and podcasts, conferences, books, white papers, and articles that they need to improve business performance, adapt to a changing workplace, and prosper in a complex and competitive business world. The AMA serves as a forum for the exchange of the latest information, ideas, and insights on management practices and business trends. The AMA disseminates content and information to a worldwide audience through multiple distribution channels and its strategic partners by offering seminars, conferences, current issues forums and briefings, books and publications, research, and online self-study courses that cover such topics as supervisory skills.

Recognition Professionals International

http://www.recognition.org/

Recognition Professionals International is dedicated to the enhancement of employee performance through recognition and education, including its strategies and related initiatives. The association provides a forum for information and best practices sharing as well as education to foster the use, excitement, effectiveness, and enthusiasm of recognition.

The American Occupational Therapy Association

http://www.aota.org/

The stated mission of AOTA advances the quality, availability, use, and support of occupational therapy through standard setting, advocacy, education, and research on behalf of its members and the public. AOTA provides its members with a variety of resources related to the supervision of occupational therapy personnel, including a number of papers that provide guidelines for the occupational therapy supervisor; access to special interest sections (SISs) that provide Listservs and quarterly newsletters, including the administration and management SIS; and continuing education options. AOTA also has the Coordinated Online Opportunities for Leadership (COOL) program, which is a database to help match members with potential volunteer leadership opportunities.

Miscellaneous Resources

Work911

http://www.work911.com

Work911 is a commercial website operated by Bacal & Associates in Ontario, Canada. In addition to commercial products, it includes a wide range of free-access features, including articles on topics related to supervision, management, and organizational development.

Reference List

American Occupational Therapy Association. (2014). *Guidelines for supervision, roles, and responsibilities during the delivery of occupational therapy services.* Retrieved from http://www.aota.org/-/media/Corporate/Files/Secure/Practice/OfficialDocs/Guidelines/Guidelines-for-Supervision-edited-2014.PDF

American Physical Therapy Association. (2012). Levels of supervision (Position statement HOD P06-00-15-26). Retrieved from http://www.apta.org/uploadedFiles/APTAorg/About_Us/Policies/Terminology/LevelsSupervision.pdf#search=%22levels%20of%20supervision%22

Bauer, T., & Erdogan, B. (2009). *Introduction to organizational behavior.* Washington, DC: Flat World Knowledge.

Bernard, J. M., & Goodyear, R. K. (2014). *Fundamentals of clinical supervision.* Boston, MA: Allyn & Bacon.

Bliss, W. (2013). *The cost of employee turnover.* Retrieved from Small Business Advisor website: http://www.isquare.com/turnover.cfm

Case-Smith, J. (2003). Using the AOTA professional development tool (PDT). *OT Practice, 8,* 1–7.

Ewen, A. J. (1994). Multi-source assessment increases healthcare employee satisfaction. *Journal of Ahima, 65,* 56–58.

Gowda, N. M. (1997). Factors associated with burnout and turnover intention among case managers who work with older adults. *Dissertation Abstracts International. B: The Physical Sciences & Engineering, 57,* 4760.

Harvey, V. S., & Struzziero, J. (2000). *Effective supervision in school psychology.* Bethesda, MD: National Association of School Psychologists.

Hawkins, H., & Shohet, R. (2006). *Supervision in the helping professions* (3rd ed.). Berkshire, UK: Open University Press.

Haynes, R., Corey, G., & Moulton, P. (2003). *Clinical supervision of the helping profession: A practical guide.* Pacific Grove, CA: Brooks/Cole Thompson.

Irvine, D. M., & Evans, M. G. (1995). Job satisfaction and turnover among nurses: Integrating research findings across studies. *Nursing Research, 44,* 246–253.

Kadushin, A. (2002). *Supervision in social work* (3rd ed.). New York, NY: Columbia University Press.

Keller, J. J. (2012). *Supervision training: A battle plan* [White paper]. Retrieved from http://www.jjkeller.com/wcsstore/CVCatalogAssetStore/whitepapers/hr/EmployeeandSupervisorTraining_2012_TD_PVA.pdf

Lawler, E. E. I. (1994). *Motivation in work organizations.* San Francisco, CA: Jossey-Bass.

Leddick, G. R. (2004). Models of clinical supervision. *ERIC Digests.* Retrieved from http://www.ericfacility.net/databases/ERIC_Digests/ed372340.html

Liebler, J. G., Levine, R. E., & Rothman, J. (2011). *Management principles for health professionals.* Sudbury, MA: Jones and Bartlett.

MacLeod, D., & Clarke, N. (2008). *Engaging for success: Enhancing performance through employee engagement.* Retrieved from http://www.engageforsuccess.org/ideas-tools/employee-engagement-the-macleod-report

Maslow, A. E. (1970). *Motivation and personality.* New York, NY: Harper & Row.

Nicklin, P. (1995). Super supervision. *Nursing Management, 2,* 24–25.

Nosse, L. J., Friberg, D. G., & Kovacek, P. R. (2009). *Managerial and supervisory principles for physical therapists.* Baltimore, MD: Lippincott Williams & Wilkins.

Patterson, C. H. (1986). *Theories of counseling and psychotherapy* (4th ed.). New York, NY: Harper & Row.

Salancik, G. R., & Pfeffer, J. (2003). Expectancy models of job satisfaction, occupational preference, and effort: A theoretical, methodological and empirical appraisal. *Administrative Science Quarterly, 23,* 224–253.

Scanlan, J. N., Still, M., Stewart, K., & Croaker, J. (2010). Recruitment and retention issues for occupational therapists in mental health: Balancing the push and the pull. *Australian Occupational Therapy Journal, 57,* 102–110.

Sladyk, K., & Ryan, S. (2005). *Ryan's occupational therapy assistant: Principles, practice issues, and techniques* (4th ed.). Thorofare, NJ: Slack.

Smith, K. (2009). *A brief summary of supervision models.* Retrieved from http://citeseerx.ist.psu.edu/viewdoc/summary?doi=10.1.1.549.7796

Smith, P., Schiller, M. R., Grant, K., & Sachs, L. (1995). Recruitment and retention strategies used by occupational therapy directors in acute care, rehabilitation, and long-term-care settings. *American Journal of Occupational Therapy, 49,* 412–419.

Stoltenberg, C. D., & McNeill, B. W. (2010). *IDM supervision: An integrative developmental model for supervising counselors and therapists* (3rd ed.). New York, NY: Taylor & Smith.

Sutton, B. (2013). Three hallmarks of good performance evaluation. Retrieved from 8 http://bobsutton.typepad.com/my_weblog/2013/11/three-hallmarks-of-good-performance-evaluations.html

Toolpack Consulting LLC. (2002). *Effective performance appraisals and evaluation.* Retrieved from http://www.toolpack.com/performance.html

Vorhauser-Smith, S. (2013). How the best places to work are nailing employee engagement. *Forbes.* Retrieved from www.forbes.com/sites/sylviavorhausersmith/2013/08/14/how-the-best-places-to-work-are-nailing-employee-engagement/

Vornholt, K., Uitdewilligen, S., & Nijhuis, F. J. N. (2013). Factors affecting the acceptance of people with disabilities at work: A literature review. *Journal of Occupational Rehabilitation, 23*(4), 463–475.

Vroom, V. H. (1964). *Work and motivation.* New York, NY: John Wiley & Sons.

Whetten, D. A., & Cameron, K. S. (2011). *Developing managerial skills* (8th ed.). Upper Saddle River, NJ: Prentice Hall.

Will, J. B. (1995). An analysis of attitudes toward measures of job satisfaction related to identified factors of paramedic education. *Dissertation Abstracts International. B: The Physical Sciences & Engineering, 60,* 2050.

Wood, L., Hassell, A., Whitehouse, A., Bullock, A., & Wall, D. (2006). A literature review of multi-source feedback systems within and without health services, leading to 10 tips for their successful design. *Medical Teacher, 28*(7), e185–e191.

World at Work. (2013). *Trends in employee recognition.* Retrieved from http://www.worldatwork.org/waw/adimLink?id=72689

Zangaro, G. A., & Soeken, K. L. (2007). Meta-analysis of studies of nurses' job satisfaction. *Research in Nursing and Health, 30,* 445–458.

CHAPTER 8

Professional Teams, Interprofessional Education, and Collaborative Practice

Brent Braveman, PhD, OTR/L, FAOTA

■ Real-Life Management

Kathryn is an occupational therapy practitioner with 9 years of experience who has practiced in several different settings and has worked with various client populations. She graduated with a master's degree in occupational therapy and has recently been considering returning to school to further her education. Until recently, she assumed that she would need to obtain a PhD or similar research doctorate and found the idea of spending a lot of time in research courses and the potential of completing a dissertation daunting. Kathryn is drawn to academic environments and finds the potential of becoming an adjunct faculty member or a clinical faculty member in an occupational therapy educational program very appealing.

A colleague suggested that Kathryn explore postprofessional clinical doctoral programs in order to obtain her doctor of occupational therapy degree (OTD). This would allow Kathryn to pursue clinical faculty opportunities and to gain advanced practice skills that would further her career as a developing expert clinician. She recently reviewed several OTD programs and became quite interested in one program that had a heavy focus

on interprofessional education and collaborative interdisciplinary practice. Kathryn was somewhat familiar with the concepts of different types of health-care teams such as *multidisciplinary* and *interdisciplinary* teams but was not familiar with the term *interprofessional team*. She was also not sure what interprofessional education really meant and what the benefits of attending a program with such a focus might be for her in gaining new knowledge, developing advanced skills, and exploring academic roles.

Kathryn started a basic Internet search using the terms "interprofessional education" and "interprofessional teams" separately, then together, and was surprised at the extent of citations that she found. She was intrigued that organizations like the World Health Organization (WHO) seemed involved with and concerned about interprofessional education. She became interested in learning about interprofessional core competencies, high-performing teams, and collaborative interprofessional practice, which were all terms she found in her basic search. Kathryn committed to reading some of the materials she found and performed a new Internet search to begin to locate journal articles from various professional disciplines. She wondered where these new findings might take her next.

Critical Thinking Questions

As you read this chapter, consider the following questions:

- What are the various types of professional teams on which occupational therapy practitioners serve and what are the similarities and differences between the types of teams?

- What are the key differences between a group and a team?

- What is a high-performing team and what contributes to effective teams?

- What is interprofessional education and what is an interprofessional team? What is important about these concepts for the occupational therapy manager to understand?

- What is the relationship between interprofessional education, collaborative practice, and the provision of optimal health services?

Glossary

- **Competencies**: explicit measures, indicators, or statements that define specific areas of knowledge, skills, and abilities related to essential functions and assigned duties within a job or role.

- **Cross-functional teams**: teams composed of persons with specific expertise and knowledge from different functional areas who work together to achieve an assigned goal or fulfill a specific purpose for the organization.

- **Functional work teams**: teams composed of persons from several vertical levels of the organization who perform specific organizational functions such as finance, marketing, community outreach, or human resources.

- **Groups**: collection of individuals who have regular contact and frequent interaction, mutual influence, common feeling of camaraderie, and who work together to achieve a common goal.

- **Interdisciplinary teams**: teams composed of members from several disciplines working interdependently in the same setting and who coordinate work and communicate more formally to contribute to an interdisciplinary plan of care.

- **Interprofessional education**: when students from two or more professions learn about, from,

and with each other to enable effective collaboration and improve health outcomes.

- **Multidisciplinary teams**: teams composed of members from more than one discipline so that the team can offer a greater breadth of services to patients. Team members work independently and interact formally.

- **Self-directed work teams**: teams that operate with a high level of autonomy and responsibility, although the teams are still held accountable for outcomes and projects assigned to the teams and they are still held to common conceptions about how work is performed within the particular organization.

- **Teams**: groups of people focused on completion of a shared goal who operate with a high degree of interdependence, share authority and responsibility for self-management, are responsible for collective performance, and work toward a common goal and shared rewards.

- **Transdisciplinary teams**: teams that engage in teaching and learning across disciplinary boundaries and entrust, prepare, and supervise the sharing of disciplinary functions while retaining ultimate responsibility for services provided in their place by other team members.

Introduction

Throughout your occupational therapy education and clinical training you will likely receive a lot of information on **groups** and on **teams.** Occupational therapy students and practitioners are often involved in groups as they work on projects with others or as the leader of a therapeutic group. There is much information and many resources available on running therapeutic groups; although it is a critical piece of your education to become an occupational therapy practitioner, this information is not the focus of this chapter.

There are a number of ways of conceptualizing different types of teams both from a clinical perspective and from a management perspective. In Chapter 13 you will be introduced to some of the classical thinking about team formation including the four commonly identified phases of team formation and functioning: (1) forming, (2) storming, (3) norming, and (4) performing. Chapter 13 will also introduce you to continuous quality improvement (CQI) teams and provide tips for working in teams, such as running effective meetings.

Occupational therapy practitioners are often part of a team of persons involved in providing service to a client. These types of teams, commonly found in the delivery of health-care services, may be referred to as multidisciplinary teams, interdisciplinary teams, or transdisciplinary teams (Choi & Pak, 2006; Falk-Kessler, 2014). Although each of these types of teams include persons from more than one discipline (e.g., occupational therapy, physical therapy, speech–language pathology, social work, etc.), they function differently because of the context of the organization and factors that influence daily work, such as the pace of decision-making and the level of dependence upon each other in order to complete their work. A **multidisciplinary team** is composed of members from several disciplines, allowing clients to get all of the individual services that they need. Work is coordinated in a broad sense and team members cooperate and contribute to common goals such as safe discharge but work independently. Each discipline may have its own plan of care that is established and carried out independently. This type of team may be commonly found in community acute care hospitals where the length of stay for patients is short and the occupational therapy practitioner may only see each patient a few times. In noncomplex cases, each professional carries his or her own plan of care in a complementary manner but with little explicit collaboration.

An **interdisciplinary team** is also composed of members from several disciplines working interdependently in the same setting; however, they coordinate work more formally. Each discipline may complete its own evaluation process and may develop separate plans of care, but can also cooperate and may contribute to an interdisciplinary plan of care. Information is communicated and problems are solved in a systematic way among team members; this often happens during team meetings. An example of such a team may be found in most inpatient rehabilitation facilities (IRFs). An interdisciplinary plan of care may be a requirement for accreditation or for payment, and even noncomplex cases in such an environment may require increased collaboration between multiple disciplines in order to effectively plan for discharge.

A **transdisciplinary team** is a team without discipline-centered boundaries, although each team member is still limited in the services that can be provided by the scope of practice included in the state regulatory act. In addition to collaborating with other team members, transdisciplinary team members prepare and supervise the sharing of disciplinary functions while retaining ultimate responsibility for services provided in their place by other team members (Falk-Kessler, 2014). For example, team members may train team members from other disciplines to complete some work tasks or functions in their absence. In a transitional living facility for persons in recovery from substance abuse, the occupational therapy practitioner may be responsible for helping a new resident establish a weekly schedule and plan transportation to recovery meetings. If the occupational therapy practitioner is absent, another professional who has been oriented by the occupational therapy practitioner will step in and perform this function. This type of team may be more common in community-based settings or settings where there may only be one representative from each discipline.

Another common way of conceptualizing teams in organizations is to identify them as one of three types of work teams: (1) functional work teams, (2) cross-functional work teams, or (3) self-directed teams (Education Portal, 2014). **Functional work teams** are composed of persons from several vertical levels of the organization who perform specific organizational functions such as finance, marketing, community outreach, or human resources. Functional teams are coordinated by managers whose direct reports help to work both internally and externally to provide services and manage internal and external customer relations. Functional team members usually have different responsibilities, but all work to perform the same departmental function. **Cross-functional teams** are composed of persons with specific expertise and knowledge from different functional areas and work together to achieve an assigned goal or fulfill a specific purpose for the organization. Each member brings his or her expertise together and contributes in a unique way to the team's functioning and outcomes. An example of a cross-functional team might be a steering committee that is formed to identify new communication strategies, as well as policies and procedures to streamline and standardize a set of work processes. **Self-directed work teams** operate with a high level of autonomy and responsibility; however, the team is still held accountable for outcomes and projects assigned to the team, and the team is still held to common conceptions about how work is performed within the particular organization. An example of a self-directed team might be a team given responsibility for organizing employee recognition events within a certain budget and within established boundaries, but who work independently once the task is clearly defined.

The Difference Between a Group and a Team

Although there are similarities between groups and teams, it is useful for the leader and occupational therapy manager to differentiate between them. A *group* may be defined simply as "a collection of individuals who have regular contact and frequent interaction, mutual influence, common feeling of camaraderie, and who work together to achieve a common goal" (BusinessDictionary.com, 2014a), whereas a *team* may be defined as "a group of people focused on completion of a shared goal who operate with a high degree of interdependence, share authority and responsibility for self-management, are responsible for collective performance and work toward a common goal and shared rewards" (BusinessDictionary.com, 2014b). Both groups and teams share "having a goal" in common, although Hoyt and Forsyth (2010, p. 782) noted that, "Groups are generally task focused; members are usually united in their pursuit of goals. Teams in particular, stress task performance to such an extent that their very existence is threatened should

they fail to achieve their common goals." Weiss, Tilin, and Morgan (2014) suggest that the difference between a group and a team can be conceptualized along a continuum with one end being simply a number of people who have something in common and the other end being people who *must* work together to achieve a common and agreed upon goal or outcome.

Because the stakes are high in terms of goal achievement for work teams, especially in health care, it is helpful to take the differentiation further. For example, West and Lyubovnikova (2013, p. 135) stated that "Organizations therefore need advice on how to develop authentic and effective teamwork that facilitates a culture for safety and quality, rather than relying on the dangerous illusion that simply labeling a group of healthcare professionals a 'team' will produce the coordination, clear role allocation and powerful shared responsibility the notion of 'teamwork' implies."

Characteristics of High-Performing Teams

Although most health-care professionals work as members of some type of team composed of persons from more than one discipline, it may be commonly assumed that not all teams are equally effective. If true, then we may wonder: What are the characteristics of a high-performing team? The high-performing team is now widely recognized as an essential tool for constructing a more patient-centered, coordinated, and effective health-care delivery system (Mitchell et al, 2012). Reviewing the literature over the last few decades reveals a number of characteristics often identified with effective or high-performing teams, even though the context of health care has changed considerably. John P. Kotter (1996) asserted that teams with sufficient trust can be effective even in times of dramatic change and can sustain their high performance if they possess the following characteristics:

- Shared vision and goals
- Shared leadership and accountability
- Continuous learning and development
- A customer focus
- Capability to gather and use feedback and data

More recently, Mitchell et al (2012) identified five principles of effective team-based care that are similar to those identified by Kotter (see Box 8-1). Themes of

---

BOX 8-1

Principles of Team-Based Health Care

- **Shared goals:** The team works to establish shared goals that reflect patient and family priorities, and can be clearly articulated, understood, and supported by all team members.
- **Clear roles:** There are clear expectations for each team member's functions, responsibilities, and accountabilities.
- **Mutual trust:** Team members earn each other's trust, creating strong norms of reciprocity and greater opportunities for shared achievement.
- **Effective communication:** The team prioritizes and continuously refines its communication skills.
- **Measurable processes and outcomes:** The team agrees on and implements reliable and timely feedback on successes and failures in both the team's functioning and achievement of the team's goals.

BOX 8-2

Personal Values of Effective Members of High-Functioning Health-Care Teams

- **Honesty:** Members value honesty and transparency about aims, decisions, uncertainty, and mistakes.
- **Discipline:** Members carry out roles and responsibilities with discipline even when it is not convenient or comfortable.
- **Creativity:** Members are excited about tackling new problems in creative manners even if mistakes are made.
- **Humility:** Members value each other's training and do not believe that one perspective is always superior to another, relying on each other to avoid mistakes.

---

shared vision and goals, trust, and clear roles and accountability appear to withstand the test of time.

Mitchell et al (2012) also identified the personal values commonly held by individual members of higher-functioning health-care teams. These personal values are briefly summarized in Box 8-2.

The History of Interprofessional Education and Interprofessional Teams

Although occupational therapy and other health-care providers work to become more globally connected, they also work in fragmented health-care systems around the world that are struggling to meet their citizens' needs. Shortages of qualified health-care professionals, limited resources, and more complex situations—including pandemic diseases such as HIV-AIDS, tuberculosis, or malaria; aging populations; and conditions such as delirium, mental health, and emerging illnesses—are taxing health systems worldwide. As

health care and health-care delivery have become more complex and more sophisticated, there has been increased focus not only on what characterizes a high-performing team but also on what team members have in common in terms of education and competencies.

A report of an expert panel organized by the Interprofessional Educational Collaborative (International Education Collaborative Expert Panel [IPEC], 2011) noted that interest in promoting more team-based education for U.S. health professions is not new. The report noted that, "At the first IOM Conference, *Interrelationships of Educational Programs for Health Professionals*, and in the related report *Educating for the Health Team* (IOM [Institute of Medicine], 1972), 120 leaders from allied health, dentistry, medicine, nursing, and pharmacy considered key questions at the forefront of contemporary national discussions about interprofessional education" (IPEC Expert Panel, 2011, p. 3). The World Health Organization (2010) published the *Framework for Action on Interprofessional Education and Collaborative Practice*, noting that successful interprofessional education is context specific and that the framework sought to provide policy makers with ideas on how to implement interprofessional education and collaborative practice within their current context. Passage of legislation such as the Recovery and Investment Act of 2009 and the Patient Protection and Affordable Care Act of 2010 has been the impetus for new approaches such as the patient-centered medical home that have kept the interest in interprofessional education keen (IPEC Expert Panel, 2011; Moyers & Metzler, 2014).

What Is Interprofessional Education?

In the United States and in many countries around the world, health care and health-care services are provided by an interdisciplinary team; however, the team's makeup and roles of individual professionals and disciplines may vary greatly. Universities and educational programs are committed to preparing graduates to function effectively on these teams and work collaboratively and independently in quickly changing health-care environments. Most formal education of health professionals is delivered within existing disciplinary silos and existing programs, which limits the system's capacity to provide graduates with the knowledge, skills, and attitudes to promote the most effective collaboration and function on an interdisciplinary team (Lapkin, Levett-Jones, & Gilligan (2013). An alternative approach to educating and preparing health professionals for interdisciplinary practice is interprofessional education. As noted earlier, this is not a new concept and has received wide support, including support from WHO, since 1973. However, definitions and approaches to interprofessional education vary, and despite its wide promotion there is varying evidence to support its effectiveness.

A simple definition of **interprofessional education** is that "Interprofessional education occurs when students from two or more professions learn about, from and with each other to enable effective collaboration and improve health outcomes" (Center for the Advancement of Interprofessional Education, 2002). The focus of interprofessional education is to assist students to understand the value of working within interprofessional teams before they engage in traditional clinical educational experiences (Moyers & Metzler, 2014). In 2010, WHO published the *Framework for Action on Interprofessional Education and Collaborative Practice* as the work product of a study group on interprofessional education and collaborative practice. According to the authors, "The framework highlighted the status of interprofessional collaboration around the world, identified the mechanisms that shape successful collaborative teamwork and outlines

a series of action items that policy-makers can apply within their local health system. The goal of the Framework is to provide strategies and ideas that will help health policy-makers implement the elements of interprofessional education and collaborative practice that will be most beneficial in their own jurisdiction" (WHO, 2010, p. 9). Key concepts from the WHO framework are included in Box 8-3.

The WHO framework also outlines the relationship between preparation of the present and future workforces through interprofessional education and ultimately the delivery of optimal health services. Understanding these key relationships can provide critical guidance for persons responsible for the development and implementation of interprofessional education. These relationships are demonstrated in Figure 8-1.

Interprofessional education efforts are becoming realities and are being implemented as best models of health education. For example, the Medical University of South Carolina (MUSC) (2007) has implemented a quality enhancement plan focused on interprofessional education involving its programs in dentistry, nursing, medicine, pharmacy, graduate studies, and the health professions entitled *Creating Collaborative Care (C^3)*. The plan includes four stated goals that represent the plan's conceptual underpinnings. The goals are:

- Goal 1: Students will acquire teamwork competencies.
- Goal 2: Students will acquire knowledge, including the values and beliefs, of health that will enable them to define interprofessional health-care delivery or research.
- Goal 3: Students will apply their teamwork competencies in a collaborative interprofessional health-care delivery or research learning setting.
- Goal 4: Students will demonstrate their teamwork competencies in collaborative interprofessional health-care delivery or translational research contexts. (p. 11)

MUSC's C^3 program describes learning as a dynamic process of engaging in increasingly more sophisticated and expansive opportunities. Competencies for teamwork develop along a continuum. Learners move from preparing themselves to be a team member, to thinking as a team member, to practicing

Key Concepts of the WHO *Framework for Action on Interprofessional Education and Collaborative Practice* (2010)

- Health worker is "a wholly inclusive term which refers to all people engaged in actions whose primary intent is to enhance health. Included in this definition are those who promote and preserve health, those who diagnose and treat disease, health management and support workers, professionals with discrete/unique areas of competence, whether regulated or non-regulated, conventional or complementary" (p. 13).
- Interprofessional education occurs when two or more professions learn about, from, and with each other to enable effective collaboration and improve health outcomes (p. 7).
- Professional is an all-encompassing term that includes individuals with the knowledge or skills to contribute to the physical, mental, and social well-being of a community.
- Collaborative practice in health care occurs when multiple health workers from different professional backgrounds provide comprehensive services by working with patients, their families, care providers, and communities to deliver the highest quality of care across settings.
- Practice includes both clinical and nonclinical health-related work, such as diagnosis, treatment, surveillance, health communications, management, and sanitation engineering.
- Health and education systems consist of all the organizations, people, and actions whose primary intent is to promote, restore, or maintain health and facilitate learning, respectively. They include efforts to influence the determinants of health, direct health-improving activities, and provide learning opportunities at any stage of a health worker's career.

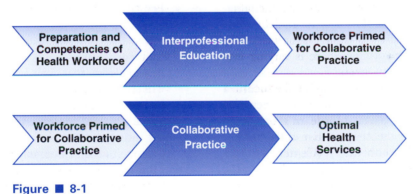

Figure ■ 8-1
Interprofessional Education, Collaborative Practice, and Optimal Health Services.

as a team member, and finally to learning to act as a team member. At the same time, learners undergo a transformational process in which they move along a simultaneous continuum from the most absolute ways of knowing, to transitional knowing, to independent knowing, and finally to knowing in context. Learners move along each of the continuum by learning and acquiring competencies, applying them, and then demonstrating them in practice. As learners move along each of these developmental continua their experiences reinforce prior learning, allowing them to move to higher levels of learning and more complex application of skills; in turn, these are implemented in collaborative care.

What Are Interprofessional Teams?

Earlier in the chapter the terms *multidisciplinary teams*, *interdisciplinary teams*, and *transdisciplinary teams* were introduced. More recently, the term *interprofessional team* has been used and is gaining popularity as a result of the changing dynamics in who provides health care and where and how it is provided. For some time concepts of health-care teams have included the patient and family members as part of the team. Yet this has not always meant that professionals from more than one professional discipline are involved in the teams. For example, trends in specialization in the health professions have led toward teams with people possessing the same basic education or degree but who have a specialty. As an example, orthopedists, physiatrists, and psychiatrists are all physicians who have the same license but are specialized in their practice (Weiss, Tilin, & Morgan, 2014). In addition, in today's changing and complex health system, others—including colleagues with non-medical or technical training—may also be part of the team, including representatives from community-based programs and resources, health educators, or others. Mitchell, Parker, and Giles (2011, p. 1322) describe this by stating, "Interprofessional composition is related to other forms of compositional variation, including functional diversity; however, while functional diversity depicts member variation on the basis of occupation or specialization, it is a broader compositional frame than professional diversity. Of course, in today's environment, we are concerned not only about the composition of teams but also their effectiveness." This is explored in more detail in the next sections of the chapter, but in brief effective interprofessional health-care teams may be characterized by the following (Memorial University, n.d.):

- Members provide care to a common group of patient or clients.
- Members develop common goals for patient or client outcomes and work toward those goals.
- Appropriate roles and functions are assigned to each member, and each member understands the roles of the other members.
- The team possesses a mechanism for sharing information.
- The team possesses a mechanism to oversee the carrying out of plans, to assess outcomes, and to

make adjustments based on the results of those outcomes.

Core Competencies for the Interprofessional Team

Chapter 12 explores the development and assessment of competencies in detail. **Competencies** are defined as *explicit measures, indicators, or statements that define specific areas of knowledge, skills, and abilities related to essential functions and assigned duties within a job or role.* The IPEC Expert Panel identified that core competencies are necessary in today's health-care environment in order to achieve multiple aims (IPEC Expert Panel, 2011). These aims include:

1. Create a coordinated effort across the health professions to embed essential content in all health professions' education curricula.
2. Guide professional and institutional curricular development of learning approaches and assessment strategies to achieve productive outcomes.
3. Provide the foundation for a learning continuum in interprofessional competency development across the professions and the lifelong learning trajectory.
4. Acknowledge that evaluation and research work will strengthen the scholarship in this area.
5. Prompt dialogue to evaluate the "fit" between educationally identified core competencies for interprofessional collaborative practice and practice needs or demands.
6. Find opportunities to integrate essential interprofessional education content consistent with current accreditation expectations for each health profession's education program (see University of Minnesota, Academic Health Center, Office of Education, 2009).
7. Offer information to accreditors of educational programs across the health professions that they can use to set common accreditation standards for interprofessional education, and to know where to look in institutional settings for examples of implementation of those standards (see Accreditation of Interprofessional Health Education, 2009a, 2009b).

8. Inform professional licensing and credentialing bodies in defining potential testing content for interprofessional collaborative practice.

Further, the IPEC panel of experts identified the desired principles underlying interprofessional competencies. These underlying principles included that interprofessional competencies should be:

- Patient or family centered
- Community or population oriented
- Relationship focused
- Process oriented
- Linked to learning activities, educational strategies, and behavioral assessments that are developmentally appropriate for the learner
- Able to be integrated across the learning continuum
- Sensitive to the system's context and applicable across practice settings
- Applicable across professions
- Stated in language common and meaningful across the professions
- Outcome driven

Barr (1998) examined different types of competence from an interprofessional viewpoint and identified overlapping competencies that are expected of all health professionals (see Figure 8-2). It is important to note that competencies may be overlapping between one or more professions but not necessarily universal. For example, occupational therapy and physical therapy both must achieve certain competencies, such as the ability to assess mobility during various types of transfers and instruct patients, caregivers, and families in techniques. This competency does not extend to other health professions such as audiology or pharmacy. Barr pointed out that this overlap can be a source of interprofessional tensions, such as in the debate about overlapping competencies between primary care physicians and nurse practitioners. *Collaborative competencies* may be defined as those that each profession needs to work together with others, such as other specialties within a profession, between professions, with patients and families, with nonprofessionals and volunteers, within and between organizations, within communities, and at a broader policy level (IPEC Expert Panel, 2011).

The IPEC report identified four domains for the core competencies for interprofessional collaborative

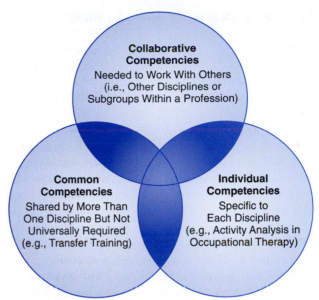

Figure ■ 8-2 Three Types of Professional Competencies.

practice (IPEC Expert Panel, 2011): (1) values and ethics for interprofessional practice, (2) roles and responsibilities, (3) interprofessional communication, and (4) teams and teamwork. Each of the domains will be briefly described next.

Competency Domain 1: Values and Ethics for Interprofessional Practice

Professions typically have sets of stated values and codes of ethics to guide their practice and to help articulate their professional identity. For example, the American Occupational Therapy Association (AOTA), the American Physical Therapy Association (APTA), and the American Speech Language Hearing Association (ASHA) all include information regarding their core values and their codes of ethics on their websites (AOTA, 2014; APTA, 2014a, 2014b; ASHA, 2014a, 2014b).

Various approaches to articulating interprofessional values and ethics have been proposed, but the IPEC Expert Panel suggested a particular focus: "the values that should undergird *relationships* among the professions, joint relationships with patients, the quality of cross-professional exchanges, and interprofessional ethical considerations in delivering health care and in formulating public health policies, programs, and services" (IPEC Expert Panel, 2011, p. 18).

Competency Domain 2: Roles and Responsibilities

In order to be an effective member of an interprofessional team, a practitioner must be able to (a) articulate his or her own role and responsibilities as a member of a profession on the team and (b) be able to understand the roles and responsibilities of the representatives from other disciplines as team members. Understanding how the roles and responsibilities of the various team members complement each other is also critical to team performance. The IPEC competencies in this domain specifically state that, "The need to address complex health promotion and illness problems, in the context of complex care delivery systems and community factors, calls for recognizing the limits of professional expertise, and the need for cooperation, coordination, and collaboration across the professions in order to promote health and treat illness. However, effective coordination and collaboration can occur only when each profession knows and uses the others' expertise and capabilities in a patient-centered way" (IPEC Expert Panel, 2011, p. 20). Recognizing and effectively understanding roles and responsibilities includes understanding the ways that practice and contributions to the interprofessional team may vary and be impacted by regulatory statutes such as licensure laws.

Competency Domain 3: Interprofessional Communication

Effective interpersonal communication is a critical element to high-performing interprofessional teams, and each team member must demonstrate a commitment to achieving competencies in this area. Effective communication promotes collaboration with members of the interprofessional team, including the patient and family members. Recognizing factors that can limit effectiveness such as the use of jargon or unnecessarily complex medical terms is an example of a competency that contribute to a high-performing team. Effective communication includes both verbal communication and written or electronic communica-tion that is common in today's electronic health records. Demonstrating respect and recognizing one's uniqueness and awareness of cultural issues in communication are examples of the content of this competency area. Training in effective communication is common in the education of most health professionals (IPEC Expert Panel, 2011).

Competency Domain 4: Teams and Teamwork

Valuing teamwork and the importance of being a constructive member of a team is naturally part of the core competencies for the interprofessional team. Teamwork includes cooperation, working to avoid duplication of efforts, working toward consensus when differences in opinion arise, recognizing the expertise of others, assuming shared accountability, and working to maintain positive interpersonal relationships. The IPEC competencies acknowledge that conflict is possible because of the diversity of expertise and professional abilities present on most interprofessional teams. For example, it is noted in this area of the competencies that, "Conflicts may arise over leadership, especially when status or power is confused with authority based on professional expertise. Whatever the source, staying focused on patient-centered goals and dealing with the conflict openly and constructively through effective interprofessional communication and shared problem solving strengthen the ability to work together and create a more effective team" (IPEC Expert Panel, 2011, p. 24).

Effectiveness of Interprofessional Education

In 2008, the WHO Study Group on Interprofessional Education and Collaborative Practice conducted an international environmental scan examining current interprofessional activities at a global level. The aim of this scan was to determine the current status of interprofessional education globally; identify best practices; and illuminate examples of successes, barriers, and enabling factors in interprofessional education. A total of 396 respondents, representing 42 countries from each of the six WHO regions, provided insight about their respective interprofessional education programs. The respondents represented various fields including practice (14.1%), administration (10.6%), education (50.4%), and research (11.6%). Despite this, respondents reported that they had experienced many educational and health policy benefits from implementing interprofessional education. For example, the study respondents identified the following benefits (WHO, 2010).

Educational Benefits

- Students have real-world experience and insight.
- Staff from a range of professions provide input into program development.
- Students learn about the work of other practitioners.

Health Policy Benefits

- Improved workplace practices and productivity
- Improved patient outcomes
- Raised staff morale
- Improved patient safety
- Better access to health care

A number of recent studies and systematic reviews have examined the effectiveness of interprofessional education. Shoemaker, Platko, Cleghorn, and Booth (2014) examined a virtual interprofessional education effort for physician assistants, as well as physical therapy and occupational therapy students. Their study aimed to evaluate the experiences of students in relation to the interprofessional teaching and learning, measure the level of students' self-reported readiness for interprofessional learning, and measure the level of students' self-reported achievement of intended learning outcomes. Both qualitative and quantitative data were collected and the students' readiness for interprofessional education was measured. Significant differences were found, with occupational therapy students having significantly higher scores in relation to interprofessional readiness, although the gap narrowed at postassessment. Occupational therapy students also showed a trend to become less positive about the benefits of interprofessional education after their experience. The authors noted that the limited experience of study participants before the use of virtual environments may have had

an impact on the students' experiences and their perceptions.

A second study in 2013 by Reeves, Perrier, Goldman, Freeth, and Zwarenstein assessed the effectiveness of interprofessional education (IPE) interventions compared with separate, profession-specific education interventions; in addition, they assessed the effectiveness of IPE interventions compared with no education intervention through review of 15 studies. Seven studies indicated that IPE produced positive outcomes in the following areas: diabetes care, emergency department culture, and patient satisfaction; collaborative team behavior and reduction of clinical error rates for emergency department teams; collaborative team behavior in operating rooms; management of care delivered in cases of domestic violence; and mental health practitioner competencies related to the delivery of patient care. In addition, four of the studies reported mixed outcomes (positive and neutral) and four studies reported that the IPE interventions had no impact on either professional practice or patient care.

Lapkin, Levett-Jones, and Gilligan (2013) completed a three-stage comprehensive search of 10 electronic databases and conducted a search of grey literature as well. Nine published studies consisting of three randomized controlled trials, five controlled before-and-after studies, and one controlled longitudinal study were included in the review. These investigators found that students' attitudes and perceptions toward interprofessional collaboration and clinical decision-making can be potentially enhanced through interprofessional education. However, like most other reviewers they noted that evidence for using interprofessional education to teach communication skills and clinical skills remains inconclusive and requires further investigation.

Hammick, Freeth, Koppel, Reeves, and Barr (2007) completed a search of bibliographic databases, including Medline 1966–2003, CINAHL 1982–2001, BEI 1964–2001, and ASSIA 1990–2003. In addition the authors hand searched (2003–2005 issues) 21 journals known to have published two or more higher-quality studies from a previous review. Their conclusions were that staff development is a key influence on the effectiveness of IPE for learners who all have unique values about themselves and others. They also concluded that authenticity and customization of IPE are important mechanisms for positive outcomes of IPE. Interprofessional education is generally well received, enabling

TABLE 8-1

Summary of Selected Evidence on the Effectiveness of Interprofessional Education

Author	Study Type	N (Sample Size)	Level of Evidence	Results
Shoemaker, Platko, Cleghorn, & Booth (2014)	Retrospective qualitative case report	Completion of a virtual patient case by 30 physician assistant, 45 physical therapy students, and 24 occupational therapy students.	Fair	Occupational therapy students had higher scores in interprofessional readiness but were less positive about the benefits of interprofessional education after an experience.
Reeves, Perrier, Goldman, Freeth, & Zwarenstein (2013)	Literature review	15 studies	Fair	Seven studies indicated positive results of interprofessional education in a number of areas. Four of the studies had mixed outcomes and four studies showed no impact on practice or patient care.
Lapkin, Levett-Jones, & Gilligan (2013)	Literature review	9 studies	Fair	Students' attitudes toward interprofessional education and clinical decision-making can be enhanced through interprofessional education.
Hammick, Freeth, Koppel, Reeves, & Barr (2007)	Literature review	9 studies	Fair	Staff development is a key influence on the effectiveness of interprofessional education, and authenticity and customization are key mechanisms for positive outcomes.

knowledge and skills necessary for collaborative working to be learned; it is less able to positively influence attitudes and perceptions toward others in the service delivery team. Table 8-1 summarizes the selected evidence on the effectiveness of interprofessional education.

Collaborative Practice

Collaborative practice happens when multiple health workers from different professional backgrounds work together with patients, families, care providers, and communities to deliver the highest quality of care. Effective interprofessional collaboration includes an understanding of the roles of other team members and their unique contributions, as well as a demonstration of respect for these contributions; these allow each team member to step forward and lead when appropriate (Interprofessional Health Collaborative, 2010). It allows health workers to engage any individual whose skills can help achieve local health goals. Collaborative practice strengthens health systems and improves health outcomes (WHO, 2010).

Collaborative practice can improve:

- Access to and coordination of health services
- Appropriate use of specialist clinical resources
- Health outcomes for people with chronic diseases
- Patient care and safety

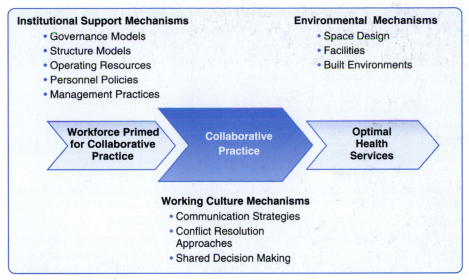

Institutional Support Mechanisms
- Governance Models
- Structure Models
- Operating Resources
- Personnel Policies
- Management Practices

Environmental Mechanisms
- Space Design
- Facilities
- Built Environments

Workforce Primed for Collaborative Practice → Collaborative Practice → Optimal Health Services

Working Culture Mechanisms
- Communication Strategies
- Conflict Resolution Approaches
- Shared Decision Making

Figure ■ 8-3 External Mechanisms That Shape Collaboration at the Practice Level.

Collaborative practice can decrease:

- Total patient complications
- Length of hospital stay
- Tension and conflict among caregivers
- Staff turnover
- Hospital admissions
- Clinical error rates and mortality rates

Figure 8-3 highlights external mechanisms in institutions, in the working culture, and in the environment that influence collaborative practice and therefore the provision of optimal health-care services.

Moyers and Metzler (2014, p. 502) note that, "accreditation organizations are creating standards for appropriate design and implementation of collaborative practice and coordination mainly through certification of primary care medical homes." The American College of Physicians defines the patient-centered medical home as "a care delivery model whereby patient treatment is coordinated through their primary care physician to ensure they receive the necessary care when and where they need it, in a manner they can understand" (American College of Physicians, 2014). The objective of patient-centered medical homes is to have a centralized setting that facilitates partnerships between individual patients, their personal physicians, and, when appropriate, the patient's family. Although the physician often plays a central leadership role in patient-centered medical homes,

other professionals—including occupational therapy practitioners—have the skills to assume leadership positions and decrease the burden on a stressed primary care physician system. In a health policy article entitled "Interprofessional Collaborative Practice in Care Coordination" in the *American Journal of Occupational Therapy*, Moyers and Metzler (2014) cite Bodenheimer (2006) in noting that, "some research shows that if other professionals are used appropriately, 24% of the physician or related professionals can be freed up, making better use of resources and competencies."

Leadership and Interprofessional Teams

Chapter 1 introduced you to a range of information on leadership including theories of leadership and evidence related to what helps leaders be perceived as effective. Although the evidence has generally demonstrated that interprofessional teams can be effective, it also has indicated that there are complications including boundary issues, issues related to organizational hierarchy, and power and status inequalities (Reeves, Macmillan, & Van Soeren, 2010). Leadership of interprofessional teams can be complicated by the needs for shifting boundaries that allow the team member who possesses the specific knowledge needed at a particular time to step forward and assume more responsibility for leading, even if in an informal way. For example, in acute hospitals the patient's medical care may appear routine, but his or her discharge planning needs and psychosocial needs may be very complex. Physician leaders who are not comfortable with stepping to the background and allowing case managers or social workers to take the lead may face many challenges to their status and credibility. The roles adopted by team members, their level of participation, and their influence in the team may vary according to the team's composition and status of the team members in the organization. However, Thylefors (2012, p. 506) reported that "despite these factors, the majority of studies in past years report a somewhat uneven distribution across different professions when it comes to influence and status, mainly explained by degree of professionalization, length of professional education and formal responsibilities."

Themes in the literature on interprofessional teams and leadership center on collaboration and communication. For example, Lingard et al (2012, p. 1762) stated the following, "The growing body of literature on interprofessional care emphasizes the essential nature of collaboration and contains a strong discourse of partnership, shared leadership, and team interactions that are horizontal, relational, and situational." Another theme included in the literature is flexibility and the ability to adapt. Successful adaptation includes adapting to different styles of leadership in different situations (see Chapter 1 on situational leadership). This can include flexibly allowing different team members to exert influence or changing styles when new or less experienced team members join the team (Hammick, Olckers, & Campion-Smith, 2009).

Although leading an interprofessional team may be complicated, there is little in the literature that suggests that being an effective leader of an interprofessional team requires any skills that are different from team leadership in general.

Chapter Summary

This chapter reviewed the various types of familiar interdisciplinary teams and the type of work teams commonly encountered in settings where occupational therapy practitioners work. The differences between groups and teams were reviewed, as were the characteristics of high-performing teams. In addition, you were introduced to the term *interprofessional*; the chapter then explored interprofessional education and the relationship of interprofessional education to collaborative care.

An important topic in this chapter was the increasing focus on interprofessional teams and effective collaborative practice globally, including by organizations such as WHO. As health-care and health professionals, such as occupational therapists, become more globally connected and face increasingly complex and shared concerns such as chronic illness, pandemic illnesses such as HIV/AIDS and influenza, and common challenges such as caring for aging populations, it is likely that interprofessional education and collaborative practice will continue to receive focused attention. Occupational therapy managers can develop the skills and competencies to perform as effective team members and to lead the interprofessional team.

■ **Real-Life Solutions**

Kathryn started her learning with a basic Internet search on the terms "interprofessional education" and "interprofessional teams." She quickly found that there was much literature and many resources on both interprofessional education and interprofessional teams. She was intrigued by the value of interprofessional education because so much of her

education occurred only with other occupational therapy students. She remembered that it was difficult as an entry-level practitioner to become confident in her own role as an occupational therapist while at the same time learning about the roles of others. She had struggled to assert herself as a professional and an important member of the team and yet remain collaborative. She was particularly excited to see that the occupational therapy literature included information on interprofessional

■ **Real-Life Solutions—cont'd**

education, interprofessional teams, and collaborative practice.

As Kathryn continued to explore, she started keeping notes about strategies that could apply to her own work environment to promote the development of interprofessional core competencies, high-performing teams, and collaborative interprofessional practice. She became more convinced that pursuing a postprofessional doctorate in an OTD program was a good fit to support her interests in developing more as an expert practitioner and as an occupational therapy educator. She was excited because she could easily imagine several applied projects that she could complete in her doctoral work that would be relevant for her everyday practice. She was also excited about the potential of contributing to the development of the profession in evolving models of service delivery such as primary care and the patient-centered medical home.

Study Questions

1. **Which of the following best names a team without discipline-centered boundaries on which team members collaborate, prepare, and supervise the sharing of disciplinary functions while retaining ultimate responsibility for services provided in their place by other team members?**

   a. Interdisciplinary team
   b. Multidisciplinary team
   c. Transdisciplinary team
   d. Interprofessional team

2. **Which of the following best names a team composed of persons with specific expertise and knowledge from different functional areas who work together to achieve an assigned goal or fulfill a specific purpose for the organization, where each member brings his or her expertise and contributes in a unique way to the team's functioning and outcomes?**

   a. Functional work team
   b. Cross-functional work team
   c. Multiprofessional team
   d. Self-directed team

3. **Which of the following is a key difference between a *group* and a *team*?**

   a. Teams work collaboratively, whereas groups are typically self-focused.
   b. Although both are task focused, teams can emphasize performance to a much more significant extent.

   c. The key distinguishing factor between a group and a team is the frequency and duration of interaction.
   d. Groups pursue individual awards via individual performance and teams pursue collective rewards.

4. **Which of the following is an impetus for the increased focus on interprofessional teams?**

   a. A complex globally connected health system
   b. Shortage of health professionals and limited resources
   c. Legislation that promotes increasingly coordinated care
   d. All of the above

5. **Which of the following is the most accurate definition of interprofessional education?**

   a. Students from two or more professions learn about, from, and with each other to enable effective collaboration and improve health outcomes.
   b. Students from two or more professions are educated in the same university or college to gain efficiencies in space and faculty.
   c. Students from two or more professions are placed in the same setting for their clinical field-work education following completion of their classroom education.
   d. Students from two or more professions have educational programs with similar curricular elements such as basic science courses (e.g., biology or anatomy).

6. **Which of the following best describes the relationship between interprofessional education and the provision of optimal health services?**

   a. Existing health-care teams are spurred to provide optimal health services when they are the beneficiaries of interprofessional continuing education.

   b. Interprofessional education helps to prepare a workforce ready for collaborative practice that then promotes the provision of optimal health services.

   c. The provision of optimal health-care services promotes increased collaboration between team members on an interprofessional team.

   d. There is no proven relationship between interprofessional education and the provision of optimal health services.

7. **Which of the following best defines the term** *collaborative competencies*?

   a. Competencies that each profession identifies as its own in order to promote more effective teamwork and prevent conflict by delineating clear professional roles.

   b. Competencies that each profession identifies that other professions must develop in order to most effectively work with others, with patients and families, with nonprofessionals and volunteers, within communities, and at a broader policy level.

   c. Competencies specifically focused on interpersonal communication, such as effective conflict resolution, and that promote teamwork.

   d. Competencies that each profession needs to work together with others, such as other specialties within a profession, between professions, with patients and families, with nonprofessionals and volunteers, within and between organizations, within communities, and at a broader policy level.

8. **Which of the following best describes the skills necessary for effectively leading an interprofessional team?**

   a. The skills for effectively leading an interprofessional team are substantially different from those required to effectively lead other types of teams.

   b. The skills for effectively leading an interprofessional team are broad, such that they encompass all of the necessary skills for effective leadership of other teams and include several other areas of competency.

   c. The skills for effectively leading an interprofessional team are very similar to those of leading other types of health-care teams and there is little difference in general.

   d. The skills for effectively leading an interprofessional team are narrower than those required for effectively leading other types of teams and are essentially a subset of skills.

Resources for Learning More About Professional Teams, Interprofessional Education, and Interprofessional Competencies

Journals Related to Professional Teams, Interprofessional Education, and Interprofessional Competencies

Journal of Interprofessional Care

http://informahealthcare.com/journal/jic

The *Journal of Interprofessional Care* includes research and new developments in the field of interprofessional education and practice. Articles include an interprofessional focus, and involve a range of settings, professions, and fields. Areas of practice covered include primary, community, and hospital care; health education and public health; and beyond health and social care into fields such as criminal justice and primary or elementary education.

Journal of Research in Interprofessional Practice and Education

http://www.jripe.org/index.php/journal

The *Journal of Research in Interprofessional Practice and Education* (JRIPE) is an open-access journal that disseminates theoretical perspectives, methodologies, and evidence-based knowledge to inform interprofessional practice, education, and research to improve health-care delivery, quality of care, and health status for individuals, families, and communities.

Associations and Organizations Related to Professional Teams, Interprofessional Education, and Interprofessional Competencies

The Interprofessional Education Collaborative (IPEC)

https://ipecollaborative.org

The IPEC seeks to promote and encourage constituent efforts that would advance substantive interprofessional learning experiences to help prepare future clinicians for team-based care of patients. The organizations included in the collaborative represent higher education in allopathic and osteopathic medicine, dentistry, nursing, pharmacy, and public health. IPEC also seeks to create core competencies for interprofessional collaborative practice that can guide curricula development at all health professions' schools.

The National Center for Interprofessional Practice and Education

https://nexusipe.org

The National Center for Interprofessional Practice and Education is a public–private partnership that contributes to the transformation of health care by identifying ways to improve health, enhance patient care, and control costs through integrating interprofessional practice and education. The center seeks to align and integrate the needs and interests of health professions' education with practice to incubate ideas, define the field, and guide program development and research. The center's work is focused on five core domains: leadership; collaborative practice and health system transformation; education and training; research, evaluation, and scholarship; and innovative and novel models.

Reference List

Accreditation of Interprofessional Health Education. (2009a). *National forum. Ottawa: Health Canada.* Retrieved from http://www.cihc.ca/static/docs/aiphe/AIPHE_National_Forum_Report.pdf

Accreditation of Interprofessional Health Education. (2009b). *Principles and practices for integrating interprofessional education into the accreditation standards for six health professions in Canada. Health Canada.* Retrieved from http://www.cihc.ca/files/AIPHE_Principles_and_Implementation_Guide_EN.pdf

American College of Physicians. (2014). *What is the patient-centered medical home?* Retrieved from http://www.acponline.org/running_practice/delivery_and_payment_models/pcmh/understanding/what.htm

American Occupational Therapy Association. (2014). *Ethics.* Retrieved from http://www.aota.org/Practice/Ethics.aspx

American Physical Therapy Association. (2014a). *Code of ethics for the physical therapist.* Retrieved from http://www.apta.org/uploadedFiles/APTAorg/About_Us/Policies/Ethics/CodeofEthics.pdf#search=%22code%20of%20ethics%22

American Physical Therapy Association. (2014b). *Strategic plan.* Retrieved from http://www.apta.org/StrategicPlan/Plan/

American Speech Language Hearing Association. (2014a). *Code of ethics.* Retrieved from http://www.asha.org/About/Strategic-Pathway/

American Speech Language Hearing Association. (2014b). *Strategic pathway to excellence.* Retrieved from http://www.asha.org/Code-of-Ethics/

Barr, H. (1998). Competent to collaborate: Towards a competency-based model for interprofessional education. *Journal of Interprofessional Care, 12*(2), 181–187.

Bodenheimer, T. (2006). Primary care—Will it survive? *New England Journal of Medicine, 355*, 861–864.

BusinessDictionary.com. (2014a). *Group.* Retrieved from http://www.businessdictionary.com/definition/group.html

BusinessDictionary.com. (2014b). *Team.* Retrieved from http://www.businessdictionary.com/definition/team.html

Center for the Advancement of Interprofessional Education. (2002). *Defining IPE.* Retrieved from http://www.caipe.org.uk/about-us/defining-ipe/

Choi, B. C., & Pak, A. W. (2006). Multidisciplinarity, interdisciplinarity and transdisciplinarity in health research, services, education and policy: Definitions, objectives, and evidence of effectiveness. *Clinical and Investigative Medicine. Medecine clinique et experimentale, 29*(6), 351–364.

Education Portal. (2014). *Types of work teams: Functional, cross-functional and self-directed.* Retrieved from http://education-portal.com/academy/lesson/types-of-work-teams-functional-cross-functional-self-directed.html#lesson

Falk-Kessler, J. (2014). Professionalism, communication and teamwork. In B. A. Schell, G. Gillen, M. Scaffa, & E. S. Cohn (Eds.), *Willard and Spackman's occupational therapy* (pp. 452–465). Philadelphia, PA: Lippincott Williams & Wilkins.

Hammick, M., Freeth, D., Koppel, I., Reeves, S., & Barr, H. (2007). A best evidence systematic review of interprofessional education: BEME Guide no. 9. *Medical Teacher, 29*(8), 735–751.

Hammick, M., Olckers, L., & Campion-Smith, C. (2009). Learning in interprofessional teams: AMEE Guide no. 38. *Medical Teacher, 31*(1), 1–12.

Hoyt, C. L., & Forsyth, D. R. (2010). Groups and teams. In R. A. Couto (Ed.), *Political and civic leadership: A reference handbook* (Vol. 2, pp. 781–789). Los Angeles, CA: Sage.

Institute of Medicine. (1972). *Educating for the health team.* Retrieved from National Center for Interprofessional Practice and Education website: https://nexusipe.org/resource-exchange/iom-1972-report-educating-health-team

International Education Collaborative Expert Panel. (2011). *Core competencies for interprofessional collaborative practice: Report of an expert panel.* Washington, DC: Interprofessional Education Collaborative.

Interprofessional Health Collaborative. (2010). A national interprofessional competency framework. Retrieved from: http://www.cihc.ca/files/CIHC_IPCompetencies_Feb1210.pdf.

Kotter, J. P. (1996). *Leading change.* Boston, MA: Harvard Business Press.

Lapkin, S., Levett-Jones, T., & Gilligan, C. (2013). A systematic review of the effectiveness of interprofessional education in health professional programs. *Nurse Education Today, 33*(2), 90–102.

Lingard, L., Vanstone, M., Durrant, M., Fleming-Carroll, B., Lowe, M., Rashotte, J., . . . Tallett, S. (2012). Conflicting messages: Examining the dynamics of leadership on interprofessional teams. *Academic Medicine, 87*(12), 1762–1767.

Medical University of South Carolina. (2007). *Creating collaborative care (C³): A quality enhancement plan (QEP).* Retrieved from http://academicdepartments.musc.edu/c3/publications/qep_final.pdf

Memorial University. (n.d.). *Interprofessional healthcare teams.* Retrieved from https://www.med.mun.ca/getdoc/601a16b5-7a06-4447-8840-60af3fa494cd/Interprofessional-Health-Care-Teams.aspx

Mitchell, P., Wynia, M., Golden, R., McNellis, B., Okun, S., Webb, C. E., . . . Von Kohorn, I. (2012). *Core principles & values of effective team-based health care.* Washington, DC: Institute of Medicine.

Mitchell, R. J., Parker, V., & Giles, M. (2011). When do interprofessional teams succeed? Investigating the moderating roles of team and professional identity in interprofessional effectiveness. *Human Relations, 64*(10), 1321–1343.

Moyers, P. A., & Metzler, C. A. (2014). Interprofessional collaborative practice in care coordination. *American Journal of Occupational Therapy, 68*(5), 500–505.

Reeves, S., Macmillan, K., & Van Soeren, M. (2010). Leadership of interprofessional health and social care teams: A sociohistorical analysis. *Journal of Nursing Management, 18*(3), 258–264.

Reeves, S., Perrier, L., Goldman, J., Freeth, D., & Zwarenstein, M. (2013). Interprofessional education: Effects on professional practice and healthcare outcomes (update). *Cochrane Database of Systematic Reviews, 3.*

Shoemaker, M. J., Platko, C. M., Cleghorn, S. M., & Booth, A. (2014). Virtual patient care: An interprofessional education approach for physician assistant, physical therapy and occupational therapy students. *Journal of Interprofessional Care, 28*(4), 365–367.

Thylefors, I. (2012). All professionals are equal but some professionals are more equal than others? Dominance, status and efficiency in Swedish interprofessional teams. *Scandinavian Journal of Caring Sciences, 26*(3), 505–512.

University of Minnesota, Academic Health Center, Office of Education. (2009). *Comparison study of health professional health accreditation standards.* Minneapolis, MN: Author.

Weiss, D., Tilin, F., & Morgan, M. (2014). *The interprofessional health care team.* Burlington, MA: Jones & Bartlett Learning.

West, M. A., & Lyubovnikova, J. (2013). Illusions of team working in health care. *Journal of Health Organization and Management, 27*(1), 134–142.

World Health Organization. (2010). *Framework for action on interprofessional education and collaborative practice.* Geneva, Switzerland: Health Professions Network Nursing and Midwifery Office, Department of Human Resources for Health, World Health Organization. Retrieved from http://apps.who.int/iris/bitstream/10665/70185/1/WHO_HRH_HPN_10.3_eng.pdf

Managerial Skills, Responsibilities, and Competencies

CHAPTER 9

Strategic Planning

Brent Braveman, PhD, OTR/L, FAOTA
Shawn Phipps, PhD, MS, OTR/L, FAOTA

■ Real-Life Management

The University of Texas MD Anderson Cancer Center (MD Anderson), created in 1941 as a part of the University of Texas System, is one of the nation's original three comprehensive cancer centers. Designated as such by the National Cancer Act of 1971, it is currently one of 45 facilities designated by the National Cancer Institute as a comprehensive cancer center. In 2015, *U.S. News & World Report*'s "Best Hospitals" survey ranked MD Anderson the nation's top hospital for cancer care. MD Anderson has been ranked the nation's leading cancer hospital 11 of 14 years. The institution has been named one of the nation's top two hospitals for cancer care every year since the survey began in 1990 (MD Anderson Cancer Center, 2015). During fiscal year 2014, MD Anderson provided cancer care for over 27,000 inpatients and 1.3 million outpatient clinic visits. About a third of the patients come to Houston from outside Texas, seeking the knowledge-based care that has made MD Anderson so widely respected. There were over 10,000 registrants in clinical trials exploring novel therapies and diagnostic tests, making it the largest such program in the nation.

The Department of Rehabilitation Services, including occupational therapy and physical therapy, at MD Anderson was initially established in 1952 as a section of the Division of Surgery and remained so until it gained sufficient recognition to become an independent department in 1967. Up until the mid-1990s there were fewer than 20 staff members. There is a separate Department of Audiology and Speech Language Pathology that developed as part of the Department of Head and Neck Oncology. The demand for rehabilitation services progressively increased as the impact of rehabilitation on the quality of lives of persons with cancer was more clearly recognized. Since 2008, the number of permanent staff in rehabilitation services has almost doubled, and in 2015 there were 125 full-time equivalent staff, including occupational therapists (OTs), occupational therapy assistants (OTAs), physical therapists (PTs), and physical therapist assistants (PTAs), as well as support staff, including rehabilitation technicians, administrative assistants, and business staff. Concurrent with this expansion and the retirement of the director, the department was led by an interim director, supported by a leadership team consisting of four clinical supervisors, a business manager, and a research coordinator. This administrative structure remained in place for 2 years until a permanent director of rehabilitation services was hired in January 2011. During fiscal year 2014, the department treated over 17,000 patients with gross revenue of over 22 million dollars.

One of the first priorities of the new director and the leadership team was designing a comprehensive strategic visioning and planning process consistent with the performance improvement culture of MD Anderson. They also sought to establish a formal

Continued

■ Real-Life Management—cont'd

strategic plan. No such plan had existed in recent years. The team agreed to begin this process by examining the existing organizational culture of rehabilitation services. This meant identifying and evaluating staff member behaviors and the underlying values and beliefs that drove those behaviors. The leadership team needed to understand how the MD Anderson organizational values of caring, integrity, and discovery were at play in the department, as well as other values that influenced the everyday decisions that staff members made related to patient care and interactions with their peers.

Critical Thinking Questions

As you read this chapter, consider the following questions:

- What is strategic planning and what types of skills does it require?

- Why is strategic planning critical in promoting departmental and organizational effectiveness?

- What are the differences between the SWOT analysis and the SOAR analysis in strategic planning?

- What value does each step of the strategic planning process bring in understanding your current operations and the environments in which you operate?

Glossary

- **Appreciative inquiry (AI):** positive approach to organizational change that begins by identifying what is positive about a department or organization when it is at its best, and then leverages these qualities for the future.
- **Business plan:** document that is focused on the actions and investment necessary to generate income from a specific program or service; includes information about an organization's products, the competitive environment, and revenue generation assumptions.
- **Case statement:** statement that is geared toward marketing and fundraising rather than planning. It describes the organization's goals, capabilities, and strengths, and the benefits it provides.
- **Contingency assessment:** assessment of all those things that might reasonably be anticipated to go wrong and the impact of these events.
- **Departmental or organizational profile:** document that identifies the customers and other key stakeholders, spotlights the processes and procedures that lead to the central products and outcomes of the business, and summarizes the internal and external environments in which the department or organization operates.
- **Mission statement:** statement of the reason for existence of a department or organization that indicates what the department or organization does, whom it does it for, and possibly how it is accomplished.
- **Operating plan:** coordinated set of tasks for carrying out the goals delineated in a strategic plan. It goes into greater detail than the strategic plan and identifies specific time frames and deadlines for activities, as well as assigns activities to specific organizational members to aid accountability.
- **Planning:** the process of deciding what to do by setting performance objectives and identifying the activities needed to accomplish these activities.

Glossary—cont'd

- **SOAR analysis:** drawn from an appreciative inquiry perspective that recognizes the value of emphasizing the positive before focusing on the negative; it stands for strengths, opportunities, aspirations, and results, and represents an alternative to the traditional SWOT analysis process.
- **Strategic plan:** document that provides guidance in fulfilling the articulated mission of a department or an organization. It articulates specific goals and describes the action steps and resources needed to accomplish them.
- **Strategic planning:** the process of determining the organization's long-term goals, establishing concrete measures of success, and formulating the strategies and general action plans to accomplish these goals.
- **SWOT analysis:** process used to examine both the organization's internal and external environments to aid with operational and strategic planning through an analysis of the organization's strengths, opportunities, weaknesses, and threats.
- **Vision statement:** statement that paints an aspirational picture of the future of a department or organization by indicating what it will look like at its best.

Introduction

Chapter 6 introduced you to the four classic functions associated with managers in organizations: planning, organizing and staffing, directing, and controlling. You were also briefly introduced to some of the planning activities that managers carry out, including operational planning; financial planning; planning for facilities, space, and equipment; and strategic planning. This chapter focuses on strategic planning and associated processes such as the development of a mission statement and the visioning process. These activities are integral when conducting strategic or long-term planning.

In Chapter 6, you were introduced to planning as the process of establishing short-term and long-term goals, measurable objectives, and action plans related to the organization's mission. Goals are usually distinguished from objectives in terms of the scope of the accomplishment. Objectives are measurable steps that are taken to reach a goal, which is a major accomplishment related to the organization's or system's output. In addition to establishing goals and objectives, planning includes determining the needs for the human resources, materials, supplies, facilities, and equipment required to meet goals and objectives. Sometimes the words *goals* and *objectives* can be interchangeable; in this case, the objective is the longer-term outcome and the goals are the measurable steps taken to reach an objective.

Operational Planning Versus Strategic Planning

Managers are responsible for planning for the day-to-day activities within a department and organization, but are also responsible for longer-term planning. This longer-term planning, commonly referred to as **strategic planning**, is the process of determining the organization's long-term goals, concrete measures of success, and achievement, and then formulating the strategies and general action plans to accomplish these goals. Over the last several decades, strategic planning has come in and out of favor as organizations have struggled to keep up with the frenetic changes in technology and the economy. And yet, operating in an environment fraught with change may be when long-term planning, especially the processes of mission statement review and visioning, becomes most important.

Given the demands for high productivity in most of today's workplaces, it is sometimes difficult to convince managers and staff members to take time from their busy schedules to think creatively about the future. A precursor to beginning or revising a strategic plan should be to spend some time reviewing and perhaps revising a department's mission and vision statements. A **mission statement** is a setting forth of an organization's or department's purpose, including definitions, products, and services. A **vision statement** expresses the aspirational and inspirational messages about what a department or organization would like to become as it seeks to fulfill its mission.

An organization's mission is typically established by the organization's founders and remains relatively stable, although updates may be needed. The mission is often operationalized through a statement that sets forth the organization's purpose, including definition, products, and services. An accompanying vision statement expresses the aspirational and inspirational messages about what a department or organization would like to become as it seeks to fulfil its mission (Braveman, 2006, 2009; Hoyle, 1995).

Strategic Planning Across the Decades

Strategic planning in organizations originated in the 1950s and was very popular between the mid-1960s and mid-1970s. However, during the late 1970s and the 1980s strategic planning was largely ignored. Strategic planning reemerged in the 1990s and became recognized as a "process with particular benefits in particular contexts" (Mintzberg, 1994, p. 64). The current context makes strategic planning necessary as rapid changes in health care require the need to set new strategic directions. Strategic planning remains popular today and is reflected in standards established by accrediting bodies such as the Commission on Accreditation of Rehabilitation Facilities (CARF) (http://www.carf.org/Accreditation/QualityStandards/ASPIREtoExcellence/) and the Accreditation Council for Occupational Therapy Education (ACOTE) (http://www.aota.org/Education-Careers/Accreditation/StandardsReview.aspx), and by quality-focused programs such as the Baldrige Criteria for Performance Excellence (National Institute of Standards and Technology [NIST], 2015).

Mittenthal (2002) provided a helpful comparison between strategic planning and other types of planning processes. This comparison is highlighted through the presentation of the following definitions:

- A **strategic plan** provides guidance in fulfilling the articulated mission of a department or an organization. It articulates specific goals and describes the action steps and resources needed to accomplish them. Strategic plans are typically reviewed and updated every 3 to 5 years.

- An **operating plan** is a coordinated set of tasks for carrying out the goals delineated in a strategic plan. It goes into greater detail than the strategic plan, identifies specific time frames and deadlines for activities, and assigns activities to specific organizational members to aid accountability.
- A **business plan** is focused on the actions and investment necessary to generate income from a specific program or service and includes information about an organization's products, the competitive environment, and revenue generation assumptions.
- A **case statement** is geared toward marketing and fundraising rather than planning. It describes the organization's goals, capabilities, and strengths, as well as the benefits it provides.

New Directions in Strategic Planning: SWOT Versus SOAR

Examination of the organization's internal environment and the multiple external environments (e.g., financial, political, regulatory, etc.) is often a first step in planning strategically. A traditional process used to examine both the internal and external environments of an organization to aid with operational and strategic planning is a **SWOT analysis.** The acronym SWOT stands for strengths, weaknesses, opportunities, and threats (McKonkey, 1976). Traditionally, completion of a SWOT analysis is understood as a balanced methodology to identify a department or organization's primary strengths and opportunities while assessing the weaknesses and threats that could hold back the department or organization from progressing. SWOT analyses help to examine the current state of the department or organization (e.g., strengths and weaknesses) and to project possible external future states (e.g., opportunities and threats).

It is certainly true that conducting a traditional SWOT analysis guides you to identify weaknesses and threats, and in this process also helps you identify options to address them. A limitation of this approach is that it has the potential of creating a lens of focus on what the organization does wrong and why, which emphasizes the negative. A concern has been identified that this can affect both the underlying culture of work and planning groups and their performance. Edwin Thomas (2006, p. 1) described the challenge in the following statement:

The traditional approach to change is problem solving in nature. It starts off from a negative perspective—something is broken, something could be done better, something needs to be fixed. Thus we engage in problem identification, root cause analysis, brainstorming possible solutions, action planning, implementation of changes, and hopefully evaluation of the results. Indeed, this is precisely what managers are trained to do—identify problems and fix them all.

Stavros, Cooperrider, and Kelley (2003) described a more contemporary approach to strategic planning utilizing a conceptual approach called **appreciative inquiry (AI).** AI is a vision-based approach of open dialogue that is designed to help organizations and their partners create a shared view for the future and a mission for operating in the present (Srivastva & Cooperrider, 1990). The AI approach to strategic planning begins by focusing on the strengths of an organization and its stakeholders' values, as well as their shared vision (Stavros et al, 2003). The following is how Stavros et al (2003, p. 2) describe the rationale for using an AI approach to strategic planning:

Think about this: Change requires action. Action requires a plan. A plan requires a strategy. A strategy requires goals and enabling objectives. Goals and objectives require a mission. A mission is defined by a vision. A vision is set by one's values. And, the appreciative inquiry (AI) approach to strategic planning starts by focusing on the strengths of an organization and its stakeholders' values.

The 4 D Model of AI was developed in 1977 and is summarized in Table 9-1 (Bushe, 2011).

There are cautions about relying too heavily on an AI approach and creating an "either-or" dynamic between problem-solving and the positive focus of AI. Bushe (2011) noted that it is possible to polarize approaches stimulated by AI and typical problem-solving approaches and that transformational change will not occur through AI approaches unless real problems of real concern to the organization's members are identified.

The acronym SOAR in the **SOAR analysis** process stands for strengths, opportunities, aspirations, and results, and represents an alternative to the traditional SWOT analysis process. The SOAR approach is drawn from an AI perspective that recognizes the value of emphasizing the positive before focusing on the negative. The more traditional SWOT approach helps you to identify a balanced view including your current weaknesses. Both approaches can be used together to avoid getting stuck in the negative while not overlooking the realities that all departments and organizations have problems, weaknesses, and threats. However, it is important to consider your department from all perspectives in the organization's context to help you shape your future direction and to know where to start and what actions to prioritize.

TABLE 9-1

Summary of the 4 D Model of Appreciative Inquiry

Discovery	Participants reflect and discuss what a work group or organization is best at, or when they were at their best. Discussion is focused on discovering and describing the positive core and the group's strengths. Key stakeholders should be involved in this process to assure that you capture a broad view and multiple perspectives.
Dream	Participants imagine their group or organization at its best and identify their common aspirations. The dream phase results in symbolic results such as graphical representations rather than concrete outcomes such as a mission statement.
Design	Participants are asked to develop concrete proposals for creating a new state for the work group or organization. The future state reflects those elements representing when the group was at its best.
Delivery or Destiny	Participants focus on the difficult task of implementing the proposals that were chosen and refined during the design phase. A major challenge is maintaining the energy and drive created in earlier phases.

Why Plan Strategically?

Given the discussion to this point, you may still be wondering if there is true value in planning in a strategic manner. You might be asking for a straightforward answer to the straightforward question, "What will a strategic plan do for me as a manager?" Here are some answers and critical points to keep in mind:

- Strategic plans create bridges between organizational goals and the key customers and stakeholders of services provided by departments and organizations.
- Strategic planning is most importantly a process that guides you through imagining a new future and not a document (although documentation is helpful and necessary!).
- Plans change and things happen along any road, but you don't start a major journey without some sort of map!
- There are many accessible approaches and models that lay out the steps in strategic planning, so most importantly, do what fits with your organizational culture.
- Remember, strategic planning takes time, commitment, and flexibility!

After reading the prior chapters on leadership, as well as the roles and functions of the manager and supervisor, you may also be wondering what sorts of skills are required to take on a strategic planning process. A nonexhaustive list of skills that support strategic planning is included in Box 9-1.

How Do You Prepare for Strategic Planning?

As noted, many accessible step-by-step models found in the business or organizational development literature lay out the steps of strategic planning. One of these models is presented in the next section of this chapter. Planning is important; in fact, "planning to plan" is sometimes a step included in the models. This includes (1) identifying the types of data and information you will need to gather and arranging for access to data sources, (2) determining who will be involved

> **BOX 9-1**
>
> **Leadership and Management Skills That Support Strategic Planning**
>
> - Transformational and transactional leadership skills
> - Long-range planning and ability to think down multiple tracks at once
> - Problem-solving and change management skills
> - Tolerance for uncertainty
> - Group process skills
> - Ability to see and help others see the big picture AND manage fine details
> - Environmental scanning and analysis skills
> - Project management

in the process itself as well as key stakeholders who will be invested in the outcome of your plan, and (3) steps that you might take to prepare your department and organization for the process itself. Some questions you might ask as part of the process of planning to plan are listed in Box 9-2. The answers to these questions may identify work that you want to accomplish before you jump into the process of strategic planning. For example, the staff in your department may have experience with strategic planning and may be excited to begin the process, but if your supervisor or "one-up" is newer to the organization and not prepared to support you in the process it may well be worth delaying your start until you and your one-up are on the same page.

The questions in Box 9-2 can be answered as part of the process of conducting an internal assessment of your environment and the process of starting to develop a department or an organizational profile. A department or organizational profile and the process of creating a profile can be helpful for strategic planning, marketing, business planning, and measuring customer satisfaction. A **departmental or organizational profile** is a document that lays out key information about who you are and how you operate in your internal and external environments. For example, some of the first important questions you might answer are listed in Box 9-3.

The Steps of Strategic Planning

The eight steps of strategic planning are represented in Figure 9-1 (Goodstein, 1992). It should be noted that the steps involved in planning, whether for long-term strategy or for day-to-day activities, are typically not completed for the purpose of planning alone. The information gathered on the environments that influence an organization, the analysis of the clients' and customers' needs, and assessment of the organization's

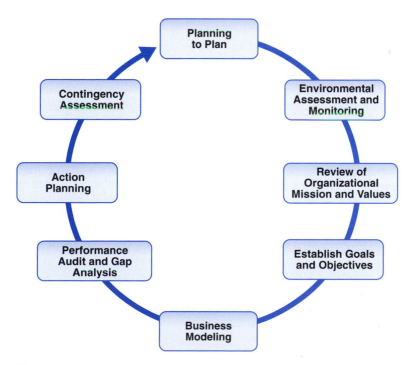

Figure ■ 9-1 The Eight Steps of a Strategic Planning Process.

internal environment are also useful for the management functions of marketing and program development, which are discussed in other chapters of this book. The steps are represented in a cycle to indicate that the process is ongoing. Like many processes, you may not complete the steps in a simple lock-step fashion. For example, you might gain additional information later in the process that would cause you to return to an earlier step to make some adjustments. It is also important to note that there are many models and frameworks to guide strategic planning. The steps presented in this chapter represent just one approach, and it is important to focus on key elements and outcomes of the process. Finally, it is important to recognize that the steps are described briefly, focusing on the purpose and key accomplishments in each step; any occupational therapy manager who finds himself or herself responsible for strategic planning should seek more detailed resources.

Planning to Plan

Planning to plan includes consideration of who needs to be involved in the planning process, establishing or discovering communication mechanisms for keeping key stakeholders informed, and identifying constraints or roadblocks to the planning process that may be encountered so that alternatives or *contingencies* may be established. Most importantly, you must identify who might create roadblocks or sabotage your plan if they are not included in the planning process and establish communication systems with them to determine how they wish to be involved. Customers including patients, clients, caregivers, family members, physicians, mid-level providers, and other referral sources are certainly one group of stakeholders, as are other internal customers such as the other members of your team. Other stakeholders might include vendors that provide you with critical products, payers who purchase or reimburse you for your services, and community members who rely on the services that you provide to maintain community health. The following is a short list of questions that you would want to answer clearly as part of your departmental or organizational profile and to complete the step of planning to plan:

- Who are your key customers?
- What are your customers' expectations (and how do you know this)?

- Who are other key stakeholders and do their expectations differ?
- Who are key suppliers, partners, or collaborators?
- Are your relationships with customers and other key stakeholders stable and healthy?

Environmental Assessment and Monitoring

Occupational therapy managers must constantly scan both the internal and the external environments of their organizations for information and events that will impact short-term operational planning and strategic planning. The internal environment is monitored for changes such as increases or decreases in resources, loss of key personnel, changes in programming, or other changes that might support or detract from the organization's ability to pursue its goals. The external environment is monitored for changes in policies or laws that affect reimbursement or practice, the addition or loss of competitors, changes related to key populations served, or new technological developments that again will support or detract from the organization's pursuit of its mission.

Data, information, and other forms of evidence described in Chapter 2 assist with the process of environmental assessment, as do answers to the following questions:

1. What are the primary factors that determine your department's and your organization's success (what contributes most to your success or failure)?
2. What critical changes are taking place that affect (or likely will affect) your organization's success?
3. What sources of comparative data exist for your organization from other member organizations (or other types of organizations)?
4. What limitations, if any, are there in your ability to obtain comparative data? (How can you compare?)
5. If you "compete" for customers, with whom are you competing (who's your competition)?
6. What are your key operational and human resource strategic challenges and advantages? (What keeps you up at night and what gives you an edge?)

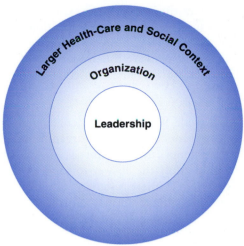

Figure ■ 9-2 The Layers of the Environment to Assess in Strategic Planning.

Strengths
- Clinical expertise
- Patient-centeredness
- Evidence-based

Opportunities
- Collaboration with universities on clinical research and outcomes studies
- Serve as a resource to the interdisciplinary team
- Expand services to a community-based model

Aspirations
- Powerful leadership
- Influence policy for persons with disabilities
- International recognition for effectiveness of clinical programs

Results
- Excellent outcomes for increasing quality of life for persons with disabilities
- Increased revenue generation for the department
- Increased budgeted and allocated positions to support departmental expansion

Figure 9-2 shows the layers of the environment that you must consider during the process of assessing the internal and the external environments. Leadership is at the core of the environment and has its own culture and ways of operating that must be assessed. Leadership operates within the context of the organizational environment. Finally, both of these environments are influenced by the larger health-care and social contexts in which they operate.

This is also the phase of strategic planning where you would start your *SOAR* (strengths, opportunities, aspirations, and results) and your *SWOT* (strengths, weaknesses, opportunities, and threats) analyses. If you have planned sufficiently and have the necessary stakeholders involved in the planning process, conducting SOAR and SWOT analyses can be relatively easy, can produce invaluable information, and can also be a reaffirming process to the participants. Reviews are conducted by combining a review of key documents or reports (financial reports, outcome statistics, program evaluation, or accreditation reports) with staff interviews, discussions, or a structured brainstorming exercise as described in Chapter 13. Sample results of SOAR and SWOT analyses identified for an occupational therapy department are presented in Boxes 9-4 and 9-5. In real life, the results of these analyses would most likely be longer and the items would be presented in more detail. Also, a single item might be listed as both a weakness and an opportunity, and this would indicate an important point for discussion among you, your staff, and others involved in planning for the department's future.

Review of Organizational Mission and Values

Mission statements are typically established by an organization's founders and usually remain fairly stable over time, although they can sometimes become diluted or lose focus as organizations age and come to serve not only the purpose for which they were created, but also the practical purpose of providing a source of income for their employees. Although most organizations have established mission statements, many individual departments do not have one. The process of writing a departmental mission statement can help to refocus and reenergize staff members by helping them better understand the role they serve within an organization and the beliefs and values they hold in common. These beliefs and values are what hold them together as a community of practice. The concept of a community of practice is explored in more depth in Chapter 17.

Mission statements often communicate the answer to four questions that provide an organization's internal and external publics with an understanding of the organization's role in society:

1. Why does the organization exist?
2. What function does the organization perform?
3. For whom does the organization perform this function or who are the primary beneficiaries?
4. How does the organization go about filling this function?

There is wide variety in the length and style of mission statements for different organizations. Some mission statements can be as short as a single sentence and may only imply the answer to some of the questions listed here, whereas others can be relatively lengthy and provide additional information. Regardless, a mission statement should be used often as a management tool to guide planning and to direct resources. Time and other resources are not limitless, and choosing to invest them in one direction means they cannot be invested in another. By asking the question, "Is this central to our mission?" you can use your mission statement as a tool in carry out your daily functions as a manager.

As an example, the mission statement of the Department of Rehabilitation Services at the University of Texas MD Anderson Cancer Center is presented. In 2011, there was an existing departmental mission statement for occupational therapy but few of the staff were aware of its existence or could state its focus. The language of the statement had also become outdated and did not reflect the full scope of service of both occupational therapy and physical therapy provided as part of best practice oncology rehabilitation services. For example, the statement focused on "impairment" rather than the broader concept of participation that reflects contemporary thinking about the impact of impairment on function. The original mission statement was reviewed; although its primary meaning was not changed, the language was updated and the following mission statement was developed. The mission of the Department of Rehabilitation Services at the University of Texas MD Anderson Cancer Center now reads:

To optimize participation and quality of life of people affected by cancer through the development, application and evaluation of best practices in oncology rehabilitation.

From this mission statement, you can tell something about the nature of this particular rehabilitation services department. It not only indicates the reason for the department's existence and its primary functions, but also provides the reader with an indication of how this department is different from the departments of rehabilitation services at other medical centers. For example, a rehabilitation services department that provides similar clinical services but that is located in a small acute care medical center not affiliated with a nationally and globally recognized cancer center might not include the development and evaluation of best practices and rather focus solely on the delivery of quality care.

Whether at the organizational or departmental level, a mission statement should be thought of as a management tool. Too often mission statements are simply a page in a policies and procedures manual or are hung on the wall without having real impact on the day-to-day work of employees. Instead, mission statements can be used as evaluation criteria that help you make decisions about how to prioritize work and the use of resources. In other words, if activities do not relate to your mission (e.g., your reason for existing), why should you spend your time and the organization's human and financial resources on these activities? A basic economic principle is that of opportunity costs, or the idea that whenever you invest resources, the opportunity cost is the next best thing that is given up because you no longer have enough resources to invest. Using your mission statement as a management tool helps you to minimize opportunity costs.

When writing a department mission statement, you may want to follow the steps suggested in Box 9-6. In addition to review of the mission statement, reviewing espoused departmental and organizational values and how they are demonstrated in everyday work helps to appreciate the function of the department in the specific setting. For example, the shared values of the University of Texas MD Anderson Cancer Center and associated behaviors are included in Box 9-7.

Vision Statements and the Visioning Process

Elaine Hom (2013, n.p.) described the nature and importance of vision statements to organizations. She stated, "Aspirational in nature, vision statements lay out the most important primary goals for a company. Not to be confused with business plans, vision statements generally don't outline a plan to achieve those goals. By outlining the key objectives for a company, they enable the company's employees to develop business strategies to achieve the stated goals. With a

---

BOX 9-6

Suggested Steps in Writing a Departmental Mission Statement

1. Inform your boss of your intention and ask for his or her support, assistance, and blessing on taking your department through this process.
2. Gather all relevant documents, including your organization's mission and vision statements and the organization's strategic plan, and distribute these to your staff.
3. Ask someone from the organization's leadership to come and speak to the staff about the organization's mission, his or her vision of the future, and where your department fits in that future.
4. Distribute a list of questions to your staff and have your staff identify key concepts to be represented in your mission statement. You may want to use the nominal group technique (described in Chapter 13) to share responses.
5. Consider asking another department director or someone from the human resources department to facilitate group discussions for you so you can participate as a member.
6. Ask for a small group of volunteers to write draft statements based on group discussions. Set ground rules for sharing feedback, and share all drafts with your boss and other important leaders (e.g., other department directors with whom you work closely).

---

single unifying vision statement, employees are all on the same page and can be more productive."

The process of "visioning" can be a fun, creative, and motivating process that communicates the valuable role that employees can play in helping a department or organization to survive and thrive. At the same time, it is important for the person leading employees in a visioning exercise to set clear and appropriate boundaries for the exercise so employees do not become frustrated or waste time. An effective vision statement reflects a vision or dream of a future state that is both sufficiently clear and powerful to arouse and sustain the actions necessary for that dream

---

BOX 9-7

Core Values and Behaviors of the University of Texas MD Anderson Cancer Center

Caring: By our words and actions we create a caring environment for everyone.

- We are sensitive to the concerns of our patients and our coworkers.
- We are respectful and courteous to each other at all times.
- We promote and reward teamwork and inclusiveness.

Integrity: We work together to merit the trust of our colleagues and those we serve.

- We hold ourselves, and each other, accountable for practicing our values.
- We communicate frequently, honestly and openly.
- By our actions, we create an environment of trust.

Discovery: We embrace creativity and seek new knowledge.

- We help each other to identify and solve problems.
- We seek personal growth and enable others to do so.
- We encourage learning, creativity, and new ideas.

BOX 9-8

Sample Portions of Vision Statements

- To become the health-care provider and employer of choice in the city of Boston
- To be a global leader in innovation in providing high-quality, cost-effective service
- To become a national model for provision of creative and highly effective fieldwork education

---

to become a reality. However, it could be said that a vision that is not based in reality is a mirage. Sample portions of vision statements are listed in Box 9-8. The process of developing a vision statement may take a number of meetings and a number of weeks or even months if done in a thoughtful manner. Some sample steps in the visioning process are outlined in Box 9-9.

Establishing Short-Term and Long-Term Goals and Objectives

Establishing short-term and long-term goals and objectives related to the organization's mission is the next step of strategic planning. It should be recognized that involvement in **planning** (e.g., analyzing the factors influencing a situation and identifying a range of possible future actions that are appropriate and contribute toward achievement of organizational objectives) is not the same at all organizational levels. The persons who are involved in planning and daily decision-making should vary according to the type of work being accomplished by those involved. Delegation of authority to personnel at lower organizational levels has gained increased favor in recent decades and may be effective at times, especially in areas of the organization in which work processes and technologies remain fairly stable. However, we must be careful not to overdelegate authority in areas of the organization calling for creativity or in which work processes must continually be revised, because this can result in the best designers, researchers, explorers, and creators being pulled from what they do best to become involved in the management of an organization or department. Careful consideration of whom to involve means balancing concern over leaving people out of the process with inappropriately pulling people from critical work assignments.

Business Modeling

Once goals and objectives are established, the current or possible structures for staffing and for lines of authority and accountability are examined. This process is referred to as *business modeling*. In many situations, occupational therapy managers may feel as if the structures of an organization are well established and therefore might tend to overlook this step of the strategic planning process. However, remaining open to change and examining new ways of organizing to

BOX 9-9

Sample Steps in a Visioning Process for Members of an Occupational Therapy Department

1. Set the boundaries for the visioning exercise (e.g., "Assuming similar levels of staffing as we have today, what is the best that you can imagine for our department in 5 years?"; "What is your dream for what you hope we can accomplish over the next 5 years?").
2. Explain the steps of nominal group technique:
   a. Clarify the group objective.
   b. Individually list as many ideas as possible (or you may want to set a limit of two to three ideas per person).
   c. Go around the group and have each member state one idea on his or her list. Individuals may pass if they have an idea that has already been stated.
   d. Record each idea on a flip chart.
   e. After all ideas are listed, clarify each idea and eliminate exact duplicates.
   f. Identify and eliminate items that do not fit the purpose of the exercise or those that may not be realistic within the agreed-upon time frame.
3. Identify common themes in the ideas that were presented through facilitated discussion (consider getting a manager from another department to lead the exercise so that you as a manager may participate in the exercise on an equal level with other department members).
4. Have a subgroup representing different types of employees volunteer to form a statement of a few sentences in length that represents the group's vision.
5. Distribute the draft statement to department members and key external stakeholders (e.g., managers from other departments, organizational leadership, customers) for feedback.
6. Continue review and revision of the vision statement until consensus is reached that the statement reflects a clear, powerful, and realistic goal for the department's future.

support goal obtainment is critical. Establishing cross-functional teams, hiring part-time or per diem (as needed) employees, or creating a new product line (moving staff from various disciplines into a single cost center) may be options supported by top administration if managers can show that significant cost savings or revenue enhancements may occur. In the case of a new business, department, or service, business modeling is a critical step beyond the scope of an introductory text on management. New managers who find themselves faced with the opportunity to create a new service should seek consultation with managers in the organization with experience in business planning or seek other resources. For example, the American Occupational Therapy Association (AOTA) has groups of practitioners referred to as "special interest sections" (SISs) (see http://www.aota.org/). One SIS, the Administration and Management Special Interest Section, has a subsection specifically for leaders, managers, administrators, private practitioners, and entrepreneurs. This subsection, like all the SISs, has online forums available to all AOTA members on the social media site OTConnections© that allow for the sharing of resources and dialogue about challenges faced.

Performance Audit and Gap Analysis

Once goals and objectives with quantifiable or measurable targets are established and you know where you want to be in the future, you need to establish where you are at present by conducting an audit of current performance. A *performance audit* is conducted by comparing your current performance against measurable quantitative and qualitative outcome indicators of success related to the departmental or organizational mission. Like many of the strategic planning process steps, the performance audit is really ongoing and not a one-time discrete activity. Managers who are effective strategic planners will develop systems to regularly check the progress of the implementation of actions related to their strategic plan. Examples of indicators that might be used would be increases in patient volume, the impact of new activities such as new orientation materials, or the provision of new services or measures of the impact of activities on employee or customer satisfaction. Performance audits help you to understand whether you are on target with the timeline of implementing your strategic plan and whether the quality of your performance is meeting expectations.

The performance audit and gap analysis identifies the gap between the current and desired indicators of performance. The performance audit and gap analysis is also best completed as an ongoing activity and can be focused on the time frame for implementation of activities or whether the quality of performance meets expectations. Few strategic plans are implemented exactly as first developed because of the dynamic nature of the environments in which health care and other types of organizations operate. Unexpected challenges, such as vacancies in key positions or an economic downturn, may result in changes to plans. Gap analyses can also spur you to reexamine plans and take new steps when they identify that the quality or quantity of performance is not meeting expectations. The performance audit and gap analysis provides quantitative measures of the completion of milestones or effectiveness, whereas the gap analysis is focused on understanding why your performance is higher or lower than expected and what you might do to get back on track if you are not meeting your expectations.

Action Planning

Action planning is the stage of planning that involves deciding exactly what you are going to do to get to where you want to be and to attain the goals and objectives established earlier in the planning process. As with the first step of "planning to plan," and in fact in each step of the process, developing an action plan that has a high chance of success is more likely if the right people are involved. Engaging in careful consideration of the key stakeholders in processes central to your plan and effectively communicating plans to those who can play roles in supporting or obstructing progress can make the difference between success and failure. A thorough action plan will include specific steps to achieve goals and objectives but will also include target dates for completion and will identify who is responsible for each action. Identifying dates to review progress on the action plan and who will be involved in these reviews is also recommended.

Contingency Assessment

Finally, an assessment of all those things that might reasonably be anticipated to go wrong and the impact of these events are conducted as part of a **contingency assessment.** In other words, this is the phase of planning in which as many of the "What ifs?" are identified as possible. A critical element of this step is imagining any event that, if it occurred, would result in having to abandon key goals and objectives. This is not as complicated or as abstract as it may sound; often some of our key fears are about those things we know might happen but we might want to otherwise avoid. For example, at one facility I started a hand therapy program and hired a certified hand therapist (CHT), who quickly helped to develop a robust program. Knowing that the CHT had specialized skills that other staff members did not have, I soon began to worry about what would happen if the therapist left the facility or needed to take a leave of absence. By making the contingency assessment a formal and visible step in the planning process, I was able to involve key stakeholders such as referring physicians in the hand therapy program, allowing me to gain support and financial resources to train additional staff in treating hand injuries. As a result, a second therapist eventually became a CHT. This not only solved the "What if the CHT leaves?" problem, but also helped to retain a second valued staff member who was looking for a new challenge.

Chapter Summary

This chapter focused on the process and outcomes of strategic planning and explained the contribution of a department's or organization's values, mission, and vision to the process. Other portions of the process, such as conducting a SWOT or SOAR analysis, were described, and sample mission and vision statements were provided.

The process of developing or revising a strategic plan and its component parts can be complicated and take time, but it can also provide extraordinary value to improving services. The key components of an effective strategic plan are summarized in Box 9-10.

At MD Anderson, the existing mission statement was evaluated by the department's leadership team using input from the staff gathered through multiple channels, including the use of an online survey with one question—"What is missing from our mission statement?"—and small-group discussions at staff meetings. These data were used by the leadership team to draft a revised mission statement that was

BOX 9-10
Key Components of an Effective Strategic Plan

1. A mission statement that clearly identifies the reason the organization exists and the primary beneficiary of the organization's efforts
2. A definition of major goals or accomplishments related to the organization's primary outputs
3. An action plan, including specific objectives detailing how the organization's goals will be achieved
4. A description of the human, material, and financial resources needed to meet the identified goals and objectives
5. A procedure for monitoring performance and identifying deviations from expected performance so alterations in the action plan can be made
6. An evaluation system to determine if goals have been met

BOX 9-11
The Mission and Vision Statements of the MD Anderson Cancer Center Department of Rehabilitation Services

The mission of the MD Anderson Department of Rehabilitation Services is to optimize participation and quality of life of people affected by cancer through the development, application and evaluation of best practices in oncology rehabilitation.

The vision of the MD Anderson Department of Rehabilitation Services is to be the globally recognized leader in the development, implementation and promotion of best practices in oncology rehabilitation, education and research.

thought to be more contemporary and reflective of current terminology while remaining consistent with MD Anderson values. This draft revision was intended to address all clients (i.e., families and caregivers in addition to patients) and incorporate an expanded departmental role in supporting cancer prevention and wellness by identifying the community as a customer. Additionally, the following steps were also taken to assess the draft: (a) review and feedback from all levels of staff in multiple forums, (b) intensive review by multiple layers of organizational leadership, and (c) sharing the revised mission with all staff and key stakeholders (i.e., physicians or nurses) for feedback before wide distribution of the revised mission statement.

Following review and distribution of the revised mission statement and the vision 2021 statement (see Box 9-11), the next step was the development of strategic objectives (broad statements that articulate our aims or responses to address major change or improvement, competitiveness or social issues, and health-care advantages) and strategic goals (specific and measurable statements about a future condition or performance level that we intend to attain). We utilized the information obtained from our SOAR analysis, our mission and vision review, and our traditional SWOT analysis.

Developing a departmental culture of openness and honesty to fully support achievement of an ambitious mission and vision for the future was a time-intensive effort that will continue for many years into the future. Based on our experiences so far, some of the "lessons learned" would include:

- Using small-group discussions is more effective than large groups. Using external facilitators helps to broaden staff discussions and participation.
- Educating the staff about the process and its goals before initiating it leads to faster results.
- The process of developing mission and vision statements facilitates the development of group cohesiveness as you move toward a single goal.
- The staff must always have a clear view of what we are doing and why it is being done during the process to allow for buy-in.
- Building trust in a department of this size is a key issue toward establishing a more positive working environment.
- Focusing on improving our processes and providing the tools for staff to do their work will result in overall effective and efficient delivery of patient care services.

■ Real-Life Solutions

The new Department of Rehabilitation Services director determined that the first step needed was an analysis of the department's and organization's current culture. The primary strategy for evaluating the organization's culture focused on using direct communication across all departmental levels. Work groups were identified (e.g., the leadership team, inpatient therapists), with each group participating in several exercises, including a *continue, start, and stop* exercise. In this exercise, work groups were asked to identify behaviors that they (a) wished to continue because they were beneficial for patient care and the health of the work group, (b) wished to start to improve patient care and working relationships, and (c) wished to stop because they detracted from patient care and positive working relationships. A second exercise was organized by the department's communication professional action coordinating team (PACT) in conjunction with the Department of Organizational Development. PACTs are a form of work team commonly used to address organizational issues at MD Anderson, and this department-specific PACT included members of the rehabilitation services staff. The activity involved staff working in small teams reflecting on and articulating current behaviors specific to the culture. This facilitated team interactions that promoted a focus on accountability for current behaviors and also identification of behavioral changes that would promote a culture of openness and honest communication. The focus on direct communication and the examination of values and their connection to everyday behavior will be ongoing in the department, but initial activities suggested the following:

- One must expect some initial uneasiness from all levels of the staff until trust is established.
- Honest discussions of specific behaviors help group members hold each other accountable for their daily actions.
- Establishing ground rules for meetings and group activities facilitates consistent behavior but is new to many group members and requires careful introduction.
- Mixing newcomers to the organization with veterans helps identify behaviors that have been acculturated. Change in culture requires the participation of all staff members and is slow to occur.
- Realistic expectations should be established regarding the pace of change to incorporate behaviors into daily routines (it will not happen overnight).

Having established a process for assessing the current departmental culture and to begin to envision the future, the director and the leadership team proceeded with steps to revise the mission statement and create a vision statement and corresponding strategic goals and objectives. They used an approach that (a) recognized and validated the existing mission statement as well as the important past work and achievements, (b) considered the tolerance for pace of change of the organization and its staff members, and (c) ensured the process was flexible enough to accommodate the daily work demands and any unexpected events that might have derailed the process. The Department of Rehabilitation Services' leadership chose to update its mission over a 6-month period. This period of time allowed the new director to get acquainted with his staff and to involve the entire department in a meaningful assessment of its culture and a discussion of how they could work together more effectively.

■ Vision 2021

Both the department director and organizational leadership at MD Anderson Cancer Center have a strong commitment to a future orientation. The Department of Rehabilitation Services director initiated strategic visioning and planning during the first month of his arrival but a systematic requirement for strategic planning in the department's division soon followed. Effective leaders must be able to create and articulate a clear and compelling

■ **Vision 2021—cont'd**

picture of where a department and its staff are headed in order to actively engage staff in actions needed to achieve strategic goals. The visioning process initiated in the department coincided with the evaluation of culture and focused on developing more direct and open communication in the department. Staff members and key stakeholders (i.e., physicians and other customers) were engaged in a process of imagining what the department's state might be in 2021. The time period of a decade was chosen because the new director had communicated to staff during his interview that he was looking to make a long-term commitment and would likely be around a decade or more if hired. The director chose to play off the news that MD Anderson had been named the number one cancer hospital in the country by *U.S. News and World Report* (*U.S. News and World Report*, 2011). He asked departmental members to imagine that in 2021 *U.S. News and World Report* has expanded its organizational rankings to include rehabilitation departments and that the MD Anderson Department of Rehabilitation Services has been ranked number one in the country. He asked, "Now imagine that the marketing department came to rehabilitation services to do an exposé on practices that led to the number one designation. What would you say?"

Study Questions

1. **A statement that sets forth an organization's or department's purpose, including definitions, products, and services, is best called a:**

   a. Vision statement.
   b. Mission statement.
   c. Purpose statement.
   d. Business statement.

2. **In strategic planning, a SWOT analysis includes all of the following domains of analysis except which of the following?**

   a. Strengths
   b. Weaknesses
   c. Operations
   d. Threats

3. **As an alternative to the traditional SWOT analysis, a SOAR analysis includes all except which of the following elements?**

   a. Strengths
   b. Opportunities
   c. Aspirations
   d. Research

4. **A document that includes a coordinated set of tasks for carrying out the goals delineated in a** strategic plan, goes into greater detail specifying specific time frames and deadlines for activities, and assigns activities to specific organizational members to aid accountability would best be called a(n):

   a. Business plan.
   b. Operational plan.
   c. Case statement.
   d. SOAR plan.

5. **Appreciative inquiries include which of the following?**

   a. Discovery
   b. Dream
   c. Design
   d. All of the above

6. **The stage of strategic planning in which you identify your key customers and their expectations; identify other key stakeholders and their expectations; identify your key suppliers, partners, and collaborators; and assess the health of your relationships with all of these persons would best be called:**

   a. Planning to plan.
   b. Environmental assessment and monitoring.
   c. Business modeling.
   d. Action planning.

7. **Which of the following best describes the purpose of the performance audit and gap analysis stage of strategic planning?**

   a. It compares current performance against measurable quantitative and qualitative outcome indicators of success related to the departmental or organizational mission.
   b. It identifies the gap between the current and desired indicators of performance.
   c. It substantiates the needed financial resources for budget planning.
   d. Both A and B.

8. **The stage of strategic planning that includes deciding exactly what you are going to do to get to where you want to be and to attain the goals and objectives established earlier in the planning process would best be called:**

   a. Planning to plan.
   b. Environmental assessment and monitoring.
   c. Business modeling.
   d. Action planning.

Resources for Learning More About Strategic Planning

Journals Related to Strategic Planning

Long Range Planning

http://www.journals.elsevier.com/long-range-planning/

Long Range Planning, the journal of the Strategic Planning Society (www.sps.org.uk), is the leading international journal in the field of strategic management. The journal publishes original research and theoretical articles including studies using primary survey data, case studies, and other approaches to data collection.

General Resources on Strategic Planning

Balanced Scorecard & Strategy Management Institute

www.balancedscorecard.org/BSCResources/StrategicPlanningBasics/tabid/459

The Balanced Scorecard & Strategy Management Institute (BSI) provides training, certification, and consulting services to commercial, government, and nonprofit organizations. BSI helps clients increase their focus on strategy and results, improve organizational performance by measuring what matters, align the work people do on a day-to-day basis with strategy, focus on the drivers of future performance, and improve communication of the organization's vision and strategy.

Baldrige Performance Excellence Program

http://www.nist.gov/baldrige/

The Baldrige Program is the nation's public–private partnership dedicated to performance excellence. To improve the competitiveness and performance of U.S. organizations for the benefit of all U.S. residents, the Baldrige Performance Excellence Program is a customer-focused federal change agent that
- Develops and disseminates evaluation criteria
- Manages the Malcom Baldrige National Quality Award
- Promotes performance excellence
- Provides global leadership in the learning and sharing of successful strategies and performance practices, principles, and methodologies

Associations Concerned With Strategic Planning

Association for Strategic Planning (ASP)

www.strategyplus.org

ASP was founded in 1999 as a not-for-profit professional association dedicated to advancing thought and practice in strategy development and deployment for business, nonprofit, and government organizations. ASP provides opportunities to explore cutting-edge strategic planning principles and practices that enhance organizational success and advance members' and organizations' knowledge, capability, capacity for innovation, and professionalism.

Strategic Planning Society

www.sps.org.uk

The Strategic Planning Society was formed in 1967 as an international network of strategists dedicated to the development of strategic thinking, strategic management, and strategic leadership, with the mission of improving the practice, development, and recognition of strategic management.

Reference List

Braveman, B. (2006). *Leading and managing occupational therapy services: An evidence-based approach*. Philadelphia, PA: F.A. Davis.

Braveman, B. (2009). Management of occupational therapy services. In E. B. Crepeau, E. S. Cohn, & B. A. B. Schell (Eds.), *Willard & Spackman's occupational therapy* (11th ed., pp. 914–928). Philadelphia, PA: Lippincott Williams & Wilkins.

Bushe, G. R. (2011). Appreciative inquiry: Theory and critique. In D. Boje, B. Burnes, & J. Hassard (Eds.), *The Routledge companion to organizational change* (pp. 87–103). Oxford, UK: Routledge.

Goodstein, K. L. (1992). *Applied strategic planning*. San Diego, CA: Pfeiffer & Company.

Hom, E. J. (2013). What is a vision statement? *Business News Daily*. Retrieved from http://www.businessnewsdaily.com/3882-vision-statement.html

Hoyle, J. R. (1995). *Leadership and futuring: Making visions happen*. Thousand Oaks, CA: Corwin Press.

McKonkey, D. D. (1976). *How to manage by results* (3rd ed.). New York, NY: AMACOM.

MD Anderson Cancer Center. (2015). *MD Anderson Cancer Center profile*. Retrieved from http://www.mdanderson.org/about-us/facts-and-history/institutional-profile/index.html

Mintzberg, H. (1994). *The rise and fall of strategic planning*. Englewood Cliffs, NJ: Prentice Hall.

Mittenthal, R. A. (2002). *Ten keys to successful strategic planning and nonprofit and foundation leaders. TCC Group: Strategies to achieve social impact*. Retrieved from http://www.tccgrp.com/pdfs/per_brief_tenkeys.pdf

National Institute of Standards and Technology. (2015). *2015–2016 criteria for performance excellence*. Retrieved from http://www.nist.gov/baldrige/publications/hc_criteria.cfm

Srivastva, J., & Cooperrider, D. (1990). *Appreciative management and leadership: The power of positive thought and action in organizations*. Cleveland, OH: Lakeshore Communications.

Stavros, J., Cooperrider, D., & Kelley, D. L. (2003). *Strategic inquiry, appreciative intent: Inspiration to SOAR*. Retrieved from http://design-n.oit.umn.edu/about/intranet/documents/Strategic_Inquiry_Appreciative_Intent.pdf

Thomas, E. (2006). *Appreciative inquiry: A positive approach to change*. Retrieved from http://www.ipspr.sc.edu/ejournal/ejournal0611/appreciative%20inquiry.pdf

U.S. News & World Report. (2011). *U.S. News best hospitals: Cancer*. Retrieved from http://health.usnews.com/best-hospitals/rankings/cancer

CHAPTER 10

Managing Change and Solving Problems

Shawn Phipps, PhD, MS, OTR/L, FAOTA

■ Real-Life Management

As a new director entering a department in turmoil and forming a new team, Shawn had numerous concerns about policies, procedures, and expectations of staff that he felt needed to be addressed right away. Shawn's team was excited about the opportunity to work with the staff members and the organization to rebuild the department and came armed with many ideas about how to begin the process. Although the staff members appreciated Shawn and his team's enthusiasm and optimism, their plans to introduce additional changes to the department were not appreciated.

As Shawn and his team began to introduce new policies, procedures, and increased performance expectations for staff, they encountered varying levels of resistance. They found it very confusing that the staff had many complaints about the current state of the department but resisted the efforts they were making to respond to those concerns. Shawn had been introduced to theories and models of "change management" in graduate school but had not made any explicit use of the information. He decided to review the literature and utilize strategies that his team could use to foster change and decrease the resistance that he was experiencing.

Critical Thinking Questions

As you read this chapter, consider the following questions:

- Why are managers concerned with creating, fostering, and managing change within individuals, groups, departments, and organizations?

- How do effective leaders and managers identify an organizational problem and implement effective strategies to enhance organizational effectiveness?

- How does data collection and evidence-based decision-making enhance the manager's ability to solve problems effectively?

- How do effective leaders and managers incorporate strategies to motivate employees within the context of generational differences?

Glossary

- **Analytical skills:** abilities that allow you to understand the whole of something by breaking it down into its component parts and in turn allow you to better understand the whole.
- **Biomedical informatics:** emerging discipline that has been defined as the study, invention, and implementation of structures and algorithms to improve communication, understanding, and management of medical information.
- **Business skills:** strategic planning, human resources, marketing, and budgeting abilities that involve solving a problem and identifying, evaluating, and implementing potential solutions.
- **Change agent:** an individual, internal or external to the organization, who plays a significant role in fostering and promoting change within organizations.
- **Change management:** the process of utilizing evidence-based approaches and tools for creating and managing change.
- **Consensus:** type of decision in which all parties have agreed to support the plan of action fully even if it is not how they would act if they were acting alone.
- **Driving forces:** forces that are pushing in the direction of change.
- **Force-field analysis:** management technique that examines the variables involved in determining the effectiveness of planning and implementing a change management strategy.
- **Health behaviors:** behaviors that we choose to perform or avoid in the course of our daily lives that have a positive or negative effect on our health.
- **People skills:** skills involved with motivating others in ways that show respect and recognize their efforts and contributions.
- **Political skills:** an understanding of the real and imagined fears, desires, and consequences of action as perceived by others in the organization and environments in which you interact.
- **Problem setting:** the process of naming the problem to be solved as specifically as possible and then implementing effective strategies to enhancing the problem-solving process.
- **Process flow diagrams:** visual representations of work processes that identify the boundaries of a work process, the major stakeholders of the process, and the steps to complete the process.
- **Protected health information:** information that could lead to the identification of patients.
- **Resistance to change:** behaviors that discredit, delay, or prevent the implementation of a work change.
- **Restraining forces:** forces that are working against change and work to maintain the status quo.

Glossary—cont'd

- **System skills:** abilities that include learning to develop, coordinate, and effectively use technical systems related to information management and general systems related to people and organizations.
- **Transactional change:** related to everyday issues, such as management practices, overseeing employee satisfaction within a work unit, or job and task assignments.
- **Transformational change:** evolution related to organizational issues, such as mission, leadership, and organizational culture.

- **Transtheoretical model of change:** a model that has been applied to understanding how change occurs in discrete health behaviors and can be useful in providing a general framework for considering how other change processes occur in a person's behavior.
- **Valence:** the capacity of a force to unite or join with other forces to cause action.

Introduction

Undoubtedly you have heard someone say, "Change is the only constant." Occupational therapy practitioners face continuous changes within any health-care organization (Campbell, 2008). Change also frequently occurs within the local, state, and national environments in terms of legislative and reimbursement policy, and within the many health-care professions as standards on practice shift. Sometimes it seems difficult to keep up with the rate of change. For example, in occupational therapy, the requirement for entry-level education for occupational therapists changed so that all educational programs needed to be at the postbaccalaureate level by the year 2007. Yet, even before many educational programs made that change, much discussion and focus on education within the profession shifted to discussion of clinical doctoral programs and whether that should be the mandated entry-level education for occupational therapists. Clinical doctoral programs, or "OTD" programs, are indeed being introduced at universities all over the country, and in 2014 the American Occupational Therapy Board of Directors issued a position statement that the profession should move to a single point of entry at the OTD by 2025 (American Occupational Therapy Association [AOTA], 2014). While this position was not endorsed by the Accreditation Council on Occupational Therapy Education (ACOTE), the number of new OTD programs and the number of master's programs transitioning to the OTD is increasing significantly.

As an occupational therapy manager, you will be responsible not only for responding to change within your department and your organization, as well as the range of external influences that affect your organization, but also for facilitating and creating change. The term **change management** has often been used to describe this function. Literature on change addresses four principles of change management: (1) theoretical models and frameworks that guide organization members' and researchers' thinking about organizational change, (2) approaches and tools for creating and managing change, (3) factors important to successful change management, and (4) the outcomes of the process of change management (Branch, 2002). In addition, literature and empirical research on change have addressed change in terms of the individual both at the level of the work group or team and at the level of the organization.

Scholarship related to change has included the development of a number of models for explaining how change occurs in individuals, groups, and organizations, as well as developed effective models for creating change (Arndt & Bigelow, 2009). Major areas of empirical investigation related to change have included change within organizations, promoting change or acting as a change agent, and resistance to change.

Solving problems is often involved in creating and managing change, and scholarship on this topic has included investigation of effective negotiation strategies and clinical and procedural reasoning in the health professions as well as in business and economics literature.

The idea that managers should make decisions based upon data and information is commonly discussed. However, many managers might admit to feeling pressured to make decisions and solve problems quickly regardless of the amount or accuracy of the data or information they have to guide these processes. Unfortunately, making decisions quickly rather than making data-driven decisions is taken as the sign of a skilled manager and is rewarded all too often. The skills related to finding and evaluating evidence are critical for effectively managing change and solving problems. This chapter focuses on the knowledge and strategies related specifically to fostering and managing change and on strategies to help solve problems.

Layers of Change

When you consider the topic of change management, you should recognize that change might occur within multiple layers of the environments in which we interact. Consider the figure first shown in Chapter 4 representing organizations as open systems (shown again in Figure 10-1). Figures similar to this have been used to represent individuals in society as well as larger organizational systems themselves. If we view an individual as an open system, then we must recognize that the input, throughput, and output relate to change within that person just as they relate to change within organizations.

Occupational therapists (OTs), occupational therapy assistants (OTAs), and occupational therapy students are typically concerned with facilitating some type of change for, and within, the individuals with whom we work. Occupational therapy managers are concerned with change both within individuals (i.e., staff development) and within larger organizational units such as a therapy department.

A number of models have been presented within the public health literature that address change within individuals as it relates to **health behaviors** (e.g., starting, stopping, or continuing to perform some health-promoting action). Health behaviors are the behaviors that we choose to perform or avoid in the course of our daily lives that have a positive or negative effect on our health. For example, each of the following would be considered a health behavior:

- Starting to exercise
- Stopping smoking
- Continuing to eat a well-balanced diet

Other considerations include the following:

- Input for the individual may include data, experiences, or observations.
- Throughput involves the processing of information and experiences, including health-related information.
- Output may include health behaviors such as starting, stopping, or continuing a behavior that may improve or negatively affect health status.

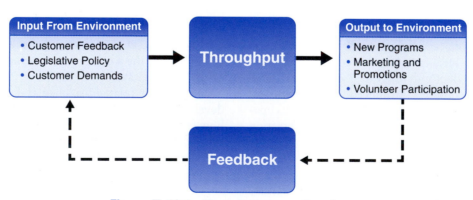

Figure ■ 10-1   The Individual as an Open System.

These models are reviewed in Chapter 15 because they are often used when developing occupational therapy programming. The most relevant model of change management is the **transtheoretical model of change**, in which change behavior is considered through a series of stages (Prochaska & DiClemente, 1993). This classic model has most often been applied to understanding how change occurs in discrete health behaviors and can be useful in providing a general framework for considering how other change processes occur in a person's behavior. The five stages are presented in Box 10-1.

In this chapter, as we consider change, we focus on change theory and models as they relate to accepting or adopting new behaviors, practices, or systems within the work environment as an individual, a department, or a work unit, such as an interdisciplinary team or an entire organization.

Bennis, Benne, and Chin (1985) identified three strategies for fostering individual change that are still commonly cited in the literature: (1) educative or empirical-rational, (2) normative or persuasive, and (3) power-coercive. These strategies, along with examples of each, are presented in Box 10-2 as applied to a common problem faced by occupational therapy managers in medical-model settings: convincing staff to adopt practices related to charging for services provided and to documenting those services.

Different situations may call for a different change strategy or for the use of more than one of these strategies in combination. The choice of strategy or strategies for any given situation may be influenced by a

---

BOX 10-1

The Five Stages of Change

- **Precontemplation:** Individuals are unaware or underaware of a problem or the need to change
- **Contemplation:** Individuals are aware of a problem and the need to change and considering taking action, but have made no commitment to any specific action
- **Preparation:** Intention to begin change is combined with criteria for action that include a time frame to begin acting
- **Action:** Individuals attempt to incorporate new behavior into their routine
- **Maintenance:** New behaviors are successfully incorporated into daily routines so that the behaviors become habitual

---

BOX 10-2

Three Strategies for Fostering Individual Change

Educative or Empirical-Rational
- If individuals are educated and guided by information, they will use logic and reason to make rational choices and behave accordingly.
- *Example:* Providing an in-service program on productivity and documentation stressing the negative impact on staffing and the ability to fill vacant positions if staff members do not charge and document according to policy.

Normative or Persuasive
- If knowledge about technology and systems is balanced with knowledge of noncognitive determinants of behavior, such as the processes of persuasion and collaboration, then individuals will be guided by internalized meanings, habits, and values and change behavior accordingly.
- *Example:* Creating a culture in which staff members support each other and remind each other to charge patients and document services, and establishing a norm in which staff members remind each other frequently to follow procedures related to charging for services and documenting appropriately.

Power-Coercive
- Individuals are exposed to strategies that emphasize political, economic, or regulatory sanctions. If they do not support change, then behavior will change accordingly.
- *Example:* Imposing penalties or removing rewards such as merit pay raises if staff do not follow policies and procedures related to charging for services and documenting.

number of factors (Nickols, 2004). These factors include:

- *Degree of resistance:* Strong resistance calls for use of more power, whereas weaker resistance allows for the use of rational strategies or education.
- *Target population:* Larger populations may require a mix of strategies, whereas smaller populations allow more limited choice of strategies.
- *The stakes:* When stakes are high, a mixture of strategies may lead to a greater likelihood of success.
- *The time frame:* Shorter time frames call for increased reliance on power; longer time frames allow more rational or educative approaches to be used.
- *Expertise:* Having considerable expertise available allows for more of a mixture of strategies, whereas limited expertise may force reliance on power.
- *Dependency:* One party being dependent upon another affects the extent to which that party may rely on power versus other strategies.

Kurt Lewin (1997) suggested what is now considered a classic and simple model of change that is related to both the individual and the organization. This model views change as occurring in three phases: (1) unfreeze, (2) change, and (3) refreeze (see Figure 10-2). The largest contribution of this simple model is that you may think about change as a staged process that can be broken down and analyzed, with different strategies being used at each of the phases. This simple approach is helpful for the new manager without extensive experience in creating and managing change processes. By focusing on each of the three phases, you can choose and plan strategies for introducing change, guiding staff through the change, and institutionalizing the new and desired state. Many of the continuous quality improvement (CQI) concepts, strategies, tools, and techniques discussed in Chapter 13 can be very helpful throughout the three phases.

The limitations of this model are that it does not consider that change often begins within an organization already in flux or unfrozen, or that organizations may need to remain frozen for extended periods of time (Nickols, 2004). In essence, the model may oversimplify how change really occurs in many situations. Often you will find yourself dealing with processes or situations that were not stable to begin with and it may not be possible to completely stabilize the process or situation. Lewin suggested that change could occur within organizations in one of three ways (Branch, 2002):

1. Change the individuals who work within the organization (skills, values, attitudes) and eventually behavior.
2. Change various organizational structures and systems such as rewards, reporting relationships, and work designs.
3. Change the organizational climate or interpersonal style (rate of interaction, conflict management, etc.).

These methods of change can be combined so that you facilitate change at both the individual and organizational levels. An example might be introducing a change to the process of completing seating assessments and recommending wheelchairs and seating systems on a rehabilitation unit. In the past, perhaps only one discipline has conducted the assessment; in the new approach, you are changing the process so that occupational therapy and physical therapy will collaborate on the assessment and must come to agreement and present one recommendation. Such a recommendation might be met with resistance because of concerns over loss of control or power. Change might be fostered at the individual level by acting to change the knowledge, skills, and attitudes of staff. The knowledge of both disciplines could be addressed by providing factual information about the education and training of each discipline, the areas of overlap, and the areas of differences so that staff members could

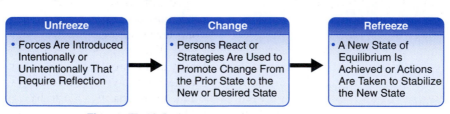

Figure ■ 10-2 Lewin's Three-Stage Model of Change.

understand how, by collaborating, the knowledge brought to the assessment process would be greater than either discipline could possess alone. Skills could be addressed by developing competencies and a training program for seating assessments specific to both disciplines. Finally, attitudes might be addressed by a number of strategies, including team-building activities to increase the personal comfort level of staff in interacting with each other, activities focusing on customer needs and what might not be adequately addressed if either discipline did not participate, and having leaders from each discipline model effective teamwork.

In addition to fostering change at the individual level, change could be fostered at the departmental and organizational levels by providing rewards and recognitions for staff members who effectively team together and by creating a climate in which open discussion of concerns is encouraged and welcomed. Other strategies for fostering this change process might include examining forms to require communication and to avoid separate processes being completed, and thinking about where assessments are conducted so that the power relationship between the two disciplines might be equalized.

Within organizations, two levels of intentional change have been identified and are discussed within the literature (Bridges, 1995; Burke, 2010; Burke & Trahant, 2000). Change related to organizational issues, such as mission, leadership, organizational culture, or other "big picture" issues, has been referred to as **transformational change**. Change related to everyday "how to get things done" issues, such as management practices, overseeing employee satisfaction within a work unit, or job and task assignments, has been referred to as **transactional change**.

Large-scale organizational change is tremendously complicated, and there is a large and varied body of work presented in the organizational development, organizational behavior, and human resources literature, some of which is addressed in other chapters (see Chapter 4 regarding learning organizations and Chapter 13 regarding CQI). Occupational therapy managers will seldom be solely responsible for leading such a change, although the number of OTs who own and operate their own business or engage in entrepreneurial ventures is increasing. Those who become involved in higher levels of organizational administration or who start their own business are encouraged to pursue a business education that will include

---

BOX 10-3

Eight Common Reasons Organizational Change Efforts Fail

1. Allowing too much complacency
2. Failing to create a sufficiently powerful guiding coalition
3. Underestimating the power of vision
4. Undercommunicating the vision
5. Permitting obstacles to block the vision
6. Failing to create short-term wins
7. Declaring victory too soon
8. Neglecting to anchor changes firmly in the new organizational culture

---

strategies for organizational management and change. Many organizations are successful in implementing large-scale changes; however, many others do not succeed. John Kotter (2012) identified eight common reasons that organizational change efforts fail in his book *Leading Change*. These eight reasons are listed in Box 10-3. Kotter argued that the biggest mistake people make when trying to change organizations is moving ahead without establishing a sense of urgency about what needs to be changed. In today's business environment, change happens quickly and organizations and managers must be prepared to react in kind. However, quick reaction does not mean acting without gathering sufficient data to make an informed and evidence-based decision. For Kotter, *complacency* means underestimating how difficult it is to move people out of their "comfort zones" and overestimating the amount of control they have over an organization.

Throughout organizational change efforts, communication is a key to success. Communication must be frequent and aimed at communicating not only what change is needed but also why, how, and when it is expected to occur. Most importantly, a vision of the future must be communicated in clear and sufficiently strong terms so that employees know where they are headed. Finally, it is the manager's responsibility to identify and remove obstacles that will get in the way of achieving the vision or desired state.

The term **change agent** has been used to refer to those individuals, internal or external to the organization, who play a significant role in fostering and promoting change within organizations. The term is typically used to refer to those individuals who foster change with an organization's best interest in mind. Internal change agents may be formal or informal leaders, whereas external change agents are typically paid consultants to an organization. Being an effective change agent requires that you (a) remain alert to situations that require change, (b) stay open to new ideas, and (c) become skilled in supporting the implementation of new ideas into everyday practice (Schermerhorn, Hunt, & Osborn, 1994).

In a review of the empirical literature on change agency, Caldwell (2003) identified four models of change agency that he advocated would encompass most of the existing literature. He emphasized that there is no universal or single model of change agency and provided a brief description of the four models of change agency as a heuristic tool. These four models are described in Box 10-4.

BOX 10-4

Four Models of Change Agency

- **Leadership models:** Change agents are identified as leaders or senior executives at the very top of the organization who envision, initiate, or sponsor strategic change of a far-reaching or transformational nature.
- **Management models:** Change agents are conceived as middle-level managers and functional specialists who adapt, carry forward, or build support for strategic change within business units or key functions.
- **Consultancy models:** Change agents are conceived of as external or internal consultants who operate at a strategic, operational, task, or process level within an organization, providing advice, expertise, project management, change program coordination, or process skills in facilitating change.
- **Team models:** Change agents are conceived of as teams that may operate at a strategic, operational, task, or process level within an organization and may include managers, functional specialists, and employees at all levels, as well as internal and external consultants.

Skills for Creating and Managing Change

Because change is created, encountered, and needs to be managed within *open systems*, a wide variety of skill sets are required. Nickols (2004) identified what he believed were the most critical skill sets related to change management: (a) political skills, (b) analytical skills, (c) people skills, (d) system skills, and (e) business skills. Each of these skill sets and its relationship to creating and managing change is briefly discussed.

Political skills involve understanding the real and imagined fears, desires, and consequences of action as perceived by others in the organization and environments in which you interact. Although the term *office politics* is often perceived as pejorative, it may also be thought to mean that persons are simply acting in a shrewd and socially aware manner. None of us wants to feel bullied or embarrassed into taking action or changing, and developing more effective political skills means that you create and manage change in ways that show awareness that all employees want to be viewed favorably by their peers. Good politicians are leaders, effective communicators, facilitators, negotiators, marketers, advocates, motivators, visionaries, and, last but not least, "doers" (Gioia & Andersen, 2003). Political skills that will help you be effective in creating and managing change include:

- Learning to recognize the unwritten rules involved in organizational culture.
- Understanding the importance of when to become more visible within meetings or projects and when to defer attention or credit to organizational leaders, your boss, and subordinates.
- Understanding your assumptions and learning to recognize the assumptions of others about work, success, and change.
- Becoming comfortable with talking to a wide variety of people in a wide variety of contexts.
- Becoming an effective communicator and skilled at giving feedback and delivering communication in nonconfrontational ways that maintain the dignity of others.

Analytical skills include the skills that allow you to understand the whole of something by breaking it down into its component parts, which in turn allow you to better understand the whole. One group of analytical skills includes those related to the evidence-based practice process of gathering and evaluating data and information. Nickols (2004) identified two important subsets of analytical skills: (1) workflow operations and (2) financial analysis. Workflow operations require that you be able to identify the start and finish of a process and the interim steps. Process analysis, including the use of **process flow diagrams**, is a central quality improvement strategy. Process flow diagrams are visual representations of work processes that identify the boundaries of a work process, the major stakeholders of the process, and the steps to complete the process. Process flow diagrams are very useful in identifying places where the process breaks down, where rework occurs, or where undesired variation may be introduced to a process. These and other workflow operation tools and techniques are discussed in depth in Chapter 13. Managers must also be able to identify the financial impact of changing a process or implementing a new process. For solutions to problems to be accepted and to be effective, they must also be cost effective. Skilled managers will complete financial analysis and recognize the financial impact of possible solutions before suggesting them.

People skills are those involved with motivating others in ways that show respect and recognize their efforts and contributions; these skills are mostly associated with communicating with others. People skills include verbal, written, and nonverbal communication skills (see Chapter 5). Creating a positive culture and learning to develop and manage effective teams, in addition to supervising individuals, are also important subsets of people skills. As noted earlier, change can create a range of negative emotions; learning to anticipate and recognize the emotional needs of employees in addition to other needs, such as training, will make the facilitation of change much easier. Managers face the difficult challenge of balancing tasks and people. During times of stress or when work processes are breaking down, attention to tasks often seems paramount. However, it is exactly those times when attending to people may be most important. **System skills** include learning to develop, coordinate, and effectively use technical systems related to information management (e.g., charge systems, documentation systems, management of data for outcomes measurement) and general systems related to people and organizations (Nickols, 2004). **Biomedical informatics** is an emerging interdisciplinary, scientific field that studies and pursues the effective uses of biomedical data, information, and knowledge for scientific inquiry,

problem-solving, and decision-making, motivated by efforts to improve human health (American Medical Informatics Association, 2013). With the rapid changes and improvements in technology, management of information has become very sophisticated. In addition, biomedical informatics has become increasingly complex with the advent of laws such as the Health Insurance Portability and Accountability Act (HIPAA) of 1996, which includes regulations and proposes fines for mishandling of **protected health information** or information that could lead to the identification of patients. See resources at the U.S. Department of Health and Human Services on privacy (http://www.hhs.gov/ocr/privacy/) and at the U.S. Department of Labor on insurance provisions (http://www.dol.gov/ebsa/newsroom/fshipaa.html). In larger organizations, the occupational therapy manager will need to become skilled in collaborating with informatics specialists. In smaller organizations, such as a private practice, business owners are encouraged to examine closely and compare the advantages and costs of purchasing commercial systems or the time of a consultant with those of trying to manage information on their own. Similarly, most large organizations handle general systems, such as personnel, through hiring staff specialists to manage these functions. Managers or owners of businesses may have to develop a wide variety of skills, including general systems knowledge, that are handled by others in larger organizations; however, caution is recommended, especially in areas such as human resources, where mistakes can be costly in terms of litigation and wasted resources.

Business skills include the various skill sets related to how business, and in particular a health-related business, works. Skills such as strategic planning, human resources, marketing, and budgeting can all become part of solving a problem and identifying, evaluating, and implementing potential solutions. Much of the learning that occurs for many occupational therapy managers ends up being on the job; however, as the health-care system and social systems in which we operate continue to become more complex, expectations for managers are increasing. As expectations for entry-level education also increase, graduates will be expected to have more advanced skill sets as they enter the profession. Still, most occupational therapy graduates will have had only one or two courses in administration and management that cover the full range of managerial tasks. Considering additional business-related graduate education or formal training in business-related and leadership skills development is recommended for occupational therapy graduates who intend to focus on management as their area of practice or who plan to own and operate their own business.

Resistance to Change

Resistance to change refers to behaviors that discredit, delay, or prevent the implementation of a work change (Newstrom, 2010). Change can elicit a wide range of feelings in individuals, including fear, uncertainty, excitement, anger, or worry over loss. Even when change is cognitively perceived as needed or beneficial, mixed feelings over experiencing the change process can cause individuals to resist. Curtis and White (2002) reviewed empirical literature from the fields of management and psychology and identified the most common reasons for resistance to change. These are summarized in Box 10-5.

Resistance to change has been the focus of much research and scholarship in the organizational development and management literature. Closely related research and scholarship has focused on ways of increasing receptivity to change. A classic and sustaining example is work conducted by Pettigrew, Ferlie, and McKee (1992) examining receptivity to change in the British National Health Service. They identified eight factors associated with receptivity to change. More recently, others have identified similar factors (van Doom, 2011). Common factors associated with receptivity to change are summarized in Table 10-1.

It is also important to recognize that often individuals who are asked to change may experience conflicting feelings. Even while recognizing and valuing the advantages of adopting some change behavior, they may also recognize and fear negative effects. You may be able to tip the balance in favor of your desired change by (a) identifying the positive outcomes of change, (b) increasing the value of those outcomes, (c) making the path to achieving those outcomes easier, (d) identifying the negative outcomes of change, and (e) decreasing the perceived impact of negative outcomes and making them less likely to occur. One often-cited method of accomplishing this is **force-field analysis**. Force-field analysis, a management technique developed by Kurt Lewin, is useful when looking at the variables involved in determining the effectiveness of—and when planning

---

BOX 10-5

Common Reasons for Resistance to Change

- **Increased stress:** Resistance can be focused not toward the change itself but toward the consequences of such change, such as loss of status or comfort, and the resulting feelings of stress that make it difficult for individuals to adjust.
- **Denial:** Denial of the need to change can be a natural reaction to perceived stress or other negative reactions to stress. Denial is recognized as a common defense mechanism used to deal with anxiety and is often thought of as a natural reaction that might be expected when individuals are initially confronted with change.
- **Self-interest:** Change often results in a shift in power or the addition of benefits to some members of an organization while other members' benefits remain the same or are decreased. Fear of personal loss has been identified as a major obstacle to change in organizations.
- **Lack of understanding, trust, and ownership:** People are less likely to accept and support change if they do not understand the purpose behind it or distrust those who are initiating change.
- **Uncertainty:** The lack of information about future events can increase feelings of lack of control and anxiety.
- **Motivation:** Motivation refers to the drive to meet our needs. When various types of needs (safety, security, belonging, or self-esteem) are threatened by the prospect of change, resistance may increase.
- **Different assessments or perceptions:** Resistance may increase when perceptions of a situation, the need for change, or the impact of change differ between persons at various levels of an organization.

TABLE 10-1
Eight Factors Commonly Associated With Receptivity to Change

Factor	Definition
Coherent and effective policies and procedures	The extent to which policies and procedures are linked to each other and to the work that must be completed
Continuity in key leadership positions	Maintaining consistency in the approaches and skills of those leading change efforts
Environmental monitoring	Awareness of external factors in triggering change
Supportive organizational culture	Values, beliefs, and behaviors that support the achievement of change goals
Effective relationships between managers and clinicians	Managers and clinicians learning about each others' perspectives and making efforts to appreciate the challenges faced by others
Effective relationships with key organizational collaborators	Productive relations with related organizations, such as social services and voluntary organizations
Simplicity and clarity of goals	Establishing key priorities for the change agenda and articulating them to all in a clear and concise manner
The fit between the change agenda and the locale	Awareness that particular features of the locality may inhibit or accelerate change

and implementing—a change management strategy (Accel-Team, 2004; National Health Service Institute, 2013).

Conducting a force-field analysis with your staff or a group of those who will be impacted by change is a great way of developing a sense of involvement. The first step in conducting a force-field analysis is to identify **driving forces** and **restraining forces**. *Driving forces* can be thought of as forces that are pushing in the direction of change. Examples of such forces might be changes in reimbursement, new competition, requests from customers, or demands for increased productivity from organizational leadership. *Restraining forces* can be thought of as forces that are working against change and work to maintain the status quo. When driving forces and restraining forces are equalized, a state of equilibrium is achieved and change is less likely to occur. However, when driving forces outweigh restraining forces, change may be inevitable. Another important concept is that of **valence**, or the capacity of a force to unite or join with other forces to cause action. In other words, not all driving forces or restraining forces are equal. Conducting a force-field analysis enables you to identify the smaller driving and restraining forces that might have otherwise gone unconsidered.

As an example, an organizational leader might ask your staff to implement new customer service protocols aimed at improving customer satisfaction. You might find one very strong driving force, such as the encouragement and support of a respected leader whom your staff does not want to disappoint. However, there may be several restraining forces that, when examined individually, do not seem strong enough to prevent change. For example, there may be minor staff resistance to taking time to learn new procedures, limited concern over the impact of new procedures on workload and productivity, and some discomfort regarding skill levels related to dealing with disgruntled customers. If you were presented with any one of these restraining forces separately, and paid attention to how strongly staff members felt and their level of concern over that single issue, it might be difficult to understand why staff members were resistant to change. However, through the process of conducting a force-field analysis and involving your staff, you might identify that there are several concerns (restraining forces) that, when combined, are sufficiently strong

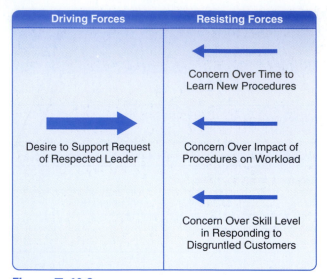

Driving Forces	Resisting Forces
Desire to Support Request of Respected Leader	Concern Over Time to Learn New Procedures
	Concern Over Impact of Procedures on Workload
	Concern Over Skill Level in Responding to Disgruntled Customers

Figure ■ 10-3
A Force-Field Analysis of Forces Affecting Adoption of New Customer Service Procedures.

to act against the staff's desire to change. Thus, the value in conducting a force-field analysis is in both the process and the outcome. This example is represented in Figure 10-3. The relative size of the arrows represents the *valance* of the individual force.

One set of behaviors that may be encountered during and after change efforts may be referred to as victim behavior (Balestracci, 2003). Victim behavior is likely to arise when individuals perceive that they have no influence over whether to change or how to change. They are likely to focus on what is happening to them as individuals and are unlikely to recognize what is happening in the environment around them or to other individuals. Victim behavior can be very frustrating to encounter as a manager, and what can be even more frustrating is that sometimes confronting it directly will only result in its increasing. Victim behavior may include complaining, lowered productivity, or missed workdays, or in worst cases can include behavior that works to sabotage the change efforts. At some point, such behavior must be dealt with directly, but other less confrontational strategies that can be used to overcome victim behavior and facilitate change include the following:

- Admit openly that change is difficult and that you also have difficulty with change at times; be empathetic and show your human side.

- Model acceptance of change by being the first to follow new procedures, attending trainings required, or adopting new ways of working.
- Be flexible when you can. Stay true to the main purpose of the intended change but recognize when you can adapt to make staff see that you are listening to them.
- Ask the staff member's advice on how to proceed with the change; invite him or her to help you identify specific actions to take to increase the likelihood of the change being successfully implemented.
- Complete a force-field analysis and enlist the staff member by assigning him or her (alone or with a small group) the task of drafting a list of driving forces to present to you or a larger group.
- Try having a face-to-face conversation in which the focus is not on the staff member's behavior; instead, use the opportunity to acknowledge that you are aware of his or her concerns and that you want to explain why change is needed. People may be open to change if they understand why it is needed, and this may act to dispel irrational fears or inaccurate information.

Laframboise, Nelson, and Schmaltz (2003) suggested that resistance to change could be managed by envisioning change as a staged process similar to the commonly identified stages of grieving (i.e., denial, anger, bargaining, and acceptance). The four stages they suggested are (1) discovery, (2) denial, (3) resistance, and (4) acceptance. These four stages, as well as strategies for each stage, are briefly summarized in Table 10-2. As with many stage models, it is important to realize that not everyone will experience every stage; some may move forward and then fall back to an earlier stage, and not everyone will eventually get to the final stage of acceptance.

Top-Down and Bottom-Up Change

Conventionally, change management has been viewed as a function of management in which organizational leaders are responsible for identifying desired change and leading, or forcing, those whom they supervise to change. Top-down theories of change management assume that the focus of theory and research should be the creation of more effective models to support the traditional hierarchical system found in most

TABLE 10-2
Four Stages of Change and Related Strategies

Stage of Change	Strategies
Discovery: when and how persons learn about the change	• Plan communication carefully so that all hear the same information at the same time. • For large-scale changes, develop a formal and written communication plan. • Put any facts, dates, or other concrete information that will help staff understand and be clear on what is to happen in writing.
Denial: when persons don't really believe that a change will occur or believe that, after a time, things will return to the way they were	• Continue wide communication in writing and in person. • Offer "town hall" meetings or allow time for questions and answers at a staff meeting. • Continue to express why the change is occurring and when. • Include persons in planning and implementing change so that they see that it will indeed occur.
Resistance: persons express frustration or anger and may avoid helping to implement change or work against it	• Continue to stress why change is occurring. • Allow opportunities to express concerns in writing and in person by using suggestion boxes or town hall meetings. • Make sure that communication includes details, and that persons are kept informed of steps as they happen. • Stress accomplishments.
Acceptance: persons understand what change will occur and agree to support it even if it is not how they would act if acting alone	• Celebrate accomplishments. • Recognize those instrumental in the change but thank all persons involved in the department or organization for their support. • Plan a review of the impact of change and assure that the change is not temporary. • Review what went well and what did not go so well to help prepare for future changes.

organizations (Lavasseur, 2001). More recent approaches to fostering and managing change within organizations have included bottom-up approaches, including those typically used within CQI process improvement efforts. Bottom-up change management approaches focus on tapping into the knowledge and expertise of those who are most familiar with work processes and may also be most familiar with the causes of rework, waste, and roadblocks within organizational processes.

Effective Delegation to Facilitate Organizational Change

Delegating responsibilities to employees contributes to their professional development by providing unique opportunities to build new skills and develop new competencies (Reinhard & Dickhauser, 2009). Dele-

gation can also provide the added benefit of motivating employees toward action, as they become the drivers of change through engagement in work responsibilities that have meaning (Honold, 1997). Empowering leadership has been shown to positively affect psychological empowerment, which influences higher levels of intrinsic motivation and creative process engagement (Hekman, Steensma, Bigley, & Hereford, 2009; Zhang & Bartol, 2010). Delegation is a leadership skill that requires an astute understanding of which tasks will challenge the employee and provide him or her with an opportunity to engage fully in shaping the organization's future. The manager can effectively empower the employee to higher levels of confidence and self-efficacy toward future-oriented organizational goals (Bandura & Locke, 2003). Delegation also allows for supportive autonomy, where the employee has an opportunity to define how a delegated task is accomplished. For example, an OT was supervising an OTA who demonstrated a high level of creativity and potential for contributing to the department. The OT delegated a program development opportunity to the OTA that allowed her to use her creativity to develop a program flyer and presentation promoting occupational therapy for distribution to physicians and the public.

Motivating Employees in Challenging Times

Motivating employees during challenging times, whether because of a down economy or rapid organizational change, can present the occupational therapy manager with opportunities for innovative leadership approaches to motivation. An effective leader consistently prepares employees for inevitable change (Nohria, Groysberg, & Lee, 2008). Leaders must ensure that employees understand why a change is necessary. Employees also need to feel that their ideas are valued as part of the solution to organizational challenges. Effective leaders inspire employees toward a more optimistic future by actively engaging the employees in solution-driven activity, despite the threat of layoffs and budgetary cutbacks (Wang, 2007). High morale, employee satisfaction, and the achievement of high levels of motivation are possible during challenging times when employees view their team's work as ultimately contributing to making others' lives more fulfilling.

Change as a Problem and Problem-Solving

Often change is initiated because a problem arises that requires that new action be taken because existing procedures or circumstances are no longer satisfactory. If you view a problem as an opportunity for planning change, then you can apply frameworks for change discussed earlier, including seeing change as moving from one state to another, specifically from the problem state to the solved state (Nickols, 2004). Interestingly, although managers spend a considerable portion of time solving routine everyday problems as well as much more complex problems, problem-solving itself is seldom taught.

A first step in problem-solving is naming the problem, or **problem setting**. Problem setting is a critical first step because it only makes sense that, as you consider solutions and alternatives, you will pay attention to information that you identify as relating to the problem and ignore information that you feel is extraneous. You attend only to information related to the problem you set. In naming or setting the problem, it is helpful if you set the problem to be as specific as possible. The more specific the problem set, the easier it is to tell when the problem is solved. Setting a problem specifically also helps in ruling out unrelated causes. For example, knowing that a fuse blows in the occupational therapy kitchen every time the microwave and any other countertop appliance are in use at the same time is a more specific problem than simply knowing that a fuse occasionally blows. By identifying the key elements of a problem and setting it as narrowly as possible, you can avoid wasted efforts.

Problem setting is not an idea new to health care or to occupational therapy. Donald Schön introduced the idea in his investigations of reflective practitioners and the logic that practitioners used to solve problems (Schön, 1983). Schön described problem setting as a process through which we name the things to which we will pay attention and frame the context in which we will attend to them. The problem-solver or practitioner then reframes the situation to fit his or her previous experiences and tacit knowledge about that type of practical situation. Mattingly and Fleming (1994) further developed these concepts in regard to the clinical reasoning and reflective practice of occupational therapy practitioners in their influential book *Clinical Reasoning: Forms of Inquiry in a Therapeutic Practice*. Often managers solve problems requiring a range of reasoning, but the works of Schön, Mattingly and Fleming, and others in regard to clinical reasoning are worth investigating to help managers with problems that involve human interaction.

Nickols (2004) suggested that the analysis of a change problem will focus on defining the outcomes of a change effort, on identifying the changes necessary to produce these outcomes, and on finding and implementing ways and means of making the required changes. Thus, a change problem may be broken into smaller problems that may be named "how problems," "what problems," and "why problems."

A second key element of problem-solving, especially in regard to more complex problems related to human interactions, is to identify the assumptions you are making about a situation. Assumptions are necessary for three reasons (Harris, 2002). First, they set limits to the problem. Second, they may reflect desired but unstated values. Third, assumptions help to simplify the problem and make it more manageable by giving us fewer things to consider. However, at times we make assumptions about a situation, a process, or people that are inaccurate. By identifying the assumptions you hold in regard to any given problem, you can seek to validate the assumptions or let them go.

For example, a common problem that occupational therapy managers face in hospital settings is scheduling staff for weekend coverage. Often in facilities where daily coverage is needed, some type of rotation system is used so that staff members take turns working weekend days and in turn take a day off during the week before or following the weekend. One manager struggled considerably with setting up a rotation system because there were several staff vacancies and the manager assumed that working weekends was not desirable to staff. It was quite accidental that the manager learned that one staff member liked working on the weekends because her fiancé typically had to work on the weekends and took days off during the week. Discovering that his assumptions about preferences for weekend scheduling might not be accurate prompted the manager to bring the problem back to the staff and look for more flexible solutions. As a result, staff members were not scheduled evenly for weekends. Rather, some staff members were scheduled more often and everyone ended up being happier. Harris (2002) provided a helpful checklist to identify some types of assumptions. The types of assumptions on his checklist are briefly presented in Box 10-6.

Another step that should be completed before jumping into problem-solving is to identify criteria for a successful and satisfactory solution. Too often, it is tempting to jump into problem-solving by beginning to identify alternatives as solutions. In fact, alternative swapping, or a group of individuals who have a problem in common proposing first one solution, and then another, and then another, is one of the most common roadblocks to successful problem-solving. Rather than beginning by proposing solutions, groups should first focus on identifying the goals or objectives for a satisfactory solution. In other words, you should identify a set of criteria against which potential solutions can be evaluated. The perfect solution that makes all parties happy may not exist, but by identifying objective criteria to evaluate solutions first, you may not only identify the best solution, but may also prevent conflict among the problem-solvers and limit individual agendas. One helpful tool that assists problem-solvers in comparing possible options to solve a

---

BOX 10-6

A Checklist of Assumption Areas Related to Solving Problems

- **Time:** You may have more time to solve a problem than you assume. Can you work with those who need to be involved to gain additional time to work on a satisfactory solution? If people are aware that you are working to solve a problem, they may be willing to wait for it to be solved, especially if allowing more time means a more effective solution.
- **Money:** Can you find more financial resources to invest in solving a problem *correctly* the first time? More importantly, do you need to spend *all* of the funds to which you have access? Sometimes simple solutions are the most effective and don't always cost a lot of money. You can win extra points for solving a problem *and* saving money.
- **Cooperation:** Have you made inaccurate assumptions about who will support you or your proposed solutions? Are there people whom you can recruit that you have not thought of? Do you need to confirm that those whom you believe are with you really support you?
- **Law:** Have you assumed that you are limited by laws without consulting legal experts, or are there legal solutions you may not have considered?
- **Energy:** Is the benefit of solving the problem worth the time and energy you will need to invest to solve the problem at this time? Would it make more sense to have all involved recognize that you will live with the problem for the time being? Are you investing enough energy, or are you just putting a temporary "Band-Aid" on the problem? Does it make more sense to invest energy in fixing the problem correctly the first time than to come back to the problem again and again?
- **Information:** Do you have all the information you need to solve the problem? Do you need to begin by gathering more information, and is the information you have correct?

problem by comparing them against a set of predetermined criteria such as cost, feasibility of implementation, and anticipated effectiveness is a proposed options matrix. This type of matrix includes the potential solution options down the left side of the matrix and the predetermined criteria for rating the options along the top of the matrix. Each cell is then rated using a numerical scale or other scale such as strong, neutral, or weak.

A key concept in decision-making and problem-solving is that of **consensus**. Reaching consensus does not mean that there is full agreement among all parties involved in making a decision or in choosing a response to a problem (Fitzgerald & Schutte, 2010). Consensus does indicate, however, that all parties have agreed to support the plan of action fully even if it is not how they would act if they were acting alone. This means that everyone commits to acting in ways that do not sabotage progress and that there is no saying "I told you so" if something goes wrong. A difficulty with reaching consensus is that it often takes time to reach real consensus, and managers are often under pressure to make decisions and solve problems quickly. However, as noted earlier, making the right decision the first time, even if it takes a little longer, often requires fewer resources than making the wrong decision multiple times! Once you have set the problem as specifically as possible, have identified those assumptions that are accurate and that you want to maintain and use, and have established criteria against which to evaluate your possible solutions, you can decide upon the appropriate problem-solving strategies. Strategies should be chosen based upon the nature of the problem to be solved, and different strategies may be needed at different points in solving the problem. For example, John Malouff (2014) identified 50 different problem-solving strategies and categorized them into eight groups. These groups are listed in Box 10-7.

Some strategies will help you gather information to more specifically set the problem, some will help you identify the problem's root causes, others will aid you in gathering information to identify and evaluate potential solutions, and still others will help you decide how to implement solutions.

Generational Considerations

Generational differences in the work setting challenge the occupational therapy manager to incorporate

BOX 10-7

Types of Problem-Solving Strategies

- Strategies to help you understand the problem
- Strategies to help you simplify the task
- Strategies to help you determine the course of the problem
- Strategies involving the use of external aids to help identify possible solutions
- Strategies involving the use of logic to help you identify possible solutions
- Strategies using a possible solution as a starting point to help you solve a problem
- Strategies to help you determine which possible solution is best
- Strategies to help you function optimally while problem-solving

innovative motivational strategies to leadership and supervision. Research indicates that differences in attitudes, preferences, and dispositions exist among various generational groups, creating rich organizational diversity and challenging managers to infuse a variety of approaches in motivating employees across generations (Arsenault, 2004).

For example, baby boomers (born between 1946 and 1964) like to set and achieve shared goals, value loyalty to the organization, and balance work with caring for children and aging parents (Frandsen, 2009). Generation X (born between 1965 and 1980) value autonomy, independence, and immediate results (Wieck, 2007). Generation Y (born between 1981 and 2000), also known as the millennial generation, are team-oriented, technologically savvy, extremely effective with multitasking, and value flexible schedules and work that contributes to a socially responsible goal (Hershatter & Epstein, 2010).

Although these generational descriptions are broad, they have implications for occupational therapy managers who must relate to each group by identifying what they value and finding creative strategies for incorporating motivation strategies to achieve the highest level of organizational productivity and effectiveness (Frandsen, 2009). As generations work together, conflict may arise because they may approach their work from different perspectives (Zacher,

Heusner, Schmitz, Zwierzanska, & Frese, 2010). For example, there may be differences in expectations around pitching in and helping others when workload is high or there are staff vacancies. There also may be differences in expectations of managers and supervisors in terms of giving feedback and providing direction. Conceptualizations of what it means to work independently or to be part of the team may also vary across generations. The occupational therapy manager is challenged to blend these perspectives into a leadership approach that motivates the team toward a shared vision.

Chapter Summary

This chapter provided an introduction to change management and problem-solving. The chapter presented a number of models and frameworks for conceptualizing change, as well as strategies for fostering change and dealing with resistance to change. Thinking about change as a process or problem that might be broken down into component parts was suggested as a way of recognizing that it is necessary to use different change or problem-solving strategies at different times. It was also recognized that managers must deal with change occurring within individuals, departments, organiza-

tions, and environments and that successfully managing change requires that we balance task needs with people needs (Cravens, Oliver, & Stewart, 2010).

It was suggested in this chapter that managing change and solving problems requires that a manager develop a broad range of skills, including political skills, analytical skills, people skills, system skills, and business skills. Many of these skill sets must be developed over time, and the knowledge underlying these skills typically is learned through on-the-job experience, although it may also be developed by pursuing graduate business education or taking advantage of the many formal training opportunities that are offered related to health care or business in general.

You were introduced to several tools and techniques that can be helpful in managing change and solving problems, including process flow diagrams, proposed options matrices, and force-field analysis. Several of the tools and techniques are discussed in more depth in other chapters of this book. In addition, you were encouraged to use the evidence-based practice strategies that you are learning to find current and more in-depth information specific to the situations you will encounter, because there are many helpful resources available on the Internet, in the professional literature, and from various professional and scholarly associations and organizations.

■ Real-Life Solutions

Initially, as Shawn and his team set about the various projects and activities that they envisioned would help to rebuild the occupational therapy department, they encountered considerable resistance to further change. Shawn had been introduced to change management and strategies for creating change in his graduate program in human resources development but had not yet made any formal use of that information. Shawn and his team began by returning to this literature and by enlisting the help of staff specialists within the human resources department and of managers in other departments who had lived through many of the changes themselves. Doing this helped them first and foremost to understand the resistance that they were encoun-

tering and to recognize the fears, uncertainty, and concerns shared by many of the staff members. By doing this, they were also able to see the various aspects of resistance as problems to be solved and, perhaps more importantly, they were able to frame the process of working with staff members to overcome their resistance as an opportunity rather than a problem.

Shawn was encouraged by his mentors and peers to see the human side of what the staff was experiencing and to pay as much attention to staff members' emotional and psychological needs as he was to the procedural and technical task needs he had identified. By consciously using people skills to enlist the help of staff members as partners in the change process, Shawn and his team were slowly able to begin to use strategies and tools such as process flow diagrams. In doing so, staff members

Continued

■ Real-Life Solutions—cont'd

were able to recognize the "how, why, and what" of change problems they faced and were able to become active partners in identifying the needed changes and strategies for creating those changes.

One key strategy was to provide training and education to staff members related to change itself as well as some of the tools and techniques they would be using. Although tacit use was made of the transtheoretical model to plan strategies for increasing staff members' awareness for the need to change and to ready them for it, the staff found Lewin's simple three-stage model of change helpful to frame their experience. By recognizing that, as a result of the turmoil they had experienced, they had essentially become "frozen" in some nonproductive ways, they were able to ready themselves for additional and intentional change.

Over the next few years, many changes in policies, procedures, and philosophy were created, and at numerous points Shawn found that he and his team did not possess the skills or knowledge needed to be successful on their own. However, as team members pursued doctoral study, they were able to take advantage of educational opportunities to gain new knowledge. Furthermore, by developing a network of peers both within and outside of the occupational therapy profession, they developed a ready bank of resources of which they took frequent advantage. Shawn also set ambitious goals to increase his skills in business, information management, and general systems. Whenever possible, on the advice of his mentors, he volunteered for various organizational task forces; as a result, he received more advanced training in quality improvement and other change management skill sets.

Study Questions

1. **Principles of change management that are commonly cited in the literature include which of the following?**

   a. Theoretical models and frameworks that guide organization members' and researchers' thinking about organizational change
   b. Approaches and tools for creating and managing change
   c. Outcomes of the process of change management
   d. All of the above

2. **According to the transtheoretical model of change, which of the following is not a specific stage of change?**

   a. Precontemplation
   b. Contemplation
   c. Avoidance
   d. Action

3. **Which of the following is not one of the three strategies for fostering individual change identified by Bennis, Benne, and Chin and still commonly cited in the literature?**

   a. Educative or empirical-rational
   b. Consultative-negotiation
   c. Normative or persuasive
   d. Power-coercive

4. **Which of the following best describes force-field analysis?**

   a. It involves an analysis of both driving and restraining forces to change.
   b. It is likely to arise when individuals perceive that they have no influence over whether to change or how to change.
   c. It involves learning to recognize the unwritten rules involved in organizational culture.
   d. It involves understanding your assumptions and learning to recognize the assumptions of others about change.

5. An individual, internal or external to the organization, who plays a significant role in fostering and promoting change within an organization and who fosters change with an organization's best interest in mind might best be called a:

   a. Driving force.
   b. Change agent.
   c. Transactional agent.
   d. Restraining force.

6. The process of clearly defining a problem or naming the problem so that you will pay attention to information that you identify as relating to the problem and ignore information that you feel is extraneous might best be called:

   a. Change management.
   b. Process flow.
   c. Obstacle definition.
   d. Problem setting.

7. A type of decision in which all parties have agreed to support the plan of action fully even if it is not how they would act if they were acting alone might best be called:

   a. Negotiation.
   b. Problem resolution.
   c. Consensus.
   d. Problem setting.

8. Which of the following describes members of Generation Y, also known as the millennial generation?

   a. They like to set and achieve shared goals, value loyalty to the organization, and balance work with caring for children and aging parents.
   b. They are team-oriented, technologically savvy, extremely effective with multitasking, and value flexible schedules and work that contributes to a socially responsible goal.
   c. They value autonomy, independence, and immediate results.
   d. None of the above.

Resources for Learning More About Change and Solving Problems

Journals That Often Address Change or Solving Problems

Journal of Organizational Change Management

http://www.emeraldinsight.com/journal/jocm

Articles published in the *Journal of Organizational Change Management* address theories, philosophies, and evidence related to managerial practices and strategies that create and foster successful organizational change. Topics often addressed in the journal include strategic planning, leadership research, CQI, and the psychology of change in the workplace.

The Learning Organization

http://www.emeraldinsight.com/loi/tlo

The Learning Organization is one of the few sources of information to deal exclusively with the philosophy and practice of continual organizational improvement. The journal publishes articles related to understanding the learning organization and ways in which organizations can adopt learning strategies and apply theories of organizational learning.

Associations That Are Concerned With Change or Solving Problems

The Change Management Association

http://www.cmassociation.org/

The main goal of the Change Management Association is to provide a forum for discussion of change management best practices. The association provides a forum for the exchange of ideas between members in order to promote identification of the most effective change management strategies for use within organizations. The Change Management Association is a global organization that includes members from varied professions who are affected by, or involved in, change management.

Other Resources

Business.com "The Business Search Engine"

http://www.business.com

Business.com is a leading business search engine and business directory designed to help its users find the companies, products, services, and information they need to make business decisions. The site includes links to articles, business sites, and other resources on managing change.

Change Management Resource Library

http://www.pmi.org/Learning/change-management/ resource-library.aspx

This site includes links to four areas related to change management that include articles, books, best practices, and training. The site is sponsored by ProSci, a commercial process design and change management research company. The company website (http://www .prosci.com) includes links to several management-related online learning centers.

Reference List

Accel-Team. (2004). *Team building—force-field analysis.* Retrieved from http://www.accel-team.com/

American Medical Informatics Association. (2013). *Definition of biomedical informatics.* Retrieved from https://www.amia.org/ biomedical-informatics-core-competencies

American Occupational Therapy Association. (2014). *AOTA board of directors position statement on entry-level degree for the occupational therapist.* Retrieved from http://www.aota.org/About AOTA/Get-Involved/BOD/OTD-Statement.aspx

Arndt, M., & Bigelow, B. (2009). Evidence-based management in health care organizations: A cautionary note. *Health Care Management Review, 34*(3), 206–213.

Arsenault, P. M. (2004). Validating generational differences: A legitimate diversity and leadership issue. *Leadership & Organization Development Journal, 25,* 124–141.

Balestracci, D. (2003). Change management: Handling the human side of change. *Quality Progress,* November, 38–45.

Bandura, A., & Locke, E. A. (2003). Negative self-efficacy and goal effects revisited. *Journal of Applied Psychology, 88*(1), 87–99.

Bennis, W., Benne, K. D., & Chin, R. (1985). *The planning of change.* New York, NY: Holt, Rinehart and Winston.

Branch, K. M. (2002). Change management. In E. L. Malone, K. M. Branch, and K. A. Baker (Eds.), *Managing science as a public good: Overseeing publicly-funded science.* Washington, DC: U.S. Department of Energy.

Bridges, W. (1995). Managing organizational transitions. In Burke, W. W. (Ed.), *Managing organizational change* (pp. 20–28). New York, NY: American Management Association

Burke, W. W. (2010). *Organization change: Theory and practice* (3rd ed.). Thousand Oaks, CA: Sage Publishing.

Burke, W. W., & Trahant, W. (2000). *Business climate shifts: Profiles of change makers.* Boston, MA: Butterworth Heinemann.

Caldwell, R. (2003). Models of change agency: A fourfold classification. *British Academy of Management, 14,* 131–142.

Campbell, R. J. (2008). Change management in health care. *Health Care Manager, 27*(1), 23–29.

Cravens, K. S., Oliver, E. G., & Stewart, J. S. (2010). Can a positive approach to performance evaluation help accomplish your goals? *Business Horizons, 53,* 269.

Curtis, E., & White, P. D. (2002). Resistance to change: Causes and solutions. *Nursing Management, 8,* 15–20.

Fitzgerald, S., & Schutte, N. S. (2010). Increasing transformational leadership through enhancing self-efficacy. *Journal of Management Development, 29,* 495–505.

Frandsen, B. M. (2009). Leading by recognizing generational differences. *Long-Term Living, 58,* 34–35.

Gioia, E., & Andersen, A. (2003). *Project managers need sharp political skills.* Retrieved from Federaltimes.com website: http://www. portfoliomgt.org/read.asp?ItemID=172

Harris, R. (2002). *Problem solving techniques.* Retrieved from VirtualSalt.com website: http://www.virtualsalt.com/crebook4.htm

Hekman, D., Steensma, H., Bigley, G., & Hereford, J. (2009). Effects of organizational and professional identification on the relationship between administrators' social influence and professional employees' adoption of new work behavior. *Journal of Applied Psychology, 94*(5), 1325.

Hershatter, A., & Epstein, M. (2010). Millennials and the world of work: An organization and management perspective. *Journal of Business Psychology, 25,* 211–223.

Honold, L. (1997). A review of the literature on employee empowerment. *Empowerment in Organizations, 5,* 202–212.

Kotter, J. P. (2012). *Leading change.* Boston, MA: Harvard Business School Press.

Laframboise, D., Nelson, R. L., & Schmaltz, J. (2003). Managing resistance to change in workplace accommodation. *Journals of Facilities Management, 1,* 306–321.

Lavasseur, R. E. (2001). People skills: Change management tools— Lewin's change model. *Interfaces, 31,* 71–73.

Lewin, K. (1997). *Resolving social conflict and field theory in social sciences.* Washington, DC: American Psychological Association.

Malouff, J. (2014). *Fifty problem solving strategies explained.* Retrieved from http://www.une.edu.au/about-une/academic -schools/bcss/news-and-events/psychology-community-activities/ over-fifty-problem-solving-strategies-explained

Mattingly, C., & Fleming, M. (1994). *Clinical reasoning: Forms of inquiry in a therapeutic practice.* Philadelphia, PA: F.A. Davis.

National Health Service Institute. (2013). *What is a force-field analysis?* Retrieved from http://www.institute.nhs.uk/quality _and_service_improvement_tools/quality_and_service _improvement_tools/force_field_analysis.html

Newstrom, J. W. (2010). *Organizational behavior: Human behavior at work.* Boston, MA: McGraw-Hill.

Nickols, F. (2004). *Change management 101: A primer.* Retrieved from Distance Consulting website: http://www.nickols.us/ change.htm

Nohria, N., Groysberg, B., & Lee, L. (2008). Employee motivation: A powerful new model. *Harvard Business Review, 86*, 78–84.

Pettigrew, A. M., Ferlie, E., & McKee, L. (1992). *Shaping strategic change: The case of the NHS*. London, UK: Sage Publishing.

Prochaska, J. O., & DiClemente, J. C. (1993). In search of how people change: Applications to addictive behavior. *American Psychologist, 47*, 1102–1114.

Reinhard, M., & Dickhauser, O. (2009). Need for cognition, task difficulty, and the formation of performance expectancies. *Journal of Personality and Social Psychology, 96*, 1062–1076.

Schermerhorn, J. R., Hunt, J. G., & Osborn, R. N. (1994). *Managing organizational behavior* (5th ed.). New York, NY: John Wiley & Sons.

Schön, D. (1983). *The reflective practitioner: How professionals think in action*. New York, NY: Basic Books.

Van Doom, K. (2011). *Readiness for change*. Saarbrücken, Germany: Lambert Academic Publishing.

Wang, L. (2007). Sources of leadership self-efficacy: Follower feedback and group performance outcomes. *International Journal of Business Research, 7*, 140–148.

Wieck, K. L. (2007). Motivating an intergenerational workforce: Scenarios for success. *Orthopaedic Nursing, 26*, 366–371.

Zacher, H., Heusner, S., Schmitz, M., Zwierzanska, M. M., & Frese, M. (2010). Focus on opportunities as a mediator of the relationships between age, job complexity, and work performance. *Journal of Vocational Behavior, 76*, 374.

Zhang, X., & Bartol, K. M. (2010). Linking empowering leadership and employee creativity: The influence of psychological empowerment, intrinsic motivation, and creative process engagement. *Academy of Management Journal, 53*, 107.

CHAPTER 11

Financial Planning, Management, and Budgeting

Brent Braveman, PhD, OTR/L, FAOTA

■ Real-Life Management

Catrina, after reexamining her career goals, thinks she is ready to move into a role as an occupational therapy department director, or even serve as director of the department of rehabilitation overseeing multiple disciplines. She currently serves as associate director of occupational therapy, but spends most of her time on program development, staff supervision, overseeing the student program, and supporting clinical performance improvement. As Catrina begins to think about what she would need to do to be ready for the next step in her career, she realizes that she does not have much experience with financial planning, management, and budgeting.

Catrina has great respect for her boss, Raymond, who is the director of rehabilitation services. He is responsible for managing over 40 staff members from occupational therapy, physical therapy, and speech language pathology. Raymond has been in his role for over 15 years and demonstrates a high level of competency in financial planning, management, and budgeting. Raymond graduated with a bachelor's degree in occupational therapy as his entry-level degree and has a master's degree in education. He has shared with Catrina that most of what he has learned about financial planning, management, and budgeting occurred "on the job" or in continuing education courses he has attended over the years. He also received mentoring from his boss and a colleague in the finance office. Catrina's entry-level occupational therapy degree was at the master's level in 2010; although her course on management covered financial planning, management, and budgeting, she does not feel ready to "go it alone" when it comes to preparing and managing an annual budget for a department. Because Catrina has always had a positive relationship with Raymond and he has offered her professional mentoring in the past, she decides to set up a meeting and share her career aspirations with him. She hopes to discuss how she might gain some exposure to the financial aspects of running a therapy department.

Critical Thinking Questions

As you read this chapter, consider the following questions:

- What is the relationship between financial planning, management, budgeting, and other management functions and duties such as strategic planning?

- What skill sets and knowledge would you need to gain to be an effective financial planner that you probably will not be pro-vided in your entry-level occupational therapy program?

- What are ways that you could begin to learn about financial planning, management, and budgeting during your first years of practice?

- Why would it be helpful to understand the financial planning, management, and budgeting processes even if you never intend to move into a management role?

Glossary

- **Bad debt:** revenue or charges that are billed but are not anticipated to be collected and must be written off.
- **Capital equipment:** generally defined as a single piece of equipment that exceeds a predetermined amount (e.g., $5,000) and a life span of longer than a predetermined period (e.g., 1 year).
- **Capital improvements:** additions or improvements in facilities costing more than a preestablished cost limit.
- **Depreciation:** a way of allocating the cost of a major asset such as a piece of capital equipment over its useful life for tax and accounting purposes.
- **Direct costs:** expenses that can be directly attributable to the activities related to production of your primary services, such as salaries, benefits, and materials.
- **Fiscal year:** a time period (typically 12 months) that represents one full budget cycle of an organization; it can be a calendar year or another predetermined cycle, such as July 1 to June 30.
- **Fixed costs:** costs that do not change with the volume of services provided.
- **Full-time equivalent (FTE):** the ratio of the total number of paid hours in a defined period (e.g., 1 week) to the number of hours defined as full-time.

- **Gross revenue:** the total revenue before any deductions or allowances are applied.
- **Indirect costs:** expenses that are not directly attributable to the activities related to production of your primary services and support the general operation of the organization, such as rent, utilities, or salaries for personnel such as human resources that support your service but are accounted separately.
- **Net profit or operating margin:** the amount of revenue that remains after deduction of all expenses, deductions, and allowances.
- **Net revenue:** the total remaining revenue after any deductions or allowances are applied.
- **Overhead:** accounting term representing costs not including direct labor costs, such as heat, electricity, or the costs of malpractice insurance, which are covered in another budget separate from direct care departments.
- **Productivity:** the number of units of care billed or the percentage of time spent in billable activity during a predetermined period, often based on an 8-hour day.
- **Units of care:** the basic unit of measure upon which services are billed, such as a 15-minute unit of care, a 1-hour group, a unit defined by the Centers for Medicare and Medicaid (CMS) "8-minute rule," or a day of treatment.
- **Variable costs:** costs that change as more or less volume of services is provided.

Introduction

One important function of many occupational therapy and interdisciplinary managers is financial planning, management, and the development and oversight of a department budget. Budgeting is both a planning and a controlling function; it involves planning because you must project the financial impact of meeting clients' needs, and it involves controlling because you must set limits on the everyday activity of staff and the salary and other forms of compensation and rewards you provide them for doing their jobs. Developing and managing a budget can be a complex process; occupational therapy practitioners who have the goal of becoming a departmental manager or director are encouraged to obtain knowledge and develop skills far beyond what they will learn in an entry-level occupational therapy program.

Advanced skill development in financial planning, management, and budgeting may be more difficult to obtain than you might imagine. It can require attending multiple continuing education events, pursuing graduate courses on financial planning and management, or even earning another graduate degree such as a master's degree in business or health-care administration. Planning and managing a budget that can include millions of dollars of revenue and expenses in larger departments requires a working knowledge of:

- Health-care systems, including city, county, state, and national systems
- Payment and reimbursement structures such as Medicare, Medicaid, workers' compensation, private insurance, and grant and foundation support
- Human resources systems and costs, including salary and benefit administration, training and educational costs and systems, and recruitment and retention structures
- Equipment and materials purchasing and management; this may include medical supplies such as splinting, assistive and adaptive equipment, and office and other supportive supplies
- Facilities management and improvement systems, including cleaning and maintenance of physical plant structures

Often a new manager may accept a role where a budget is already in place; he or she can rely on historical budgeting data to help him or her with the process of projecting work volume, revenue, and expenses. However, projecting revenue, expenses, and activity (e.g., the amount of therapy provided using a specific measurement of service provision) for new programs can be surprisingly complicated. When planning a new program, you will benefit greatly by having a network of outside sources and peers to help you gather and analyze the various forms of data, information, and other evidence that you will need.

The size and complexity of department budgets and the resources devoted to the process varies a great deal. Managers in school systems or community-based organizations may have input into grants or other forms of revenue and input on staffing and equipment needs but may not have direct responsibility for day-to-day management of a budget. A first-time manager in a small community hospital may have only a few staff members as part of the department and may rely on employees in human resources or financial management to determine salaries and other benefits, set prices for services, and determine what to charge for materials such as splints, adaptive equipment, or medical supplies. Managers in large departments may be responsible for oversight of over 100 employees, and although they also often rely on departments such as human resources or finance, they may have much more responsibility in making day-to-day financial decisions. Other times much of the budget—including salaries, benefits, and equipment—may be centrally managed in another part of the organization, and the occupational therapy management role may be more limited and focused on clinical decision-making. Finally, managers who are also the owner, such as the case of some private practice settings, may need to learn about a variety of issues that don't concern the hospital-based manager, such as taxes, property **depreciation,** or real estate principles.

The Relationship of Financial Planning and Management and Strategic Planning

In Chapter 9, you learned about the process of strategic planning, which is the process of determining an organization's long-term goals, establishing concrete measures of success, and formulating the strategies and general action plans needed to accomplish these goals. Managers use strategic plans to translate the methods the organization chooses to achieve its mission and vision to staff and to guide their involvement in key organizational activities.

Frezatti, Aguiar, Guerreiro, and Gouvea (2011, p. 243) and Steiner (1979) note that the strategic planning concept is:

1) "Related to the future consequences of current decisions;
2) A process that begins by setting organizational objectives, then defines the strategies and policies to reach them, and, finally, develops detailed plans to guarantee that the strategies are implemented;
3) An attitude so that it is not just an intellectual exercise; and
4) Responsible for the links among long-term strategic plans, medium-term programs, short-term budgets, and operational plans."

The budget is a tool that managers use to plan, organize, and apply the organization's financial resources to carry out activities needed to achieve the planned objectives. Moving back and forth between the strategic plan and the budget both helps the manager stay focused and requires that the manager determine priorities for action. As discussed in more detail later in the chapter, a typical financial planning process guides the manager to develop the budget based upon a determined plan, as well as report performance and analyze variances between the plan and results. This can be a challenging and stressful process for a number of reasons. Unplanned events such as breakdowns in critical equipment or unexpected opportunities can arise that may require shifting funds from your plan. It is difficult at times to make these decisions and to fully anticipate the risks and benefits of deviating from your plans. In addition, a manager must be mindful of opportunity costs. Opportunity costs are "those opportunities that must be bypassed in order to pursue one business strategy rather than another" (Nosse & Friberg, 2010, p. 356). Whatever course of action you choose, it means that you do not have the human or other types of resources to do something else. Close alignment between your mission, vision, strategic plan, and budget prevents these opportunity costs from becoming major regrets.

Basic Accounting Principles

Accounting can be defined as "a set of concepts and techniques that are used to measure and report financial information about an economic unit" (Principlesofaccounting.com, 2013). The economic unit in health care is typically a separate department such as a department of occupational therapy, a department of physical therapy, or a department of rehabilitation. The financial information is reported to a variety of different types of stakeholders, including whomever the director reports to as well as persons responsible for oversight of the organization's finances. Others include owners, boards of directors, creditors, governmental units, financial analysts, and even employees. Financial accounting gathers and summarizes financial data to prepare financial reports such as the balance sheet and income statement for the organization's management, investors, lenders, suppliers, tax authorities, and other stakeholders (Businessdictionary.com, 2014).

Ellexson (2011) identified the basic principles of accounting as (a) tracking accounts payable and receivable, (b) monitoring cash flow, (c) developing a budget, and (d) managing risk for profitability. These basic concepts are highlighted and explained further in Table 11-1.

This explanation of basic accounting principles is both brief and relatively simplistic. Accounting functions are complex and require mathematical and economic tracking and forecasting skills that are typically beyond the scope of an entry-level occupational therapy education.

The Financial Planning Process

Budgets are typically planned through a financial planning process that spans either a calendar year or **fiscal year.** A fiscal year is a time period (typically 12 months) that represents one full budget cycle of an organization; it can be a calendar year or another predetermined cycle such as July 1 to June 30. The fiscal year for school therapists or for those working in hospitals affiliated with universities may be the academic year (i.e., September 1 to August 31). In most organizations, the process is structured so that certain activities happen on a schedule at about the same time each year. These activities must be coordinated between all the

TABLE 11-1		
The Four Basic Principles of Accounting		
Accounting Principle	**Explanation**	**Outcome for the Manager**
Tracking Accounts Payable and Receivable	Monitoring the funds owed you (accounts receivable) and the funds you owe others (accounts payable). This may be based on when funds are actually received or paid out or when the services are rendered or received.	Provides an understanding of the resources coming into the organization and those going out in the short and long term by organizing them in categories or accounts to help you understand if you are meeting the assumptions and projections you built into your budget.
Monitoring Cash Flow	"Cash on hand" or credit is the amount of money available to you to pay expenses and bills such as salaries or the purchase of equipment and supplies.	Provides an understanding of your ability to meet your financial commitments or to have resources available to obtain new resources to accomplish your most important work.
Developing a Budget	A budget is a projection of how all of the various types of revenue and expenses will combine to result in some amount of financial gain or loss at the end of a preidentified time period, typically called a fiscal year.	Provides an understanding of the financial impact of delivering your services in order to meet client needs. Budgets align activities and the resources required to carry them out with your key goals and objectives related to your mission, vision, and values.
Managing Risk for Profitability	Making daily decisions about the activities that will contribute to a positive "bottom line," including the charge per unit of service, exactly what service will be delivered, and the quality and quantity of materials needed to carry out this work.	Provides an understanding of when you will pass your "breakeven point." Ultimately any business must bring in more money (revenue) than it pays out (expenses) in order to continue to exist and fulfill its mission.

departments that have budgetary planning and control responsibility so that ultimately a budget is determined for the organization as a whole. Nosse, Friberg, and Kovacek (2005) described the financial planning process as having four steps, which are described next and are reflected in Figure 11-1.

Financial Management Planning

As mentioned previously, managers working in existing organizations have the benefit of relying on historical data from the organization and the department to establish a financial plan that may span a period of several years. The typical occupational therapy or interdisciplinary manager coordinates the depart-

ment's financial planning goals with those of the organization through the development of the annual budget.

Longer-term financial planning and coordination of department and organization strategies and actions require managers to move out of their departments and scan their external environments. The organization's overall financial health, the economic trends occurring in the industry or primary market in which the organization functions, and trends in the U.S. and global economies all can influence the financial plan. The types of health policy and system changes described in Chapter 3 are good examples of environmental trends and influences that can affect financial planning. For example, John Holahan (2014) of the Urban Institute examined the impact of Medicaid

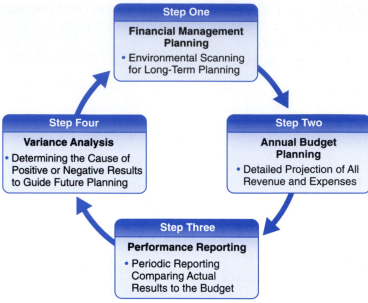

Figure ■ 11-1 The Four Steps of the Financial Planning Process.

expansion in the Patient Protection and Affordable Care Act (ACA) on states and concluded that

> States expanding Medicaid will receive significantly larger inflows of federal dollars than those that do not. Medicaid expansion will bring in large amounts of federal dollars that will offset cuts in the ACA to Medicare provider payment rates and Medicaid and Medicare disproportionate share hospital payments. States that do not expand Medicaid will experience the ACA cuts but will have much smaller inflows of federal revenues. All states will experience some new spending but much can be offset by savings in other parts of state budgets.

In hospital settings, this type of environmental influence will ultimately have an impact not only on the organization but also on the financial planning and budgeting process of the occupational therapy or rehabilitation services department.

Annual Budget Planning

Planning and developing the annual budget is a detailed process of identifying all sources of revenue and expense. Planning revenue requires that you

project total work volume and then multiply by the gross charge associated with all **units of care** (e.g., 15-minute work unit, a group, a single visit, or a day of care). There often are different charges associated with different types of units of care. For example, a unit of "self-care management training" in a hospital setting may be charged at a set rate such as $106 per 15 minutes of intervention, whereas "group therapeutic procedures" on a mental health unit may be charged at a "per group" rate such as $60 per group attended. Combining the total number of individual and group intervention units allows you to identify both total volume and subsequently **gross revenue**. Charges for units of care are determined in various ways. In hospital settings, they are often based upon the relative value and complexity of various types of interventions established by third-party payers, including Medicare, Medicaid, and private insurances. Rates per unit of care in private practices are influenced by third-party payment as well as the market value of the service to individuals willing to pay "out of pocket" for service or through contracts with companies or other agencies contracting for service.

The **net revenue** is then calculated by deducting any discounts or allowances, uncompensated care, and any budgeted plan for **"bad debt"** or revenue that is charged but is not anticipated to be collected. There is variation in whether and how discounts are included in departmental budgets in various organizations. For example, a discount may be uniformly applied to all categories of revenue if the organization discounts an average across all payers. The discount may represent the impact of various rates of payment, with lower rates negotiated with certain payers as well as the cost of uncompensated care or charity care. Discounts to gross revenue can be 52% or higher, meaning that of every dollar charged only 48 cents (or less) is collected. This reflects a significant challenge that organizations experience in collecting billed services. Other organizations may not apply discounts to departmental budgets but may apply the discounts when the budgets of multiple cost centers are "rolled up" into a summary report for a division or group of related cost centers. An example of the calculation of total volume and gross revenue for a given period is provided in Box 11-1.

Many budgets include both revenue and expenses, although it is not uncommon in settings such as a community-based organization for a manager to have oversight of only expenses with no direct sources of revenue. Revenues may include third-party payment for services from private and public insurers, grants from government agencies or private foundations, and gifts from individuals or foundations. Expenses typically include costs associated with personnel, supplies,

facilities management, and equipment. Some key concepts related to revenues and expenses are defined in Box 11-2.

Planning expenses requires that you project the volume for all types of costs charged to your cost center. The types of expenses charged to your budget will also vary from organization to organization. Expenses typically will include all **direct costs** and **indirect costs** that can be isolated and applied to the costs of running your department. Other expenses related to the cost of doing business may not be reflected in a departmental budget even if they are influenced by changes in your work volume. For example, many hospitals have separate transportation departments responsible for transporting patients from one location to another in the facility. The salary and equipment costs for this service are directly influenced by the work volume of departments such as occupational therapy or physical therapy, but may not be reflected in those departments' budgets. Often these and other expenses—commonly referred to as **overhead,** or costs not including direct labor costs such as heat, electricity, or the costs of malpractice insurance—are covered in another budget separate from direct care departments. It is *critically* important that you remain aware of such budgeting and accounting practices so that you do not make any claims or assertions that damage your credibility as a manager.

For example, it could be possible to mistakenly talk about your department's "profit" when, after applying discounts and associated costs such as transportation or reception salaries not reflected in your budget, your department actually operates at a loss. Another common mistake might be not recognizing that it is your organization's practice to not account for services paid on a per-stay basis, such as those covered under Medicare Diagnosis-Related Groups (DRGs) within departmental budgets. A DRG is a method of payment that Medicare uses for inpatient acute medical services and is based on a payment for the hospital stay based on the diagnosis. Boasting that you have intensified services, resulting in increased profits, when these patients are paid under a Medicare DRG would be an embarrassing mistake because you have in fact increased costs to your organization by intensifying services to this group of patients. Naturally, if you could show that intensified occupational therapy services contributed to shorter lengths of stay for patients covered under a DRG, you might be able to show a positive financial impact because expenses would

---

BOX 11-1

Sample Calculation of Total Volume and Gross and Net Revenue

Total individual units of care (15 minutes) = 13,240

Total group units of care (1 hour) = 2,210

Charge per 15-minute individual unit of care = $106

Charge per 1-hour group intervention = $60

Total gross revenue = (13,240 × $106) + (2,210 × $60) = $1,536,040

Net revenue = $1,536,040 × 0.48 = $737,299 (gross revenue minus example of 52% deduction)

BOX 11-2

Key Concepts Related to Revenues and Expenses

- **Cost centers:** A manner of referring to the grouped costs associated with a set of activities within the organizational structure (e.g., the occupational therapy department, the behavioral health day treatment program, or the human resources department).
- **Gross revenues:** The aggregate, cumulative, or total sum of revenue before any deductions (e.g., the total work volume multiplied by billed charges before any deductions are made).
- **Allowances or deductions:** A percentage of fees that is negotiated with a payer to be deducted or discounted from the gross charge for services.
- **Net revenues:** The amount of revenue that you expect to collect after deductions, such as discounts for managed care payers, are applied.
- **Net profit or operating margin:** The amount of revenue that remains after deduction of all expenses, deductions, and allowances.
- **Direct costs:** Costs such as salaries, services, contracts, and equipment directly related to operation of a department.

- **Indirect costs (sometimes called operating expenses):** Costs associated with running an organization that may be spread across departments according to a predetermined rate or formula and that are not influenced by work volume, such as secretarial support, or overhead costs, such as electricity.
- **Cost per unit of care:** The ratio of all expenses to total work volume such that the cost to produce one unit of care (e.g., 15-minute work unit, day of care) is represented and can be tracked over time or compared with costs of other programs or organizations.
- **Full-time equivalent (FTE):** The number of hours paid to a full-time employee during a designated time period, including payment of vacation or other benefit time. For example, payment for a typical 40-hour workweek multiplied by 52 weeks is 2,080 hours.
- **Capital equipment:** Nonconsumable equipment with a cost and life span over an amount set by the organization (e.g., any single piece of equipment costing more than $500 and with a life span of greater than 12 months).

---

decrease even though there was no change in revenues.

Projection of salary expenses is completed by multiplying the number of **full-time equivalent (FTE)** employees required by your work volume by each employee's hourly rate of salary. Calculating the work that an FTE can handle requires that you identify both the number of hours per year that a typical employee devotes to provision of care during an identified period (often 1 work day) and the number of days that each employee will work. The number 2,080 is commonly recognized as equivalent to one FTE (40 hours per week × 52 weeks per year). Obviously, employees do not work 5 days a week year round. Rather, in order to accurately predict the volume of work for an employee you must deduct expected vacation leave, sick leave, family and medical leave, holiday leave, and

other planned time for which the employee will be paid but not expected to produce work (e.g., paid leave for continuing education).

A sample calculation of the expected number of *paid and worked hours* for an occupational therapy practitioner is included in Box 11-3. To identify the number of FTEs needed to handle the work volume shown you would begin by dividing the total number of hours of care by the total number of worked hours. This calculation is shown in Box 11-4.

The 3.02 FTE figure does not mean that you would only need to plan to hire three occupational therapy practitioners (FTEs), however, because this number assumes that all 8 hours worked per day are *productive* or spent in activities for which you can charge. In fact, there are numerous aspects of the workday for which you cannot charge (assuming you work in a setting

BOX 11-3

Sample Calculation of Paid and Worked Hours for an Occupational Therapy Practitioner

Category of Pay	Number of Hours Per Year
Paid hours	2,080
Vacation (3 weeks used)	−120
Sick days (4 days used)	−32
Paid holidays (11 days)	−88
Paid continuing education leave	−16
Worked hours	1,824

BOX 11-4

Sample Calculation of Required Number of Full-Time Equivalents (FTEs)

13,240 treatments/4 = 3,310 hours of direct care

3,310 hours of direct care + 2,210 group hours = 5,520 hours of care

5,520 hours of care/1,824 worked hours per FTE = 3.02 FTEs

that charges for services at all). These activities include meetings, such as staff meetings, team or family conferences, or meetings of continuous quality improvement teams. Time spent waiting for inpatients who are late or for outpatients who do not keep their appointments, or the time wasted traveling to a patient's room only to find that he or she is off the patient care unit for a test, is *nonbillable or unproductive* time, which is experienced in all organizations. Other common examples include time spent documenting or reviewing a patient's medical record before initiation of an evaluation.

Nonpersonnel expenses must also be projected and include both **fixed costs** and **variable costs** or expenses. Fixed costs are those expenses that are not directly influenced by changes in volume, such as the cost to lease space or equipment. Variable costs are those expenses that are directly influenced by changes in volume, such as some types of office supplies, food used for meal preparation activities, or the costs for splinting and medical supplies used with the most commonly seen types of clients. Salaries and benefits such as health-care costs may be treated as fixed or variable depending on the organization. In some organizations, the assumption is that staffing is relatively

stable; unless there are unanticipated events requiring adding staff or reducing staff, the costs for each employee are assumed to be fixed throughout the budget period. Other organizations may rely on overtime or variable part-time or per diem employees; therefore, salaries and some benefits may increase as more staff members are needed to meet volume and then be reduced during slower times. Although there may not always be a direct correlation, over time you will be able to estimate how an increase or decrease in volume might affect these categories of expenses. An abbreviated sample of a calculation of expenses is included in Box 11-5.

Reporting Financial Performance

A budget is a financial plan for a period of time, often a 12-month fiscal year. Throughout the fiscal year, periodic reports are typically generated to compare and summarize the actual revenue and expenses to budgeted revenue and expenses and to determine the extent of the organization's profit or loss. Reports are generated in various ways and vary a great deal in their level of detail and complexity. In multimillion-dollar departments, sometimes located in multibillion-dollar organizations, there can be computerized financial systems that allow you to design and run customized financial reports for any period you designate. It is also common for managers in smaller organizations to have more limited access to data and information and to rely only on routine reports designed and generated by a financial office.

The most typical reports include data related to volume or the amount of work completed as well as

---

BOX 11-5

An Abbreviated Sample of Calculation of Expenses

Category of Expense	Total Cost
Direct Expenses	
Salaries (3.5 FTE × $48,000 average salary)	$168,000
Medical supplies (average $1.74 per hour of care)	$9,604
Office supplies (average 50.7 cents per hour of care)	$2,800
Food supplies (7 cents per hour of care)	$400
Indirect Expenses	
Phones (16.3 cents per hour of care)	$900
Postage (3 cents per hour of care)	$200
Equipment repair and service contracts	$2,200
Continuing education ($600/employee)	$2,100
Total Expenses	$186,204

---

the revenue generated and expenses incurred. Results are often reported for a month and compare the actual results to budgeted results. Results are also often reported for the "year to date" (all results from the start of the fiscal year to the last day of the most recent month), and sometimes they compare the current year against a previous year's performance. Four common types of financial reports are described in the following list:

1. Income statements report the revenue minus the expenses and show how this income was generated.

2. Expense statements report the amount and categories of expenses incurred during the budget period.
3. The balance sheet or statement of operations summarizes the assets and limitations of the department or organization.
4. The statement of cash flows tells you how much cash came into and out of your department or private business during a specific time frame, such as a quarter or a year. It differs from the income and expense statements because the organization may show revenue that is not yet collected or expenses that are committed but not yet paid.

Variance Analysis

After reading a description of the process of planning a budget and of all of the data and information included in reports commonly received by managers, it may seem as if analyzing the results would be a simple process. However, although the reports provide information on the positive or negative *variance* in actual performance from projected or budgeted performance, they often provide no or limited insight into the "why." If volume or revenue are lower than anticipated or if expenses are higher than anticipated, it may lead to a negative variance or less **net profit** than expected. If volume or revenue are higher than anticipated or if expenses are lower than anticipated, if may lead to a positive variance or more net profit than expected. Although the latter may typically be seen as a good thing, managers are expected to be able to analyze what led to this result and determine if it forecasts additional future results. The real challenge for a manager is to manage revenue and expense to achieve a net gain, but also to predict this accurately. It is not uncommon for managers to be rated as poorly on their financial performance if they budget substantially less profit than achieved as if they do not obtain projected results and budget more profit than is realized.

Setting Expectations and Measuring Work: Productivity

In order to set reasonable targets for elements of your budget, you must accurately project the amount of work that an employee is going to complete. Some of the services provided by occupational therapy practitioners are deemed as *billable service;* in other words, you can charge for the associated time and perhaps some of the associated materials. As noted previously, not all services provided by practitioners can be included as billed services; whether you can or cannot is determined by guidelines and rules provided by third-party payers.

The most stringent rules for what can and cannot be billed are typically those provided by the Centers for Medicare and Medicaid (CMS) for services provided in any setting where Medicare and Medicaid covers occupational therapy (www.cms.gov). The settings that commonly include Medicare and Medicaid as payers include inpatient and outpatient hospitals; inpatient, outpatient, and partial hospitalization mental health care; skilled nursing facilities; inpatient rehabilitation settings; intermediate care facilities; home health services; and hospice care. Although the rules provided by private insurers or workers' compensation insurers may cover services that Medicare or Medicaid do not, it is not unusual to apply the most stringent rules to all patients regardless of who is paying the bill.

To determine if services are covered, there are often two key conditions that must be satisfied. These are demonstrating that services are *medically necessary* and that services meet criteria to deem them as *skilled service* (CMS, 2012). These following two terms are defined here:

- Services can be deemed medically necessary and reasonable if:
  - The potential for rehabilitation is significant in relation to the extent and duration of services.
  - You can expect improvement in a reasonable and predictable period of time.
  - You can show improvement through objective measurements.
  - Therapy is not necessary to improve function where spontaneous recovery is expected or where loss of function is easily reversed or temporary.
- Skilled services must not only be *provided* by the qualified professional (or by qualified personnel for incident to services), *but they must require* the expertise, knowledge, clinical judgment, decision-making and abilities of a therapist that assistants, qualified personnel, caretakers, or the patient cannot provide independently. Skilled services include:
  - Evaluating and reevaluating
  - Establishing treatment goals
  - Designing a plan of care
  - Performing ongoing assessment and analysis
  - Providing instruction leading to development of compensatory skills
  - Selecting devices to replace or augment a function
  - Training patients and caregivers

Many activities related to patient care that you might expect to be deemed as skilled and necessary are still not allowed as billable care. Examples of nonbillable care include time spent in a family conference, time in interdisciplinary rounds, time discussing a case with a physician or case manager, and time spent documenting an evaluation or intervention in the medical record. Time spent on the phone or online ordering equipment for a patient is typically not deemed a billable service, either.

The fact that these valuable services require the involvement of occupational therapy practitioners and cannot be delegated to administrative personnel is often frustrating for clinical staff. Practitioners who know they are spending time in an activity that is very important to the outcome of the intervention and yet for which they cannot charge can react negatively. This is especially true because this time is often accounted for outside of their "productive" time, because once the organization determines which services are billable and which services are not billable, an expectation is established for how much billable care is provided each day. This amount is commonly referred to as **productivity,** or the number of units of care billed or the percentage of time spent in billable activity during a predetermined period, often based on an 8-hour day.

The manager must set reasonable expectations for productivity and clearly communicate these expectations to all staff so they can be enforced in a fair, consistent, and equitable manner. In large complex environments where staff may be working on various floors of a large building or in different locations, this may be challenging. Meeting productivity expectations for a department overall is one of the most common problems faced by managers; providing the supervision, support, and direction to help staff improve their daily productivity can be both challenging and frustrating for the manager.

Expectations for productivity vary a great deal from setting to setting. The factors that influence this include:

1. Do you bill a third-party payer for care? If so, are units of work defined according to what is billable? Not all settings rely on third-party payers directly (e.g., school settings or many community-based settings) and measure units of work in some manner other than billed units.

2. Are staff members exempt, nonexempt, or a mixture of both types of staff? Exempt staff members are those who are exempt from U.S. labor laws dictating that persons who work more than a prescribed number of hours in a day or week receive additional compensation (United States Department of Labor, 2014). This affects productivity because the denominator (e.g., number of billed units/number of hours worked) may be counted as 8 even if the staff member really works 9 or more hours to achieve his or her target for billable service. Occupational therapists are often classified as exempt, whereas occupational therapy assistants (OTAs) are often classified as nonexempt.

3. How much control do you have over how staff spend their time and will you be able to limit the amount of time spent in nonbillable activities such as interdisciplinary rounds, even if you perceive that participation is highly valuable to patient care.

4. What is the department's culture and history? Expecting exempt employees to work frequent long days beyond 8 or 9 hours will increase revenue but may have a negative impact on staff morale and may result in increased turnover which, in turn, is very expensive.

Productivity levels are commonly expressed as percentages, such that an expectation of 75% productivity means that each FTE is expected to spend 6 hours of each 8-hour day performing activities that are billable or otherwise defined as productive by the department. Productivity targets vary by setting; comparing targets with others or benchmarking can help you determine your expectations. You can benchmark by contacting other managers directly or finding data in surveys or other methods provided by professional groups.

For example, the Health Policy and Administration section of the American Physical Therapy Association (APTA) published a survey of 171 respondents on the productivity expectations for physical therapy practitioners across five settings: acute care, skilled nursing, inpatient rehab, home health, and outpatient. The expected level of productivity for 48% of respondents was nearly 23 billed time units, which equates to 72% productivity. The minutes of billable service was 67% using a denominator of 450 potential minutes (7.5-hour day); if assuming skilled nursing, this level appears low based upon managers' class surveys noting 80% to 90% billable time (Dobrzykowski, 2012).

Productivity expectations for occupational therapy practitioners and physical therapy practitioners are often parallel in the same setting but can vary. Expectation standards may be higher in outpatient settings where patients are scheduled for the practitioner (8 to 9 patients per day) and practitioners are expected to document and complete nonbillable activities when patients do not arrive (e.g., no shows), at lunch, or before or after scheduled hours. Expectations are often also very high in skilled nursing facilities and in private practices. Expectations may be lower in acute care medical settings where there may be more interruptions to care or it may be more difficult to find patients who are both in their room and feeling well enough to participate. Still, expectations in these settings may be as high as 70%, or 22 to 23 billed units per day.

As noted, managing billed service and productivity is a common, difficult, and sometimes frustrating challenge for managers. It is difficult to balance the organization's financial needs and handle the pressures you may feel to achieve financial targets while also considering the needs of your staff and of the patients or clients in your setting. Many of the skills described in other chapters of this book, such as process improvement and effective supervision, are necessary to effectively manage workload and maintain the high morale of your staff.

Two other important concepts in regard to budget planning are budget periods and that of variance, which was mentioned previously. It is common practice to spread a yearly budget across 12 months and to be asked to project volume, revenue, and expenses for the year, as well as project each of these figures for each month of the fiscal year. In most organizations, you will receive a monthly budget summary or report that compares the *actual* volume, revenue, and expenses to the *projected or budgeted* volume, revenue, and expenses. The difference between the actual and projected or budgeted figures is the *variance*, which can either be positive or negative.

A positive variance for volume or revenue means that the actual figures are higher than projected or budgeted; a positive variance for expenses means that the actual figures are lower than projected or budgeted. A negative variance indicates just the opposite relationships. This might sound confusing at first, but simply think in terms of your own personal budget. A variance that means you end up with more money than expected (either because more money came in or you spent less than expected) is a positive variance. On the contrary, if you earned less money than expected or spent more than you had budgeted, it is a negative variance.

Small variances are expected (less than 5%), because it is seldom possible to precisely predict volume for any single budget period. However, large variances in either direction may be an indication of a problem. It is easy to understand why a large negative variance in volume, revenue, or expenses would be of concern to organizational leaders, but you should recognize that the ability to accurately plan a budget is what will be rewarded most often, and consistently underestimating volume or revenue or overestimating expenses will likely been seen as indicative of poor management skills.

A simplified budget sheet for one budget period is shown in Table 11-2. For the sake of simplicity, this table assumes that all volume, revenue, and expenses are spread evenly across the 12 budget periods. In real life, this is hardly ever the case; experienced managers will plan for increases and decreases based on historical patterns. For example, in an acute care hospital you might expect December to be a lower month for volume because fewer people will schedule elective surgeries near the holidays. In a pediatric private practice, you might expect volume to drop during the summer months when families commonly take vacations and increase in September when school is in session again.

When you review Table 11-2, please note the following points:

- This report is for the month of March, which would be the third budget period for an organization that uses the calendar year as its fiscal year. The report indicates figures for both the budget period and the *year to date (YTD)*, or the sum of all activity for the months of January, February, and March combined.
- When a figure in the variance column indicates that the *actual amount* is lower than the *projected or budgeted amount*, it is presented in parentheses such as "(1,962)," whether the variance is positive or negative. This is a common accounting practice in many organizations.
- The figures in the "% Variance" columns indicate the relationship between *actual amounts* and *projected or budgeted amounts*, so a positive or negative number can represent a positive or negative variance depending upon whether you are discussing a revenue item or an expense item.

Capital Equipment and Improvements

New managers must become familiar with the process of planning for a *capital equipment* budget. Capital equipment is often requested during a planning and budgeting process that occurs separately but concurrently with the planning and submission for approval of departmental budgets. The definition of **capital equipment** is determined by the organization, but typically includes a minimum cost (e.g., single items over $500) and a minimum life span (e.g., nonconsumable equipment with a life span of over 12 months). Sometimes **capital improvements**, or additions or improvements in buildings and facilities costing more than a preestablished cost threshold, are considered in the same process.

Depending on the nature of the equipment being requested, its cost, and the organization's financial health, obtaining approval for a capital equipment request can be easy or very difficult. Items that are critically important to the provision of intervention or daily work, such as a refrigerator for storage of patient food used in meal preparation activities or an ultrasound machine used in treating persons with hand injuries, may be more easily justified. Equipment that may result in increased revenue or contributes to bringing new referrals and business to an organization may also be more likely to be approved if you can write a sufficient justification showing that the initial outlay of resources is warranted given the increased net revenue (the change needs to be a real increase in *net revenue* and not just in nonreimbursed charges). Examples of such equipment would include a work simulator used in intervention with persons with

TABLE 11-2

Sample Budget Report for Budget Period 3—March

Budget Activity	Actual	Budget	Variance	% Variance	YTD Actual	YTD Budget	Variance	% Variance
Revenue								
Individual treatment	33,344	35,306	(1,962)	−5.55	109,184	105,918	3,266	3.00
Group treatment	15,390	16,575	(1,185)	−7.15	43,830	49,725	(5,895)	−11.86
Total revenue	48,734	51,881	(3,147)	−6.00	153,014	155,643	(2,629)	−1.69
Direct Expenses								
Salaries	14,883	14,000	883	6.31	36,000	42,000	(6,000)	14.29
Medical supplies	615	800	(185)	23.13	2,000	2,400	(400)	16.67
Office supplies	187	233	(46)	19.74	600	699	(99)	14.16
Food	31	33	(2)	6.06	80	99	(19)	19.19
Indirect Expenses								
Phones	75	75	0	0	220	225	(5)	2.22
Postage	14	17	(3)	17.65	47	51	(4)	7.84
Equipment Contracts	183	183	0	0	549	549	0	0
Continuing education	0	150	(150)	0	200	450	(250)	55.55
Total Expenses	15,988	15,491	386	2.49	39,696	46,473	(6,777)	14.58
Net Profit or Operating Margin	32,746	36,390	(3,644)	−11.00	113,318	109,170	4,148	3.88

various types of physical impairments or a driving simulator used to evaluate the capacity of persons with various types of disabilities to return to driving.

In writing a justification for a piece of capital equipment, the following points might be considered:

- Initial cost of purchase
- Cost of supplies and maintenance associated with the equipment's use (paper, parts, repairs, routine calibration, etc.)

- Space required for operation and installation costs
- Revenue associated with direct charge for use of the equipment or with intervention facilitated by purchase of the equipment
- Estimated life of the equipment
- Training costs for employees to learn to use the equipment
- Potential liabilities or safety issues in use of the equipment

Coding and Billing

Coding

Coding medical services including occupational therapy services is the first step in preparing the medical bill that will be sent to a third-party payer such as Medicare, Medicaid, or a private insurance company. Various types of codes must be attached to the bill and supported in the documentation provided by the occupational therapy practitioner or other health-care worker (i.e., physician, physical therapist (PT), mid-level provider such as physician assistants or advanced practice nurses, etc.). Coding is complex; in addition, the persons involved and the roles of each person may vary. Professional medical coders receive specialized training to become certified coders and code the complex medical care and procedures provided in hospital settings (www.aapc.com). Occupational therapy practitioners may be involved in the coding process by choosing the code that represents the rehabilitation diagnosis being treated and the codes that indicate what service was provided. This involves ICD codes, CPT codes, and HCPCS codes as well as other types of "modifiers" to codes. Each of these is briefly explained next.

- *ICD codes* are drawn from the International Classification of Diseases (ICD), which is the guideline used to code and classify mortality data from death certificates. The International Classification of Diseases, Clinical Modification (ICD-CM) is used to code and classify morbidity data from the inpatient and outpatient records, physician offices, and most National Center for Health Statistics (NCHS) surveys (Centers for Disease Control and Prevention, 2014). The classification of codes used in the United States is scheduled to be upgraded from ICD-9 to ICD-10 in 2015. Each code indicates a specific disease or impairment.
- *CPT codes*, or current procedural terminology codes, are published by the American Medical Association (AMA). This 5-digit numeric code is used to describe medical, surgical, radiology, laboratory, anesthesiology, and evaluation or management services of physicians, hospitals, and other health-care providers. There are approximately 7,800 CPT codes ranging from 00100 through 99499 (University of Florida Office of Physician Billing Compliance, 2014). There are codes used by occupational therapy, physical therapy, and speech–language pathology that indicate the service provided, as well as timed codes (representing a timed unit of service) and untimed codes (one code for the service no matter how long it takes). For example, the code 97003 is the code for an occupational therapy evaluation and the code 97533 is used to indicate sensory integrative techniques were used. Up-to-date information on occupational therapy coding can be found at the AOTA website at http://www.AOTA.org.
- *HCPCS* (commonly pronounced as "hick picks") stands for Health Care Common Procedures Coding System and includes two levels of codes. HCPCS Level I codes are the CPT codes just described, and HCPCS Level II codes are alphanumeric codes used to report supplies, equipment, and devices provided to patients.
- *Other coding modifiers such as "G-codes"* are sometimes required and regulations can be added or changed. For example, according to the American Occupational Therapy Association (AOTA), "effective July 1, 2013 practitioners billing for outpatient therapy services under Medicare Part B must now report functional data on their claims in order to be reimbursed. Functional data reporting takes the form of new G-codes, which identify the primary issue being addressed by therapy, and modifiers that reflect the patient's impairment, limitation or restriction. All Medicare outpatient billing must include this new functional data, which will be used to track patient achievement of goals over time" (AOTA, 2014). G-codes must also be reported on some other types of patients, such as those on observation units who may be transferred to inpatient care if their condition warrants an admission.

Billing

Although the process of medical coding assigns the various types of codes to the diagnoses and procedures found in documentation, the process of medical billing organizes and uses the codes and other information to submit medical claims to insurers or other payers. The billing process includes recording the medical codes on the claim forms sent to payers, providing examples of some of the medical documentation to support the claims, assuring that accurate and complete patient insurance information is included, and appealing denials of billed services.

Although it is common for occupational therapy practitioners to be involved in the coding process by selecting ICD and CPT codes that accurately reflect the patient's diagnosis or condition and the services provided, it is less common for them to be involved in the billing process unless they are a private practitioner or business owner. In hospitals and other larger settings, professionals with specialized training complete the billing and even much of the coding. This is done because of the complexity and because of the importance of submitting accurate claims to increase the likelihood that payment will be received. Claims are sometimes denied because the documentation is not complete or sufficiently detailed and accurate to substantiate that the services provided were medically necessary and reasonable, and that they required the skilled service of an occupational therapy practitioner.

Payment Models

Earlier in the chapter, the process of projecting gross revenue by identifying the volume of work to be completed and multiplying it by the various charges applied to each type of service was described. Net revenue was distinguished from gross revenue by noting that certain types of allowances, deductions, and "bad debt" were subtracted from the gross revenue. The types of payment structures in place affect these deductions and allowances. Some forms of payment use the treatment unit as the unit of service delivery, whereas at other times payment may be on the basis of a per-day fee or a predetermined rate for all care provided. Casto and Layman (2006) provided a review of the traditional and common forms of payment. These include:

- Fee-for-service reimbursement in which the provider bills and receives payment for each service provided (e.g., a set fee for each unit of occupational therapy).
- Self-pay is a type of fee-for-service because the patients or whoever has accepted responsibility

for the bill agrees to pay a specific amount for each service received. Patients may choose self-pay because they do not have insurance or the services they desire are not covered services.

- Retrospective reimbursement is a type of fee-for-service in which the insurer or other payer provides reimbursement providers for costs or charges previously incurred.
- Managed care reimbursement methods involve close management of approved services by the insurer or payer as well as management of the outcomes of care through strategies to control the costs of health care while maintaining quality. For example, visits to specialists may have to be preapproved by a generalist or some other type of "gate-keeper."
- Capitation includes providers allowing a fixed, per capita amount for a predetermined time period. "Per capita" means "per head" or "per person."
- Prospective payment methods set payments in advance of services for a specific time period. The predetermined rates are based on average levels of resource use for certain types of health care such as per diem (per day) or per case.
- Pay for coordination involves payment for specified care coordination services such as the medical or health-care home model, whereby the medical home receives a monthly payment in exchange for the delivery of care coordination services that are not otherwise provided and reimbursed.
- Pay for performance includes a financial incentive for achieving defined and measurable goals related to care processes and outcomes, patient experience, or resource use.
- Bundled payments are single payments for a group of services related to a treatment or condition that may involve multiple providers in multiple settings (CMS, 2014).

Other types of payment systems and structures continue to evolve, with most seeking to help achieve what has been referred to as the "triple aim" of health-care reform. The triple aim is (1) improving the experience of care, (2) improving the health of populations, and (3) reducing the costs of health care (Berwick, Nolan, & Whittington, 2008). It is likely that other models will evolve that have not been included at the time of this text's publication. (Silversmith, 2011).

Chapter Summary

This chapter reviewed the critical management functions of financial planning, management, and budgeting. The relationship between financial planning, management, and budgeting and other management responsibilities such as strategic planning or program development were described. You were introduced to a variety of key terms and concepts that must be understood in order to effectively project and plan volume, revenue, and expenses that influence the establishment and management of a department budget.

A key message included in this chapter is the importance of recognizing the limitations of what you will be provided in terms of knowledge and skills in many entry-level occupational therapy educational programs. Although you may be exposed to basic concepts of financial planning, management, and budgeting, such as those covered in this chapter, most occupational therapy managers will need some type of additional education or training to become a competent and effective steward of a department's resources. You are encouraged to develop a professional network early in your career and to watch for opportunities to learn from others. Financial planning, management, and budgeting can be complex processes, but they are also a rewarding part of being an occupational therapy manager.

■ Real-Life Solutions

Catrina approached Raymond and shared her developing career aspirations to move into the role of director of a department. Raymond was happy to hear that Catrina was planning ahead for the next step in her career and responded by offering to involve Catrina in the department's budgeting and financial planning and management activities. He suggested that she begin by reading a few introductory chapters on financial planning and management and that she begin to familiarize herself with basic concepts of budgeting such as the typical categories of revenue and expense. He also offered to begin to review the financial reports that he received each month.

Raymond explained to Catrina that they were right at the half-way point of their current fiscal year, which started the first of each July and ended on the last day of June. This meant that it was already time for him to begin to organize the data and information that he would need to complete the budgeting process for the next fiscal year. He offered to begin to review the monthly reports that summarized the department's gross revenue, deductions to revenue, net revenue, and all of the expenses. He explained that the process of projecting the amount of work (e.g., volume) completed in the department was complex and that it was tied to other management functions including strategic planning, staff development, and ensuring patients received theory-based and evidence-based care. Raymond also suggested that Catrina join in on several networking opportunities such as the Administration and Management Special Interest Section (AMSIS) of AOTA and begin to monitor discussions on OTConnections©. He also recommended beginning to develop a personal network of contacts whom she could rely on as she started to develop her financial skills.

Study Questions

1. **Basic principles of accounting as identified by Ellexson include which of the following?**

   a. Tracking accounts
   b. Managing risk
   c. Monitoring cash flow
   d. All of the above

2. **Which of the following best defines the term** *fiscal year*?

   a. A period of time representing one full budget cycle
   b. A period of time representing a federal tax period
   c. A period of time representing a staff recruitment cycle based on graduation dates

d. A period of time representing a year of performance used to determine staff merit increases (pay increases)

3. **Which of the following best defines the term** *net revenue***?**

   a. The total revenue charged after multiplying total units provided by charge per unit during a specific period
   b. The total revenue charged minus any expenses such as salary, rent, and equipment purchased
   c. Gross revenue minus any allowances, deductions, and anticipated bad debt that are applied
   d. The revenue that varies according to the volume of work produced

4. **Which of the following best defines the term** *full-time equivalent* **(FTE)?**

   a. The number of hours paid to a full-time employee during a designated time period, including payment of vacation or other benefit time
   b. The productive hours paid to a full-time employee equivalent to one caseload in a particular setting
   c. The volume of work produced by one FTE who is meeting established productivity expectations
   d. The number of hours used to determine if a full-time employee has reached "exempt" status and must be paid overtime

5. **The term** *productivity* **can best defined as:**

   a. Care that is provided that proves to be beneficial to the patient in retrospective reviews.
   b. The number of rehabilitation treatments provided to a patient during a Medicare approved acute hospital stay.
   c. Care that is provided that is medically necessary and deemed as a skilled service.
   d. The number of units of billed care or the percentage of time spent in billable activity during a predetermined period of time.

6. **The two concepts that are used to determine if services provided under Medicare in hospital settings are appropriate as billed services are:**

   a. The correct ICD code and the correct CPT code.
   b. Medical necessity and the correct CPT code.

   c. Medical necessity and qualifying as skilled service.
   d. Qualifying as skilled service and the correct ICD code.

7. **A single piece of equipment that exceeds a predetermined amount (e.g., $5,000) and has a life span of longer than a predetermined period (e.g., 1 year) would best be called which of the following?**

   a. Capital improvements
   b. Capital equipment
   c. Capital investments
   d. Capital depreciation

8. **A type of code used by an occupational therapy practitioner to describe the type of services provided by an occupational therapy practitioner, a physical therapy practitioner, a physician, or other health-care provider would best be called a(n):**

   a. ICD code.
   b. HCPCS code.
   c. CPT code.
   d. G-code.

Resources for Learning More About Financial Planning, Management, and Budgeting

Journals Related to Financial Planning, Management, and Budgeting

Health Economics

http://onlinelibrary.wiley.com/journal/10.1002/ (ISSN)1099-1050

This journal publishes articles on all aspects of health economics, ranging from the theoretical to empirical studies as well as analyses of health policy from the economic perspective. Its scope includes the determinants of health and its definition and valuation, as well as the demand for and supply of health care, planning and market mechanisms, microeconomic evaluation of individual procedures and treatments, and evaluation of the performance of health-care systems.

Organizations Related to Financial Planning, Management, and Budgeting

The Healthcare Financial Management Association (HMFA)

https://www.hfma.org/

The HFMA has more than 40,000 members and promotes itself as the leading membership organization for health-care financial management executives and leaders. The HMFA has national and regional chapters and provides member resources and development opportunities through conferences, eLearning, and certification programs. The HFMA website includes free access to introductory materials on a wide range of health-care financial management topics.

The American College of Healthcare Executives (ACHE)

http://www.ache.org/aboutache.cfm

The ACHE is an international professional society with 80 chapters and more than 40,000 health-care executives who lead hospitals, health-care systems, and other health-care organizations. Although not focused solely on financial planning and management, ACHE provides access to networking, education, and career development at the local level. Resources include courses and continuing education on all aspects of financial planning and management and helps members complete the environmental scanning necessary to stay on top of policy and other influences on the health-care arena.

Networks and Newsletters Related to Financial Planning, Management, and Budgeting

The American Occupational Therapy Association—Administration and Management Special Interest Section (AMSIS)

www.aota.org

AOTA's special interest sections (SISs) provide networking opportunities and resources by specialty area. There are 11 SISs, including the Administration and Management SIS, whose members are a resource on financial planning, management, and budgeting. Resources include quarterly newsletters, discussion forums (http://otconnections.aota .org), and professional networking communities. As an AOTA member, you can join up to three SISs, and designate one as your primary SIS to receive a print newsletter. There is also a coding, billing, and reimbursement section of the member's only area of the AOTA website.

Reference List

American Occupational Therapy Association. (2014). *Resources for G code functional data reporting*. Retrieved from https://www.aota .org/en/Advocacy-Policy/Federal-Reg-Affairs/Coding/G -Code.aspx

Berwick, D. M., Nolan, T. W., & Whittington, J. (2008). The triple aim: Care, health and cost. *Health Affairs, 27*(3), 759–769.

Businessdictionary.com. (2014). *Financial accounting*. Retrieved from http://www.businessdictionary.com/definition/financial -accounting.html

Casto, A. B., & Layman, E. (2006). *Principles of healthcare reimbursement*. Chicago, IL: American Health Information Management Association. Retrieved from http://www.bilozix .com/hcreimburesement.pdf

Centers for Disease Control and Prevention. (2014). *Classes of diseases, functioning and disability*. Retrieved from http://www.cdc .gov/nchs/icd.htm

Centers for Medicare and Medicaid. (2012). *Physical, occupational and speech services*. Retrieved from http://www.cms.gov/ Research-Statistics-Data-and-Systems/Monitoring-Programs/ Medical-Review/Downloads/TherapyCapSlidesv10_09052012 .pdf

Centers for Medicare and Medicaid. (2014). *Bundled payments for care improvement (BPCI) initiative: General information*. Retrieved from http://innovation.cms.gov/initiatives/bundled -payments/

Dobrzykowski, E. (2012). Measurement of productivity. Retrieved from Health Policy and Administration Section of the American Physical Therapy Association website: http://hpaapta .wordpress.com/2012/01/09/measurement-of-productivity/

Ellexson, M. T. (2011). Financial planning and budgeting. In K. Jacobs & G. L. McCormack, (Eds.), *The occupational therapy manager* (5th ed., pp. 113–125). Bethesda, MD: AOTA Press.

Frezatti, F., Aguiar, A. B., Guerreiro, R., & Gouvea, M. A. (2011). Does management accounting play role in planning process? *Journal of Business Research, 64*, 242–249.

Holahan, J. (2014). *The launch of the Affordable Care Act in selected states: The financial impact on state from the Affordable Care Act*. Retrieved from http://www.urban.org/publications/ 413037.html.

Nosse, L. J., & Friberg, D. G. (2010). *Managerial and supervisory principles for physical therapists* (3rd ed.). Baltimore, MD: Lippincott, Williams & Wilkins.

Nosse, L. J., Friberg, D. G., & Kovacek, P. R. (2005). *Managerial and supervisory principles for physical therapists* (2nd ed.). Baltimore, MD: Lippincott, Williams & Wilkins.

Principlesofaccounting.com. (2013). *Chapter one: Welcome to the world of accounting*. Retrieved from http://www.principlesofaccounting.com/chapter1/chapter1.html

Silversmith, J. (2011, February). Five payment models: The pros, the cons, the potential. *Minnesota Medicine*. Retrieved from http://www.minnesotamedicine.com/Past-Issues/Past-Issues-2011/February-2011/Five-Payment-Models-The-Pros-the-Cons

Steiner, G. A. (1979). *Strategic planning*. New York, NY: The Free Press.

United States Department of Labor. (2014). *Fair Labor Standards Act advisor: Exemptions*. Retrieved from http://www.dol.gov/elaws/esa/flsa/screen75.asp

University of Florida Office of Physician Billing Compliance. (2014). What is a CPT code? Retrieved from http://compliance.med.ufl.edu/compliance-tips/what-is-a-cpt-code/

CHAPTER 12

Assessing and Promoting Clinical and Managerial Competency

Brent Braveman, PhD, OTR/L, FAOTA

■ Real-Life Management

Emily has worked as an occupational therapy assistant (OTA) for more than 20 years in a number of different settings, but has specialized in spinal cord injury rehabilitation for the last 8 years and has developed specialized skills in a number of areas. Recently, Emily and her spouse relocated and she began working within a spinal cord injury program at a different rehabilitation facility. Most of the program's components are very similar to those of the program in which she was working, and, in her interview, it seemed that her job tasks would be almost identical to those she had been completing. It seemed that she would need to learn relatively little new information to return to the independent style of working she had adopted.

Given her experience, she was surprised by the very formal and in-depth orientation program she was expected to complete before she began treating patients without "line of sight" supervision. Because the facility was accredited by The Joint Commission (TJC) and the Commission on Accreditation of Rehabilitation Facilities (CARF), she could understand having to review videotapes and take written examinations on fire and electrical safety and even on hand washing (although she assumed everyone knew the importance of hand washing).

However, Emily did not understand why she had to spend time reviewing orientation information on aspects of intervention that she considered basic, such as techniques for safely transferring patients or completing "skin checks" to prevent pressure sores. She had to admit privately that she was somewhat insulted to be supervised so closely given the excellent references she had received from her prior supervisors. Moreover, she could not understand why her supervisors were being so slow to assign her patients when her new supervisor reported that the facility was short staffed and had several vacancies. Emily had offered to jump in and suggested that she could help by beginning to treat patients in their rooms for activities of daily living (ADL) sessions or to complete portions of the assessment

Continued

■ **Real-Life Management—cont'd**

appropriate for the OTA. However, her supervisor had responded that they took the "assessment of competencies" for new employees very seriously and did not cut any corners.

Emily had been excited about beginning to work at the facility because the other OTAs who worked there reported feeling highly valued and respected by all of the occupational therapists (OTs), but all of this attention to her level of "competency" made her wonder if she had made a mistake. She decided to confront her supervisor during their next meeting and express her dissatisfaction at the close level of scrutiny she was under. She decided to make a list of the competencies noted on her orientation checklist that she had been completing independently for more than 5 years and to ask that she be able to forgo the rest of the orientation period.

Critical Thinking Questions

As you read this chapter, consider the following questions:

- What are the differences in common terminology related to assessment of competencies, competency, and continued competence of which we must be aware?

- What is the relationship between the process of conducting assessment of competencies and other management functions, including employee recruitment, orientation, performance planning, and accreditation reviews?

- Are occupational therapy practitioners and managers good judges of their own level of competence?

- What role do occupational therapy managers play in the assessment of competencies, continued competence, and the development of specialized and advanced skills recognized through processes such as certification?

Glossary

- **Advanced practice competencies:** competencies that require complex critical reasoning based upon prior clinical experience, which entry-level practitioners are not expected to be able to demonstrate.
- **Certification** (noun): formal recognition that an individual has proficiency within, and a comprehension of, a specified body of knowledge.
- **Competence** (noun): the knowledge, critical thinking, motives, traits, characteristics, or skills to achieve a specific goal or perform job responsibilities.
- **Competencies** (plural of competency): explicit measures, indicators, or statements that define specific areas of knowledge, skills, and abilities related to essential functions and assigned duties within a job or role.
- **Competency** (noun): an individual's actual performance in a particular situation.
- **Competent** (adjective): defined as successfully performing a behavior or task as measured according to a specific criterion.
- **Continued or continuing competence:** dynamic and multidimensional processes in

Glossary—cont'd

which occupational therapy practitioners develop and maintain the knowledge, performance skills, interpersonal abilities, critical reasoning, and ethical reasoning skills necessary to perform current and future roles and responsibilities within the profession.

- **Entry-level competence:** the level of competency expected of all entry-level practitioners to a given profession.
- **Portfolios:** collection of documents, artifacts, and evidence of learning, as well as learning activities, that serves as an assessment instrument and learning tool for the development and documentation of competence.

- **Professional development:** approach that may include a program of continuing competence, but also includes a focus on one's career development in terms of achieving excellence or achieving independent practitioner and expert role status, and in terms of assuming new, more complex roles and responsibilities.
- **Specialized practice competencies:** competencies that relate to abilities that are not expected to be reflected in the entry-level practice of all professionals but that do not require advanced clinical judgment, prior experience, or complex clinical reasoning in order to demonstrate competence.

Introduction

The importance of identifying and documenting the initial and ongoing competence of health-care workers has evolved over several decades. Concerns regarding competency-related issues for occupational therapy practitioners span over a period of time from which a health professional is judged to be **competent** to practice as an entry-level practitioner (e.g., National Board for Certification in Occupational Therapy, Inc. [NBCOT] certification), through the process of hiring and orienting staff, to fostering continued competence of health professionals across entire careers.

Occupational therapy managers often play critical roles in determining whether an individual has met or can meet the competency standards to practice within a particular setting through a review of an applicant's credentials and experiences. Upon hiring a new employee, the manager must assess the individual's ability to perform specific skills or recall specific information by assessing his or her performance against a set of **competencies,** or specific statements of action representing competency in a skill or procedure. The manager also can facilitate the continued competence of staff through a variety of professional development activities.

Increased attention to issues related to the competence of occupational therapy practitioners and other health professionals has come about because of a variety of factors. The increased sophistication of health-care consumers has led to increased scrutiny of the entry-level competence of health-care professionals as well as a call for more severe penalties and consequences for lapses in competence. As a result, the process of certifying the entry-level competence of practitioners has also become more sophisticated. The rapid rate of technology change has had a dramatic impact on the rate at which new knowledge is developed and communicated. The workforce has become more mobile, and with personnel shortages in fields such as occupational therapy, physical therapy, and nursing, recruitment of personnel has become more competitive. Economic influences have resulted in expectations for higher productivity and flexibility on the part of workers. These factors and others have contributed to an increased need to assess employees' competencies as they enter a job or demonstrate various skills, as well as perform **continued or continuing competence** assessment as employees progress.

This chapter overviews the key organizations involved in the assessment of competency and the promotion of continued competence, examines the reasons why these processes are important to any health profession, and introduces you to the components and tools of basic systems for assessing competencies and promoting continued competence of occupational therapy personnel. The chapter also introduces advanced certification and specialty certification as methods of indicating competency in particular areas of practice.

Why Do We Need to Worry About Competency?

The answer to the question, "Why worry about assessing the competency of occupational therapy personnel?" might seem simple, and in fact there are some readily identifiable reasons. These reasons include the following:

- We want to promote the provision of the best possible quality of intervention for our patients and clients.
- We want to avoid litigation that comes with allegations of malpractice and incompetence.
- Lifelong learning, practice based upon evidence, and keeping pace with the introduction of new knowledge and changing technology are commonly recognized values of the profession.

However, there are additional reasons for developing an ongoing and integrated system for the assessment of competencies and the promotion of continued competence. First, a fully integrated system will relate strategies and efforts to assess competencies to strategies and efforts for hiring, orienting, supervising, and evaluating staff. A system for assessing competencies can help you recruit and hire the right person with the right skills or identify the skills you need to develop in current staff. Second, evidence suggests you cannot fully rely on persons to accurately assess their own skills or to accurately identify their own learning needs for the present or for the future (Davis et al, 2006; Dickson, Engelberg, Back, Ford, & Curtis, 2012; Dunning, 2013; McManus, Rakovshik, Kennerley, Fennell, & Westbrook, 2012). Limited evidence exists on the self-assessment accuracy of occupational therapy practitioners specifically, but other disciplines have conducted multiple studies of student self-perception versus external assessments of competency, and these suggest that we should have cautioned confidence in the self-assessment of competency (Blanch-Hartigan, 2011). Moreover, there is not always a high

level of agreement between the subordinate's self-assessment of his or her level of competence and the manager's assessment of that subordinate's level of competence (Meretoja & Leino-Kilpi, 2003). In fact, staff members may underestimate their level of competence as often as they overestimate it. In either case, inaccurate assessment of level of competence may lead to poor utilization of resources, rework, lowered levels of staff satisfaction, and decreased quality of care.

Finally, occupational therapy managers play an important role in retaining staff once hired. In times of personnel shortage, competition for available personnel increases, and retaining staff and avoiding the costs of recruiting and orienting new staff becomes even more important. One key strategy for staff retention is continuing education and staff development, including the provision of free in-service education or funds and time off to pursue graduate education and attend courses or other forms of continuing education. Evidence from multiple types of organizations suggests that managers utilize this strategy often and view it as one of the most effective retention strategies (Govaerts, Kyndt, Dochy, & Baert, 2011; Scanlan, Still, Stewart, & Croaker, 2010; Tran, Davis, McGillis Hall, & Jaglal, 2012). Initiating planned efforts to help staff members develop specialized and advanced competencies (sometimes leading to formal certification) is one method of implementing this strategy.

Key Terms, Concepts, and Players

Multiple organizations related to health-care delivery are concerned with developing and maintaining the "competency" of staff; as noted, competency-related issues arise at various points in the entrée of a professional to a profession. The American Occupational Therapy Association (AOTA), the NBCOT, TJC, CARF, and many state professional regulatory boards, among other organizations, have programs, policies, or efforts under way related to competency issues (Moyers-Cleveland & Hinojosa, 2011). Because of the many organizations and bodies involved and because of the range of points in the careers of professionals at which competency issues arise, the terminology involved can be confusing. Focusing on the context in which terminology is used can be a useful way of keeping the terminology straight.

For example, AOTA distinguishes between the terms **competence** ("an individual's capacity to perform job responsibilities") and continuing competency ("a dynamic and multidimensional process in which the occupational therapy practitioner develops and maintains the knowledge, performance skills, interpersonal abilities, critical reasoning, and ethical reasoning skills necessary to perform current and future roles and responsibilities within the profession") (AOTA, 2010a). Box 12-1 includes the definitions of some key terms that are used throughout this chapter.

The process of establishing that a professional meets requirements representing **entry-level competence** (the level of competency expected of all entry-level practitioners to a given profession) includes multiple steps that are overseen by a variety of types of organizations. Often, NBCOT is thought of as having primary responsibility for establishing that an individual meets standards related to initial competency through administration of the certification examination. As stated on its website (http://www.nbcot.org), "The National Board for Certification in Occupational Therapy, Inc. (NBCOT®) is a

---

BOX 12-1
Key Terms

- **Competent** (adjective): Successfully performing a behavior or task as measured according to a specific criterion (Hinojosa et al, 2000).
  - *Example:* "Based on the established criterion, I am competent to take range-of-motion measurements."
- **Competency** (noun): An individual's actual performance in a particular situation (McConnell, 2001). Competency implies a determination that one is competent.
  - *Example:* "During my orientation to my job, my supervisor observed me and determined that I demonstrated competency in taking range-of-motion measurements."
- **Competencies** (plural of competency): Explicit measures, indicators, or statements that define specific areas of knowledge, skills, and abilities related to essential functions and assigned duties within a job or role.
  - *Example:* "New employees are required to demonstrate a range of competencies before they are allowed to treat patients without direct supervision, such as taking range-of-motion measurements, transferring patients, and making basic splints. These competencies are listed on an orientation check sheet."
- **Competence** (noun): The knowledge, critical thinking, motives, traits, characteristics, or skills to achieve a specific goal or perform job responsibilities (Hickerson-Crist, 2014).

- *Example:* "My performance appraisal indicates that I demonstrate competence in assessing range of motion."
- **Continued or continuing competence:** A dynamic and multidimensional process in which the OT and OTA develop and maintain the knowledge, performance skills, interpersonal abilities, critical reasoning, and ethical reasoning skills necessary to perform current and future roles and responsibilities within the profession. (AOTA, 2010a).
  - *Example:* "Because I do not take range-of-motion measurements every day, I need to do periodic reviews to maintain my continued competence; as new information is developed related to strategies for managing joint contractures, I will need to develop and demonstrate new competencies."
- **Professional development:** May include a program of continuing competence, but also includes a focus on one's career development in terms of achieving excellence or achieving independent practitioner and expert role status, and in terms of assuming new, more complex roles and responsibilities.
  - *Example:* "Because I hope to one day become a college instructor, I plan to begin supervising fieldwork students to learn more about the process of teaching others skills such as taking range-of-motion measurements."

not-for-profit credentialing agency that provides certification for the occupational therapy profession. NBCOT also works with state regulatory authorities and employers, providing information on credentials, professional conduct, and regulatory and certification renewal issues" (NBCOT, 2015). The mission statement of the NBCOT is as follows:

Serving the public interest by advancing client care and professional practice through evidence-based certification standards and the validation of knowledge essential for effective practice in occupational therapy. (NBCOT, 2015)

Undoubtedly, NBCOT does play a vital role in the process of establishing the entry-level competence of occupational therapy practitioners. However, it is important to recognize that there are multiple steps in determining initial competence that occur before an OT or OTA reaches the point of taking the NBCOT certification examination.

Before candidates may sit for the certification examination, they must graduate from an educational program accredited by the Accreditation Council on Occupational Therapy Education (ACOTE). To graduate from such a program, students must not only receive a passing grade in a large number of courses by demonstrating competencies in multiple domains of learning but also successfully complete mandated full-time clinical fieldwork. Graduating from an accredited occupational therapy program is in fact the first step toward certifying initial competence. The process that NBCOT oversees is referred to as **certification**. Certification is defined as "formal recognition that an individual has proficiency within, and a comprehension of, a specified body of knowledge" (American Society for Quality, 2014). Certification is the process by which a professional certification agency grants a person permission to use a certain title if that person has attained entry-level competence. Certification is intended to assure the public that a professional has completed an approved educational program and has passed an examination that assesses the knowledge, skills, and experience needed to provide quality care (DeLisa, 2000). Professional certification agencies:

- Serve the credentialing needs of the profession regardless of membership status (meaning that membership in the profession's association is not

required to become certified or to maintain certification).
- Develop professional standards and measure compliance.
- Promote a vision to improve the overall performance of a profession through a quality certification system.

The NBCOT develops a certification examination through a process they call *practice analysis* that is completed every 5 years. The practice analysis is a method for determining key components required for entry-level occupational therapy practice across three levels: (1) domains, (2) tasks, and (3) knowledge. Domains broadly define the major performance components of the profession (e.g., evaluation; intervention planning; implementing intervention; identifying and implementing performance needs of populations; and managing, organizing, and promoting occupational therapy services). Tasks describe activities that are performed in each domain (e.g., job duties performed by an entry-level practitioner). Knowledge statements reflect the information required to perform each task (e.g., knowledge of sources for staying current in legislative changes influencing practice). These levels are used to develop an *examination blueprint* that guides the percentage of the certification examination related to each domain. For example, beginning in 2013, the examination blueprint calls for 10% of examination questions to relate to the domain of "Manage and direct occupational therapy services to promote quality in practice" (NBCOT, 2014).

State professional regulatory agencies are also involved in establishing initial competence of professionals through licensure, the process by which an agency of government grants an individual permission to engage in a given occupation upon finding that the applicant has attained the minimal degree of competence required to ensure that the public health, safety, and welfare will be reasonably well protected. Professional regulatory agencies serve a number of purposes, including:

- Serving the public by legally monitoring entrée to public practice
- Establishing minimum standards to protect the public in a particular jurisdiction
- Monitoring minimal standards of practice via a practice act and ongoing disciplinary process

In Chapter 3, you learned that it is common to refer to any type of state regulation of who may practice within a profession as "licensure," although there are actually a number of different types of regulation often grouped under that term. According to AOTA, as of 2014 "occupational therapy is currently regulated in all 50 states, the District of Columbia, Puerto Rico, and Guam. Different states have various types of regulation that range from licensure, the strongest form of regulation, to title protection or trademark law, the weakest form of regulation" (AOTA, 2015, n.p.). Certification laws simply regulate who may refer to themselves as OTs or OTAs and may or may not provide a definition of occupational therapy. In some cases, persons may practice as long as they do not refer to themselves as occupational therapy practitioners. Similarly, registration laws prevent nonregistered persons from stating that they are providing occupational therapy services, and trademark laws simply limit who may refer to themselves as OTs or OTAs (AOTA, 2015).

Generally, unlike certification, registration, and trademark laws, a licensure law defines a lawful scope of practice for practitioners. Defining a scope of practice legally articulates the domain of practice and provides guidance to facilities, providers, consumers, and major public and private health and education facilities on the appropriate use of services and practitioners. Defining practice can further ensure important patient protections by offering guidance on appropriate care, particularly in the investigation and resolution of consumer complaints involving fraudulent or negligent delivery of services.

Competency, Skill Acquisition, and Theory

David McClelland, a Harvard University psychologist and founder of the Hay-McBer Company, is credited with founding the competency movement in the United States (Manley & Garbett, 2000). McClelland set out to define competency variables that could be used in predicting job performance and that were not biased by race, gender, or socioeconomic factors. **Competency** was thought to be a broader term than *skill* because it related to performance on the job that required integration of a number of skills. McClelland's colleague, Richard Boyatzis, furthered this work. He focused on identifying competencies

that could differentiate superior performance from average or poor performance by focusing on a person who does the job well and the characteristics and qualities that enable that person to do a superior job, rather than focusing on the job itself (Boyatzis, 1982; Manley & Garbett, 2000). During the 1980s and 1990s, refinement of assessment of competencies continued in the human resources field and began to gain acceptance in other fields, including health care.

One commonly cited model related to the development of competence and competencies in health care is the *Dreyfus Model of Skill Acquisition* that was originally based on the study of U.S. Air Force pilots (Dreyfus, 1981). In the 1980s, Patricia Benner adapted the Dreyfus model to nursing and published an often-cited book, *From Novice to Expert* (Benner, 1984). This model frames skill acquisition as moving through various stages (Driscoll, 2002; Leach, 2002):

- *Novice:* Learners focus on learning the rules of a particular skill.
- *Advanced beginner:* Learners focus on applying the rules of a skill in specific situations that become increasingly dependent on the particular context of the situation.
- *Competency:* Learners see actions in terms of long-range goals or plans and are consciously aware of their skills.
- *Proficiency:* Learners perceive situations as "wholes" rather than "aspects," and their performance is guided by intuitive behavior.
- *Expert:* Learners integrate mastered skills with their own personal styles.

Applications of the Benner model have been widely reported within the nursing literature and to some extent within the literature of other health professions, often in relation to clinical decision-making, education, and development of training programs or career ladders (Crook, 2001; Hargreaves & Lane, 2001; Manley & Garbett, 2000; Nichol, Fox-Hiley, Bavin, & Sheng, 1996; Nuccio et al, 1996; Winchcombe, 2000).

Traditional models of learning such as the Dreyfus model that focus upon the acquisition of knowledge and skills have been challenged by models of learning that emphasize social participation and communities of practice. You will read more about communities of practice in Chapter 17. Learning theories have shifted their focus from individual learning to social learning in new and emerging pedagogies. The emphasis in these new theories moves from learning as a passive and content-driven process to one that is dynamic and active, and requires reflexivity (Berragan, 2011).

In the last decade, numerous disciplines, including medicine and nursing, have investigated simulated activity as a way of training, as well as developing and assessing competency. There are mixed results. Ahmed et al (2011) found that simulation models are valid and reliable in the early phases of training and assessment but were not appropriate for assessment of advanced or specialist competencies. Issenberg, McGaghie, Petrusa, Gordon, and Scalese (2005) conducted a systematic review of 109 journal articles and found that overall high-fidelity medical simulations are educationally effective and simulation-based education complements education in patient care settings. Knecht-Sabres, Kovic, Wallingford, and St. Amand (2013) reported results of a mixed methods exploratory study on the effectiveness of the use of standard patients (a well person trained to simulate a patient's illness in a standardized way or an actual patient using his or her own story in a standardized way) in an adult occupational therapy practice course. They found that the use of standard patients in combination with a sequential, semistructured, and progressively complex series of client cases improved the students' self-perception of their level of comfort and skill on various foundational occupational therapy–related competencies. Bradley, Whittington, and Mottram (2013) reported positive results of the use of simulated activities for final year occupational therapy students that were planned around an assessment scenario that required reasoning about readiness for hospital discharge or safety to remain at home. Finally, McNulty, Price, Cardell, and Dunn (2013) reported the results of a study that revealed 90% of the students involved in a standard patient experience with a paid actor enabled them to demonstrate skills that they could not do on a strictly paper-and-pencil test, and that 74% of students agreed or strongly agreed that the experience significantly contributed to the development of their professional competencies.

Interestingly, relatively little discussion appears in the occupational therapy literature on competency and assessment of competencies regarding exactly *how* one comes to acquire a particular competency. Reference is often made to learning theories, and the assumption seems to be that managers should rely on bodies of knowledge related to education and skill development to guide training or education efforts aimed to help staff develop competencies. Discussion widely seems to focus on the roles of the individual, the manager, the organization, regulatory and accrediting bodies, and the profession in facilitating the development of competence through processes such as self-assessment, reflective practice, or professional development strategies (e.g., continuing education, portfolio development and use, or specialty or advanced certification) (Hickerson-Crist, 2014; Moyers-Cleveland & Hinojosa, 2011). Hinojosa et al (2000) presented an approach for self-assessment, identification of needs, development and implementation of a plan, and implementation of changes in professional behavior as part of AOTA's continuing education products titled "Self-Initiated Continuing Competence," which is included in AOTA's professional development tool (AOTA, 2014a).

Assessment of Competencies and Other Functions of the Occupational Therapy Manager

Occupational therapy managers complete a range of functions that relate to the assessment of specific competencies. As described earlier, competency issues span the period from entry into the profession to working with staff to try to assure that they maintain continued competence as they accept new responsibilities and as the profession's knowledge base rapidly grows and changes. Skilled managers will look across the various discrete management functions they perform and create bridges from one management function to another to establish a system that ties the assessment of competencies to other management tasks. This section briefly overviews some of the most important management functions to which the assessment of competencies is related.

Creating Job Descriptions

A job description is described in Chapter 7 as "the core personnel document that serves to codify best practice." It does this by establishing the essential functions that a particular employee or class of employees performs (e.g., OTs versus OTAs). In Chapter 7, you were introduced to the components of job descriptions and strategies for developing job descriptions. To review, these components include the requirements for the job (e.g., eligibility for state licensure), the relationship of the employee to others in the organization, and the essential functions of the position or the fundamental job duties that the employee must be able to complete independently with or without a reasonable accommodation.

The essential functions performed by each employee should be reflected in specific competencies developed in relation to each function. The process of developing competencies may also help you reexamine the job descriptions of personnel to assure that they are accurate and complete. For example, including "Assists clients to develop positive support mechanisms to prevent relapse" in a job description for an occupational therapy practitioner in a community mental health setting might indicate the need for development of competencies related to understanding addiction to substances and the recovery process. In turn, knowing that a staff member often intervenes to help clients develop leisure activities and social supports that foster sobriety might indicate the need to add related tasks as essential functions within the individual's job description.

Recruitment of New Employees

Well-written job descriptions that accurately and completely identify the essential functions of a position and the related set of competencies can make the process of recruiting and hiring new employees easier and can increase the likelihood of recruiting an employee who is a good match for the position. Assessment of specific competencies may be useful in determining the skills, training, and education required for persons being hired to fill a specific vacancy, and can therefore guide the manager or supervisor in writing recruitment materials and screening and interviewing applicants (Braveman, Gentile, Stafford, Berthelette, & Learnard, 2004). Additionally, job offers can be made contingent upon the ability to demonstrate competency in the essential job functions as identified in the job description. Job descriptions and statements of competencies should be reviewed each time a vacancy occurs, because the knowledge required for successful performance can change, sometimes over relatively short periods of time.

Initial Assessment of Competencies

The initial assessment of competencies is often associated with settings that undergo organizational accreditation by bodies such as TJC. Such bodies often do require documentation of a comprehensive orientation of new employees, and initial assessment of competencies for essential job functions is an important part of a comprehensive employee orientation. However, documentation of initial assessment of competencies is not important only in settings subject to an accreditation process. In addition, managers should consider initial assessment of competencies in any setting in which they wish to assure provision of quality care and to safeguard to whatever extent possible against malpractice litigation (Braveman et al, 2004).

Initial assessment of competencies related to essential job functions, high-risk job tasks (e.g., transferring patients, working with a patient with cardiac precautions), and job functions requiring performance of specialized competencies (e.g., use of physical agent modalities) or advanced competencies (e.g., comprehensive cognitive evaluation of patients with neurological conditions) should occur before the employee independently completes these job tasks (Braveman et al, 2004). Determination that an employee cannot demonstrate competence in an essential job function as part of the orientation process allows the manager or supervisor to safeguard consumers by taking steps to assist the staff member to develop competence in essential job functions before the end of the orientation period.

It is often assumed that if a practitioner has obtained initial certification, he or she will indeed be able to adequately perform the functions expected of an entry-level practitioner. Although this is typically the case, there are exceptions. At times, a manager may hire an OT or OTA, or may encounter staff members hired by previous managers, who in fact are not able to demonstrate all of the required competencies for adequate performance. If comprehensive job descriptions and statements of initial competencies exist, they can guide assessment of the staff member's level of competency. Hopefully the practitioner will be able to develop the skills, knowledge, and attitude required to demonstrate the necessary competencies. In worst-case situations, staff members who cannot demonstrate competencies at the end of an orientation period—or in some cases later in their employment—may have to be terminated. Situations such as this are rare, but they highlight the seriousness of managerial tasks and the importance of having structures and tools such as job descriptions and statements of competencies in place.

Annual Assessment of Competencies

In addition to the initial assessment of competencies conducted when a new employee begins work, there are some competencies that should or must be assessed on an annual basis. Competencies such as those required by the Occupational Safety and Health Administration (OSHA), which is a government agency that seeks to help employers and employees reduce on the job injuries, illnesses, and deaths, can be documented as part of the process of conducting an annual performance appraisal (for more information on OSHA, see http://www.osha.gov). Often managers think that assessment of competencies differs vastly from performance appraisal. In fact, assessment of competencies is simply part of a performance appraisal based on defined skills and performance criteria. To reflect this single process and reduce paperwork, some organizations have reengineered their job descriptions and performance appraisal systems. By basing the job description on the specific skills that are required, forms that previously did "double duty" as performance evaluations can serve also as the assessment of competencies documentation tool (LaDuke, 2001).

Examples of competencies assessed on an annual basis would include those related to fire safety and electrical safety or to blood-borne pathogen precautions, such as knowledge of effective hand washing and infection control techniques. Competency statements included in an annual assessment of competence might also include competencies related to a specific employee's job tasks or skills (e.g., competencies related to specialized practice skills such as conducting an evaluation for driver safety or the provision of low vision services) or to general skills such as customer service. Assessment of age-specific competencies is typically completed both at hire and on an annual basis. Age-specific competencies relate to the knowledge and skills of practitioners specific to understanding age-related capacities across the age span. These competencies assure that a practitioner has the necessary knowledge and skills to intervene with the population with which he or she is assigned to work. We must not

assume, for instance, that a pediatric occupational therapy practitioner has the knowledge and skills to be moved to cover for a practitioner working with older adults.

Competencies included in annual assessments may build on established knowledge, skills, and capacities reflecting the ever-changing nature of some jobs in light of an organization's mission and goals. Braveman et al (2004) noted that these competencies might reflect new, changing, high-risk, or problem-prone aspects of the job as it evolves over time. Examples of when the need for such competencies might come about include the following:

- Competencies based on new initiatives, procedures, technologies, policies, or practices are identified.
- Competencies based on changes in procedures, technologies, policies, or practices occur.
- Competencies related to high-risk job functions are identified or added to a job description.
- Competencies related to problematic job functions are identified through continuous quality improvement (CQI) efforts, consumer or staff surveys, incident reports, or any other formal or informal evaluation processes.

Professional Development and Portfolios

As a result of implementing a comprehensive system for assessment of competencies, a manager may become aware of the acute or long-term **professional development** needs of staff. Through the process of assessing competencies, you may identify learning needs that can be met through your department's in-service education program or through continuing education or training. Tying the staff's development goals to needs identified during the initial or annual assessment of competencies, as well as the annual performance appraisal, creates a synergy of effort that can save you time and help you identify the most effective strategies for using limited continuing education resources. For example, the need for a newer staff member to develop splinting skills could guide your choice of how to spend continuing education funds in the coming year.

One approach to professional development that relates to continued competence is the development and use of **portfolios.** Portfolios have become popular as assessment instruments, as well as learning tools for the development of competence, because they provide opportunities to monitor and appraise changes in performance (Alsop, 2002; College of Physiotherapists of Ontario, 2013: Smith & Tillema, 1998). Portfolios contribute to the process of assessing competency (note that the more general term *competency* is used here rather than *competencies*) by compiling evidence about performance and relevant feedback about individual practices (Tillema, 2001). A portfolio may also be a useful tool in gathering and organizing information about an individual's involvement in professional development activities to satisfy the requirements for professional development for NBCOT recertification, for maintaining advanced certification such as AOTA Board certifications, or for maintaining state licensure (Alsop, 2001).

Several types of portfolios have been identified and each type has advantages if designed for a specific purpose (Forde, McMahon, & Reeves, 2009). You may consider a combination of elements or copying items and having more than one portfolio. The general types of portfolios include the following:

- *Course content portfolios* contain items that have significant relevance to a course.
- *Continuing professional development portfolios* contain a record of professional development with reflections and evaluations.
- *Competence-based portfolios* record achievement against specific criteria.
- *Accreditation for prior learning portfolios* contain evidence related to prior learning.
- *Project portfolios* contain resources and reflections of groups related to a specific topic.

Regardless of the type of portfolio used, the advantages of developing and using portfolios include (College of Physiotherapists of Ontario, 2013; Tillema, 2001):

- Assistance in identifying strengths and weaknesses in performance
- Fostering development of awareness of competence
- Assistance in setting learning goals
- Resolving discrepancies between external standards and achieved performance
- Assistance with planning for future growth

- Documenting evidence of reflection and integration of learning
- Capturing achievements under realistic circumstances and recording them using authentic evidence and tangible products
- Documenting experience and growth across jobs and practice areas

Staffing Plans, Including Per Diem or Registry Staff

According to the Bureau of Labor Statistics and AOTA, employment of OTs is projected to grow 29% from 2012 to 2022, much faster than the average for all occupations. In addition, the demand for occupational therapy practitioners will be high (AOTA, 2010b; Bureau of Labor Statistics, 2014). With continued high vacancy rates, many organizations have pursued a variety of strategies to respond to the shortage. One strategy is to purchase personnel services (referred to as contract staff) from an outside agency or vendor or maintain their own registry of per diem staff (i.e., staff who are on call to occasionally work as needed). In this situation, the organization must obtain information from that outside vendor to assure that the contracted staff members have the proper credentials (e.g., licensure as required by a state practice act).

Contract or per diem staff members are typically held to the same standards for demonstrating both initial and annual competencies as permanent staff. For example, TJC has stated that, "The standards in the human resource chapter apply to direct, contract, and volunteer personnel providing patient care and/or services on behalf of an organization, regardless of whether the contracted organization is accredited" (TJC, 2012, n.p.). Assessing competencies for these staff members can be costly. Often, the human resources department will verify basic credentials such as licensure, whereas the occupational therapy manager is typically responsible for verifying that the contract or per diem staff can demonstrate competencies related to essential job functions. To minimize expense, documentation of some competencies before beginning work (e.g., cardiopulmonary resuscitation [CPR] certification, blood-borne pathogen training) might be written into contracts with agencies or may be made the responsibility of per diem staff to be completed during nonpaid time. However, it is the responsibility of the organization using these staff to assure that the per diem staff have actually completed the training and that documentation is available. Additionally, by making adjustments in how caseloads are assigned and assigning contract or per diem staff only patients within a specified age range and with a limited variety of conditions, you may be able to limit the scope of competencies that must be assessed initially.

A system for the assessment of competencies is a key component in the development of a department's overall staffing plan. In settings accredited by TJC, these plans are required, but such plans can help you identify the number of staff necessary and the competencies they must be able to demonstrate to meet the care needs of any setting. For example, identifying your department's needs for providing specialized types of intervention based on competencies would alert you that, because of staff turnover, you employ only a single staff member who has documented competencies related to treating patients with wound care needs. Competency-based staffing plans can help you identify that additional training must be provided to other staff to assure adequate coverage when employees who have demonstrated competency are not working. Accrediting bodies may require that the same level of care be provided regardless of the day of the week patients are admitted to your facility.

Agency Accreditation and Licensure

Both accrediting bodies and state regulatory agencies have increased their focus on the assessment of competencies and on continuing competency. Increasingly, state regulatory agencies are including requirements for continuing education as part of an effort to promote continued competence, and AOTA has responded with the development and maintenance of standards for continuing competence (AOTA, 2010a). Managers working in accredited and licensed facilities and programs must ensure that their programs for assessment of competencies meet all accrediting and licensing standards. You should be aware that standards related to competency may vary from one accrediting body to another and may change over time, so you must be vigilant in monitoring these changes.

Licensure laws often include what are referred to as "sunset" provisions, meaning that a provision of the law is automatically repealed on a specific date, unless the appropriate legislative body reenacts the law. This means that state licensure regulations often have to be reenacted on a regular cycle. State professional associations often see sunset provisions as an opportunity to change provisions or add new provisions to the regulation, and updated versions of the regulation may have an impact on what competencies should be assessed or how, or the requirements for documenting efforts to maintain continued competence.

The most common accrediting bodies occupational therapy managers may be involved with are TJC and the CARF. Standards related to the assessment of competencies for both TJC Leadership and CARF Business Practices are primarily found in the human resources section of their manuals. Managers should carefully review these standards when developing competency programs for their staff.

Quality Control and Continuous Quality Improvement Efforts

Chapter 13 provides an in-depth discussion of quality control and continuous quality improvement (CQI). Assessment of competencies and efforts to promote continued competence are natural fits with CQI initiatives. For example, the use of quality control measures such as "check sheets" to determine the level of conformance to preestablished standards for interventions such as splint fabrication, use of modalities, or documentation can flag the need for education or training of staff. Similarly, CQI efforts focusing on process improvement may indicate the need to establish new competencies or revisit established measures of competency by providing targeted training for staff.

As a result of a CQI effort, processes may be changed or new processes may be implemented. Introducing a changed or new process and assuring that it becomes "institutionalized" so all staff members are aware of the process and complete it in the same manner is a key final step in any CQI effort. Identifying the key competencies and developing assessment methods can help measure the extent of compliance to new procedures.

Outcomes Evaluation and Management

Many factors influence the outcomes of occupational therapy intervention, and the assessment of competencies will not automatically assure desired outcomes. Other factors related to patients or clients, their support, their medical condition, and the length and type of intervention provided might all impact the outcome of occupational therapy intervention. You must be aware that evaluating outcomes of interventions with individual clients calls for very different procedures than evaluating outcomes of occupational therapy intervention at the program level. Systems to assess competencies related to essential job functions can help to prevent unusual cases or "outliers" from influencing the overall variability found in outcome measures (Braveman et al, 2004). It is important to recognize that not all outliers in a process are negative events. Sometimes we should attend to an outlier because it signifies that someone has found a more effective way of doing something or might be our most skilled employee, and we would benefit from others adopting that employee's procedures. Again, the process of developing statements of competencies can help guide the institutionalization of new and improved procedures.

Domains of Knowledge, Competency, and Assessment of Competencies

Traditionally, Bloom's Taxonomy of learning and the three domains of performance included within it have been identified to guide programming related to education, training, and the development of competency. These three domains are the cognitive domain (knowing), the affective domain (appreciating and valuing), and the psychomotor domain (physical performance) (Munzenmaier & Rubin, 2013). In addition, two other domains of performance for OTs have been identified: ethical reasoning and critical reasoning. These domains were identified as related to competency by the AOTA's Commission on Continuing Competency in the "Standards for Continuing Competence," which are intended to assist occupational therapy practitioners to assess, maintain, and document competence in all the roles they assume (AOTA, 2010a). The standards address the following five

domains: (1) knowledge, (2) critical reasoning, (3) interpersonal attitudes, (4) performance skills, and (5) ethical practice. Table 12-1 includes examples of competency statements related to the cognitive, critical reasoning, affective, psychomotor, and ethical reasoning domains for an OT involved in work-related occupational therapy practice.

Examples of Types of Competencies

Competencies can be generic to clinical practice in any setting (basic), specific to a clinical specialty, or reflective of specialized knowledge or advanced practice. In most practice settings, a manager will have to identify a wide range of types of competencies related to the setting, the population seen, a variety of personnel and staffing processes, and specific interventions and types of equipment. This section provides a brief introduction to the most common types of competencies that must be assessed.

Age-Specific Competencies

The age-specific category of competencies documents that employees have the knowledge and skills to work with a specific age group. It also documents that the special needs of age-specific populations are addressed when developing the job descriptions, orientation, performance appraisal tools, and competence assessment tools for the staff members who care for them. For example, employees who work in a neonatal intensive care unit require one set of knowledge and skills specific to that age group, whereas employees who work with adolescents in an outpatient psychiatric program and those who work with older adults in a skilled nursing facility require different sets of knowledge and skills specific to those age groups. With the frequent shortages in occupational therapy personnel, it may be tempting to move experienced staff from one program to another to accommodate vacations, vacancies, or fluctuations in work volume. You must remember in those situations, however, that when staff is rotated to different units or programs and is asked to provide intervention to a different age group, staff members should be assessed on competencies for this new group before they intervene

TABLE 12-1	
Examples of Competency Statements From the Cognitive, Critical Reasoning, Affective, Psychomotor, and Ethical Reasoning Domains	
Cognitive Domain (Knowing)	• The therapist will be able to identify various physical, cognitive, and environmental factors that can affect performance within the worker role. • The therapist will be able to identify resources available to assist workers and employers in accessing services in their community.
Critical Reasoning Domain	• The therapist will integrate knowledge from multiple sources to formulate a comprehensive description of prior work performance. • The therapist will reflect on prior practice and be able to identify strategies that have not been effective in the past.
Affective Domain (Appreciating and Valuing)	• The therapist will document in a manner that reflects an appreciation for cultural influences on personal values related to worker identity. • The therapist demonstrates valuing the involvement of parents in the process of planning occupational therapy intervention by asking their opinions and using information-seeking behaviors.
Psychomotor Domain (Physical Performance)	• The therapist will be able to attach and detach all basic attachments to a work simulator. • The therapist will be able to demonstrate proper lifting techniques to clients when lifting up to 50 pounds.
Ethical Reasoning Domain	• The therapist will be able to identify ethical principles and their relationship to reporting to workers' compensation payers, employers, and others. • The therapist will be able to identify limits in knowledge and understanding of ethical principles in order to know when to seek guidance from others.

independently. Such age-specific competencies are commonly accepted as part of a TJC requirement (i.e., 2014 standard HR.01.07.01: The hospital evaluates staff performance) that when a hospital defines specific competencies it should consider the needs of its patient population, they types of procedures conducted, conditions or diseases treated, and the kinds of equipment it uses (TJC, 2014). The use of the following five-step method is recommended to help you meet this standard: (1) reflect age-specific competence when developing job descriptions, (2) reflect age-specific competence when developing performance appraisal tools, (3) develop age-specific competencies for specific job titles, (4) provide age-specific education and training, and (5) provide evidence of age-specific care. As suggested earlier, although you might most commonly implement a process such as that just described because of the regulations of an outside accrediting agency, assuring that staff members have the knowledge and can demonstrate competencies specifically related to the age group to which you assign them is a mark of ethical managerial practice in any setting.

Equipment-Related Competencies

Assessment of equipment-related competencies may overlap with other competencies and relates to performance of skills, knowledge, attitudes, or critical or ethical reasoning involved with the use of specific equipment. These competencies may be part of the initial assessment of competencies in some settings (e.g., use of mobile arm supports on a spinal cord injury unit) or of assessment of specialized or advanced competencies in other settings (e.g., the use of a computerized work simulation unit or cognitive assessment of a person with a brain injury). When purchasing some types of equipment, especially if the cost is significant, vendors may be able to assist you with the development of competencies. Often training materials for the equipment may include tests or checklists that can be easily adapted.

Specialized Practice Competencies and Advanced Practice Competencies

There is often confusion over the difference between **specialized practice competencies** and **advanced practice competencies**. Specialized practice competencies relate to abilities that are not expected to be reflected in the entry-level practice of all professionals but that do not require advanced clinical judgment, prior experience, or complex clinical reasoning in order to demonstrate competence. Specialized practice competencies require specific education and training but may not require the type of complex clinical reasoning only expected from an experienced practitioner. New graduates might be expected to demonstrate competencies related to specialized practice after appropriate training. An example of specialized practice might be the use of physical agent modalities such as ultrasound. Licensure laws and other forms of practice regulation vary from state to state as to whether the use of physical agent modalities is within the domain of occupational therapy practice. AOTA's position is that "physical agent modalities may be used by an occupational therapist or occupational therapy assistant as an adjunct or preparation for intervention that ultimately enhances engagement in occupation" (AOTA, 2012, n.p.). AOTA further stipulates that "physical agent modalities may only be applied by occupational therapists and occupational therapy assistants who have documented evidence of possessing the theoretical background and technical skills for safe and competent integration of the modality into an occupational therapy intervention plan" (AOTA, 2012, n.p.). Other examples of specialized practice competencies might relate to the provision of low vision services or wound care.

Advanced practice competencies are those that require complex critical reasoning based upon prior clinical experience that is not expected to be demonstrated by entry-level practitioners. An example of advanced practice skills might be the application of advanced neurological rehabilitation techniques that require the assessment and integration of complex knowledge and clinical judgments based on prior experience.

Employees who use specialized practice skills or advanced practice skills should be evaluated specifically for competencies in these skills. Documentation of assessment of these competencies should become a formal part of employee records. This documentation should include the competency assessed, the method of assessment, the person determining competency, and an indication if it is an initial or annual competency, including the date it was performed. Because techniques and equipment change frequently, specialized or advanced practice competencies should be reevaluated for appropriateness and be updated frequently.

Competencies Related to Specific Skills or Procedures

In most settings, occupational therapy practitioners perform specific procedures related to the process of assessing and intervening with clients for which specific assessment of competencies might be appropriate. These differ from the specialized practice competencies just discussed in that it might be expected that any entry-level practitioner would be able to quickly learn to demonstrate these competencies without first undergoing extensive training or education. These competencies simply reflect the common types of interventions carried out in a specific setting. For example, in most pediatric settings, competencies related to the administration of standardized assessments to identify developmental milestones might be appropriate. In other settings, competencies related to procedures routinely performed, such as the fabrication of certain types of splints, serial casting, or procedures related to safety precautions (such as on a mental health unit) may be appropriate.

Reviews of job descriptions, documentation procedures, and common referrals are some simple ways to screen for common procedures for which you might develop competencies. Having experienced practitioners keep simple time logs in which they note the primary activities in which they are involved and the common procedures that they complete is another way of identifying competencies for which assessments might be developed. You may also do a review in which you involve staff in identifying high-risk procedures or interventions that were not typically completed but are occurring more often to determine if any of these might be appropriate to incorporate in your system for assessment of competencies.

Documenting Assessment of Competencies

A critical part of any system for assessing competencies is to assure that the assessment results, as well as any action taken if the results are not to full satisfaction, are documented. You must realize that, as far as an accreditation reviewer or legal entity is concerned, assessments of competencies that are not documented in a permanent written format may as well have not have occurred at all. Assessments of competencies should be documented by a formal and standardized method, and it is recommended that such documentation become a permanent part of each employee's personnel file (Braveman et al, 2004). Documentation of assessments of competencies may be completed in concert with or as part of other elements of managerial documentation, including

- New employee orientation forms
- Annual performance appraisal forms
- Personnel development and in-service education plans and posttests
- Staffing plans
- Quality control and improvement forms, including check sheets and audits

Elements of Effective Documentation

Documentation of assessment of competencies should include the following elements:

- Written specific statements reflecting essential job functions that identify specific and measurable tasks or behaviors
- The method(s) to assess each competency
- The person(s) who assessed each competency
- The date(s) on which a competency was assessed
- An action plan for competencies for which the employee is deemed less than fully competent
- The date for the next assessment of the competency if it is to be repeated

One observation regarding establishing time frames for reassessment is that it is not uncommon for a practitioner in a setting to go for long periods of time without completing a particular aspect of evaluation or intervention, and that skills can become rusty over time when not practiced. A potential mistake that can be made by a manager is assuming that once a competency is demonstrated, it need not be repeated. That may be the case for skills that are used frequently, but may not hold true for other skills, such as splinting, use of some types of equipment, or even transferring patients safely. Including some type of review of work assignments and the need for reassessment of competencies is highly recommended. A good time for such a review is at the annual employee performance appraisal.

Writing Assessment of Competencies Statements

The primary question you must be able to ask before beginning to write an effective assessment of competencies statement is, "What is it that you expect a person to know or do in order to demonstrate the competency?" This question must be answered such that an assessment of competencies statement can be written in clear, concise, and unambiguous terms so both the person expected to demonstrate the competency and the person conducting the assessment interpret the competency statement in exactly the same way. There should be no doubt as to when performance is adequate and when continued practice or learning is required. Box 12-2 includes four criteria for

---

BOX 12-2

Four Criteria for Assessment of Competencies Statements

1. Begin each critical element with a verb that succinctly identifies the mandatory aspect of the skills to be demonstrated.
2. Use language that is clear and unambiguous and has a commonly accepted, uniform interpretation.
3. Include behaviors (actions) at the higher end of the thinking and action spectrum.
4. Include only actions (behaviors) that are essential for documenting competence.

evaluating assessment of competencies statements, presented as part of the Competency Outcomes and Performance Assessment (COPA) model described in the nursing literature (Lenburg, Abdur-Rahman, Spencer, Boyer, & Klein, 2011).

Methods of Assessing Competencies

The methods of assessing various competencies must be matched to the domains of learning being evaluated (e.g., cognitive, affective, psychomotor, critical reasoning, and ethical reasoning). In most cases, the completion of a specific intervention may require competency in multiple domains, so the comprehensive assessment of competency may require that you develop multiple competency statements and consider assessing the competency using more than one strategy. Some competencies (e.g., CPR or responding to ethical dilemmas) may not easily be assessed in "real-life" situations and may need to be assessed through case studies, role-playing, or drills that simulate situations that might be encountered. For example, you are likely familiar with fire drills or mock simulations of disasters used to estimate an organization's or system's readiness to respond to an emergency. Similar exercises can be used as part of an assessment of competencies system.

Any assessment of competencies program should be based upon sound adult learning principles, including those of Malcom Knowles (Knowles, Holton, & Swanson, 2012). Box 12-3 lists some of these principles.

A variety of methods can be used when assessing competencies, and each method has its advantages in terms of the resources needed for administration, such as the time it takes or whether you can assess one person or multiple persons at a time. These methods can be categorized into one of three types: (1) simulated tests, (2) objective tests, and (3) observational tests. Simulated tests usually involve a video presentation or a written scenario. The person being tested watches a videotape or reads the scenario and then answers questions. Objective tests can contain true-or-false, multiple-choice, and matching questions. Observational tests require the person being tested to be observed by a skilled assessor in a natural setting, and these tests typically list observable, objective measures (Barney, Long, McCall, Watts, & Cash, 2000).

The method you choose for assessing competencies should match the domain of knowledge related to each

---

BOX 12-3

Principles of Adult Learning to Incorporate in an Assessment of Competencies Program

- Adults perform better when they understand why they need to know specific information or to be able to demonstrate specific skills.
- Adults bring prior learning and experience to all learning situations and build on their prior experience.
- Some persons may require more time to learn a skill than others.
- New material should be presented in multiple formats (e.g., oral, written, and observation).
- Self-directed learning should be allowed as a learning option when possible, especially with assessment of competencies related to advanced skills such as equipment or physical agent modality.

---

competency. Whenever possible, you should use multiple methods to assure that you have adequately addressed each domain of performance. Table 12-2 lists a variety of methods for assessment of competencies and factors to consider in their use.

Synthesizing Assessment of Competencies and Documentation

Developing an effective and comprehensive system for assessment of competencies requires that you identify categories of competencies, develop appropriate competency statements, match appropriate assessment methods to each competency, and select a method of documenting the results of the assessment and follow-up of actions taken if the result of the assessment of competencies is not satisfactory.

Table 12-3 includes examples to illustrate how a sample of categories of competencies, specific competency statements, methods of assessing competencies, and documenting assessment are combined. Sample forms for the documentation of the assessment of competencies are included as appendices at the end of this chapter.

TABLE 12-2

Methods for Assessment of Competencies and Factors to Consider in Their Use

Posttests (written tests, oral examinations, or worksheets)	• Measure cognitive skills (an individual's comprehension of basic knowledge) • Ineffective to measure behavioral performance (psychomotor skills)
Return demonstration (demonstrating a set of skills to another skilled assessor)	• Appropriate for measuring behavioral performance (psychomotor domain) • May occur in an artificial environment (skills lab) or in a real-world setting • Must go beyond description—describing an action may reflect the cognitive domain (knowing), but performance is required to assess competencies in the psychomotor domain • Most effective if a standard set of criteria for evaluation (competency checklist) is used • The assessor must be familiar with the criteria for evaluation and have demonstrated the indicated competency to another trained assessor
Observation of daily work	• Appropriate for measuring skills in the psychomotor and affective domains • Both supervisors and peers can be used for these types of observation
Case studies (provide individuals with a situation and ask them to explain their responses or choices in that situation)	• Appropriate for assessing critical thinking skills • Manager or supervisor must create a check sheet or other evaluation tool to document specific competencies that are based on predetermined criteria related to the case content • Can be prepared in many different ways • Can be used with individuals or discussion groups to facilitate team building and group problem-solving
Exemplars (a story describing a situation you have experienced or describing a rationale you thought about and choices you made in a situation)	• Appropriate to measure critical thinking skills and interpersonal skills • Captures actions NOT taken as well as those chosen • Appropriate for use with a variety of personnel, including staff and leadership • Very useful for personnel who must establish trust with a client, provide customer service, or deal with sensitive issues
Peer reviews	• Appropriate for assessment of interpersonal skills and critical thinking skills • Staff should be prepared via a thorough orientation to the process, including suggestions for giving constructive feedback so that receiving feedback from peers is viewed as a positive experience • May use a written format or verbal "face-to-face" format
Self-assessment	• Appropriate for assessment of critical thinking skills • Appropriate for assessment of values, beliefs, opinions, and attitudes because it engages the individual in a reflective exercise that allows him or her to put into words his or her conscious and unconscious thoughts • Has limited utility for assessment of psychomotor skills, and an additional method should always be used for high-risk procedures or skills that could result in harm to patients or clients

Managerial Competencies

To this point, our discussion has focused primarily on competency and the assessment of competencies for those you might supervise. In addition, you may have asked the question: "What about my competency as an occupational therapy manager?" Although the assessment of competencies for managers has not received the same attention by bodies such as accrediting agencies, competency development and the assessment of competencies for managers have been addressed by a number of professions, and some empirical investigation of managerial competencies has been conducted. This information is useful in considering the major areas in which specific managerial competencies might be developed or for conducting

TABLE 12-3			
Examples of Synthesis of Assessment and Documentation of Competencies			
Category of Competency	**Example of Competency Statement**	**Example of Assessment Method(s)**	**Documentation Methodology**
Initial evaluation of competence	Accurately reads a cardiac rehabilitation patient's blood pressure before engaging the patient in ADLs	• Observation by supervisor using a check sheet • Check of accuracy by supervisor, who also takes the patient's blood pressure	Checklist of initial competencies and observation form showing "competent" or need for intervention and action taken is dated and placed in file.
Annual evaluation of competence	Is able to state the steps taken if a fire occurs in a patient area with patients present	• Videotape viewing combined with a posttest • Mock drills twice yearly	Copy of posttest placed in personnel record signed by qualified reviewer. Results of drills reviewed at staff meeting.
Age-related competence	Identifies physical and cognitive changes experienced during puberty	• Written test based upon a filmed case • Verbal discussion after assessment of adolescent with peers using a check sheet	Test results and peer evaluation form signed by employee, observer, and supervisor, including any intervention plan, placed in the personnel file.
Equipment-related competence	Completes monthly safety check of fluidotherapy machine	Self-review using checklist	Checklist turned into supervisor and placed in personnel record.
Physical agent modality competence	Identifies all contraindications for use of heat and cold	Posttest after training module	Copy of posttest placed in personnel record, signed by qualified reviewer.

self-assessment of managerial competencies as part of a professional development plan.

Some competencies might be considered "universal" for managers. One traditional method of identifying competencies is to use the commonly identified managerial functions (e.g., planning, organizing and staffing, directing, and controlling) as a guide. For example, Box 12-4 lists these traditional management functions and the related categories of competencies identified by Anderson and Pulich (2002).

Other managerial competencies will be more dependent upon the nature of your job. Just as you would identify competencies specific to any clinical environment, some competencies for the occupational therapy manager will need to be developed with the specific organizational context in mind, although some common core competencies for health-care managers have been identified.

The Healthcare Leadership Alliance is a consortium of major professional membership organizations including the American College of Healthcare Executives, the American Organization of Nurse Executives, the Healthcare Financial Management Association, the Healthcare Information and Management Systems Society, and the Medical Group Management Society. The Alliance has over 140,000 members and has identified five common competency domains for health-care managers based on research on the credentialing processes of each organization (Stefl, 2008). These five competency domains are:

1. Communication and relationship management
2. Professionalism
3. Leadership
4. Knowledge of the health-care system
5. Business knowledge and skills

Others have also developed sets of competencies and competency assessment for high-performance leadership as well as high-performance management.

BOX 12-4

Traditional Management Functions and Managerial Competencies

Planning
- Using goal setting
- Understanding the changing health-care environment
- Making effective decisions

Organizing and Staffing
- Understanding team structure and flexible work design
- Using cooperation techniques
- Applying coordination techniques

Directing
- Interpersonal competencies
  - Communication skills
  - Communicating with the boss
  - Communicating with peers and others
  - Communicating with employees
- Being politically astute
- Managing conflict
- Managing diversity
- Role model competencies
- Demonstrating professionalism in conduct and demeanor
- Enhancing technical competence

Controlling
- Using employee empowerment
- Applying CQI efforts

For example, the Schroder High Performance Leadership Competencies include competency categories of (Spangenberg & Theron, 2003):

1. Informational capability
2. Conceptual capability
3. Strategic capability
4. Developmental capability
5. Interpersonal learning
6. Cross-boundary learning
7. Purpose building
8. Confidence building
9. Proactive capability
10. Achievement capability

Competencies cannot be isolated from the institutional surroundings and must be defined by taking day-to-day "real-life" behavior into account (Noordegraaf, 2000). They should reflect the nature of what you do in the course of everyday work, including some of the activities that might be taken for granted. For example, most managers would agree that they spend a tremendous amount of their time in meetings. Running effective meetings, recognizing the power dynamics of meetings, preparing adequately and differently depending on the type and agenda of a meeting, or even organizing a room or seating to affect interactions in a meeting are all examples of competencies that you might identify for yourself as a manager.

Another way of considering competencies for managers is to distinguish between what have been referred to as *threshold competencies* and *high-performance competencies*. This approach draws on the work of McClelland and Boyatzis described earlier. A threshold competency is a cluster of related behaviors that is used by managers but that has not been empirically associated with superior job performance. A high-performance managerial competency is a cluster of related behaviors that has been found empirically to distinguish high-performing from average-performing managers (Cockerill, Hunt, & Schroder, 1995; Jackson, 2009; Janjua, 2013). An example of a threshold competency might be "concern with close relationships," or spending time with subordinates, whereas an example of a high-performance competency would be "concept formation," or building frameworks and models or ideas on the basis of information to become aware of patterns and cause-and-effect relationships. Table 12-4 lists a sample set of competencies based on work by Cockerill et al (1995) that continue to be associated with high-performance management today (Janua, 2013; Martina et al, 2012).

Although high-performance management and average-performance management have been distinguished based on empirical evidence in the business literature, there has been limited investigation of high-performance managerial behaviors as they relate to health-care settings, but results are promising (Fields, Roman, & Blum, 2012). It may be useful as part of a self-assessment process to identify competencies that you desire to achieve by using the underlying schema to identify behaviors that separate high-performing managers from average performers in your organization.

TABLE 12-4	
Sample High-Performance Managerial Competencies	
Gathering and Synthesizing Information	Identifies a variety of relevant sources of data, information, and evidence to guide planning and decision-making
Conceptual Flexibility	Ability to think along multiple paths at the same time to imagine different possible futures
Interpersonal Communication and Understanding	Uses a variety of communication strategies to understand how others see issues and appreciates the perspective and viewpoints of others
Team Management and Coaching	Understands the stages of team development and is effective in helping teams to develop, become high-performing teams, and contribute toward the mission and vision
Coaches from a Developmental Perspective	Applies evidence-based theories to employee development and approaches each employee from an individualized perspective to promote growth
Presentation of Ideas to Groups and Customers	Effectively addresses groups and customers in a variety of situations, is able to clearly articulate ideas, and uses technical, symbolic, nonverbal, and visual aids effectively
Proactive Orientation	Thinks ahead, anticipates problems and opportunities, and involves employees in creatively developing future-oriented goals and success plans
Quality Orientation	Continually evaluates processes and outcomes and promotes continuous improvement to achieve higher-quality results

Specialty and Advanced (Board) Certifications

Another form of indicating competency is obtaining specialty or advanced certifications. As described earlier, specialty practice relates to practice that requires specific training or education that is not expected to be part of all entry-level education, whereas advanced practice requires reliance on experience or advanced clinical or critical reasoning that would not be expected of any new graduate. Such certifications may be offered within a discipline such that only members of a specific profession are eligible for the certification.

For example, AOTA is pursuing development of both specialty certifications and advanced (board) certifications for OTs. The specialty certifications are relevant to the scope of occupational therapy practice and reflect a defined set of skills, techniques, and interventions. As of 2014, the areas offered by AOTA for specialty certification include driving and community mobility, environmental modification, feeding, eating and swallowing, and school systems. Advanced or board certifications reflect a major domain of practice with an established knowledge base in occupational therapy and reflect the scope of occupational therapy. Areas offered for advanced certification included gerontology, mental health, pediatrics, and physical rehabilitation (AOTA, 2014b).

Other certifications serve the same purpose but are open to persons from more than one professional discipline as long as they meet the criteria for the certification. For example, the American Society of Hand Therapists (ASHT) is a professional organization composed of licensed occupational and physical therapists, some of whom have earned the advanced designation certified hand therapist (CHT) and who specialize in the treatment and rehabilitation of the upper extremity. The ASHT's mission is "To build and support the community for professionals dedicated to the excellence of hand therapy" (ASHT, 2014).

Certification as a hand therapist is administered by the Hand Therapy Certification Commission (http://www.htcc.org) and the certification process includes the following requirements (Hand Therapy Certification Commission, 2014):

- Must be an OT or physical therapist (PT) with a current professional credential
- Accrual of a minimum of 4,000 hours of direct practice experience in hand therapy as an OT or PT
- A passing score on the certification examination

Although specialty and advanced certifications have become more common and are indeed indicators that practitioners have completed learning or practice experiences, they should not automatically be accepted as the sole indicator of competency. Credentials such as specialty or advanced certification are indicators of what an individual *should* be able to do based on the examination or the certification process and not what that individual *can* or *will* do in the actual job. Assessment of competencies should not automatically be waived simply because an individual has a certification.

Chapter Summary

This chapter introduced you to the concepts of competency, assessment of competencies, and continued competence and the critical role that the occupational therapy manager plays in the process of assessing and documenting competencies. You learned that numerous regulatory, certification, and professional bodies and organizations play a role in protecting the public by requiring assessment of competency using a variety of strategies. These strategies include initial certification of entry-level practitioners by NBCOT, requirements for professional development to promote continued competence by NBCOT and state regulatory boards, standards related to assessment of competencies by accrediting bodies including TJC and CARF, and specialty or advanced certification through professional associations such as AOTA or ASHT.

At the beginning of the chapter, you were introduced to Emily, an OTA with more than 20 years of experience who had just started a new job. Emily was surprised at the formal orientation she was expected to undergo, especially the amount of time she was asked to spend reviewing basic aspects of care such as hand washing and conducting skin checks for patients with spinal cord injury. Emily had decided to express her dissatisfaction at the level of scrutiny that she was under and the amount of attention that was being paid to her competency.

■ Real-Life Solutions

Emily met with her supervisor as planned for their weekly supervision session. During the session she expressed her concern over the length of time and the amount of energy that were being spent in assessment of competencies as part of her orientation. Emily explained that she had been working for more than 20 years and had worked in close collaboration with the OTs in her last job. She had established service competency with her supervisor and had been independently completing standard parts of patient evaluations and was certainly prepared to do the same in this facility. She also admitted to her supervisor that she was somewhat

offended that her skills were not being better utilized given the high caseloads in the facility and that the department had several vacancies.

Emily's supervisor, Joan, began by thanking Emily for her concern over helping to meet the department's patient care needs. She shared that she, too, was very worried over how the department was going to handle its work given the vacancies on the staff. Joan also assured Emily that she had no concerns over Emily's skill level or whether or not she was a competent OTA. She told Emily that she and the other OTs on the spinal cord injury staff were confident in Emily's skills but that prior experience and even glowing reports from other OTs could not be substituted for formal assessment of competencies. In addition to legal, licensure, and

■ **Real-Life Solutions—cont'd**

accreditation concerns, Joan saw the assessment of competencies system as an important indication of the level of professionalism and concern for quality care shared by the organization's leadership.

Joan provided Emily some readings on competency, assessment of competencies, and continued competence to help her become more familiar with how the concepts were related to each other and to other management functions. As Joan and Emily discussed Emily's concerns and experiences, they realized that all of the staff could benefit from additional information, and Joan enlisted Emily's help to develop an in-service presentation for the staff. After their discussions, although Emily remained concerned about increasing her contributions to the team as quickly as possible, she felt more comfortable that the time being taken to assess her level of competence should not be taken personally.

Study Questions

1. **Which of the following organizations has direct responsibility for assessing the entry-level competency of an occupational therapy practitioner via an examination process?**

   a. American Occupational Therapy Association
   b. American Occupational Therapy Foundation
   c. National Board for Certification of Occupational Therapy
   d. National Society for Quality

2. **Statements of explicit measures or indicators that define specific areas of knowledge, skills, and abilities related to essential functions and assigned duties within a job or role may best be named:**

   a. Competence.
   b. Certifications.
   c. Continuing competence.
   d. Competencies.

3. **Which of the following is most accurate in regard to the status of professional regulation as of 2014?**

   a. All 50 states, the District of Columbia, Puerto Rico, and Guam had some form of regulation.
   b. All 50 states, the District of Columbia, Puerto Rico, and Guam had licensure, which is the strongest form of regulation.

   c. All 50 states, the District of Columbia, Puerto Rico, and Guam had title protection, which is the strongest form of regulation.
   d. All 50 states, the District of Columbia, Puerto Rico, and Guam had certification, which is the strongest form of regulation.

4. **Which of the following is the most accurate statement summarizing the evidence on the use of simulation-based education?**

   a. There is no empirical evidence to support or not support simulation-based education.
   b. There is mixed evidence to support simulation-based education, with some positive results.
   c. The evidence clearly shows that simulation-based education is ineffective.
   d. None of the above.

5. **Which of the following employment processes is not appropriate for inclusion in an assessment system of entry-level competencies for a new employee?**

   a. Advanced competencies
   b. Orientation competencies
   c. Equipment use competencies
   d. Age-specific competencies

6. **A description of a professional portfolio that best describes its use would be as follows: A professional portfolio is an assessment and learning tool:**

   a. That is used to document readiness for the certification examination to enter the profession as an entry-level occupational therapy practitioner.

   b. That documents experience and learning and helps to identify future learning and professional development needs and goals.

   c. Appropriate for educators to identify the learning needs of students.

   d. Appropriate for a human resources department to document the learning needs of staff for accreditation.

7. **Which of the following statements is most accurate in regard to assessment and documentation of competencies for per diem or contract staff?**

   a. Organizations are not responsible for assessing or documenting competencies for per diem or contract staff.

   b. Organizations can rely on the agency providing the per diem or contract staff to handle everything related to assessing and documenting competencies.

   c. Organizations only must assess and document specialized competencies used only in their practice setting.

   d. Organizations must assure that per diem or contract staff have met all competencies required for permanent staff and must assure that these staff have documentation of appropriate training.

8. **Which is most accurate in regard to the assessment of competencies for occupational therapy managers?**

   a. The assessment of competencies is a process used only for front-line clinical staff and not for managers.

   b. Competencies for managers can be categorized according to the traditional functions of managers and threshold and high-performing competencies.

   c. Competencies for managers relate only to entry-level competency and are not helpful in identifying more advanced managerial competencies.

   d. Assessment of competencies for the manager is a new idea with little support, and we should wait to see if there is any empirical support before developing managerial competencies.

Resources for Learning More About Assessment of Competencies and Continued Competency

Journals That Often Address Assessment of Competencies and Continued Competence

Nursing Management

http://journals.lww.com/nursingmanagement/pages/default.aspx

Nursing Management is a monthly journal that focuses on applied strategies and educational information for nursing managers. Topics included in the publication include legal and ethical aspects of nursing leadership to personnel management, recruitment and retention, budget issues, product selection, and quality control. Although focused on management in nursing, many articles address issues and topics of concern to managers in any area of health care, including staff development, health-care policy, and the like.

Journal for Healthcare Quality

http://www.nahq.org/Quality-Community/journal/jhq.html

The *Journal for Healthcare Quality* targets health-care quality professionals who are responsible for promoting and monitoring quality, safe, evidence-based, cost-effective health care as its audience. Published articles focus on a variety of management-related topics, including accreditation issues and successes, administration and management, behavioral health-care quality, compliance, confidentiality, evidence-based practice, government affairs and policy making, information systems and management, health-care innovations, knowledge management, performance measurement and improvement, and health-care quality research. Additional monthly columns provide reviews and announcements of Internet sites, reports on conferences, and other resources. The journal provides coverage of state-of-the-art technology, quality management techniques, practical applications of quality improvement systems, and new and emerging trends and innovations.

Organizations and Associations Concerned With Assessment of Competencies and Continued Competence

The Joint Commission on Accreditation of Healthcare Organizations

http://www.jointcommission.org/

The mission of TJC is to continuously improve the safety and quality of care provided to the public through the provision of health-care accreditation and related services that support performance improvement in health-care organizations. TJC publishes standards related to competency in numerous health-care settings and publishes resources on promoting competency and quality care.

Commission on Accreditation of Rehabilitation Facilities

http://www.carf.org/

CARF's mission is to promote the quality, value, and optimal outcomes of services through a consultative accreditation process that centers on enhancing the lives of the persons served. CARF publishes standards related to competency in a variety of rehabilitation settings.

National Board for Certification in Occupational Therapy, Inc.

http://www.nbcot.org

NBCOT is a not-for-profit credentialing agency responsible for certification for the OT profession. NBCOT develops, administers, and continually reviews a certification process that reflects current standards of entry-level practice in occupational therapy. It also works with state regulatory authorities, providing information on credentials, disciplinary actions, and regulatory and certification renewal issues. NBCOT is responsible for establishing initial competency through its certification examination and has requirements for maintaining certification related to continuing education to promote continued competence.

American Society for Training and Development

http://www.astd.org/astd/

The ASTD is an association for human resources professionals and other fields related to training and development of employees. ASTD members represent multinational corporations, medium-sized and small businesses, government, academia, consulting firms, and product and service suppliers. Assessment of competency is a concern of human resources professionals in various fields. The ASTD publishes *T + D Magazine* and includes issues related to assessment of competency and a wide range of other topics relevant to managers.

Reference List

Ahmed, K., Jawad, M., Abboudi, M., Gavazzi, A., Darzi, A., Athanasiou, T., & Dasgupta, P. (2011). Effectiveness of procedural simulation in urology: A systematic review. *Journal of Urology*, *186*(1), 26–34.

Alsop, A. (2001). Competence unfurled: Developing portfolio practice. *Occupational Therapy International*, *8*, 126–131.

Alsop, A. (2002). Portfolios: Portraits of our professional lives. *British Journal of Occupational Therapy*, *65*(5), 201–206.

American Occupational Therapy Association. (2010a). Standards for continuing competence. *American Journal of Occupational Therapy*, *64*, S103–S105. doi:10.5014/ajot.2010.64S103

American Occupational Therapy Association. (2010b). *Workforce trends in occupational therapy*. Retrieved from http://www.aota .org/-media/Corporate/Files/EducationCareers/Prospective/ Workforce-trends-in-OT.PDF

American Occupational Therapy Association. (2012). Physical agent modalities. *American Journal of Occupational Therapy*, *66*(6), S78–S80.

American Occupational Therapy Association. (2014a). *AOTA professional development tool (PDT)*. Retrieved from http://www1.aota .org/pdt/index.asp

American Occupational Therapy Association. (2014b). *Board and specialty certifications*. Retrieved from http://www.aota .org/Education-Careers/Advance-Career/Board-Specialty -Certifications.aspx

American Occupational Therapy Association. (2015). *Issues in licensure*. Retrieved from http://www.aota.org/en/Advocacy-Policy/ State-Policy/Licensure.aspx

American Society for Quality. (2014). *What is certification?* Retrieved from http://www.asq.org/cert/faq/what-is-certification

American Society of Hand Therapists. (2014). *Mission and vision.* Retrieved from http://www.asht.org/about/leadership-and-governance/mission-and-vision.

Anderson, P., & Pulich, M. (2002). Managerial competencies necessary in today's dynamic health care environment. *The Health Care Manager, 21,* 1–11.

Barney, J. D., Long, K. G., McCall, E., Watts, J. H., & Cash, S. H. (2000). National call to test for competence: Strategies for clinical managers. *Administrative and Management Special Interest Section Quarterly, 16,* 1–3.

Benner, P. (1984). *From novice to expert.* Menlo Park, CA: Addison-Wesley.

Berragan, L. (2011). Simulation: An effective pedagogical approach for nursing? *Nurse Education Today, 31*(7), 660–663.

Blanch-Hartigan, D. (2011). Medical students' self-assessment of performance: Results from three meta-analyses. *Patient Education and Counseling, 84*(1), 3–9.

Boyatzis, R. E. (1982). *The competent manager: A model for effective performance.* New York, NY: John Wiley & Sons.

Bradley, G., Whittington, S., & Mottram, P. (2013). Enhancing occupational therapy education through simulation. *British Journal of Occupational Therapy, 76*(1), 43–46.

Braveman, B., Gentile, P. A., Stafford, J., Berthelette, M., & Learnard, L. (2004). A guide for managers and supervisors to develop a system for assessment of competencies. Retrieved from American Occupational Therapy Association website: http://www.aota.org/

Bureau of Labor Statistics. (2014). *Occupational outlook handbook: Occupational therapists.* Retrieved from http://www.bls.gov/ooh/healthcare/occupational-therapists.htm

Cockerill, T., Hunt, J., & Schroder, H. (1995). Managerial competencies: Fact or fiction? *Business Strategy Review, 6,* 1–12.

College of Physiotherapists of Ontario. (2013). *Professional portfolio guide: Quality management program.* Retrieved from http://www.collegept.org/Assets/qualitymanagement/QM%20Resources/QM_Portfolio_Guide_130222.pdf

Crook, J. A. (2001). How do expert mental health nurses make on-the-spot clinical decisions? A review of the literature. *Journal of Psychiatric and Mental Health Nursing, 8,* 1–5.

Davis, D. A., Mazmanian, P. E., Fordis, M., Van Harrison, R., Thorpe, K. E., & Perrier, L. (2006). Accuracy of physician self-assessment compared with observed measures of competence: A systematic review. *JAMA, 296*(9), 1094–1102.

DeLisa, J. A. (2000). Certifying and measuring competency in the United States. *Archives of Physical Medicine and Rehabilitation, 81,* 1236–1241.

Dickson, R. P., Engelberg, R. A., Back, A. L., Ford, D. W., & Curtis, J. R. (2012). Internal medicine trainee self-assessments of end-of-life communication skills do not predict assessments of patients, families, or clinician-evaluators. *Journal of Palliative Medicine, 15*(4), 418–426.

Dreyfus, S. E. (1981). *Four models v. human situational understanding: Inherent limitations on the modeling of business expertise* (Air Force Office of Scientific Research, USAF Contract F49620-79-C-0063). Unpublished manuscript, University of California, Berkeley.

Driscoll, J. W. (2002). Paradigms for assessment: Women's knowledge and skill attainment. *American Journal of Maternal/Child Nursing, 27,* 288–293.

Dunning, D. (2013). The problem of recognizing one's own incompetence: Implications for self-assessment and development in the workplace. In S. Highhouse, R. Dalal, & E. Salas (Eds.), *Judgment and decision making at work* (pp. 37–56). New York, NY: Routledge.

Fields, D., Roman, P. M., & Blum, T. C. (2012). Management systems, patient quality improvement, resource availability, and substance abuse treatment quality. *Health Services Research, 47*(3pt1), 1068–1090.

Forde, C., McMahon, M., & Reeves, J. (2009). *Putting together professional portfolios.* London: Sage.

Govaerts, N., Kyndt, E., Dochy, F., & Baert, H. (2011). Influence of learning and working climate on the retention of talented employees. *Journal of Workplace Learning, 23*(1), 35–55.

Hand Therapy Certification Commission. (2014). *Eligibility requirements.* Retrieved from http://www.htcc.org/certify/test-information/eligibility-requirements

Hargreaves, J., & Lane, D. (2001). Delya's story: From expert to novice, a critique of Benner's concept of context in the development of expert nursing practice. *International Journal of Nursing Studies, 38,* 389–394.

Hickerson-Crist, P. A. (2014). Competence and professional development. In B. A. Boyt-Schell, G. Gillen, & M. Scaffa (Eds.), *Willard & Spackman's occupational therapy* (pp. 989–1004). Philadelphia, PA: Wolters Kluwer: Lippincott Williams & Wilkins.

Hinojosa, J., Bowen, R., Case-Smith, J., Epstein, C., Moyers, P., & Schwope, C. (2000). Self-initiated continuing competence. Retrieved from American Occupational Therapy Association website: http://www1.aota.org/pdt/docs/CE1200InitiatingCont.pdf

Issenberg, S. B., McGaghie, W. C., Petrusa, E. R., Gordon, D., & Scalese, R. J. (2005). Features and uses of high-fidelity medical simulations that lead to effective learning: A BEME systematic review. *Medical Teacher, 27*(1), 10–28.

Jackson, D. (2009). Profiling industry-relevant management graduate competencies: The need for a fresh approach. *The International Journal of Management Education, 8*(1), 85–98.

Janjua, S. Y. (2013). The competence classes: An integrated approach to develop managers. *European Journal of Business and Social Sciences, 1*(11), 92–130.

Knecht-Sabres, L. J., Kovic, M., Wallingford, M., & St Amand, L. E. (2013). Preparing occupational therapy students for the complexities of clinical practice. *Open Journal of Occupational Therapy, 1*(3), 4.

Knowles, M. S., Holton III, E. F., & Swanson, R. A. (2012). *The adult learner.* Burlington, MA: Butterworth & Heinemann.

LaDuke, S. D. (2001). The role of staff development in assuring competence. *Journal for Nurses in Staff Development, 15,* 221–225.

Leach, D. (2002). Building and assessing competence: The potential for evidence-based graduate medical education. *Quality Management in Health Care, 11,* 39–44.

Lenburg, C. B., Abdur-Rahman, V. Z., Spencer, T. S., Boyer, S. A., & Klein, C. J. (2011). Implementing the COPA model in nursing education and practice settings: Promoting competence, quality care, and patient safety. *Nursing Education Perspectives, 32*(5), 290–296.

Manley, K., & Garbett, R. (2000). Paying Peter and Paul: Reconciling concepts of expertise with competency for a clinical career structure. *Journal of Clinical Nursing, 9,* 347–359.

Martina, K., Hana, U., Jiří, F., Iveta, Ř., Abraham, A., Jebapriya, S., & de Matos, A. C. (2012). Identification of managerial competencies in knowledge-based organizations. *Journal of Competitiveness, 4*(1), 129–142.

McConnell, E. A. (2001). Manager's fast track: Competence v. competency. *Nursing Management, 32*(5), 14.

McManus, F., Rakovshik, S., Kennerley, H., Fennell, M., & Westbrook, D. (2012). An investigation of the accuracy of therapists' self-assessment of cognitive behaviour therapy skills. *British Journal of Clinical Psychology, 51*(3), 292–306.

McNulty, T., Price, P., Cardell, B., & Dunn, L. (2013). *Standardized clients in case-based simulation: Student perceptions and relevance of an occupation-based curriculum.* Retrieved from http://commons.pacificu.edu/sso_conf/2013/3/6/

Meretoja, R., & Leino-Kilpi, H. (2003). Comparison of competence assessments made by nurse managers and practicing nurses. *Journal of Nursing Management, 11,* 404–409.

Moyers-Cleveland, P. A., & Hinojosa, J. (2011). Continuing competence and competency. In K. Jacobs & G. McCormack (Eds.), *The occupational therapy manager* (5th ed., pp. 485–502). Bethesda, MD: AOTA Press.

Munzenmaier, C., & Rubin, N. (2013). *Bloom's taxonomy: What's old is new again. Perspectives.* Santa Rosa, CA: The eLearning Guild.

National Board for Certification in Occupational Therapy, Inc. (2014). *Examination blueprints—OTR&COTA.* Retrieved from http://www.nbcot.org/exam-blueprints

National Board for Certification in Occupational Therapy, Inc. (2015). *About NBCOT.* Retrieved from http://www.nbcot.org/public

Nichol, M. J., Fox-Hiley, A., Bavin, C. J., & Sheng, R. (1996). Assessment of clinical and communication skills: Operationalizing Benner's model. *Nurse Education Today, 16,* 175–179.

Noordegraaf, M. (2000). Professional sense-makers: Managerial competencies amidst ambiguity. *Journal of Public Sector Management, 13,* 319–332.

Nuccio, S. A., Lingen, D., Burke, L. J., Kramer, A., Ladewig, N., & Raaum, J. S. B. (1996). The clinical practice development model: The transition process. *Journal of Nursing Administration, 26,* 29–37.

Scanlan, J. N., Still, M., Stewart, K., & Croaker, J. (2010). Recruitment and retention issues for occupational therapists in mental health: Balancing the pull and the push. *Australian Occupational Therapy Journal, 57*(2), 102–110.

Smith, K., & Tillema, H. H. (1998). Evaluating portfolio use as a learning tool for professionals. *Scandinavian Journal of Educational Research, 41,* 193–205.

Spangenberg, H. H., & Theron, C. C. (2003). Validation of the high performance leadership competencies as measured by an assessment centre in-basket. *South African Journal of Industrial Psychology, 29*(2), 29–38.

Stefl, M. E. (2008). Common competencies for all healthcare managers: The healthcare leadership alliance model. *Journal of Healthcare Management, 53*(6), 360–374.

The Joint Commission. (2012). *Human resources standards applicability to contracted and volunteer personnel.* Retrieved from http://www.jointcommission.org/mobile/standards_information/jcfaqdetails.aspx?StandardsFAQId=344&StandardsFAQChapterId=66

The Joint Commission. (2014). *The Joint Commission E-dition.* Release 6.0. Available for purchase at The Joint Commission website. Retrieved from https://e-dition.jcrinc.com/maincontent.aspx.

Tillema, H. H. (2001). Portfolios as developmental assessment tools. *International Journal of Training and Development, 5,* 126–135.

Tran, D., Davis, A., McGillis Hall, L., & Jaglal, S. B. (2012). Comparing recruitment and retention strategies for rehabilitation professionals among hospital and home care employers. *Physiotherapy Canada, 64*(1), 31–41.

Winchcombe, J. (2000). Competency standards in the context of infection control. *American Journal of Infection Control, 28,* 228–232.

Appendix 12-1

Sample Form for Assessment of Competency

Department of Occupational Therapy

Physical Agent Modality Assessment of Competency: Hot Packs

Name: _____   Date:_____

Reviewer: _____

Method of Assessment: *Direct Observation by Skilled Reviewer*

A.	SELECTION	YES	NO	N/A	COMMENTS
1.	Verbalizes clinical rationale for use of modality				
2.	Verbalizes contraindications for use of modality				
B.	**APPLICATION**	**YES**	**NO**	**N/A**	**COMMENTS**
1.	Conducts skin check and assesses patient sensation				
2.	Orients patient to use of hot pack, including process, impact, and complications				
3.	Matches size of pack to body part				
4.	Uses towels to wrap hot pack to sufficiently guard against burn				
5.	Positions patients for comfort and to assure that pack remains in place				
6.	Drapes hot pack correctly onto body part				
7.	Documents time of start of application and provides instruction to patient				
8.	Checks patient's skin within minutes of application				
9.	Adjusts hot pack if necessary when conducting skin check				
10.	Removes hot pack in timely manner				
11.	Checks skin within 2 minutes of removing hot pack and informs patient of outcomes				
12.	Checks impact of treatment on patient				
C.	**DOCUMENTATION**	**YES**	**NO**	**N/A**	**COMMENTS**
1.	Documents use of modality in medical record				
2.	Documentation includes reference to preparation for participation in occupational behavior				
3.	Documentation includes start time, end time, and length of treatment				
4.	Documentation includes reference to patient response and impact of treatment				

Competency Met: ☐ yes   ☐ no

If no, document action plan on reverse of form and instruct staff member not to use modality unsupervised until competency is met.

Reviewer's Signature: _____

Staff Signature: _____

Appendix 12-2

Sample Form for Annual Assessment of Competencies

Department of Occupational Therapy

Competency	High Risk	High Volume	Problem Prone	Link to Quality Plan	Professional Standard	Assessment Method
Mandatory All Employees						
Patient confidentiality (HIPAA)						
Fire safety						
Electrical safety						
Hazard communication						
Infection control						
Emergency management						
Mandatory Patient Contact						
CPR						
Age-specific care						
TB test						
Signs of abuse						
Restraints						
Blood-borne pathogens						
Job-Specific Annual Competencies						

Annual Assessment of Competencies

(To be completed and filed as part of Annual Employee Performance Appraisal)

Assessment Method Key:

1. Return demonstration
2. Cognitive test
3. Observation

4. Peer review
5. Chart review/audit
6. Other

Employee Signature: _____

Supervisor Signature: _____

Appendix 12-3

Sample form for Documentation of Assessment of Competencies

Organization Employee Competency Assessment

_____ (UNIT)

NAME: _____ JOB POSITION: _____

HIRE DATE: _____

Competency	Self-Assessment			Action Plan				Validation			
Standard of care, practice, procedure, equipment, or skill	0 = Never done 1 = Need review 2 = Can perform without review			Minimal Level of Planned Activity LEARN P&P = Review policies and procedures C = Attend class V = Video/self-learning packet		VALIDATE 1 = Once only A = Annually		This is to certify that the above individual is competent (able to perform task safely and correctly) as demonstrated in a simulated or practice setting VALIDATOR = Enter date and signature			
	0	1	2	Learn/ Practice	Validate	Target Date		First Validation	Renewal	Renewal	Renewal
A.											
B.											
C.											
D.											
E.											

CHAPTER 13

Continuous Quality Improvement

Maureen Triller, MPA, DrPH
Alanna Motzi, LCSW
Gayle Harper, MSW

■ Real-Life Management

Joan has accepted a position as an occupational therapy supervisor at Rehab-World, a new facility of a nationally recognized chain of regional occupational and physical therapy centers. This new location will provide outpatient therapy services to physician offices and hospitals in a three-county area. Although Joan functioned as a team lead (supervisor) in her previous position, this is her first official management position. One of Joan's new responsibilities is to lead the continuous quality improvement (CQI) efforts for her occupational therapy team. She participated in several performance improvement (PI) teams in her previous role and even led a couple of successful project teams. Joan feels this is her opportunity to shine.

Rehab-World has a strong corporate-level commitment to quality and high expectations for the performance of each of its locations. However, from her first day on the job, it was clear to Joan that her team at Rehab-World did not have the same positive experiences or perceptions of PI as she did. Many of her staff members were fresh out of school, and Rehab-World was their first real job. Others were just getting back to work after taking years off to raise children. Joan's challenge was to align her team's efforts to Rehab-World's goals, give her team a shared understanding and appreciation of CQI, and provide them with a set of PI tools that would allow them to make this new location a success!

Critical Thinking Questions

As you read this chapter, consider the following questions:

- Why is CQI considered to be both a management philosophy and a management method for structured problem-solving?

- How can a CQI approach coordinate the strategic alignment of improvement initiatives with organizational priorities?

- How can a CQI management philosophy as well as the tools and techniques of CQI be applied to improvement efforts at the department or business unit level?

- What are the common quality tools, concepts, and strategies that you can add to your own personal CQI "toolbox" to use in the PI efforts in which you will participate?

Glossary

- **Control chart:** type of line graph showing performance in relation to a set of upper and lower control limits. A process is typically said to be "in control" if the graphed data points continuously fall between the upper and lower control limits.
- **Fishbone diagram:** (also called a cause-and-effect diagram) a method used to identify and document causes to the problem (effect) being studied.
- **Histogram:** type of bar chart where frequency distribution is shown by means of "bars" or rectangles.
- **Multivoting or nominal group technique:** method of team voting used to decrease many choices to an important few.
- **Pareto chart:** type of bar chart (histogram) reorganized so that frequency distributions are presented in order from more to less to reflect relative frequencies.
- **Pareto principle:** the concept that 80% of the problem is caused by 20% of the contributing root causes.
- **Pilot test:** a small-scale implementation often used to test a possible solution.

- **Plan-do-study-act (PDSA):** the commonly recognized process improvement cycle often used in CQI projects.
- **Process flow diagrams:** graphic representations of the steps and decision points in any process.
- **Return on investment (ROI):** a calculation of what was gained from doing a project minus what was invested in doing the project, typically expressed in terms of dollars.
- **Root cause analysis:** a method used to analyze the underlying reason(s) for a problem. The "root cause" is what causes the problem to occur repeatedly.
- **Run chart:** type of line graph that shows changes in data over time.
- **Statistical process control:** the principle that variation from common-cause systems should be left to chance, but special causes of variation should be identified and eliminated.
- **Stratification:** breaking data into categories such as by time, date, location, referral source, and so on.

Introduction

Over the last two decades, although quality continues to be a priority in health care, perspectives on evaluating and improving health-care services have undergone considerable change. However, the focus has shifted from quality of products and services to an increased emphasis on patient safety and on "value-added" health care, with the value being the ratio of the quality of products and services compared with the cost to provide them. This focus on value-added work requires a thorough understanding of customer requirements combined with well-defined work processes. Continuous quality improvement (CQI), a structured approach to continually evaluating and improving an organization's processes and outcomes, remains relevant in the ever-changing health-care environment.

The opening sections of this chapter provide you with a brief history of the changing perceptions of quality in health care along with the application of CQI approaches in health care and some of the related key concepts. The remaining sections of the chapter will provide more detail on the concepts, strategies, tools, and techniques and how they might be applied at the department, team, or business-unit level of an organization. Just as the delivery of health care has changed dramatically over the past decade, so too has the perception of what constitutes quality in health care. Two landmark reports by the Institute of Medicine (IOM), *To Err Is Human* (2000) and *Crossing the Quality Chasm* (2001), documented unacceptably high rates of medical errors and wasted resources in health care. These problems were related to variation in treatment practices and a failure to implement known best practices. As a result, insurance payers and regulators began closely scrutinizing adverse events; now, broadly ranging quality indicators are being reported, monitored, and compared. During the last decade, the paradigm of CQI shifted from being just a managerial tactic to being a professional responsibility (Sollecito & Johnson, 2013). Despite shifts in the definition and importance of quality in health care, the application of CQI is still relevant today. In health care, CQI is defined as a structured organizational process that involves staff in planning and executing improvements to provide quality health care that meets or exceeds expectations (Sollecito & Johnson, 2013). At the organizational level, CQI typically involves a common set of characteristics that emphasize: (a) setting the direction for the organization, (b) a focus on organizational learning and people development, and (c) the application of key PI processes and tools. These characteristics are highlighted in Box 13-1.

Although organizations may vary greatly in terms of which management philosophies they use to drive improvement, the key elements of CQI can be implemented at either department or work-unit levels and still be effective.

In CQI-focused organizations, a key role of leadership is to identify the organization's priorities and use the information to set the direction of its improvement strategies. Priorities may include achieving and maintaining accreditation requirements, controlling costs, or improving the organization's competitive position in the market. Some organizations may even employ a quality council, consisting of representatives of the organization's leadership team, to review, select, and monitor major improvement initiatives to ensure their strategic alignment with resource management and performance expectations.

A key component of a successful CQI program is organizational learning. All of the staff members need

---

BOX 13-1

Characteristics of CQI

1. **Setting Direction**
   - A link to key elements of the organization's strategic plan
   - A quality council made up of the institution's top leadership
2. **People Development**
   - Training programs for personnel
3. **Key Processes and Tools**
   - Mechanisms for selecting improvement opportunities
   - Formation of PI teams
   - Staff support for process analysis and redesign
   - Personnel policies that motivate and support staff participation in PI
   - Application of the most current and rigorous techniques of the scientific method and statistical process control

to understand the elements of CQI and how they align with the organization's priorities, as well as how using appropriate tools and techniques can ensure the success of PI initiatives. Additional training in PI methods, tools, team leadership, project management, and process analysis will support the spread of CQI approaches throughout the organization.

The desired outcomes of CQI at any organization cannot be achieved until the staff is mobilized to carry out specific improvement initiatives. Mobilizing staff might involve creating personnel policies that motivate and support staff participation in PI and may even include requiring all managers and supervisors to serve as PI team leads. It could also be as simple as encouraging staff participation in PI activities as a professional growth and development opportunity. Staff participation may also be promoted through rewarding those who participate on a team or rewarding teams for achieving excellent outcomes.

The value of using a collaborative team approach in the PI process is well established. The team approach supports improved outcomes by improving team inputs and outputs and promoting multidisciplinary sharing of knowledge and ideas. Though the general priorities and goals of the CQI program may have been established at the organizational leadership level, these leaders are typically not the experts on how to address the specific problems identified at the process or operational level. Quality problems are often not visible to individuals at senior management levels; rather, the individuals who are actually doing the work are most aware of the problems and will have the greatest insights into root causes and potential solutions.

Performance improvement methodologies such as the **plan-do-study-act (PDSA)** cycle provide teams with a basic process and a set of tools that can be applied to a variety of improvement initiatives (The W. Edwards Deming Institutes, 2014). However, when projects become large and complex, even teams that are made up of subject matter experts on the problem being evaluated may not have the analytical skills needed to collect, analyze, and interpret project-related data. Some organizations with robust CQI programs may have analytical staff available to assist larger and more complex project teams.

As one considers the key characteristics of CQI, it becomes clear that CQI is both a management philosophy and a management method. As a management philosophy, CQI takes an organizational perspective:

setting direction and promoting strategically aligned improvement initiatives through leadership support, organizational learning, and resource allocation. As a management method, CQI provides a framework for identifying improvement opportunities and managing PI teams tasked with analyzing problems so that solutions can be identified and implemented; in this way, desired results are achieved.

As you read this chapter, keep in mind that the principles, tools, and approaches that comprise CQI are not limited to organization-wide implementations. CQI may be integrated on a smaller scale within a department or a business unit to obtain desired results and drive your team's continuous improvement efforts.

A Short History of Continuous Quality Improvement

A brief review of the origins of CQI may provide a useful context for understanding the movement of CQI into health care. Most histories of CQI credit Walter Shewhart, W. Edwards Deming, and Joseph Juran with providing major contributions to the CQI field that are still in use today. Such contributions include statistical process control and control charts, the plan-do-check-act (PDCA) cycle, and the Pareto chart, which are discussed later in the chapter. CQI actually has roots that go much further back in history to Sir Francis Bacon's time in the 16th century. Sir Francis Bacon believed the process of knowledge generation should follow a planned structure and proceed through observation and inductive reasoning instead of through deductive reasoning that was common during the time. This philosophy went on to influence thinkers in subsequent generations, one of which was Walter Shewhart.

Walther Shewhart was an American physicist, statistician, and engineer who worked at Bell Telephone during the early 1900s on efforts to improve reliability in the company's processes and systems. At the time, Bell Telephone was struggling with how to reduce variation in its manufacturing processes in a cost-effective manner. Although there was an inspection program in place to ensure finished goods were not defective before delivering them to consumers, the process was costly and only somewhat effective. Walter Shewhart introduced the concepts of **statistical process control** and **control charts** to monitor and

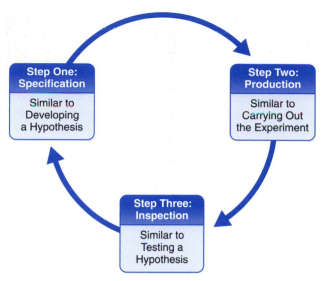

Figure ■ 13-1   The Shewhart Cycle.

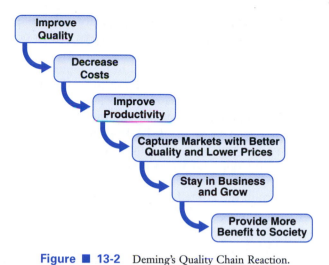

Figure ■ 13-2   Deming's Quality Chain Reaction.

more economically manage their processes. Following the belief that knowledge generation should follow a planned approach, he also developed a three-step scientific process of specification, production, and introspection (Figure 13-1) and likened the process to the scientific method of hypothesizing, carrying out an experiment, and testing the hypothesis. This process is often referred to as the Shewhart cycle (Moen & Norman, 2010).

In the 1950s, W. Edwards Deming worked in Japan on efforts to rebuild the country's industry and economy post-WWII. He implemented a statistical approach to quality improvement, expanded on the Shewhart cycle, and developed the Deming wheel or circle. The Deming wheel focuses on the interaction among four steps: design, production, sales, and research (Moen & Norman, 2010):

- *Design:* Design the product.
- *Production:* Make the product and test in the production line and in the laboratory.
- *Sales:* Sell the product.
- *Research:* Test the product in service and through market research.

Deming's concepts are widely credited with turning an industrial economy known for low-tech, low-quality, and low-priced goods into one known for producing high-tech, high-quality, and often high-priced goods. Deming introduced what he called the quality

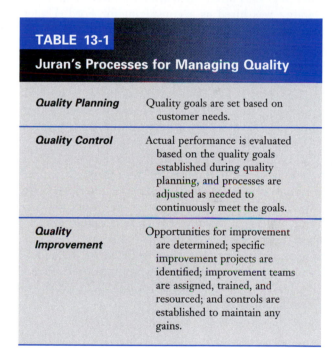

TABLE 13-1	
Juran's Processes for Managing Quality	
Quality Planning	Quality goals are set based on customer needs.
Quality Control	Actual performance is evaluated based on the quality goals established during quality planning, and processes are adjusted as needed to continuously meet the goals.
Quality Improvement	Opportunities for improvement are determined; specific improvement projects are identified; improvement teams are assigned, trained, and resourced; and controls are established to maintain any gains.

chain reaction (Figure 13-2), which drew a direct connection between an organization's improved quality and improved financial status. The Deming wheel later evolved into the PDCA cycle (Moen & Norman, 2010).

Joseph Juran was also working in post-WWII Japan independently of Deming. Juran developed additional CQI principles such as the **Pareto principle,** where 80% of the problems come from 20% of the causes, and "managing for quality" (Table 13-1), which included the three processes of quality planning, quality control, and quality improvement (Juran & Godfrey, 1999).

The Japanese also contributed to developments in CQI that continue to have an impact today (Sollecito & Johnson, 2013). For example, the fishbone cause-and-effect diagram, developed by Kaoru Ishikawa and sometimes referred to as an Ishikawa diagram, continues to be used today as a mainstay tool in CQI efforts. Although CQI was accepted and largely successful in Japanese industry, it did not gain popular acceptance in the United States until the 1980s, after American industry lost major market share for products such as automobiles and electronics between 1950 and 1980.

After a documentary entitled *If Japan Can, Why Can't We?* was aired on national television in 1980, Deming was hired as a consultant for Ford. Under his guidance, CQI principles were used and led to the production of the Ford Taurus, the car that is credited for turning Ford around. Concurrently, Juran facilitated relationships between Japan and U.S. industry leaders and founded the Juran Institute quality-consulting firm in 1979. Since that time, several other companies have adopted and profited from using a CQI approach.

In 1986, Deming amended his description of PDCA to emphasize the importance of reflecting on the meaning of, or studying, whatever metrics you're "checking," and thus the plan-do-study-act (PDSA) model emerged. With this change, Deming emphasized the importance of not just checking your new process, but using that knowledge to better understand the product or process being improved. PDSA took hold as a natural evolution of PDCA (Moen & Norman, 2010).

History of Quality Improvement in Health Care

The adoption of CQI in health care has been fostered by standards from accrediting bodies such as The Joint Commission (TJC) and the Commission on Accreditation of Rehabilitation Facilities (CARF). Many accreditation standards include elements related to customer satisfaction and quality of care. The shift to the CQI approach has also been a move away from the previously dominant quality assurance (QA) approach.

In a typical QA approach, the focus was on gathering data on what were assumed to be stable processes and taking action only when major problems were identified or when outcomes fell below predetermined target levels. In a CQI approach, the focus is not only on monitoring the performance of a process, but on identifying opportunities to improve the process, ideally before major problems occur or outcomes fall below target levels.

What Is Quality?

To this point, the term *quality* has been used numerous times without discussing what the term means. According to Joseph Juran, quality includes those features of a product or service that meet customer needs and contribute to customer satisfaction. Quality can be tied to income in that providing a higher-quality product or service increases customer satisfaction and leads to higher profit (Juran & Godfrey, 1999). A brief discussion on ways to conceptualize quality products and services will be helpful before delving further into specific CQI concepts, strategies, tools, and techniques.

When you ask someone to define quality, you will most likely be asked for further clarification of what you mean. This is because the definition of quality is greatly context-dependent. For example, how might you define quality in relation to the following products and services?

- Purchasing a piece of clothing
- Buying a meal at a restaurant
- Having your car serviced by an automotive mechanic
- Checking into a hotel for a vacation
- Going to an appointment with your primary care physician

Undoubtedly, the definition will vary for each situation, and likely more information will be needed such as:

- What sort of clothing?
- Is it a fast-food restaurant or a fine-dining establishment?
- Is it for routine auto service or is there a specific problem?
- Is it a discount hotel or a 5-star resort?

- Is it for a routine check-up or is there a specific problem?

In addition to value (the relationship between cost and quality), they would also likely consider other aspects of each product or service (i.e., performance characteristics) in determining the quality of the product or service they purchased. Performance characteristics are often tied to customer requirements and expectations and can include timeliness of service, politeness of staff, and specific product qualities (e.g., color, texture, taste, etc.). Sample performance characteristics are shown in Table 13-2.

As customer satisfaction is a key consideration on CQI, and customer requirements and expectations for quality can change over time, how might you determine what your customers want on any given day? You could do this through a concept called the "five Cs" of valid customer requirements (Box 13-2). The "five Cs" involve meeting requirements that are current, calculable, completeable, consensus-based, and consistent with your organizational goals. "Valid" is included in the concept as well, because sometimes customer requirements are unrealistic, not in line with your ideas, or unachievable because of resources or other limitations.

Consider the following example. The process of admitting a patient to a hospital inpatient unit can be measured in several ways. At the basic level, you can measure the time it takes from when the patient arrives at the hospital to when he or she is assigned to an inpatient bed. However, preparing a hospital bed to be clean and ready for a new patient is a complex process in itself that involves many departments. If you've ever arrived at a hotel only to be told that there were no clean rooms available yet, you've probably felt annoyed.

As preparing a bed in a sterilized hospital environment is probably more complicated and time-consuming than readying a hotel room for a new guest, imagine how a patient who may be in discomfort would feel knowing there was a wait for the bed. So how long is it appropriate for a patient to wait to be assigned to an inpatient bed? Although the answer may vary based on patient need (e.g., is this a planned admission? Is the patient being admitted for an urgent need?), one can use the five Cs for valid customer requirements to arrive at an answer.

In the example, the turnaround time for the admission process should be *current* with those at other facilities. You can determine the turnaround times for other facilities through the process of benchmarking (comparing a current level of performance to the performance of others) or though collecting and analyzing your own historical data. The fact that you can collect and analyze data to determine turnaround time indicates that the admission time requirement is *calculable* (i.e., measurable). Additionally, your admission time goal should be realistic and able to be reasonably accomplished or *completeable*. A patient who expects to be taken immediately to an inpatient bed without first stopping at the admission desk might have a requirement of zero wait time. In most hospitals, this is unrealistic or not reasonable, as patients need to be checked into the hospital system before being placed in an inpatient bed. In this case, the zero wait time

---

TABLE 13-2

Sample Performance Characteristics to Help Define Quality

• Timeliness	• Reliability	• Safety
• Courtesy	• Ecological impact	• Accessibility
• Availability	• Accuracy	• Professionalism
• Price	• Waste	• Follow-up
• Technical support	• Durability	• Flexibility

BOX 13-2

The Five Cs of Valid Customer Requirements

- **Current:** They are consistent with today's competitors and benchmarks.
- **Calculable:** They can be measured.
- **Completeable:** They can be reasonable and realistically accomplished.
- **Consensus-based:** They are identified and supported by key stakeholders involved in the process; includes consideration of resources and resource limitations.
- **Consistent with organizational goals:** They are consistent with the organization's mission and vision.

requirement is not a valid requirement. However, a patient with a preplanned admission might expect to complete minimal paperwork at admission, which would minimize wait time. This could be a valid customer requirement when looking for opportunities to shorten wait times.

A *consensus-based* customer requirement is usually identified by obtaining input from all internal stakeholders involved in the process. In the admission wait time example, consensus on customer requirements might be obtained through input from representatives from admission, housekeeping, and patient transportation. (Patient transportation is responsible for moving patients from place to place within a hospital system.) Gaps between customer requirements and realistic staff performance can be examined closely by those representatives, and appropriate targets can be set based on consensus. Lastly, a valid customer requirement for any organization must be in line with or *consistent* with organizational goals. In our example, the customer requirement for minimal wait time for admission is in line with most hospital goals.

In most organizations, including health-care organizations, CQI is focused mainly on measuring and improving performance in key work processes, with key work processes being repeatable elements of daily work that are critical to the organization's success. The remainder of this chapter includes common CQI concepts, strategies, and tools that are used successfully in organizations and in health-care settings.

CQI as a Management Philosophy

Successfully introducing CQI as a management philosophy and approach to quality improvement at an organization-wide level is a major endeavor. Its wide scale use requires advanced planning and investment of a great amount of organizational resources such as time and money. It is also a developmental process that must evolve over time. Integrating CQI on a smaller scale (e.g., in a rehabilitation services department within a larger organization) will require less time and fewer resources; however, it still requires advanced planning and preparation.

The process of fully integrating CQI at an organization or within a department can be conceptualized in four stages as illustrated in Figure 13-3. In the first stage, leadership must create readiness for CQI by building awareness of the need to operate differently. Highlighting current problems with organizational or departmental effectiveness or efficiency can help to create a state of readiness for process improvement. This may be accomplished by providing specific examples of customer dissatisfaction, or showing the negative impacts of process inefficiencies such as waste and rework.

Another strategy for creating a *state of readiness* is to discuss CQI success with staff. Look to your peers and the literature to find case studies of companies or organizations that have made significant process improvements. Professional organization publications such as the *American Journal of Occupational Therapy* or more CQI-focused journals such as the National Association for Healthcare Quality's *Journal for Healthcare Quality* commonly include write-ups on industry best practices and case studies of organizations that have made significant process improvements. Professional association meetings and conferences provide an opportunity to network and share performance data with peers. In the case of Rehab-World, which is part of a national chain of occupational therapy providers,

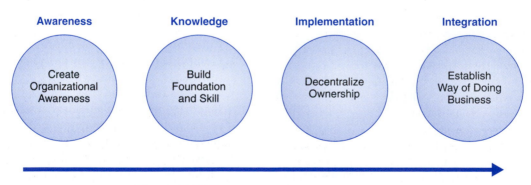

Figure ■ 13-3   The Stages of CQI Implementation.

there exists the opportunity to network and compare performance with peers within the organization. Once the organization or department is ready to explore CQI opportunities, the second stage involves building a foundation of knowledge and skills by providing education and training in CQI basics.

Depending on the level at which you are bringing CQI into your organization, careful planning for both the order and the extent of initial training is important. CQI is sometimes referred to as both a *top-down and a bottom-up* philosophy. It is considered to be a *top-down* philosophy because CQI may not be as successful in an organization if leadership does not fully buy into the CQI approach and does not role model usage of the key concepts, strategies, tools, and techniques. For this reason, it may be prudent to focus early training efforts on leadership or supervisors before training frontline staff. CQI can also be considered a *bottom-up* philosophy because it focuses on involving employees closest to the work and work processes in making the improvements regardless of the employee's level in the organization. In other words, frontline staff should be involved in CQI efforts. For this reason, providing education that focuses on the basic philosophy of CQI and presents key concepts, strategies, tools, and techniques at an introductory level for frontline staff is advisable. More in-depth training on specifics can be reserved until later and often provided just before it is needed (e.g., "just-in-time" training).

Once a foundation of knowledge and skills is built, the third stage is decentralizing ownership of CQI from organization leadership to all levels of the organization. This is achieved by setting the organization up for success. Two ways to accomplish this are to choose initial projects that are relatively simple and to be sure not to take on too many projects at one time. Taking on the organization's or department's most significant problems may be tempting. However, these types of projects are often large or complex and can contribute to frustration and disappointment if things don't go exactly as planned. Beginning with a small and easily achievable demonstration project where employees can experience success and see the value of CQI will foster confidence. Another common pitfall early on is starting more CQI teams than you can properly train and facilitate. Early excitement can lead to diffused efforts focusing in too many directions, which may result in

frustration and skepticism with the entire CQI philosophy.

After a strong foundation of skills and knowledge have been established, initial projects have been carefully implemented and supported, and all levels of the organization or department are involved, the focus can shift to the fourth stage of ongoing support of processes to fully integrate CQI into daily work, with the ultimate goal being that CQI becomes *a way of doing business*. Indicators that this is happening in your organization include:

- A constant focus on *customers and customer satisfaction* by employees at all levels,
- Staff readiness for change and process improvement,
- Application of CQI concepts, strategies, tools, and techniques within and outside of formal CQI efforts or teams becomes standard operating procedure, and
- A shared belief that taking longer to make the right decision based on data is better than making a fast decision based on speculation.

Identifying Quality Improvement Opportunities

In the previous section, we discussed the importance of selecting the right projects for your CQI teams to take on to foster a sense of confidence with their CQI skills and abilities. Moving forward on your CQI journey, it continues to be important to put a good deal of thought into the projects that are selected. Assembling a team to address a problem requires time, effort, and oftentimes additional resources, so there is always a cost involved. The goal is to ensure that the project's outcome, whether it is dollars saved, efficiencies gained, or improved patient satisfaction, is worth the investment of resources you will make to achieve that outcome.

Determining what projects to take on requires that you assess your organization's current performance in order to identify where the opportunities for improvement lie. According to Juran, "improvement" means "the organized creation of beneficial change; the attainment of unprecedented levels of performance" (Juran & Godfrey, 1999). He identified two types of beneficial change that involve *improving product features* and *freedom from deficiencies*.

Improving product features increases customer satisfaction and can be measured in terms of:

- Customer satisfaction (e.g., satisfaction with therapy practitioner knowledge, helpfulness, or courtesy)
- Reduction of cycle time (e.g., time from date of referral to date of first appointment)
- Number of complaints (e.g., patient complaints with wait times, delays, or billing errors)
- Productivity levels (e.g., billable units or therapy practitioner per day)

Freedom from deficiencies is a means by which to reduce customer dissatisfaction with a product or service and to eliminate waste. Deficiencies can be measured in terms of:

- Compliance (e.g., lack of adherence to policy or regulatory requirements)
- Patient safety (e.g., patient falls)
- Quality (e.g., undesired outcomes of care)

With a better awareness of your organization's performance, you are now ready to determine what CQI projects to focus on. As stated earlier, these types of projects require the investment of time and resources, so the projects selected must demonstrate value to the organization. Several factors should be considered when prioritizing which improvement activities will have the most impact. The alignment of improvement activities to the organization's mission and vision, department priorities, regulatory requirements, and governmental mandates allows for focus on projects that impact the organization's most critical issues. Operational performance metrics that demonstrate performance is below expectation should trigger an opportunity to investigate and develop action plans for improvement.

At this point you have some ideas for where you need to focus your CQI efforts and resources. The next step is developing a business case. Depending on how well CQI is integrated into your organization, you may be required to present a formal project business case to an organizational quality council for approval. A formal project business case includes information such as the project aim, the data that will be collected and how the data will be collected, who will be on the team, and the anticipated return on investment. In an organization where formal CQI project approval processes do not exist, you may simply use the business case as a tool to communicate to your staff why taking on this improvement is important. The business case should address the specific problem you are trying to solve, why solving this problem is important to the organization, the outcome you want to achieve, and the resources that will be required to achieve the outcome.

Building a strong business case requires bringing together the right data and supporting information. Let's assume the problem you want to address is that patients are unsatisfied with how long it takes to get an appointment. Some questions to consider are: "*Why are wait times important?*" "*How unsatisfied are they?*" "*Has it gotten worse?*" "*How do our wait times compare to Organization X?*" "*How much of an improvement do you think you can make?*" Your business case should concisely answer these kinds of questions.

Now imagine how you might answer those questions.

- "*Why are wait times important?*" Establishing itself as a leader in patient satisfaction is a strategic priority for this new Rehab-World location.
- "*How unsatisfied are they? Is it getting worse?*" Our patient satisfaction survey is showing us that only 37% of patients are satisfied with the wait time for appointments, and this score has been steadily decreasing over the past 6 months.
- "*How do our wait times compare to Organization X?*" When we look across the Rehab-World locations in our region, our patient satisfaction scores on wait time lag behind by over 40%. The Rehab-World dashboard shows our average patient wait time for an appointment to be 11 days compared with the regional Rehab-World average of 3 days.
- "*How much of an improvement do you think you can make?*" Establishing a measurable goal allows the leadership and a project team to know if the project had a measurable impact. In this example, the team's focus for measurement may be increasing patient satisfaction from 37% to 75% or reducing patient wait times for appointments from 11 days to 3 days.

If the data exist, you can even build a financial case for the project. For example, Rehab-World data show that patient satisfaction directly correlates to new patient referrals. Therefore, keeping current patients satisfied will help Rehab-World be more competitive in the local market and will drive the future business of this Rehab-World location. If you have access to the data, you can even demonstrate how the successful outcome of your project can be translated into dollars. For example, with sufficient data you might be able to state, "It has been estimated that each 5% increase in patient satisfaction translates into an addition $1.5 million in patient revenue per year."

The information provided in the business case should meet the needs of your organization's quality council and your departmental leadership, as well as your project team members. It clearly articulates to everyone the project's importance and why it is a worthwhile investment of resources. Understanding that is just as important to the regional manager who will approve the commitment of staff resources to the project as it is to the occupational therapist (OT) whom you will ask to be a member of the team because both of them, in their own way, are making a determination of whether or not this project is worth the effort.

Forming a QI Team

Once an improvement project has been identified, a project's success can be determined by including the right people on the project team. Team members should include individuals familiar with the various parts of the systems or processes that will be affected by the improvement project. To be effective, teams should also include members representing three different types of expertise with the organization: system leadership, technical expertise, and day-to-day leadership. Sometimes overlooked, but essential for each team, is to have an executive sponsor who takes responsibility for the project's success. Obtaining executive sponsorship provides the green light to proceed with project goals, helps to ensure alignment with institutional or departmental goals, and provides a top-level individual to present high-level updates on the project status to ensure awareness of project activities and focus on the stated goals. An example of a team with the right people on board can be seen in the following example.

Several nurses on the physical medicine and rehabilitation (PM&R) team noted inconsistencies regarding the response times of the physical therapy and occupational therapy practitioners to the electronic referrals for service and reported their findings to a rehabilitation services manager. The rehabilitation services manager brought the concern back to her team to conduct an analysis of what was taking place. Based on nursing feedback and rehabilitation services' initial brainstorming meeting, as well as inconsistencies with the physical and occupational therapy practitioners receiving the electronic referrals, the team noted (1) the delay of services impacted, (2) patient and PM&R team dissatisfaction, (3) problems with the system that resulted in delays or electronic referrals not being received, and (4) delays in service that impacted patient flow (patients' discharges and admissions).

The rehabilitation services recommendation was to form a team to confirm the problem and to make recommendations to address the issue. The rehabilitation services manager met with the director of rehabilitation to obtain further support and executive sponsorship. The vice president of clinical services responsible for oversight of patient throughput agreed to sponsor the project. In addition to a representative from occupational therapy, other team members invited to join the team were a PM&R nurse, the physician and administrative clerk involved in initiating a referral once the physician orders were written, an information technology (IT) representative, and a PI consultant to assist with the facilitation of meetings. All of these individuals confirmed their invitation except the PM&R physician, who had a scheduling conflict. However, she identified one of her PM&R residents to participate on the team. The membership on this team demonstrates a diverse representation that will allow the team to begin effectively conducting a **root cause analysis** of the problem. After completing a thorough analysis of the problem, the team may identify additional team members to add to the team or content expert consultants to include as needed.

To maximize the effectiveness of teams, a number of different team roles are often identified and utilized. These roles are the team leader, a facilitator, a recorder or scribe, a timekeeper, and members. The roles of team leader and facilitator typically remain relatively stable for the life of the team, but the roles of timekeeper and recorder can rotate among team members. The functions of these roles are summarized in Box 13-3. These roles are flexible; they may be combined or omitted, or may overlap, in different organizations. However, it is important that these roles be identified and addressed before the team begins meeting on a regular basis. How successful is your team likely to be if no one is in charge of leading the

BOX 13-3

Standing Roles for a CQI Team

- **Team leader:** Guides the team through the CQI process, sets meeting agendas and leads meetings, provides "just-in-time" training to the team, and liaises with organization leadership.
- **Team facilitator:** Assists team leader with his or her role; monitors group process and shares observations with the team to improve effectiveness; reminds the team of the PDSA cycle and critical concepts, strategies, tools, and techniques; helps the team stay focused within the boundaries of the process being investigated; and advises which CQI tools to use and provides training in tool use and CQI application.
- **Timekeeper:** Helps to keep the team on track by helping to assure that meetings begin and end on time and gives warnings to the team if they are running over time for an agenda topic or if the meeting is nearing the end.
- **Scribe:** Takes notes or minutes of the meeting to document team progress and distributes notes to team members for review; also writes on a board or flip chart during activities such as brainstorming.

BOX 13-4

Commonly Used Ground Rules for Meetings

- Start and end meetings on time.
- Show mutual respect.
- Arrive with between-meetings assignments completed.
- Stay on task; no side conversations should occur.
- Listen to others and don't interrupt.
- Follow an agenda.
- Operate on consensus—seek general agreements all can "live with."
- Make decisions based on clear information.
- Bring closure to decisions.
- Identify actions that result from decisions.
- Ensure committee members will support committee recommendations.
- Agree on what information goes "out" and what stays in the group.
- Accept the fact that there will be differences of opinion.
- Honor brainstorming without being attached to just one viewpoint.
- Attack the problem, not the person—no "blame game."
- Share time so that all can participate.
- Be free to speak minds without fear of reprisal.
- Don't attribute ideas to individuals.
- Put pagers, phones, and other electronic devices on vibrate and leave the room to answer a call or message.
- Realize it is okay to have fun, laugh, and enjoy the time spent at meetings.

meetings, taking minutes, or keeping the team on schedule?

To ensure that everyone is clear about the roles and responsibilities of all members during the first meeting, it is important that the team leader and facilitator review the team roles with the team members. Introducing ground rules during the first meeting is very beneficial for setting expectations for team behavior. Establishing ground rules such as starting and ending on time, respecting each other's opinions, and accepting that disagreement is a healthy part of the process provides members with a sense of confidence and security that you value them, their time, and their voice. A sample of team ground rules for meetings can be found in Box 13-4.

With your team assembled and roles defined, it is time to get down to business and to lay out the overall

plan for the project team. Unlike routine work such as seeing patients, by definition, a project is a planned set of activities designed to achieve a particular outcome. It has a distinct beginning and a distinct ending, or boundaries. This is known as the project scope. When establishing a project team, it is important to identify the project scope so that all team members understand where the project begins and the expected end of the project to prevent the project from expanding beyond the outlined scope, known as scope-creep. A project team should clearly know if the project will focus on an entire process or a portion of the project, as well as if it will impact an entire department or a smaller pilot area. Addressing these questions will help keep the project team on target regarding the project's focus and prevent expanding or unexpected project costs because of unclear project parameters.

Regardless if the teams that come together to work on improvement projects are temporary, newly formed teams or groups of members who have worked together in the past, Bruce Tuckerman's research on the theory of group dynamics suggests teams on the path to high performance experience the following stages: *forming, storming, norming,* and *performing.* Later, he added a fifth stage, *adjourning,* which some have described as *mourning.*

The *forming* stage is often short and has been described as the "honeymoon" period. Team members are anxious about what the project entails and their role on the project. They are polite and positive, still trying to figure things out regarding the project and the other team members. At this stage, individual roles and responsibilities are not clear and the team will need the leaders to provide clear aims and objectives.

The *storming* stage is where the team leader's authority may be challenged. Different ideas are competing for consideration. Tension, confrontations, and conflict can occur. This stage can make team members uncomfortable and overwhelmed with the process and the lack of clarity. If not handled appropriately, some teams are not able to develop past this stage. Although storming is difficult, it is necessary for the team's growth. The team lead will need to remain available to members, role model professional behavior, and guide them through the difficult decision-making process.

As the team members begin to respect one another and their leader's authority, the team is entering into the *norming* stage. The team feels more comfortable sharing ideas, receiving constructive feedback, and offering commitment to the project goal. This stage is where you begin to see progress. Once the team members have gotten to know one another better and establish relationships, members sometimes focus too much effort on avoiding conflict rather than sharing controversial ideas. Because the focus has been placed on group harmony or conformity to this point, the team decisions may not be based on critical evaluation of alternative ideas or viewpoints. There are several

strategies that the team leader can use to address this issue; for example, group members may rotate in the role of "devil's advocate" to ensure different perspectives are considered when making decisions.

Once the team reaches the *performing* stage, it is able to function as a unit, the team members' motivation and confidence about the task at hand is secure, and their efforts demonstrate progress. The team lead is able to delegate because the team is competent and capable of making decisions without supervision. Conflict is managed without any major problem. As new tasks come up, changes occur in leadership, and so on, some teams may revert back to storming, but at this stage it usually does not prevail.

As the project goals are completed or a team is disbanded, the team experiences the *adjourning* or *mourning* stage. The stage can be stressful for some team members, resulting in ambivalent feelings. The stress or feelings could be related to working together and developing close relationships and knowing that they will not be having that experience in the future or feeling that the team did not fully accomplish what they needed to do. It is important for the team lead to acknowledge the team's work, recognize contributions, and formally close out the project.

Effectively leading a team can be difficult, and some organizations or departments may invest considerable resources in training team leaders. An in-depth discussion of strategies for developing and leading teams effectively is beyond the scope of this chapter. However, you may find a brief introduction to the stages of team development helpful (Box 13-5). For more information on leading teams and running meetings (such as the use of ground rules to guide member behavior in meetings), you are encouraged to refer to the resources at the end of the chapter. An especially helpful resource is *The Team Handbook,* a "how to manual for inexperienced managers" (Scholtes, Joiner, & Streibel, 2003).

Plan-Do-Study-Act (PDSA)

Now that you have assembled your team, assigned roles, and clarified the scope of the project, it is time to get to the task at hand and solve your problem. The plan-do-study-act cycle (PDSA) (Figure 13-4) is a *systematic, repeatable,* and *teamwork-based* process for solving problems or realizing opportunities for enhanced performance at the organizational, system,

BOX 13-5

CQI Team Participants and Their Roles

Executive Sponsor

1. Provides support and guidance to the team at the organizational level.
2. Approves necessary resources for the team to do its work and be successful.
3. Facilitates communication and involvement of departments not included as regular team members.

Team Leader

1. Sets up job responsibility and keeps team members focused on accomplishing tasks.
2. Models all the behaviors desired in team members.
3. Guides the team through the problem-solving process.
4. Participates as an active, voting member during meetings.
5. Discusses the progress, direction, and problems of the team.
6. Obtains input concerning major activities, problem analysis, solutions, proposals, and pilot projects.
7. Arranges follow-up meeting times, locations, and agenda.

Facilitator

1. Acts as a neutral member of the team.
2. Focuses energy of the team on a common task (helps the team solve the problem).
3. Suggests alternative methods.
4. Protects individuals and their ideas from attack (with help from the team).
5. Encourages participation.
6. Helps the team find win/win situations.
7. Does not take responsibility for answering all the questions—the answers are in the team.
8. Does not pretend to know your business—does understand team building and improvement tools and concepts.
9. Speaks his or her mind and may "shoot from the hip" to increase awareness; all comments are meant to be helpful.
10. Reminds the team that it's their responsibility to use the facilitator well.

Recorder or Scribe

1. Supports the facilitator.
2. Listens, then writes.
3. Does not evaluate or edit.
4. Writes briefly.
5. Records on flip chart if needed.
6. Prepares meeting minutes.

Timekeeper

1. Helps the team keep on track with meetings by beginning and ending on time.
2. Gives warnings to the team members if they are running over time for an agenda topic or if the meeting is nearing the end.

Team Member

1. Participates as an active, voting member during meetings.
2. Takes on assignments as assigned.

process, and employee levels in order to achieve desired results. The PDSA cycle is shorthand for testing a change—by planning it, trying it, observing the results, and acting on what is learned. The beauty of the PDSA cycle is its scalability to projects of any size or complexity. At the most basic level, the PDSA cycle offers as simple four-step approach to identifying and addressing a PI issue. This model can also be applied to larger and more complex problems because it also mirrors the scientific method of hypothesizing, carrying out an experiment, and testing the hypothesis.

There are two key things you should notice about the PDSA cycle. First, it is a cycle, which means getting to the level of performance you are striving for may require "going around" the cycle more than once. For example, if you implemented a solution you believed would reduce customer complaints by 50% and your solution only achieved a 20% improvement, the team should repeat the PDSA cycle to build upon

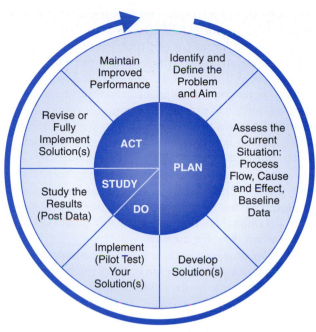

Figure ■ 13-4 The Plan-Do-Study-Act (PDSA) Cycle.

important steps. The team members will first identify the problem they are trying to solve and brainstorm potential solutions during the plan phase. The do phase involves testing a solution either as a small-scale pilot test or a full implementation. Determining the effectiveness of a solution is the focus of the study phase. Based on the outcome of the study phase, the team makes a determination of how to act or proceed forward. If the solution was effective, the team will move forward with its implementation. If it fell short, the team may need to go around the PDSA cycle again and test other potential solutions.

Plan the Change to Be Tested or Implemented

By far, the plan phase is the project's most important phase and is also the step most teams tend to underestimate. Many teams feel planning is boring and takes too long. If the team members "know" what the solution is, why can't they just dive in and start fixing the problem? When teams jump into action without having a clear understanding of the problem, the extent of the problem (data), and its key causes, it is likely that a lot of time will be spent putting Band-Aids on the problem or even having to solve the same problem over and over again because the team didn't effectively address the problem's root cause.

It may sound simple, but the first step is making sure the team has identified the problem. Having an agreed upon and common understanding of the problem is critical. That is why one of the first things a team should do is draft a *problem statement*. A problem statement concisely identifies the problem and only the problem; it is not intended to identify the problem's cause or solution. Imagine that you are the team lead and you say, "OK team, we are here to improve the problem we are having with the way the doctors are ordering our services. Let's get to work." What are the odds that everyone sitting around the table has the same mental picture of the problem? For example, Mary may be thinking it's a paperwork problem; there is always missing patient information. Joe may be thinking how frustrating it is to receive orders 5 minutes before closing. Jen is sure the problem is doctors' offices not verifying insurance before they make the referral. It may sound silly, but the reality is that the team lead must make sure the team members are all on the same page when it comes to understanding the problem they are there to address.

what has been learned about the process so far and work to design further enhancements. The second key observation is that the circle is not sliced into four equal quadrants. The cycle's planning component takes up half the circle. That's because investment in the project's planning stage will set you and your team up for future success. It is human nature to want to skip past the planning and spring into action to fix a problem. However, if the team doesn't take the time to truly understand the problem and the variables that are contributing to the problem, chances are you will find yourselves "solving" this same problem over and over again.

> *Plan:* the change to be tested or implemented
> *Do:* carry out the test or change
> *Study:* data before and after the change and reflect on what was learned
> *Act:* plan the next change cycle or full implementation

The plan-do-study-act (PDSA) cycle is a scalable model that can be used to manage improvement projects of any size. Using this four-phased model provides project teams with a road map to improvement that can be used to keep the team on track, and, most importantly, prevent the team from skipping over

Writing a problem statement is deceptively simple; after all, it is just one brief statement. However, it is important to ensure that this statement captures the problem's main focus and that it is understood and agreed upon by everyone on the team. Keep your problem statement clear and concise. Be sure not to include the causes—we will get to that—and do not include the solution. So, let's consider the problem of doctors' orders. What is the problem with the doctors' orders? Are they late? Missing? Incomplete? For the purposes of this example, let's say that the problem is "Doctors' orders are incomplete." To further clarify the problem statement, the team needs to agree on what the word *incomplete* means. This may seem like minutia, but at this point of the project, it is critical that everyone has a common understanding of the problem. It is agreed upon that "incomplete" means any missing data that will require the therapist to contact the doctor's office before being able to proceed with the patient evaluation.

Now that the team members have agreed on the problem they are working on, the next step is to assess the situation. This requires collecting data that will tell you more about the problem, such as frequency and causation. Before collecting any data, the team members should *brainstorm* ideas about what they would need to know about the problem to help them develop effective solutions, such as: How many incomplete orders do we receive? Who is sending them? When are they coming in? What data are missing? Considering these kinds of questions is critical to the development of a good data collection plan.

Brainstorming is a simple tool that can be used to generate ideas or gather feedback. It can be spontaneous, with people blurting out ideas, or it can be a formal process where the facilitator poses a question to the group and members provide ideas in an organized fashion as the facilitator captures the ideas on a flip chart. One approach is to go around the table and have each member contribute an idea to the list. Members may choose to add a new idea, piggyback or build on an existing idea, or pass if they don't have anything else to add. Continue to go around the table until you have collected all the ideas. If you find that some members on your team are not comfortable speaking up in front of the group, provide the participants with Post-it notes and allow them to place their ideas up on the flip chart. The most important rule of brainstorming is to focus on the collection, not the judgment, of ideas. Keep the ideas flowing rather than stopping to make suggestions or critique whether an idea is valid or not. Think quantity.

Measuring the extent of a problem requires having an objective measure, which means the problem is something you can observe; this is called *operationalizing*. By creating a clear problem statement and operationalizing what an incomplete order is (missing data that will require the therapist to contact the doctor's office before being able to proceed with the patient evaluation), the team can objectively identify and therefore measure when an order is incomplete. Just like the team members identified what "incomplete" meant, it is also important that they identify the specific data elements that require a call to the doctor's office when they are missing.

It's now time for the team to develop a *data collection plan*. The data collection plan outlines the what, when, who, and how of the data collection process:

- What data need to be collected?
- When will the data be collected?
- Who will collect the data?
- How will the data be collected?

Using the questions the team members brainstormed regarding what they would want to know about the incomplete orders, the team can answer the "what data need to be collected" question. The team needs to know: how many orders came in, how many were incomplete, what data element(s) were missing, where the order originated from, and the day and time the order was received.

Determining when the data will be collected is another important consideration. The goal is to ensure that the sample of data is large enough to represent what is going on within the ordering process. The team should consider if ordering patterns are fairly consistent or if some days of the week or weeks of the month are busier than others. Do all clients refer patients fairly regularly (several per week) or does their business fluctuate? Do more orders come during the morning than during the afternoon? There are many books available on data sampling and analysis. For our purposes, the goal of the data collection plan is simply to ensure that the data collected represent the ordering process.

It is important to identify who will collect the data for the purposes of consistency. Anyone involved in the data collection process needs to be trained on the data definitions, data collection plan, and how to use the data collection tools. This is particularly important if the data collection process is manual. As previously mentioned, those collecting the data need to know specifically what data elements to capture and how to capture the data. It may seem like an insignificant thing, but imagine that you are the one analyzing the data that were collected.

Consider this: You have collected data on 200 orders. One of the data elements the team wanted to look at was time of day of the order. Some of the people collecting the data used military time to collect the data, whereas other people used regular time. Someone else wrote "7" or "9" for the time. Is that 7 a.m. or 7 p.m.? Some of the data collectors rounded the time to the nearest 15-minute interval, whereas others rounded to the closest hour. So, if you want to know what time the problem orders are coming in, how do you figure that out? Collecting data manually can be a very labor-intensive process. Having a clearly defined procedure for collecting the data will prevent later problems with missing, incorrect, or just unusable data.

As you work on different projects, you will notice that *data sources* will vary. In some cases, organizational databases capture all the data you need. Getting the data can be as simple as querying the database or pulling a standardized report. In other cases, the data you need may require a manual collection process. The *check sheet* is a great tool to help standardize a manual data collection process. The check sheet is simply a standardized data collection worksheet. It should include instructions and is organized to make the data collection as consistent and easy as possible.

Once you have collected the data, it is time to analyze the data to determine what the data tell you about your problem. The first element to consider is the extent of the problem. How frequently is it occurring? This may be expressed as the number or rate of occurrences. Using our example of incomplete orders, you may want to look at how many times a day this is occurring, or what percentage of the total orders are incomplete. The data collected during the project's plan phase are your baseline data. These data tell you where you are, or how the process is functioning today. Displaying your data over time on a **run chart** (Figure 13-5) is a simple way to demonstrate current performance and shifts or trends in the data as the process is changed and improved.

Now it's time to dive more deeply into your data to determine what they reveal about the cause or causes

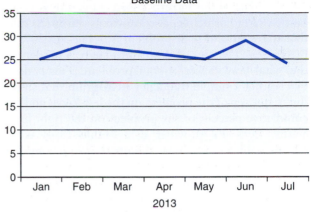

Run Chart of Number of Incomplete Orders Per Month: Baseline Data

Figure ■ 13-5   Run Chart.

TABLE 13-3	
Stratification of Data by Provider	

Provider	Number of Incomplete Orders
A	42
B	36
C	8
D	7
E	2

of your problem. **Stratification** (Table 13-3) is a way to look at your data by different groupings or categories to see if they reveal any root causes of your problem. The root cause is the fundamental, underlying reason for a problem and is what causes the problem to happen repeatedly. Remember that when you created your data collection plan for incomplete orders, you captured the data by provider, day of the week, and time of day. Look at your data and determine if there is a difference in the number of incomplete orders by day of the week, provider, or time of day. This is done simply by plotting the frequency of incomplete errors by the different strata. If, for instance, Provider A creates more incomplete orders than any other provider, the problem may reside with Provider A.

Another helpful tool to use when assessing your baseline data is the **Pareto chart**. This tool is based on the Pareto principle, also known as the 80/20 rule, that states 80% of your problem is because of 20% of the causes. The aim of the Pareto chart is to identify the "vital few" causes of your problem. This is done by creating a simple frequency **histogram** that shows the frequency of the problem on the left Y-axis and the cumulative percent of the problem on the right hand Y-axis. Let's use provider data (Table 13-4) as an example. This table shows the number of incomplete orders by provider in order of most to least.

Create a simple *frequency histogram* (Figure 13-6) using these data. Next, calculate the cumulative percent of the number of incomplete orders by provider. These data will be used to create the second Y-axis of your final Pareto chart (Figure 13-7).

The Pareto chart has given us further insight into the problem. We now know that Providers A and B have the most incomplete orders; together, they are causing 80% of our problem. What we don't know is why. What is different about Providers A and B that we receive so many incomplete orders from them? A handy tool for identifying causes for your problem is a cause-and-effect diagram, also known as a fishbone or Ishikawa diagram (Figure 13-8).

To create a **fishbone diagram,** the team begins by brainstorming all the causes of the problem you are trying to solve. In our case, the problem is "*too many incomplete orders.*" Write the problem on the right-hand side of a flip chart and draw a box around it. This is the "head" of your fish. Then draw the major "spines" of the fishbone diagram. Now it's clear to see where the name fishbone diagram comes from.

With the team, brainstorm the causes of the problem, which again is too many incomplete orders. Ask the team: "Why does this happen?" This may be done in a structured way, by giving the team categories of causes to brainstorm such as methods, machines and equipment, manpower (people), materials, measurement, and the environment. Label each of the "spines"

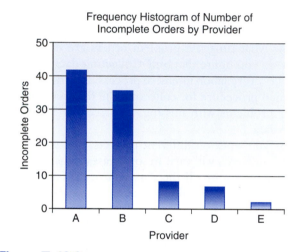

Figure ■ 13-6

Frequency Histogram of Number of Incomplete Orders by Provider.

TABLE 13-4

Cumulative Percent of the Number of Incomplete Orders by Provider

Provider	Number of Incomplete Orders	Cumulative Percent
A	42	44%
B	36	82%
C	8	89%
D	7	98%
E	2	100%
Total	95	

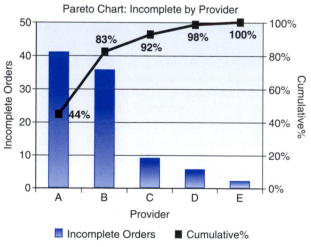

Figure ■ 13-7   Pareto Chart of Incomplete Orders by Provider.

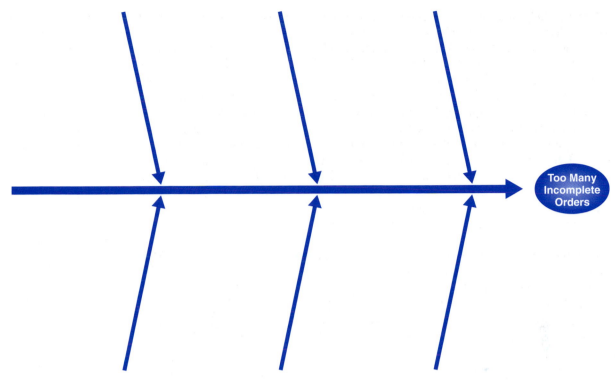

Figure ■ 13-8 Blank Cause-and-Effect (Fishbone or Ishikawa) Diagram.

of the fish with your categories, and create smaller bones to list the associated causes. For each cause, ask again: "Why does this happen?" to determine if there are any subcauses. Layers of branches off the main spines indicate the relationships of the causes and subcauses (Figure 13-9).

For example, if one identified cause of too many incomplete orders is "the ordering clinics don't understand why we need the information," ask the team: "Why does this happen?" again. The answer may be: "Because we don't train them." Keep asking "why" until you believe the team members have identified as many causes as they can.

Once the team members have brainstormed as many causes as they can and you have organized them by category onto a fishbone diagram, the team now has a clear picture of the problem and associated causes. With this information, the team can move on to the next step, which is identifying key or root causes.

Not all of the causes identified are the major drivers of your team's problem. For example, one cause of incomplete orders may have been that the form is printed on blue paper and it's hard to read all the text.

Another cause may be the lack of training among the staff that submits the orders. Although both causes may contribute to the problem, it's up to the team to determine which cause(s) are the most significant.

Sometimes identifying the most significant cause or causes is easy. Most fishbone diagrams are not balanced and causes tend to cluster around one or two categories. Sometimes the root cause is so clear that the entire team recognizes it and quickly agrees on it. Other times, there is debate over which causes are really critical and are worth pursuing. One approach to use when needing to create consensus among the team is called the **nominal group technique**, also known as **multivoting**. To use this technique, give each member of the team a set number of votes (three to five). Create a list of the options the team must choose from. Members can place all of their votes on one item on the list, or spread them among multiple items on the list. Once everyone has cast his or her votes, tally up the total number of votes. The item(s) with the highest number of votes are the ones the team has selected. Not everyone may agree, but the approach to making the selection is fair.

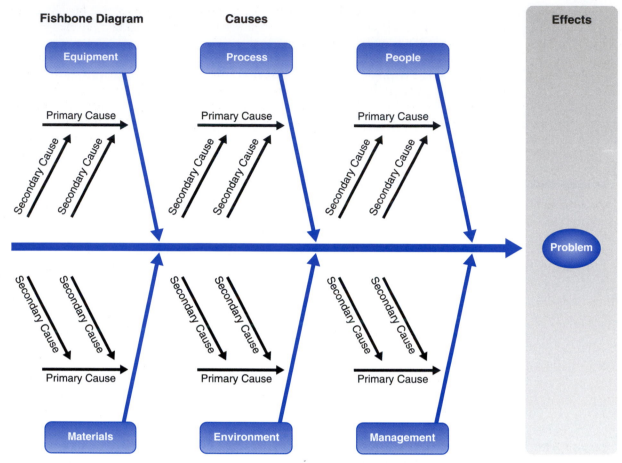

Figure ■ 13-9   Cause-and-Effect Diagram (Completed).

If the team is unsure of the problem's causes, or wants to be sure the team has not overlooked any key causes, mapping the process can be helpful. Creating a diagram of the steps in a process can help a team identify redundant steps, hand-offs, and weak spots in the process that may contribute to the problem.

In its most basic form, a **process flow diagram** consists of steps and decisions that are indicated by symbols. An oval indicates the beginning and end of a process, a square indicates a single step in the process, and a diamond indicates a decision (Figure 13-10).

The steps in the process are connected by arrows that indicate the "flow" of the process from step to step. Process flows can range from being very simple—indicating only high-level steps—to being very detailed—indicating specific steps, who completes the step, and even how long it takes to complete each step. The team members must decide the level of

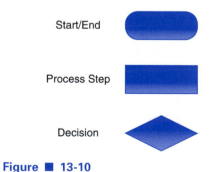

Figure ■ 13-10
Common Symbols Used in Process Flow Diagrams.

detail needed to assist them in "seeing" and understanding the causes of the problem.

At this point, the team should have a good handle on the problem and its causes. The final planning step is to develop solutions. The solution to the problem will depend on the scope and complexity of the problem the team is working on. A simple, focused problem with one identified key cause will likely require a simple solution. Larger, more complex problems with multiple causes may require multiple solutions. Using the Pareto principle, the team members may not have to address every cause of the problem; however, it is important that they address the primary cause(s) of the problem.

Developing solutions is another point in the process where the team can utilize brainstorming and multivoting. Encourage the team members to be creative in their thinking and generate as many ideas as possible.

Do—Carry Out the Test or Change

It's easy to see how the work of the "plan" phase sets the team up for success in the "do" phase. In this phase of the project, the team—now with a clear understanding of the key causes of their problems—develops and implements the solution to the problem. But before springing into action, the team needs to do a bit more work.

Based on the root causes of the problem, it is likely that the team has come up with a number of ways to solve the problem they are working on. Chances are the proposed solutions require people to make an effort to change their work processes and may possibly cost the organization money. The questions the team needs to consider at this point are:

- Is the time, effort, and resources required for this solution appropriate for the problem being addressed?
- Will the organization be receptive to the proposed changes?
- What can the team do to ensure the success of this solution?

By nature, human beings tend to resist change. Implementing changes in an organization, no matter how small, can be challenging. Therefore, it is important that the proposed solution to the problem be appropriate for the problem being addressed. For example, proposing the purchase of a new computer application that will cost tens of thousands of dollars would be met with great resistance if the impact of your problem on the organization were relatively small. The solution may be effective, but the cost to the organization would be greater than the benefit of pursuing the solution.

Even if you have identified the appropriate solution for the problem, it is important to consider how the solution will be received in the organization. Let's use the computer application example again. In this case, this solution is completely appropriate for the problem being addressed. In Organization A, where the staff is used to working with computers, bringing in a new system will likely be well received. But what if you are replacing a manual process with an automated process in Organization B that does all its work on paper? Again, implementing a new system may be the best solution to the problem; however, in each case, the team will have different organizational issues to consider when developing and implementing the solution.

What can the team do to ensure the success of this solution? The key here is to anticipate what is working against you and what is working in your favor. This requires recognizing your *barriers and aids*. Let's continue with the example of implementing a new computer application in Organization B to solve the incomplete orders problem. Why will this solution be successful? These reasons are your team's aids to success. What problems might the team run into? These answers are your team's barriers to success (see Table 13-5).

TABLE 13-5

Aids and Barrier to Success

Aids	Barriers
The regional manager is very bottom-line focused and this project will save the organization money.	The staff is used to doing everything on paper. This will be a big change for staff.
The location manager is very supportive of our team and knows this is a significant problem that needs to be addressed.	Not everyone has computer skills.
The staff members are frustrated with all the extra work the incomplete orders create for them.	Everybody is so busy, it's going to be hard to get them to take the time to learn a new work process.

Understanding the barriers and aids to a project's success is very important. Identifying the aids to success helps team members determine where they have support for moving their solution forward if they run into problems, delays, or organizational barriers. By identifying the likely barriers to success, the team members can be sure to address those barriers in their solution implementation plan. Providing the staff computer skills training and gaining their buy-in to the effort required to implement this solution is key to the team's success.

Now the team is ready to develop an implementation plan for the solution. The first key decision is whether or not to implement the solution across the entire organization, or to do a smaller-scale implementation, or **pilot test**, to make sure it will work. A pilot test is a great way to "work out the bugs" of a solution on a smaller scale. Working with a small group may allow the project team to implement the solution more quickly and provides the team the opportunity to identify and address unanticipated problems. Pilot testing is recommended for expensive or high-risk projects.

If the solution is relatively low risk, and the organization is receptive to the change, the team may opt to simultaneously implement the solution organization-wide. Full implementation may also be appropriate in smaller organizations or when the solution impacts only a small group of people.

Just as the plan phase of the PI project was critical for setting up the team for success, the implementation plan for the solution is equally important. The key elements of an implementation plan are:

- A timeline
- A project charter
- A data collection plan
- A communication plan

The timeline for the implementation plan outlines how long the implementation will take as well as key milestones along the way. The *project charter* will outline the key steps and activities that will take place along the timeline, indicating who is responsible for each step. In order to measure the success of the solution's implementation, comparative "post" data need to be collected. Who will collect the data, when, and how needs to be determined. Lastly, the team needs to develop a communication plan (Table 13-6) that outlines who needs to know about this implementa-

TABLE 13-6

Communication Plan

Who	When	What	How
Regional manager	First of the month	Project status report including project costs	E-mail project status report
Physical therapists	Weekly	Project updates	Weekly staff meetings
All clinic staff	Monthly	General project updates	Staff newsletter

tion, when they need to know about it, what they need to know, and how it will be communicated.

Study Data Before and After the Change and Reflect on What Was Learned

You have implemented your solution, and it is time to verify that you are achieving the desired results. In our example, we have been focusing on incomplete orders. Back in the plan phase, the team developed a detailed data collection plan that focused on clearly defining and measuring incomplete orders. It is important that you use that same approach to measurement during the study phase.

The goal of the study phase is to determine if the solution you implemented has had the desired impact on your problem. Think of your baseline and post-implementation data (Figure 13-11) as the "before" and "after" pictures of your project. The goal is to be able to demonstrate if your implementation was successful, and if it was successful, to what extent. If we used "number of incomplete orders" as our baseline metric, the same metric needs to be used for our post-implementation metric. In this way, we are comparing apples to apples. Displaying the data in a run chart provides a great deal of information very concisely. This chart easily conveys the extent of the problem before the implementation and the degree of impact the solution has had on the problem. It can also

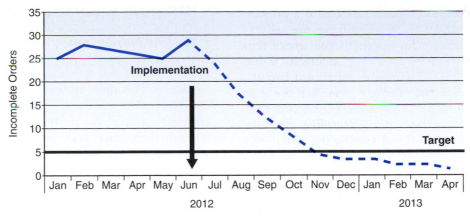

Figure ■ 13-11 Run Chart of Incomplete Orders.

demonstrate that the target level of performance has been achieved or exceeded for several months in a row, indicating that the "new and improved" level of performance is taking hold in your organization.

Based on the outcome of the study phase, the steps you will take during the act phase will vary. If the implementation of your solution was deemed to be effective in a pilot test, the solution should be spread throughout the rest of your organization. Your team may repeat the PDSA cycle (to a lesser degree) as the solution is "rolled out" in various areas of your organization. If your successful solution was implemented organization wide in lieu of a pilot test, and the outcome was successful, the team should continue to monitor performance for several months to ensure that the new level of performance has become the "new normal."

Before you disband the team after completing a successful project, there are still two important steps to take. You don't want to let the efforts of your team go unnoticed; therefore, it is important to communicate the outcome of your project to the organization and to recognize and reward your team members for their efforts.

Your project's **return on investment (ROI)** is a calculation comparing what you invested in the effort (time, resources, dollars) and what you got out of it (efficiencies, cost savings, improved customer satisfaction). Whenever possible, communicate the gains made by this project in terms of dollars.

Determine what the team invested into the project. Team time can be calculated in terms of dollars by

identifying an average hourly wage and multiplying it by the number of hours the team worked on the project. Other costs, such as consultant's fees, software, and equipment purchased, can be included if applicable.

Calculate the value of what was gained from your project in the same way. If your improvement saved the department time, determine how much time per month was saved and multiply those hours by the average hourly wage. If your improvement created efficiencies so that practitioners are now able to see more patients, determine the average revenue per patient and multiply that by the number of additional patients who can be seen. Annualizing your data (determining monthly savings and multiplying that by 12 to demonstrate what the organization will save each year) is another effective way to communicate the impact of your project to your organization's leadership.

Your project may also have achieved some intangible benefits. These are benefits that may not be easily expressed in terms of dollars, but are still important to identify. Improving a work process may result in other intangible benefits such as:

- Improved teamwork and morale among the staff
- Improved working relationships with clients
- Improved customer satisfaction
- Increased confidence of your team to engage in quality improvement efforts
- The identification of other opportunities for improvement

Finally, you need to recognize your team members for their efforts. Without their time and effort, those positive outcomes would not have been achieved. Box 13-6 outlines several items to consider when determining how to recognize and reward your team. Recognizing staff for going above and beyond their routine duties to benefit the organization is one way you make an investment in your team's future. Making the improvement process a positive and rewarding experience for staff increases the likelihood that they will be on board with you the next time an opportunity to improve a process comes up.

If your solution was implemented and found not to be successful, there may have been a flaw in your team's understanding of the problem, or development of the solution. This will require "going around" the PDSA cycle again. There are a number of reasons a solution may not have been successful:

- *Problems with the data:* Did the data truly represent the process under study?
- *Problems with the team's makeup:* Were all key areas represented?
- *Problems with how the team identified key causes and solutions:* Was there truly consensus?

During the plan phase, the team members collected data to help them better understand the extent and key causes of the problem. Review the data collection plan. Were the data collected consistently? Were the operational definitions and instructions for data collection clear? Were the data collected representative of the process?

Another consideration is the makeup of the team. Did the team membership include the people who have knowledge of all aspects of the process you were trying to improve? If not, your team may not have fully understood the process, or was "blind" to key causes of the problem because you did not have that source of knowledge or expertise on the team. Good teamwork can yield powerful results. However, a group of people sitting around a conference table does not necessarily constitute a team. Consider the decision-making process used to identify key causes and the solution that was selected. Did any team members pull rank or bully others into their way of thinking? Did brainstorming and voting methods give all team members a fair opportunity to participate?

Not achieving the desired level of results does not mean the project failed. Each time a team goes around the PDSA cycle, it deepens the understanding of the process and has the opportunity to refine the solution to be even more successful.

BOX 13-6

Keys to Determining Appropriate Rewards and Recognitions

- Consider when to recognize individual contributions and when to recognize the team as a whole.
- Consider whether all team members will receive the same reward or determine if rewards be personalized by giving each member a different but equal reward.
- Consider whether there are ways that your reward or recognition could backfire or be considered unpleasant or punishing by members of the team.
- Consider getting feedback from others on your choice of reward or recognition before presenting it publicly.
- Consider whether there are any temporary members of the team or consultants who contributed to the team's success who should be rewarded.
- Consider whether team members can be consulted in choosing their own reward or how they wish to celebrate their accomplishments within predetermined boundaries and guidelines.

Chapter Summary

In this chapter you were introduced to CQI as both a management philosophy and an approach to process improvement. CQI was contrasted with QA and quality control, and the focus of CQI on meeting and exceeding valid requirements of customers was emphasized. You were provided with an introduction to the basic concepts, strategies, tools, and techniques to begin to develop your conceptual "CQI toolkit" (see Table 13-7).

Although it might seem that the examples provided were "in depth," it is important to keep in mind that CQI initiatives in organizations that have mature

TABLE 13-7

A Continuous Quality Improvement Toolkit

Quality Tool or Term	Application
PDSA Cycle	A *systematic, repeatable, and teamwork-based* process for solving problems or realizing opportunities for enhanced performance at the organizational, system, process, and employee levels in order to achieve desired results
Problem Statement	A concise description of the problem (and only the problem) the team is addressing. Does not include elements of cause or solution.
Brainstorming	Used to generate a large number of ideas in a short period of time
Operationalize	To put a problem or issue in terms of something that can be observed and measured
Check Sheet	A standardized tool developed for manual data collection
Run Chart	A graph that shows measurement (on the vertical axis) against time (on the horizontal axis)
Stratification	Separating data into categories so that potential patterns can be seen
Root Cause(s)	The fundamental, underlying reason for a problem; the root cause is what causes the problem to occur repeatedly
Histogram	A bar graph that shows the distribution of a set of data; each bar on the horizontal axis represents a subset of your data, whereas the vertical axis indicates number or frequency
Pareto Chart	A bar graph that includes a second vertical axis to demonstrate cumulative percent; the Pareto chart is used to identify the vital few causes of a problem
Cause-and-Effect (Fishbone) Diagram	Used to relate identified causes to the problem (effect) being studied
Nominal Group Technique/ Multivoting	Team voting method
Process Flow Chart	A graphical representation of the steps and decisions in a process
Barriers and Aids	Tools that help the team consider the driving and restraining forces of ideas or options
Pilot Test	Small scale implementation often used to test a possible solution
Project Charter	A formal document recognizing the existence of the project; includes the business case for the project, the objectives, and the scope of the project
Return on Investment	Calculation of what was gained from doing a project minus what was invested in doing the project; typically expressed in terms of dollars

programs can be extraordinarily complex. Further, learning how to effectively balance the tasks at hand with the people involved requires a wide range of managerial skills from data collection and statistical analysis to managing agreement and solving conflicts. In Chapter 2, you were introduced to the strategy of evaluating different types of evidence and it was noted that evidence-based practice requires a manager to utilize good judgment in applying evidence to a problem. Gathering and analyzing data as evidence in a CQI approach also requires sound managerial judgment. The emphasis of CQI on making decisions with data does not release the manager from his or her responsibilities for coaching and nurturing staff.

■ Real-Life Solutions

Joan knew that if she was going to foster an environment that embraces CQI, she needed to set her team up for success. Fortunately, Rehab-World put a number of tools at Joan's disposal to assist her in this effort. Joan reviewed the Rehab-World strategic plan and organizational dashboard that displays key performance indicators and compares them across all Rehab-World locations. As a new location, the strategic focus for Joan's branch was to grow the client base by being a leader in patient satisfaction. Joan began to wonder how her team could impact patient satisfaction. Then she noticed that the dashboard metrics showed that the wait time to see a therapy practitioner at her location lagged behind that of her peers at the other locations.

Joan put together a business case for pursuing an effort to reduce patient wait time and presented it to the Rehab-World quality council with the support of her regional manager. The quality council blessed the project and even provided Joan with additional resources such as just-in-time training for her project team and data analysis support if she needed it.

Joan felt empowered and was ready to assemble her team. She put a lot of thought into selecting her team members and communicated how she would support the rest of her staff while the project team was away at training and working on the wait time problem. The entire team could see how improving patient wait times could benefit the patients, the therapy practitioners, and Rehab-World.

At their first team meeting, Joan and the regional manager discussed the project and why it was so important. They also noted how much they valued the efforts and inputs of every team member toward making this project a success. Joan then wrote the problem statement on the white board—*takes too long for patients to get an appointment*—and said, "Let's brainstorm." Joan's PDSA journey had begun.

Study Questions

1. **Which of the following represents the four stages teams commonly go through in correct order?**

   a. Storming, forming, performing, norming
   b. Forming, storming, norming, performing
   c. Performing, storming, reforming, norming
   d. Forming, norming, storming, performing

2. **Which of the following best describes the PDSA cycle?**

   a. It is a systematic, repeatable, and teamwork-based process for solving problems or realizing opportunities for enhanced performance.

   b. It is a set of cautions to be avoided during the cycle of CQI efforts.
   c. It is an acronym for the requirements to determine a valid customer concern.
   d. It represents the four critical tools that must be used in analyzing variation in work processes.

3. **Which of the following is true regarding the principles, tools, and approaches that comprise CQI?**

   a. They must be implemented organization-wide.
   b. They require the assistance of a consultant to implement effectively.
   c. They may be integrated on a smaller scale within a department or business unit.
   d. They must be led by a quality council.

4. **Which of the following is true regarding quality goals according to Juran?**

   a. Quality goals should be based on organizational priorities.
   b. Quality goals are set based on customer needs.
   c. Quality goals are designed to reduce variation.
   d. Quality goals are developed using the PDSA cycle.

5. **When selecting a CQI project, a leader should consider:**

   a. The alignment of the initiative to the organization's mission and vision.
   b. Whether the project relates to a regulatory requirement or government mandate.
   c. The priorities of the department.
   d. All of the above.

6. **Which of the following best describes the purpose of a fishbone diagram?**

   a. It is a method used to assist with identification and documentation of causes to the problem (effect) being studied.
   b. It is a method used to assist with variance analysis.
   c. It is a method used to order the causes of a problem from most relevant to least relevant.
   d. It is a method to help identify the most appropriate members for participation in a CQI team.

7. **Which of the following best describes the purpose of a process flow diagram?**

   a. It demonstrates the flow of revenue within an efficient and high-performing organization.
   b. It is a graphic representation of recommended decision-making processes in the PDSA cycle.
   c. It is a graphic representation of the steps and decision points in any process.
   d. It demonstrates the flow of expenses within an efficient and high-performing organization.

8. **Which of the following best describes the Pareto principle?**

   a. It is the concept stating that most of the cause of any problem is because of special cause variation.
   b. It is the concept stating that 80% of the problem is caused by 20% of the contributing root causes.
   c. It is the concept stating that most aspects of any problem can be solved by a single solution.
   d. It is the concept stating that 80% of the gain in process efficiency is created by 20% of those contributing to the solution.

Resources for Learning More About Continuous Quality Improvement

Journals That Often Address CQI or Quality

Quality Management in Health Care

http://journals.lww.com/qmhcjournal/pages/default.aspx

This peer-reviewed quarterly journal provides a forum to explore the theoretical, technical, and strategic elements of total quality management in health care. Each issue of *Quality Management in Health Care (QMHC)* features a timely symposium that addresses a key issue in health-care quality management. Also included in each issue is an in-depth interview with a key individual in health-care quality management, an educational tutorial on basic quality management tools and processes, an information clearinghouse to encourage informal communication among those involved in the field of health-care quality management, and a reference center that reviews books, journal articles, seminars, and videos of interest.

Total Quality Management and Business Excellence

http://www.tandfonline.com/loi/ctqm20

Total Quality Management and Business Excellence is an international journal that sets out to stimulate thought and research in all aspects of total quality management and to provide a natural forum for discussion and dissemination of research results. The journal is designed to encourage interest in all matters relating to total quality management and is intended to appeal to both the academic and professional community working in this area.

Journal for Healthcare Quality

http://www.nahq.org/Quality-Community/journal/jhq.html

Journal for Healthcare Quality is a professional forum that advances quality in a diverse and changing health-care environment. *Journal for Healthcare Quality (JHQ)* addresses an audience of professionals who are responsible for promoting and monitoring quality, safe, cost-effective health care. It features articles written by and for health-care quality professionals that focus on improvement, risk management, utilization review, and the latest in regulations from The Joint Commission, PROs, and payment systems. The journal also publishes reviews of publications in the field and updates on pertinent legislation. It offers coverage of state-of-the-art technology, total quality management techniques, and practical applications of quality improvement systems and innovations.

Professional Organizations Concerned With CQI or Quality

National Association for Healthcare Quality

http://www.nahq.org

The NAHQ is committed to developing and promoting professional expertise in the art and science of health-care quality. The NAHQ members include professionals in general, acute, managed, long-term, home, rehabilitation, mental health, and ambulatory care settings as well as consultants whose responsibilities include quality or risk management in a wide area of health professions.

American Society for Quality

http://www.asq.org

The American Society for Quality (ASQ), a professional association headquartered in Milwaukee, Wisconsin, aims to create better workplaces and communities worldwide by advancing learning, quality improvement, and knowledge exchange. The ASQ makes its officers and member experts available to inform and advise the U.S. Congress, government agencies, state legislatures, and other groups and individuals on quality-related topics. ASQ representatives have provided testimony on issues such as training, health-care quality, education, transportation safety, quality management in the federal government, licensing for quality professionals, and more. ASQ also works with the media on quality-related matters, providing informational resources and referrals to qualified experts from its broad member base.

Miscellaneous Resources

Carey, R. G., & Lloyd, R. C. (1995). *Measuring quality improvement in healthcare: A guide to statistical process control applications.* Milwaukee, WI: ASQ Quality Press.

http://qualitypress.asq.org/

This book provides an excellent introduction to the statistical process control applications that are most frequently used to analyze data in process improvement initiatives. Key concepts include variation, use of critical tools including run charts and control charts, and statistical thinking through the use of case examples.
Published by Quality Resources of the American Society for Quality.
ISBN 0-527-76293-8

Biemer, P. P., & Lyberg, L. E. (2003). *Introduction to survey quality.* Hoboken, NJ: John Wiley & Sons.

http://qualitypress.asq.org

As more and more professionals who are not trained as survey researchers take on tasks associated with surveys, the need has arisen for a basic introduction to current survey methods and quality issues associated with them. The authors review both well-established and recently developed principles and concepts in the field and examine important issues being currently researched. Topics include common errors in interviewing, data collection methods, and practical survey design for minimizing total survey error.

Scholtes, P. R., Joiner, B. L., & Streibel, B. J. (2003). *The team handbook.* Madison, WI: Oriel Inc.

This comprehensive resource book provides data on creating high-performance teams. Information is included on different types of teams, tools and strategies for leading change, and a variety of CQI tools and techniques.
Published by Oriel Inc.
ISBN-13: 978-1884731266

Reference List

Institute of Medicine. (2000). *To err is human*. Washington, DC: National Academy Press.

Institute of Medicine. (2001). *Crossing the quality chasm: A new health system for the 21st century*. Washington, DC: National Academy Press.

Juran, J. M., & Godfrey, A. B. (1999). *Juran's quality handbook*. New York, NY: McGraw-Hill.

Moen, R. D., & Norman, C. L. (2010, November). Circling back: Clearing up the myths about the Deming cycle and seeing how it keeps evolving. *Quality Progress*, *43*(100), 22–28.

Scholtes, P. R, Joiner, B. L., & Striebel, B. J. (2003). *The team handbook*. Madison, WI: Oriel Inc.

Sollecito, W. A, & Johnson, J. K. (2013). *Mclaughlin and Kaluzny's continuous quality improvement in health care* (4th ed.). Burlington MA: Jones & Bartlett Learning.

The W. Edwards Deming Institute. (2014). *The plan, do, study, act (PDSA) cycle*. Retrieved from https://www.deming.org/theman/theories/pdsacycle.

CHAPTE

Marketing Occupational Therapy Services

Brent Braveman, PhD, OTR/L, FAOTA
Julie Ann Nastasi, ScD, OTD, OTR/L, SCLV, FAOTA

■ Real-Life Management

Patrick is the new director of occupational therapy in a community hospital. The occupational therapy department provides a range of services, including services to the acute medical and psychiatric units and outpatient services. Although psychiatric services are provided only for adults, the acute medical services span the full age range. Patrick's supervisor, Keesha, who is the administrative director of rehabilitation services, has encouraged him to begin to explore additional services that could be developed to bring in new streams of revenue. She has stressed that any new products or services that are added cannot be focused on simply providing more service to existing populations because most of those patients are insured under some form of capitated reimbursement, such as a Medicare diagnosis-related group or negotiated discounts. However, Keesha is also concerned that the needs of occupational therapy's customers are not being met. The hospital has a strong customer focus and considers both internal and external customers. For example, internal customers include individuals such as nurses and physicians, whereas external customers include individuals such as patients, payers, and other referral sources. Keesha has requested that Patrick investigate whether existing services are adequate to meet the needs of these various customers.

Patrick was introduced to the marketing process in the management course that he took as part of his entry-level occupational therapy education. As such, he is aware that marketing is a process of assessing the needs, resources, and limitations of both an organization and the target populations served by the organization. During his course it was stressed that the marketing process can be very complicated but can also be applied in simpler ways and used by occupational therapy managers for the development and promotion of occupational therapy services. Patrick also remembers that making connections with others in the organization who are concerned with aspects of marketing or with meeting the needs of

Continued

Real-Life Management—cont'd

the same target populations is an important first step. He is excited to use the knowledge he has about the marketing process but is also worried that his department has a limited budget and very few discretionary funds that can be spent on marketing. To get the ball rolling, Patrick sets up appointments with the director of physical therapy, as well as with an associate in the publications and promotions department who he knows is involved in the organization's strategic planning activities.

Critical Thinking Questions

As you read this chapter, consider the following questions:

- How are the marketing processes of assessing needs, planning a product or program, and assessing the resources and limitations of your organization similar to the occupational therapy processes of evaluating patients and planning occupational therapy interventions?

- What are some examples of simple marketing strategies that can be employed by newer occupational therapy managers and what are some examples of complex marketing strategies that would require the assistance of people with professional marketing expertise?

- What types of data, information, and other forms of evidence would be used in the marketing process that might already be identified, collected, and analyzed by your organization for other management functions such as planning?

Glossary

- **Environmental assessment:** the examination of the data, information, and other forms of evidence, including the needs of target populations, that will guide the development and promotion of a new product or service.
- **Market analysis:** the use of the information gained during organizational and environmental assessments to validate perceptions of the wants and needs of the target populations that will receive a new product or service.
- **Marketing:** process consisting of organizational assessment, environmental assessment, market analysis, and marketing communications.
- **Marketing communications:** devising methods of communicating with your target populations to promote your products and services.

- **Organizational assessment:** the examination of the factors within an organization that will influence the development and promotion of a new product or service.
- **Packaging:** the image being presented to target populations.
- **People:** employees within the organization and internal and external customers.
- **Physical evidence:** tangible information available to consumers.
- **Place:** the location where the product is being delivered.
- **Price:** the monetary cost for the product.
- **Primary data sources:** resources that generate data that are specific to your product or service, such as existing customers or potential

Glossary—cont'd

customers, from your target markets, referral sources, payers, employees, suppliers, consultants, or other sources involved in your product or service.

- **Products:** the goods or services being delivered to the target population.
- **Promotion:** a method to inform target populations about the product being offered.
- **Secondary data sources:** research that already exists; organizations may provide the

data, information, or other forms of evidence for free or may charge for its use; examples include government census reports, economic statistics about a potential target population in a specific geographic area, information from news sources, and surveys conducted by trade associations.

- **Target populations:** any group of persons who receive, benefit from, or pay for an occupational therapy product or service.

Introduction

Over the last few decades, our dualistic health-care system has become increasingly complex. Service delivery methods have grown and health-care providers are able to meet physically and virtually with consumers to provide services (American Occupational Therapy Association [AOTA], 2013). As a result, the occupational therapy profession has been faced with both challenges and new opportunities. Among other challenges, we have faced the continued need to become highly visible and to explain who we are and what we do while competing with other health-care providers for limited resources and reimbursement. Consumers have become more sophisticated in their understanding of health services and have increased expectations of health-care providers. Consumers expect results and want to see a value for their time and money spent (Richmond, 2011). Both traditional health-care organizations and organizations in emerging practice settings have faced difficult economic times. Many organizations have flattened their administrative structures, often decreasing resources devoted to staff management functions such as planning and marketing. The remaining resources are typically focused on an organization's major revenue-producing products and service lines. Although occupational therapy services are often part of these service lines, it may be difficult to garner resources specifically for the development and promotion of a new occupational therapy product or service.

At the same time that the occupational therapy profession has been challenged, there have been opportunities to expand into new areas of practice. We have seen a return of many occupational therapists (OTs) and occupational therapy assistants (OTAs) to community-based practice, and practice has expanded in areas such as low-vision rehabilitation, telehealth, veteran and wounded warrior care, and hand transplants and bionic limbs (Yamkovenko, 2013). The occupational therapy profession has embraced emerging practice areas and has created forums, resources, and position papers in these emerging areas. As noted in other chapters, there are also opportunities for expansion of service through telehealth service, primary care, and other areas affected by implementation of the Affordable Care Act.

Although traditional occupational therapy entry-level curricula have focused on preparing graduates to provide holistic, occupation-based intervention, they have understandably fallen short of preparing practitioners in managerial skills beyond the basics. Although entry-level standards on administration and management are included in accreditation standard or occupational therapy education by the Accreditation Council on Occupational Therapy Education (ACOTE), it cannot be expected that an entry-level program adequately prepares someone for the role of manager. The marketing process can be extraordinarily complex. Occupational therapy managers and business owners who want or need to assess the needs of the target populations they serve and to design, develop, and promote new products and services to meet those needs will likely need some education or training beyond their entry-level education. Luckily, in many larger organizations there are professionals who have focused on marketing products and services as their career and can guide you in the process. However, occupational therapy managers need to have a good understanding of marketing products and services to ensure that plans created through collaboration with marketing professionals are feasible, ethically responsible, and uphold the profession's scope of practice.

The complexity of the marketing process should not deter you from thinking that you can learn the necessary skills to effectively develop and promote occupational therapy services. The marketing process can be simplified, adapted, and applied in a basic manner to even existing and traditional services such as obtaining referrals for basic activities of daily living. This chapter provides an introduction to the full marketing process and describe the synergistic relationship between marketing activities and other managerial functions described in other chapters, such as program development (see Chapter 15). The use of data, information, and other forms of evidence in the marketing process is also discussed.

Target Populations

You may notice in this book, and in other books and resources on management, that various terms are used to refer to those who benefit from occupational therapy services as well as those who pay for services. In Chapter 13, you were introduced to the concept that persons concerned with continuous quality improvement (CQI) efforts identify both internal and external *customers*. Some customers are also the direct beneficiaries of occupational therapy services and are often referred to as *clients* or *patients*. Although these individuals often are responsible for full or partial payment for services, you are likely already familiar with the term *third-party payer*. Further, the term *consumer* is sometimes used to refer to those who buy products and services (Richmond, 2011).

There is no doubt that the many terms used to describe those who receive and those who pay for occupational therapy services are potentially confusing. This is especially true as occupational therapy practitioners move into new areas of practice that are supported by new sources of revenue and payers. AOTA uses the term *client* to refer to "*persons* (including those involved in care of a client), *groups* (collec-

tives of individuals, e.g., families, workers, students, communities), and *populations* (collectives of groups of individuals living in a similar local—e.g., city, state, or country—or sharing the same or like characteristics or concerns)" (AOTA, 2014, p. S3). Terminology is important, and it is also important to distinguish between the various types of persons who receive or pay for your services in order to effectively implement the marketing process. Doing so will aid you in designing specific methods to collect data, information, and other forms of evidence on the needs, resources, and limitations of those who are the intended targets of your occupational therapy product or service without wasting valuable effort. Throughout this chapter, the term **target population(s)** will be used to refer to any group of persons who receive, benefit from, or pay for an occupational therapy product or service.

Components of the Marketing Process

A simple way to think about the marketing process is to view it as comprising four major components or steps. It is easier to understand the activities and purposes of these components if they are described separately. However, it is important to recognize that in reality the components of the marketing process are often completed simultaneously rather than in lock-step sequence. The activities from one component inform and aid with completion of other components. Also, managers use much of the data, information, and other forms of evidence obtained in the marketing process in other managerial functions, such as planning or program development and evaluation activities.

Each of the four components of the **marketing** process is briefly described in Box 14-1 and is outlined in the following sections of this chapter. As you read about each component, you should recognize that in some situations, such as in the case of a small business owner or entrepreneur, an OT or OTA might be responsible for all steps of the process or might consider hiring a marketing professional to complete parts of the process for him or her. In other situations, such as the case of a director of occupational therapy for a department in a large integrated health-care system, an occupational therapy manager may collaborate with or rely on professionals in other departments such as marketing, publications, or development to complete some of the marketing components.

Organizational Assessment

Organizational assessment is the process of collecting data, information, and other forms of evidence to examine the internal factors and influences that will impact the future development of your product or service. One common way to assist with organizational assessment is the completion of a *SWOT analysis*. This acronym stands for *strengths*, *weaknesses*, *opportunities*, and *threats*. A SWOT analysis was previously described in Chapter 9 as part of organizational and environmental assessments in the planning process. It was suggested that often SWOT analyses can be conducted by combining a review of key documents or reports (financial reports, outcome statistics, program evaluation, or accreditation reports) with staff interviews, discussions, or structured brainstorming exercises. SWOT analyses may also be completed with a focus toward development of a particular product or service. Organizational assessments examine factors such as your organization's reputation in the community, customer service, programs, the staff's qualifications, type and quality of equipment, available space, geographic location of your organization, and the level of administrative support for new programs (Richmond, 2011). The desired result of this assessment will be to have a comprehensive understanding of the resources available to aid you with development and promotion of your product as well as the challenges and constraints that you will face. You will also seek to gain an understanding of the perspectives of the key stakeholders within your organization, such as other department directors or those responsible for your organization's financial health.

The best place to start an organizational assessment is with a review of the organization's mission statement, as well as the mission statement of your department. This review establishes the context for evaluating the extent to which your planned product or service matches your organization's objectives. There is not always a perfect match between each and every product offered by organizations and their missions, but starting with a mission review will give you some indication of how a new product or service proposal might be received. If the relationship between your proposal and your organization's mission is not clearly evident, you should be prepared to provide an explanation of why valuable time and resources should be used to carry out your proposal. Similarly, as an occupational therapy manager, you may find yourself in the position of being asked to develop services for members of target populations that are not a good match for your department. In this case, a mission review will aid you in preparing a sound rationale for why you should not respond positively to such a request.

Organizations sometimes end up involved in the delivery of products or services that are not a good match with their mission for a number of reasons. At times, influential members of an organization can successfully move forward agendas or projects that are not

---

BOX 14-1

Components of the Marketing Process

- **Organizational assessment:** Examination of the factors within an organization that will influence the development and promotion of a new product or service. This includes identifying strengths and weaknesses through a SWOT analysis.
- **Environmental assessment:** Examination of the data, information, and other forms of evidence, including the needs of target populations, that will guide the development and promotion of a new product or service. This is done through analyzing changes outside of the organization.
- **Market analysis:** Use of the information gained during organizational and environmental assessments to validate perceptions of the wants and needs of the target populations that will receive a new product or service. This is the most time-consuming step, but it is vital in market management.
- **Marketing communications:** Packaging and promoting a product so the target populations and other key stakeholders in a new product or service have a clear understanding of what the product or service is and how it may be accessed. This is often done through different methods such as television, radio, print, and social media.

good matches for the mission. At other times, an organization may knowingly take on projects that are not reflective of its mission because of perceived advantages to the organization, such as a new source of revenue. However, although such products and services may bring benefits to the organization, they may also pull valuable and needed resources from other products, services, or activities that are more closely aligned with the needs of those whom the organization serves. It is important to recognize the *opportunity costs* involved in such ventures. You learned in Chapter 9 that opportunity costs are those things you cannot accomplish secondary to a lack of resources because you are investing your time and other resources in another effort. All decisions to develop a new product or service have opportunity costs associated with them. Most successful organizations develop new products and services in a planned and thoughtful manner. This means that we must be prepared to accept that a new product or service idea that we value highly may not be enough of a priority for others to devote the necessary resources to move forward on its development.

It is beneficial and important to coordinate organizational assessment activities with others in the organization who may be able to assist you and who will also benefit from information that you may learn. In addition to marketing or development departments, those involved in strategic planning in any way, such as other department directors, may be important allies in the marketing process. Other department managers may already have or might benefit from the information that you will need to assess your organization's needs, resources, and limitations.

Large organizations routinely collect various forms of data, information, and other forms of evidence that are used in planning and marketing activities. Information on referral rates, payer mix, demographic information such as the geographic location of target populations, space utilization, and staff turnover are just some examples of such information. Occupational therapy managers may find this readily available information helpful in planning new products and services as well as to aid with the evaluation of existing products. Sometimes, however, the information that you need may not be available, especially if you are seeking information related to a specific occupational therapy product or service that might not catch the attention of those concerned with larger organizational needs. A sample list of simple strategies for organizational assessment is presented in Box 14-2.

BOX 14-2

Simple Strategies for Organizational Assessment

- Conduct informational interviews with other department directors over coffee or a meal to learn more about the skills, resources, and needs of other disciplines.
- Obtain your boss's permission to make an announcement about a potential product or service that you are considering in a directors' meeting, in a newsletter, or on a Listserv and ask for input or concerns from your peers.
- Ask your boss and representatives from departments such as planning, marketing, publications, or business affairs if routine reports are produced that might be helpful to you that you are not currently receiving.
- To obtain information from physicians, nurses, or other internal customers, conduct a short survey of needs, resources, or limitations by visiting other departments' staff meetings.
- Complete a SWOT analysis with your department; enlist other department directors to do the same and share the results.
- Spend some time reviewing your own organization's Web page and make a note of relevant services offered by other departments that might have some synergy with one of your existing or future products or services.

Environmental Assessment

An **environmental assessment** focuses on examination of external data, information, and other forms of evidence, such as demographic information, sociocultural trends, health-care utilization patterns, political and regulatory issues, new technologies, or socioeconomic status of the target populations served by your organization, to help determine their needs and resources. Identification of existing products and services offered by your competitors and their strengths and weaknesses is also completed as part of the environmental assessment.

One way to think about the types of data, information, and other forms of evidence that you will collect is that market research data can be divided into two categories: **primary data sources** and **secondary data sources** (Doman, Dennison, & Doman, 2002). Primary data sources are those that generate data specific to your product or service. Such data sources can include existing customers or potential customers from your target markets, referral sources, payers, employees, suppliers, consultants, or other sources involved in your product or service. Primary data usually cost some money to generate, ranging from a few dollars for a simple in-house survey to tens of thousands of dollars for a sophisticated survey of the needs of a large target population. Secondary data sources are those that already exist. Organizations may provide data, information, or other forms of evidence for free or may charge for use of the data. Such data sources might include government census reports, economic statistics about a potential target population in a specific geographic area, information from news sources, or surveys conducted by trade associations. Your organization may already purchase or use data from some of these secondary sources.

It is interesting to note that, unfortunately, requests for some of the types of information, data, or other forms of evidence that you may wish to obtain from others in your organization, such as demographics, reimbursement patterns, and information on discounts to payers, may sometimes be met with a less-than-enthusiastic response. This type of response may result from concerns that you might be communicating inaccurate information about the organization to outsiders or that you might be duplicating the efforts of others, or may occur because others feel that their level of control or power in the organization is threatened. It may be unusual in some organizations for directors of smaller departments to initiate development of new products, programs, or services. By identifying early the others who have vested interests in marketing activities and who might also benefit from your success in the development of a new product or service and keeping them informed, you may be more likely to gain their true support.

Once you have identified others who play a role in assessing how your organization interacts with the community and your organization's or department's target populations, you can search the information available to learn more about their needs, resources, and limitations. Examples of the sorts of data, information, and other forms of evidence you might use in evaluating the needs and resources of your target populations include:

- Population demographics (age, marital status, socioeconomic data, insurance status, etc.)
- Payer mix for particular catchment areas
- Targeted areas for expansion for your organization
- Organizational plans for future space and resource allocation

As discussed in Chapter 3, some types of secondary data, information, and other forms of evidence that you might use to describe your target populations and their needs are available from sources such as federal, state, and local agencies or from nonprofit organizations. Sources such as the U.S. Census Bureau (http://www.census.gov), the Centers for Disease Control and Prevention's National Center for Health Statistics (http://www.cdc.gov/nchs), the National Institutes of Health (http://www.nih.gov/), or *Healthy People* (http://www.healthypeople.gov) may provide you with information such as demographics or incidence rates of a particular disease or condition within a geographic area. Organizations such as the National Multiple Sclerosis Society (http://www.nmss.org/) may have state or local chapters that not only can provide you with demographic data on a target population but may have also conducted needs assessments or other surveys that describe existing services and information on their use and effectiveness. Combining evidence from several sources may be necessary to piece together a complete picture of your target population.

Community needs assessments can require extensive time and resources. However, there are some efforts than can be undertaken by occupational therapy managers to collect some information about target populations that may be combined with other sources of data, information, and other forms of evidence as part of an environmental assessment. A sample list of simple strategies for environmental assessment is presented in Box 14-3.

Conducting large-scale needs assessments of communities or target populations not already served by your organization is a major effort, and describing this process in depth is well beyond the scope of this chapter. See Box 14-4 for an example of a needs assessment for starting a low-vision program. These questions are a starting point to investigate referral sources, support services, and direct competitors. It is

Simple Strategies for Environmental Assessment

- Use the Internet, phonebook, and professional association directories to identify competitors in the area who are already serving your target population and review their websites and brochures to learn about their products and services.
- Conduct information interviews with leaders of community-based organizations or public health officials concerned with the health and wellness of your target population.
- Conduct informal or formal focus groups* with members of your target population.
- Have a booth or a table at a health fair, community festival, or street fair or collaborate with others in your organization to offer free screenings where you can also collect information on your target population.
- Identify the physicians providing services to your target population and collect information by making appointments to visit their offices, conducting a mail or telephone survey, or offering a continuing education event or meeting where you might be able to collect information on their perceptions of your target population's needs, resources, and limitations.

Focus groups are a type of formal data collection and research strategy. Marketing professionals often use focus groups to collect information about a target population's needs or reaction to a product or service, and formal use of focus groups is a sophisticated process. To learn more about focus groups, see the list of references provided at the end of the chapter.

important to see what state services are being provided in the local area. In addition, it is common to refer clients with low vision to state services in order optimize the client's independence. Although occupational therapy practitioners address functional mobility, clients with low vision should be referred to orientation and mobility specialists who provide training in sight cane travel and safe travel on public transportation, sidewalks, and intersections, as well as overall travel. In addition, state vocational services often will provide adaptive equipment for clients with low vision who need adaptive equipment in order to work. Referral to vocational services can save clients out-of-pocket expense for work-related equipment. As the occupational therapy manager, you will analyze the results of your low-vision needs assessment to determine if a low-vision program is appropriate.

Market Analysis

The purpose of the **market analysis** component of the marketing process is to use the data, information, and other forms of evidence identified during your assessment of your organization and the environment to validate your perceptions of the wants and needs of the target populations with which you interact. The desired outcome of your market analysis is a *marketing plan* that coordinates and uses information about your organization, its products and services, and its objectives and strategies to guide your activities to communicate with your target populations about your occupational therapy products and services (Richmond, 2011).

Marketing firms routinely conduct sophisticated forms of market analysis. For example, trial marketing a product in target communities is a market analysis strategy. Few occupational therapy departments have the resources available to conduct these types of market analyses. However, lack of financial and human resources should not deter you from completing this vital stage of the marketing process or from relying on a little creativity. Some of the same strategies that can be used to collect primary data, information, and other forms of evidence from your target populations as part of your environmental analysis can be used in the market analysis to validate your perceptions of the needs, resources, and limitations of the same target populations.

As an example, the director of an occupational therapy department in a small acute care hospital with few financial resources and little spare time might work with the staff to identify several inexpensive and creative ways of conducting a market analysis to compare perceptions of the needs and resources of various customers, including physicians, nurses, and patients. For example, to develop a hand rehabilitation program, primary data may be collected from hand surgeons and plastic surgeons known to the hospital and that already refer clients with hand injuries. Other

BOX 14-4

Needs Assessment for a Low-Vision Program

- Is there a need to develop an outpatient low-vision program?
- How many people have low vision or blindness in the area?
  - State Services
    - What state agencies are providing low-vision services in the area?
      - Locate the names, addresses, and contact information for the agencies (this information will be important for referring clients for orientation and mobility services as well as vocational rehabilitation).
      - How do clients with visual impairment qualify for services?
      - What services are provided?
      - Who provides these services?
      - Is there a waiting list?
      - What are the hours of operation?
  - Assistive Technology
    - What organizations, agencies, or grants are available for assistive technology?
      - Locate the names, addresses, and contact information for the agencies (this information will be important for locating equipment and assisting clients with obtaining equipment).
      - How do clients with visual impairment qualify for services?
      - What services are provided?
        - Who provides these services?
      - Is there a waiting list?
      - What are the hours of operation?
  - Local Services
    - What local services are providing low-vision services? (This might be the Lion's Club providing a support group, a senior center, etc.)
      - Locate the names, addresses, and contact information for the agencies.
      - How do clients with visual impairment qualify for services?
      - What services are provided?
        - Who provides these services?
      - Is there a waiting list?
      - What are the hours of operation?
- Optometrists and Ophthalmologists
  - Identify all of the optometrists and ophthalmologists in the area.
    - Locate the names, addresses, and contact information for the doctors.
    - What areas do the doctors specialize in?
    - What services are provided?
    - Is there a waiting list?
    - What are the hours of operation?
- Other Potential Referral Sources
  - Identify all endocrinologists, neurologists, and gerontologists in the area.
    - Locate the names, addresses, and contact information for the doctors.
    - Are the doctors aware of occupational therapy's role in low vision?
    - Who are the doctors currently referring their clients to for rehabilitation?
    - What are the hours of operation?
- Direct Competition
  - Which rehabilitation programs are direct competitors?
    - Locate the names, addresses, and contact information for the competitors.
    - Do your direct competitors have a low-vision program?
    - How do clients with visual impairment qualify for services?
    - What services are provided?
    - Who provides these services?
    - Is there a waiting list?
    - What are the hours of operation?

physicians who refer clients with upper extremity conditions are also probable primary data sources. By sending a one-page needs assessment that lists common diagnoses such as arthritis and repetitive motion injuries along with the services that an occupational therapy practitioner specializing in hand rehabilitation could offer, perceptions can be validated and confirmed. The needs assessment should also include a space where physicians may note how often their clients would benefit from the services described on the assessment. The assessment is only helpful if the physicians complete and return the form. A simple strategy to increase the return rate for the assessment might be offering coffee and doughnuts in the physician's lounge at the hospital as the physicians hand in completed assessments. Through this process, the director is able to validate perceptions and establish new relationships with potential referral sources for the hand rehabilitation program.

Marketing Communications

Marketing communications is the marketing component with which you are likely most familiar. Marketing communications consists of packaging and promoting a product. Thinking of occupational therapy services as a product may be a new way of thinking for some. It is common for new practitioners who are just beginning to learn about the complexities of the health-care system and confronting issues such as reimbursement and productivity demands for the first time to feel frustrated because they "Just want to treat their patients!" Yet, it is the nature of a free-market economy and of the *dualism* present in our health-care system that services can never be provided without someone considering expenses and revenues (see Chapter 3). Even when care is provided for "free," as it is sometimes assumed to be in our welfare system or by a health-care provider's *indigent care* funding, revenues to support those services must come from some source. Thinking about occupational therapy services as a product that can be packaged and sold will help you to accomplish that aim more effectively.

Marketing communications involves devising methods of communicating with your target populations to promote your occupational therapy products and services. As noted earlier in the chapter, it may be helpful to distinguish between target populations that are payers (those who provide financial reimbursement for your services) and those that are customers (those who are the direct recipients of your services) when involved in the marketing process for a new occupational therapy product. Sometimes the payer and the customer may be one and the same, but at other times identifying the specific concerns of payers and recipients of services and devising related but separate communications can be more effective in getting the word out about your new product or service. It is also conceptually helpful to realize that often, when providing a service, we may have one payer but multiple customers, such as the patients, referring physicians, nurses, families, and others.

Strategies like the marketing mix that address product, price, place, and promotion (formally the *four Ps of marketing*), plus physical evidence, packaging, and people, have been used to combat the challenges (Richmond, 2011). Occupational therapy managers need to identify the product (program needs) and price the services so they are valuable to the consumer and profitable for the organization. In addition, by knowing the correct place to offer the services, the occupational therapy manager is able to package physical evidence of the services in a way that provides a great first impression. Finally, the occupational therapy manager values the people who provide the services as much as the message that is articulated in the promotion of the services. The manager knows that the employees play a vital role in the marketing of services (Richmond, 2011). The seven areas of mixed marketing will be briefly discussed in the following sections of this chapter.

Product

Defining your **product** clearly for all involved in product development, delivery, and marketing communications is important. This may sound simple, but a common mistake—and the fastest way to lose potential customers from your target populations—is to promise more than you can deliver. For example, consider the process of beginning to develop work-related services. At first you might have available staff members who are trained to conduct work capacity screenings if provided with specific job descriptions and the necessary duties of a classification of employees, such as the ability to lift 40 lbs. or the ability to bend repeatedly. Your plan might be to begin by conducting work capacity screenings only and offer additional services later as you are able to add more staff or send existing staff for training. As physicians or others become aware of the services that you are offering, it may be common to begin to receive calls about other related services, such as conducting assessments of worksites and making recommendations for worksite adaptations. In these situations, it is tempting to try to accommodate such requests to "grow your business" faster, but it is important to avoid the temptation of promising an enthusiastic customer a service that you are not prepared to deliver. Failing to deliver on such promises is the fastest way to squelch a program's potential.

Defining your product means knowing in advance exactly what you can and cannot deliver, as well as what you may be able to deliver but not want to deliver. Not only does this help prevent you from making promises that you cannot fulfill, but it also helps you in comparing your product or service to that being offered by competitors in your area to determine the risks involved in continuing with product or service development. See Box 14-5 for an example of how an occupational therapy manager defines the product of a work capacity screening within an organization.

Price

As a consumer of a wide range of products, chances are that you already understand more about the concept of **price** than you probably realize. Naturally, you are familiar with the monetary cost of a product; however, with most products or services there are other less obvious types of cost to a consumer that will influence the success of a new product or service. Some of these other types of costs are described in Box 14-6.

In Chapter 13, you were introduced to the concept of *value*, or the relationship between cost and quality. It was suggested that at times we might be satisfied with lower quality if the associated costs were also lower. We do not expect the quality of a fast-food cheeseburger to be the same as a cheeseburger we buy

---

BOX 14-5

Defining the Work Capacity Screening

The occupational therapy manager has decided to pilot test the work capacity screening within the organization before rolling the service out to the public. In order to define the product, the occupational therapy manager has created a memo to be sent out to the organization. See the memo below.

Memo to Organization

Our rehabilitation department is excited to announce a new service for the organization. By appointment, an occupational therapist will complete a work capacity screening for employees. In order to have a work capacity screening completed, managers must provide the following:

- Name of employee
- Times when employee works
- Title of job position
- Detailed job description
- Necessary requirements for the position (for example, lifting demands, amount of time in a required position, etc.)
- Any current concerns or issues

Once scheduled, the occupational therapist will complete the work capacity screening. The screening uses a checklist format that will identify the employee's ability to complete the required tasks, the need for adaptations to complete the tasks, and tasks that the employee will not be able to meet. Recommendations for additional services or equipment will be identified. It will be the manager's responsibility to follow up with the employee on the results of the screening as well as recommendations.

Sincerely,
The Occupational Therapy Manager

By creating a memo with bulleted requirements, the occupational therapy manager has highlighted what is expected from other managers before requesting a screening. In addition, the memo states what will be completed by the OT, and what the manager will be responsible for after the screening is completed.

- *Time costs*, such as the time involved in getting to or using your service, including the time away from paid employment or family
- *Emotional or psychological costs* associated with admitting the need for your service
- *Physical costs*, such as pain associated with a treatment
- *Monetary costs* beyond direct charges for services, such as costs for parking or travel to and from your service location

at a nicer restaurant; however, we do evaluate the cost compared with the quality of the product or service we receive and determine whether the product or service is of good value. This evaluation of cost, quality, and value does not always hold true when it comes to our health care. In fact, seldom are we willing to accept lower-quality services despite lowered costs. We need to be careful when communicating with members of our target populations about the cost and quality of our services and avoid the temptation of promising more for less. Still, even when quality is high, the perceived value of a service may be lessened when members of target populations encounter nonmonetary costs such as difficult parking, long waiting periods, or unpleasant surroundings.

Place

Place refers to where and when your product or service is available to your target populations. Again, this may seem straightforward when it comes to most occupational therapy services. However, as competition for limited health-care reimbursement has increased, health-care providers are becoming more flexible and creative to meet the needs of those they serve and increase customer satisfaction. Giving consideration to providing services on days and at times when members of your target populations are available, such as weekends and evenings, may give your product or service an edge over that of your competitors. Another example might be to develop relation-

ships and programs in which the occupational therapy practitioner brings the program to the target population rather than expecting them to come to a clinical site. The popularity of *onsite work programs* in which rehabilitative services are provided at the workplace of injured workers is an example of such programming that has become increasingly popular. In addition to the advantage for the occupational therapy practitioner in seeing the client's "real-world setting," the client misses less time from the workplace and costs may be saved for both the payer and the employer because they are able to have the injured worker return to light duty more quickly. Finally, managers need to consider providing telehealth services. As an emerging practice area, telehealth services have the potential to be another venue for providing services. Consumers in rural areas may not have access to health-care services or may have to wait to be seen by health-care providers because there are few in their geographic area. Managers need to look into their state laws, practice acts, and reimbursement guidelines in order to determine if telehealth services are an option.

Promotion

New products and services may need to be promoted both within and outside of your organization, depending on the organization's complexity and the target populations for the new programming. A first step to internal or external **promotion** is making a list of anyone else in the organization who might have an interest in your product or service, or who might have an interest in reaching the same target populations. For example, after beginning the hand rehabilitation program described earlier, the manager initiated visits to some local workers' compensation insurance representatives to persuade them to refer their clients to the program. After several visits, the importance of promoting a product or service internally became evident. On one visit the manager encountered questions about the injury tracking system that was being marketed by the manager's organization through direct mail brochures to insurers. On a second visit, the manager discovered that another representative from the organization had made a "cold call" to the insurance office just before the manager's arrival. The representative had been marketing the organization's employee assistance program services.

The manager was unprepared to answer the questions being asked, and it appeared that the manager was not familiar with all that the organization had to offer. In addition, the organization appeared disorganized; it also lost an opportunity to gain some economy of effort to impress potential payers with multiple complementary products. After these experiences, the manager contacted both representatives and they met and undertook a coordinated effort to promote several products that they thought would be attractive to a workers' compensation insurer. Often programs have to be promoted internally or to others within the organization, especially in settings in which occupational therapy is heavily dependent upon others (e.g., nurses or physicians) to identify clients who would benefit from its products and services.

External promotion also calls for a carefully coordinated effort by all stakeholders who are interested in providing products or services to the same target population. By collaborating with others in your organization, you can develop an action plan for promoting your products and services to various target populations. Answering the following questions can help you begin to develop an action plan for external promotion:

1. Who is the target population of your product or service (i.e., the consumer)?
2. Besides the consumer or direct beneficiary of your product or service, who else is either an internal or external customer (e.g., nurses, physicians, payers)?
3. What are the primary goals of your consumers and customers?
4. Who will be involved in deciding where to go for services?
5. What is the most efficient and effective way to reach your consumers and customers?

Physical Evidence

Physical evidence provides tangible information to consumers. Managers need to find ways to turn intangible services into physical evidence (Enache, 2011; Sapre & Nagpal, 2009). Client testimonials and reports of client satisfaction are some ways to provide physical evidence for services provided. Because of privacy laws, caution should be taken and appropriate release forms should be completed for client testimonials or promotional materials that use actual clients. A retrospective research study of client outcomes is another way to provide physical evidence for services

being provided. See Box 14-7 for an example of how an occupational therapy manager used testimonials as physical evidence.

The manager needs to create physical evidence that allows consumers to evaluate and compare the organization's services to those of other competing organizations. Materials should be marketed through print, radio, websites, and social media. The manager needs

---

BOX 14-7

Using Testimonials as Physical Evidence

The occupational therapy manager has decided to share client testimonials as physical evidence on the department website. The following testimonials provided on the department website.

Occupational Therapy Department
Our rehabilitation department provides skilled occupational therapists and occupational therapy assistants in a state-of-the art facility. Don't just take our word for it; see what our clients have to say.

"I loved coming for occupational therapy, my occupational therapist helped me regain the skills I needed to get back to work after my injury. I never thought I would be able to work again, but thanks to Jill I'm back to work and I feel like new!"—John Smith

"I loved coming to occupational therapy! I couldn't believe that there was a house setting! I worked with my therapist on cooking in the kitchen, and practiced getting in and out of the shower in the bathroom. I was even able to practice getting in and out of a recliner in the living room. I don't know any other outpatient rehabilitation centers that have an actual home setting!"—Jane Taylor

By using client testimonials, the occupational therapy manager provided potential consumers with physical evidence about the OTs, OTAs, and the department's facilities. The manager also included photos of the facilities on the website after the client's testimonial about the house setting.

to be aware of the advantages and disadvantages of the organization compared with other organizations in order to market services in a way that is advantageous to the organization.

Packaging

First impressions are vital to an organization. **Packaging** is the initial image that is presented to the consumer and affects how the consumer will judge and select services. For an outpatient practice, the consumer's interaction with the receptionist or secretary on the phone creates a first impression. If the consumer has to wait on the phone for a long period of time or has to leave a message in order to talk to the receptionist, the consumer will likely call a competitor's practice. However, if the consumer is greeted by a friendly voice on the phone and is walked through the process and scheduled promptly, the transaction will be completed.

Managers need to be aware of organizational practices and policies when attempting to create a good first impression. Many impressions are made before the consumer enters the actual department in the organization. Telephone services, parking, and travel distance from the car or public transportation to the department are all factors that impact a consumer's first impression. Managers need to be aware of internal and external factors to the department that make an impression on the consumer.

People

The **people** in the organization and in the department play a vital role in marketing. All employees should know the organization's mission, vision, and goals, as well as their own department's mission, vision, and goals (Richmond, 2011). When employees are knowledgeable of these guiding principles, the employees are empowered and able to act as ambassadors of the organization (Sapre & Nagpal, 2009). This strengthens the overall organization.

Managers need to provide in-services or training to employees to ensure that the employees know the mission, vision, and goals for the organization and department. By providing employees with knowledge of the organization, the employees will feel a personal connection to the organization and want to see the organization succeed. Employees also play an important role in explaining the existing and new

products that your department offers. Educating your employees about how to explain and talk about your services is an important marketing-related task for mid-level managers. For example, a common suggestion given to occupational therapy practitioners is to develop an "elevator speech" so you always have a ready answer to the question, "What is occupational therapy?" Imagine stepping into an elevator while attending a professional conference and someone riding in the elevator with you notices your name badge and asks you, "Occupational therapy; what is that?" Would you have a ready answer that would be motivational and help the person remember your reply the next time he or she heard the words *occupational therapy*?

Selecting Promotional Media

Various methods are available to deliver information about your product or service to members of your target populations; these methods are referred to as promotional media. Choosing the most effective promotional media may be straightforward or complex, depending upon whether you will be promoting your product or service internally, externally, or both. Often the time and financial resources that you have available will limit your choice of promotional strategies. Recognizing the advantages and disadvantages of each form of promotional media will also help you narrow your options and make a selection. The advantages and disadvantages of some of the most common forms of promotional media are presented in Table 14-1. In addition to the strategies listed in Table 14-1, other methods of promoting a new product or service to a target population might include making presentations at a continuing education conference and community groups; developing a newsletter; offering an in-service education program to physicians, nurses, or other target populations; or holding an open house in your department or program (Giles, 2011).

Chapter Summary

This chapter provided an introduction to the marketing process and a description of the four marketing components: organizational assessment, environmental assessment, market analysis, and marketing communications. Hopefully, you now recognize that the process

TABLE 14-1

Advantages and Disadvantages of Common Forms of Promotional Media

Communication Method	Advantages	Disadvantages
Face-to-Face Meetings	• Lower cost depending on number • Can customize message and alter based on response • Can evaluate customer reaction more easily • More personal	• Time intensive; can reach fewer contacts • May be perceived as an interruption
Brochures and Direct Mail	• Can reach larger number of contacts with one effort • Provide contact information in sustainable form for future • Time investment in development only	• Higher cost depending on number and quality • Fixed message • Difficult to evaluate customer reaction and effectiveness of effort • May be difficult to reach the "decision-maker"
Telephone Solicitations	• Lower cost • Can customize message and alter based on response • Can reach larger number of contacts	• May be perceived as an interruption • May be difficult to reach the "decision-maker"
Seminars	• Can customize message and alter based on response • Can evaluate customer reaction more easily • Establishes a relationship with attendees that can be developed	• Higher cost • Time intensive; can reach fewer contacts • Difficult to evaluate customer reaction and effectiveness of effort
TV, Radio, and Print Ads	• Can reach larger number of contacts with one effort • Provide contact information in sustainable form for future • Time investment in development only	• Higher cost • Fixed message
Website	• Can reach a large number of customers • Provide valuable information to the customers on contact information, services provided, and so on • Lower cost • Can track number of site visits	• Time intensive for initial set-up • Requires regular updates • Difficult to evaluate customer reaction and effectiveness
Social Media	• Provide an interactive environment with customers • Provide updated information quickly (written or video) • Can establish a relationship through blogs and threads	• Time intensive for set-up and monitoring of blogs and threads • Requires regular updates and posts • Requires knowledge of current trending social media • Requires strong technology skills

of identifying the needs, resources, and limitations of your organization and of various target markets can be extraordinarily complex. However, this chapter also provided a perspective on simplifying the process and applying it to the common sorts of challenges that an occupational therapy manager may face in developing a new product or service.

Throughout the chapter, the value of developing collaborative relationships with others in your organization, community, and profession that can help you with marketing functions was stressed. Such relationships not only aid in identification of resources that can be used but are also helpful in identifying the various types of data, information, and other forms of evidence available from primary and secondary sources that will help you justify the need for a new product or service. It is also critical that you become aware of the efforts of others who might be developing and promoting complementary products or services for the same target populations so that you share data, information, and other forms of evidence and avoid wasted time and effort.

At the start of the chapter, you were introduced to Patrick, who was being encouraged by his boss, Keesha, to explore and develop additional services that could bring in new streams of revenue. Although he had had some exposure to the marketing process in an administration and management course as part of his occupational therapy education, he decided to begin by reaching out to others in his organization.

■ Real-Life Solutions

After meeting with the director of physical therapy and the associate from the publications and promotions department, Patrick became energized about the process of exploring the needs, resources, and limitations of his department and hospital, as well as those of the target populations served by the department of occupational therapy. The director of physical therapy shared some of the same concerns about whether her department was meeting the needs of physicians, nurses, patients, payers, and other target populations, but had felt overwhelmed and did not know how to start investigating the situation on her own. Not only was the physical therapy director responsive but also, in addition, both she and Patrick received praise and recognition from their boss, Keesha, who appreciated their collaborative efforts.

Patrick learned that he, the director of physical therapy, and the associate from publications and promotions already collected some of the same data, information, and other forms of evidence about the effectiveness of current services and the needs and resources of various target populations. However, he also discovered that they each collected some data, information, or other forms of evidence that were not being widely shared. By combining their efforts, they would not only save valuable time and energy but would be able to develop a more complete picture of some of their key target populations. This also helped to relieve some of Patrick's concern over the limited budget and funds he had to invest in marketing efforts.

Patrick was not surprised to learn that there were few available resources to support new activities or complex and costly strategies for assessing the organization and its environment. He was optimistic that he and his new collaborators would be able to identify creative and inexpensive methods of assessing their departments and their hospital, as well as learn more about the needs, resources, and limitations of their target populations. Patrick and the director of physical therapy each agreed to start by having their staff participate in a SWOT analysis exercise and share the results with each other. They also agreed to have their staff review existing programs and their perceptions of effectiveness and identify any potential new products and services for either discipline so they could begin to collaborate with key stakeholders in the marketing process for occupational therapy and physical therapy.

Patrick, the director of physical therapy, and the associate from publications and promotions agreed to begin meeting every 2 weeks to discuss their progress. Patrick also volunteered to gather data, information, and other forms of evidence on healthcare marketing so that they could begin to develop a more sophisticated understanding of each of the four marketing components and strategies for success.

Marketing can be complex, and the novice occupational therapy manager may feel overwhelmed when first learning about the diverse range of activities that must be completed when exploring the development of a new product or service. In some situations, such as that of a business owner or entrepreneur, it may be wise to consider hiring a marketing consultant to assist with the process, but even the novice manager can rely on skills developed in related managerial functions such as planning and program development to become an active participant in the marketing process.

Study Questions

1. Your manager has asked you to complete a SWOT analysis. Which of the following components of the marketing process addresses the SWOT analysis?

   a. Organizational assessment
   b. Environmental assessment
   c. Market analysis
   d. Marketing communications

2. Which component of the marketing process best helps you to identify the needs of your external customers?

   a. Organizational assessment
   b. Environmental assessment
   c. Market analysis
   d. Marketing communications

3. Which common form of promotional media may be perceived as an interruption by customers?

   a. Direct mailings
   b. Face-to-face meetings
   c. Seminars
   d. TV ads

4. Which of the following sources of data is best categorized as a primary data source?

   a. Government census reports
   b. Economic statistics
   c. Surveys
   d. AOTA tip sheets

5. Tangible information readily available to your customers may best be called:

   a. Tangible evidence.
   b. Price.
   c. Promotion.
   d. SWOT data.

6. From a marketing perspective, the time required to take advantage of your product or service, the psychological and emotional toll of taking advantage of your product or service, and the physical pain that may be experienced when taking advantage of your product or service would best be categorized as which of the following?

   a. Price
   b. Product weaknesses

   c. Disadvantages
   d. Service dissatisfiers

7. From a marketing perspective, nurses, payers, patients, doctors, and outside referral sources may all best be categorized as which of the following?

   a. Health-care consumers
   b. Internal audiences
   c. Customers
   d. External audiences

8. Target populations include which of the following?

   a. Customers
   b. Clients
   c. Third-party payers
   d. All of the above

Resources Related to Marketing Health Services

Journals That Often Publish on Marketing Health Services

Health Marketing Quarterly

http://www.tandfonline.com/toc/whmq20/current#.VDlnLL5t6nI

Health Marketing Quarterly is a journal that targets professionals in the areas of marketing for health and human services. The journal focuses on applied strategies and resources such as "how-to" marketing tools. Each issue includes articles that demonstrate the applicability of marketing for specific health services. Health-care managers and service providers will appreciate the inclusion of articles and columns devoted to such topics as how to develop a thorough marketing approach and how marketing can improve awareness of opportunities, increase customer and patient satisfaction, and improve the cost-effectiveness of programs. The focus of the journal is broad and includes a range of contexts, including:

- Group practice marketing
- Mental health marketing
- Long-term care marketing
- The marketing of ambulatory care

- Alternative care programs
- Social services
- Hospitals
- Health maintenance organizations
- Health insurance
- Health products

Strategic Health Care Marketing

https://www.plainenglishmedia.com/plain-english
-health-care/strategic-health-care-marketing/

Strategic Health Care Marketing focuses on news, analysis, and interpretation of events affecting the ever-changing health-care services marketplace. Coverage includes

- Customer and patient satisfaction
- Wellness and prevention
- Advertising and brand management
- The Internet
- Niche marketing opportunities
- Employee recruitment and retention
- Database and relationship marketing
- Care management
- Community and public relations
- Special markets
- Report cards
- Ambulatory care development
- Market research reports
- Physician relations
- New product development
- Planning
- Service line management

Organizations Concerned With Marketing Health Services

American Marketing Association

http://www.marketingpower.com/

The American Marketing Association (AMA) has over 30,000 members representing every area of marketing, including health-related fields. For over seven decades, the AMA has served as a resource for providing marketing information. The AMA website offers a wide array of newly expanded information, including a guide for better social media security, ways to increase customer loyalty, a guide for social marketing in an online community, secrets of data-driven chief medical officers, ingredients to smarter marketing, and other resources. The AMA's prestigious marketing journals provide access to the newest developments in marketing thought, whereas the AMA has a more practical focus on the applications of marketing strategies to address daily needs on the job. In addition, the AMA offers specialty conferences to help marketers build the skills that keep them ahead of emerging trends, as well as help with long-term professional development.

Reference List

American Occupational Therapy Association. (2013). Telehealth position paper. *American Journal of Occupational Therapy, 67,* S69–S90.

American Occupational Therapy Association. (2014). Occupational therapy practice framework: Domain and process (3rd ed). *American Journal of Occupational Therapy, 68,* S1–S48.

Doman, D., Dennison, D., & Doman, M. (2002). *Market research made easy.* Bellingham, WA: Self-Counsel Press.

Enache, I.-C. (2011). Marketing higher education using the 7 Ps framework. *Bulletin of the Transilvania University of Brasov, 4,* 23–30.

Giles, G. (2011). Starting a new program, business, or practice. In K. Jacobs & G. McCormack (Eds.), *The occupational therapy manager* (5th ed., pp. 145–166). Bethesda, MD: AOTA Press.

Richmond, T. (2011). Marketing occupational therapy. In K. Jacobs & G. McCormack (Eds.), *The occupational therapy manager* (5th ed., pp. 127–143). Bethesda, MD: AOTA Press.

Sapre, A., & Nagpal, A. (2009). Viewer relationship management in Indian news channels: An analysis using the 7 Ps framework. *The Icfai University Journal of Marketing Management, 8,* 38–47.

Yamkovenko, S. (2013). *The emerging niche: What is next in your practice area?* Retrieved from American Occupational Therapy Association website: http://www.aota.org/Practice/Manage/Niche.aspx

CHAPTER 15

Developing Evidence-Based Occupational Therapy Programming

Brent Braveman, PhD, OTR/L, FAOTA

■ Real-Life Management

David recently attended the annual American Occupational Therapy Association (AOTA) Conference & Exposition, where he sat in on a number of presentations on current research, evidence-based practice, and methods of developing occupation-based programming. After the conference, he is convinced that he and the occupational therapy practitioners that he supervises need to integrate strategies for using evidence into their daily work and their ongoing program development.

Upon returning to the mental health agency where he works, David realizes that all of the presentations he attended focused on how practitioners could use evidence in making decisions about how to directly intervene with clients. Although those strategies are clear to him, he begins to wonder about how he can use evidence in his daily work. David's work often relates to making decisions at the program level as he plans, develops, implements, and evaluates occupational therapy services. For example, he has recently been asked to lead the development of a new day treatment program in conjunction with other clinical disciplines.

David and his associates, the occupational therapists (OTs) and occupational therapy assistants (OTAs) he supervises, have always been well respected by the physicians, social workers, nurses, and other professionals with whom they work for their use and application of theory. They have become skilled at combining both occupational therapy theory and conceptual practice models with theories and models developed by other disciplines.

As David begins to think about planning the new program, he identifies the following questions:

1. How can an occupational therapy manager use theory and evidence in planning, developing,

Continued

■ Real-Life Management—cont'd

implementing, and evaluating occupational therapy services?

2. What is the relationship between a program development model and a theory?

3. What kinds of theories or models are available to guide program development?

4. How are different theories and models combined as you proceed with program development using an evidence-based approach?

Critical Thinking Questions

As you read this chapter, consider the following questions:

- How can available evidence on the problem a program is meant to address be used to impact the underlying mechanisms of action in order to promote the desired change in the target population?

- How can occupational therapy conceptual practice models and related knowledge be combined in order to address all mechanisms of action required for a comprehensive program?

- How will the varying levels of evidence that exist to validate occupational therapy theories, conceptual practice models, and frames of reference (and theories from related knowledge) impact the use of these models in the development of programming?

- How can the use of a program development model guide the occupational therapy manager through the process of applying appropriate theories while assessing the needs of the target population and the environments in which programming will be delivered?

Glossary

- **Beliefs:** convictions or feelings that something is real or true that rest at some point on a body of fundamental definitions or irreducible axiomatic principles whose truth is accepted a priori; they do not require, and may not be susceptible to, proof.
- **Conceptual practice model:** tool used to help generate theory and the methods (e.g., assessments and intervention strategies) therapists use in their everyday work to apply that theory.
- **Frame of reference:** structure for guiding practice by delineating the beliefs, assump-

tions, definitions, and concepts within a specific area of practice. Frames of reference employ existing theory and focus on developing methods of applying that theory in occupational therapy.
- **Knowledge:** the condition of apprehending truth or fact; it entails the awareness that particular propositions or assertions are factual or true on the basis of some justification or evidence that sufficiently supports them.
- **Mechanisms of action:** tools that specify what changes, how change proceeds, the conditions under which an intervention achieves beneficial

---

Glossary—cont'd

results, and why a change may occur for certain groups of consumers and not others.

- **Occupational therapy paradigm:** knowledge that specifically addresses the identity and perspective of the occupational therapy profession. It articulates a shared vision of members of the field that defines the nature and purpose of the discipline.

- **Related knowledge:** knowledge from outside occupational therapy that has been developed and investigated primarily by members of another discipline.
- **Theory:** an explanation of how or why a particular phenomenon occurs and how that phenomenon might be influenced.

Introduction

Occupational therapy managers often find themselves responsible for developing, planning, implementing, and evaluating programming. Occupational therapy program development can be relatively simple, such as developing an intervention for individuals with a specific diagnosis in a familiar practice setting, for example, formalizing a protocol for educating patients undergoing a total hip replacement as part of a critical pathway within an acute care hospital.

Conversely, program development can be complicated and challenging. It can require the assessment of how complex human and environmental factors impact totally new target populations in nontraditional practice contexts, for example, developing independent living and prevocational programming for persons living with HIV/AIDS in a transitional living residence that previously operated with a hospice focus. Such program development may call for the use of multiple theories and new approaches to organizing interventions.

Regardless of the program's complexity, reliance on sound theory by evaluating and using available evidence is the best strategy for developing effective services with good outcomes. The value of evidence-based practice and strategies for finding and evaluating evidence were presented in previous chapters. This chapter focuses on strategies for integrating theory and evidence with program planning. Before beginning this discussion, the definition of a few key terms and concepts would be helpful.

How Is Knowledge Organized in Occupational Therapy? Paradigms, Theories, Conceptual Practice Models, and Related Knowledge

In occupational therapy, different authors and scholars use different terms to describe the knowledge that managers might use to guide program development. Terms such as *theory*, *model*, and *frame of reference* are sometimes used interchangeably in the field, although scholars often use these terms to refer to concepts that are quite different from each other. Moreover, the necessity of using bodies of knowledge from other disciplines (e.g., related knowledge) can lead to encounters with yet other terminology, which can cause additional confusion and frustration.

Although you should not become overly bogged down in the differences in terminology, it is useful to have some understanding of how knowledge is organized and approached by occupational therapy scholars. There are three broad categories of knowledge and related questions: (1) knowledge that seeks to answer the ontological questions related to what is most real for occupational therapy, (2) knowledge that seeks to answer the epistemological questions related to what is known and understood in occupational therapy, and (3) knowledge that seeks to answer the axiologic questions related to what is the right action to be taken by the occupational therapy practitioner (Hooper & Wood, 2014). Occupational therapy literature can often be categorized to fit one of these questions.

It is also helpful to understand why different authors and scholars use different terminology. Having a clear understanding of the differences between terms used to describe the organization of knowledge can assist you in applying this knowledge to the process of planning, developing, implementing, and evaluating occupational therapy programming. Therefore, a brief discussion of some of these terms is presented in this section as a means of highlighting the key contributions that well-developed theories and models make to guiding program development. The terms that will be defined are *theory*, *paradigm*, *conceptual practice model*, *frame of reference*, and *related knowledge*.

A **theory** provides an explanation of how or why a particular phenomenon occurs and how that phenomenon might be influenced. Theories are often composed of both general concepts that refer to larger chunks of reality and specific concepts that refer to the elements of which they are organized. Thus, the key element of a theory is explanation—that is, giving a plausible account for how something works (Kielhofner, 2009). Theories provide a way of understanding what is necessary for practice. For example, we might be interested in why people choose to participate in specific occupations while choosing not to participate in other occupations, and how this process can be influenced or used when collaborating with persons with disabilities to reestablish a full complement of roles. A theory that seeks to explain motivation and interests would be helpful in this case. It is unlikely, however, that a theory that seeks to explain motivation and interest would also seek to explain complex elements of neuromuscular function such as reflexes or motor planning. For this reason, occupational therapy managers need to draw from a wide range of theories in developing occupational therapy programming. Theory is found in the occupational therapy paradigm, in frames of reference, in conceptual practice models, and in related knowledge.

Cohn and Coster (2014, p. 482) contrast a broad definition of theory ("a plausible or scientifically acceptable general principle or body of principles offered to explain a phenomena") and a discrete definition of theory ("a hypothesis assumed for the sake of argument or investigation"). They note that, although theories in general make claims about hypothesized relationships, some theories are more developed and specific regarding how to intervene, essential features of the intervention, how they are meant to address the underlying cause of a problem,

or how they specifically address a phenomena. For example, Kielhofner (2009, p. 68) cited "kinematics" as an underlying theory of the biomechanical conceptual practice model. Kinematics seeks to explain how forces produce motion in the body. It should be noted that even though Kielhofner includes biomechanics as a conceptual practice model, others refer to it as a frame of reference. A second example provided by Kielhofner (p. 204) is that the sensory integration practice model is based on theories that explain how the brain processes sensation and how it results in motor and other responses.

The **occupational therapy paradigm** is knowledge that specifically addresses the occupational therapy profession's identity and perspective. It articulates a shared vision of members of the field that defines the discipline's nature and purpose (Kielhofner, 2009). The occupational therapy paradigm addresses the following factors:

- What human need does the service address?
- What kinds of problems does it solve?
- How does it solve these problems (i.e., what is the nature of its service)?

Paradigms include theory to address these questions, but the theory in a paradigm is broad and focused on questions such as what the focus of an occupational therapy program should be. It does not provide more concrete concepts and tools for practice and it does not provide specific guidance for the steps to take when developing occupational therapy programming.

A **conceptual practice model** generates theory and the methods (e.g., assessments and intervention strategies) that are used by practitioners in their everyday work to apply that theory. These methods are sometimes referred to as *technology for application*. Each conceptual practice model addresses some phenomenon related to occupational functioning (e.g., motivation, perception, movement) and specifies theories and tools for application pertaining to particular kinds of problems in that area. Because each conceptual practice model focuses on specific phenomena or areas of function or capacity, you will likely need to rely on a combination of conceptual practice models to develop a comprehensive program that addresses the range of factors influencing your clients' occupational functioning. A conceptual practice model often builds upon theories from a variety of disciplines to create a new unique theory that explains the problems and challenges addressed by the model. For example, the Model of Human Occupation (MOHO) integrates theories related to motivation, habits, underlying human capacities, and the environment.

A **frame of reference** is a structure for guiding practice by delineating the beliefs, assumptions, definitions, and concepts within a specific area of practice. Frames of reference employ existing theory and focus on developing methods of applying that theory in occupational therapy. So, for example, a frame of reference may delineate a function–dysfunction continuum, evaluation processes, and intervention strategies that are consistent with a theory from outside occupational therapy (e.g., behavioral theory or object relations theory) (Crepeau & Schell, 2003).

Thus, the most important distinction between the use of the terms *conceptual practice model* and *frame of reference* is that conceptual practice models generate theory unique to occupational therapy, whereas frames of reference simply apply existing theory to practice (Kielhofner, 2009). A frame of reference may borrow a theory from another discipline and apply it to occupational therapy practice without formulating unique occupational therapy theory or giving consideration to how occupational therapy practitioners would use the knowledge differently from professionals in other disciplines. For example, sensory integration is a model of practice developed by OTs. It includes theory that seeks to explain how the human nervous system perceives and processes information to guide performance. Although many of the concepts of sensory integration build on interdisciplinary theory, this model offers a unique theoretical explanation that guides occupational therapy intervention. An example of a frame of reference is object relations (Buckley, 1996). The underlying theory for this frame of reference comes from the psychoanalytic tradition of psychiatry and psychology. In occupational therapy, these concepts are applied to understanding how involvement in occupations and the relationship with the therapist can be used to achieve the kinds of personal change in occupational therapy patients that psychologists and psychiatrists seek to achieve in their psychotherapy patients.

Related knowledge comes from outside occupational therapy and thus has been developed and investigated primarily by members of other disciplines. For example, a theory of motor learning may address redundancies in neurological systems that allow individuals with a stroke or brain injury to relearn familiar tasks such as putting on a sock or opening a cabinet door. Although many occupational therapy practitioners may rely upon such knowledge to guide their interventions with these clients, occupational therapy scholars were not primarily responsible for developing this knowledge. Box 15-1 summarizes the key terms presented here and their definitions.

BOX 15-1

Definition of Key Terms

Theory: Explanation of how or why a particular phenomenon occurs and how that phenomenon might be influenced. Theories are often composed of both general concepts that refer to larger segments of reality and specific concepts that refer to the elements of which they are organized.

Frame of reference: Structure for guiding practice by delineating the beliefs, assumptions, definitions, and concepts within a specific area of practice. Frames of reference employ existing theory and focus on developing methods of applying that theory in occupational therapy.

Conceptual practice model: Model that generates theory and the methods (e.g., assessments and intervention strategies) that are used by therapists in their everyday work to apply that theory. Each model addresses some phenomenon related to occupational functioning (e.g., motivation, perception, movement) and specifies theory and tools for application pertaining to particular kinds of problems in that area.

Paradigm: Knowledge that specifically addresses the identity and perspective of the occupational therapy profession. The paradigm articulates a shared vision of members of the field that defines the nature and purpose of the discipline.

Related knowledge: Knowledge that comes from outside occupational therapy and thus has been developed and investigated primarily by members of another discipline.

In developing most occupational therapy programs (regardless of level of complexity), managers will undoubtedly rely on a combination of the occupational therapy paradigm—to guide thinking about what the service should be—and conceptual practice models and related knowledge—to define more specifically what problems are addressed, what services are provided, what outcomes will be achieved, and how they will be achieved. An example of such a combination is presented at the end of this chapter in Case Example 1, which spotlights the Enabling Self-Determination (ESD) for Persons Living With HIV/AIDS Program. In this program, the developers used an occupational therapy conceptual practice model, MOHO, as the overarching guide for program development. However, in developing the program's discrete intervention elements, reliance on multiple theories and models from related knowledge, including disability studies, Social Cognitive Theory, the Transtheoretical Model (TTM) of Change, and the Health Belief Model (HBM), helped guide decision-making (McLeroy, Bibeau, Steckler, & Glanz, 1988; Prochaska & DiClemente, 1993; Strecher, DeVillis, Becker, & Rosenstock, 1986).

Learning to become comfortable in thinking about ways in which to combine various theories and models represents an important skill set for occupational therapy managers. As with other skill sets, you will learn and develop your program development skills through application. Initially, heavy reliance on a program development model may be useful as a guide to decision-making and sequencing of tasks for the new manager who is unsure of his or her skills. However, just as with assessment skills, documentation skills, or other skill sets, over time the program development process will become more fluid as you gain confidence and will likely take on a more "organic" nature.

Program Development Models

Numerous discussions of approaches to program development and case examples of programs can be found in the occupational therapy literature (Braveman, Goldbaum, Goldstein, Karlic, & Kielhofner, 2001; Braveman, Kielhofner, Belanger, Llerena, & de las Heras, 2002; Braveman, Sen, & Kielhofner, 2001; Brownson, 2001; Giles, 2011; Grossman & Bortone,

1986; Scaffa, 2014). Parallel to the discussion earlier in this chapter of the different types of theories, this section presents a discussion of the focus of different types of program development models. Models for program development and evaluation may have different foci. Some program development models are more focused on systematic levels and are useful in guiding us in deciding where and with whom to intervene to address a particular challenge or health problem. Other models are more useful in guiding decision-making once a setting and population for an intervention are known. For example, the Ecological Model of Health Promotion describes five societal levels at which intervention could be planned (McLeroy et al, 1988; Sallis, Owen, & Fisher, 2008). These five levels are:

1. *Intrapersonal:* individual factors and characteristics such as knowledge, beliefs, and values that may influence behavior.
2. *Interpersonal:* relationships and interactions with persons such as friends, family, and peer groups that are examined for opportunities to influence behavior.
3. *Institutional:* the structures within organizations and their programs, policies, and procedures that are examined for opportunities to influence behavior.
4. *Organizational:* the interrelationships between organizations or within existing social networks that are examined for opportunities to influence behavior.
5. *Public policy:* the policies, programs, and regulations of local, state, and federal bodies that are examined for opportunities to influence or regulate behavior.

Although the Ecological Model of Health Promotion is very helpful in deciding *where* one might intervene once a particular challenge or health problem is identified, it is not useful in deciding *how* to intervene. To make this decision, reliance on a more focused model to guide decision-making regarding how to combine various theories (paradigmatic and related knowledge) and how to sequence program development actions is useful. Various models may emphasize different factors depending on the particular context in which the model is implemented. Four common processes, which are defined in Box 15-2 and illustrated in Figure 15-1, are typically involved.

BOX 15-2

The Four Steps of Program Development

- **Needs assessment:** The process of describing the target population, naming perceived and felt needs, and analyzing available resources and constraints both internal and external to the organization or context in which the program is being planned.
- **Program planning:** The process of identifying the steps and sequence of actions to be taken to plan for initiation of the program.
- **Program implementation:** The process of initiating intervention first in trial format and then in a more formal and sustained manner.
- **Program evaluation:** The ongoing process of assessing the impact and quality of program processes and outcomes and making continuous improvements in efficiency and effectiveness.

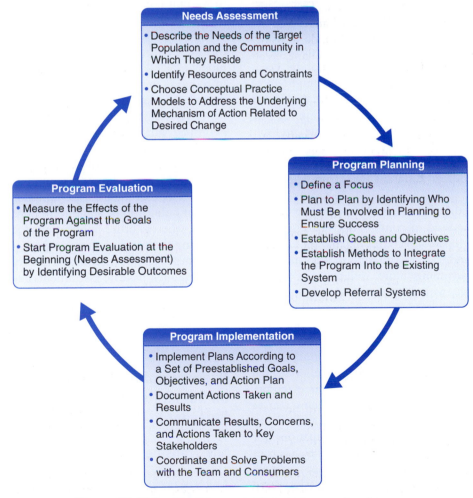

Figure ■ 15-1 Four Common Processes in Program Development.

What Are the Relationships Between Theory and a Program Development Model?

Theories or conceptual practice models and program development models are used in combination to guide decision-making about where, how, and when to intervene given a chosen problem or target population. We seldom begin the process of developing occupational therapy programming without predefining some critical variables, such as the context or organization in which the program will be delivered or the target population to whom it will be delivered. For this reason, and because no single theory or practice model typically addresses all of the factors needed to plan intervention, you should begin by identifying a program development model that will help guide the order of your managerial actions. In some cases, especially in emerging areas of practice, we may be familiar with the target population but not yet be aware of its needs, or we may be interested in addressing an area of occupational dysfunction and not be completely sure where to intervene or who might most benefit from the services. In such a case (as in the ESD Program case and the oncology programing case later in this chapter), you might combine multiple program development models in the same way you might combine several conceptual practice models that seek to address different but complementary phenomena.

To explain further, here is an example of how several models might be used in combination. Imagine that you wish to develop an intervention program for older adults living in high-rise apartment buildings in a large city who are becoming more isolated and having increased difficulty with daily activities such as getting groceries and maintaining social contacts. The Ecological Model of Health Promotion may help you decide *where* to intervene, such as at the intrapersonal, interpersonal, organizational, and community levels. The four-step program development model presented in Figure 15-1 can help you develop your program. You know that you need a model that helps you to understand motivation and why older adults may choose to become involved in various occupations; for this reason, you select MOHO. As you develop specific intervention components, you find that you need to address physical aspects of function such as decreased strength, lack of endurance, and other deficits because

of normal aging or conditions such as arthritis. To address these problems, you rely on related knowledge such as the biomechanical model and neurological model in combination with MOHO.

Whether from the occupational therapy paradigm or from related knowledge, we should recognize that different theories and models have been developed to varying extents. In other words, different levels of evidence exist. Some theories and models are well investigated, have established assessments or other technologies for application, and have substantial and growing bodies of evidence to support their use. Other theories or models have been presented in the literature, but valid assessments or other technologies for application are limited and relatively little evidence exists to support their use. In some cases, even though a theory or model may receive initial attention, interest may wane because of the lack of strong evidence to warrant continued investigations.

For example, the Ecology of Human Performance (EHP), MOHO, Occupational Adaptation (OA), and the Person-Environment-Occupational Performance model (PEOP) are all occupation-focused models introduced in the last few decades. Lee (2010) conducted a review of the literature and evaluated evidence related to each of these models. She found 503 published works: 12 related to the EHP, 433 related to MOHO, 31 related to OA, and 27 related to the PEOP model. She also noted that, although textbooks and chapters were the most commonly found form of publication, there was a wide variation in the types and focus of publications; some were purely descriptive in nature, whereas other publications focused on studies, including the psychometric property of assessment or outcomes of application of the theory. The EHP and PEOP models have no assessments designed to capture constructs of the model, OA has one assessment and MOHO has more than 20 assessments.

Overview of Evidence on Select Related Knowledge Relevant to Program Development

The Transtheoretical Model of Change

Much of occupational therapy programming is implemented with the expectation that, as a result of intervention, consumers will adopt some new behavior or change behavior in some way in order to better facilitate occupational performance. One model, the TTM of Change, suggests that change often occurs in a series of stages (Prochaska & DiClemente, 1993; Prochaska & Norcross, 2006). This model has been well investigated in relation to behaviors such as smoking cessation, weight control, and exercise. It has not yet been studied in regard to adoption of behaviors that might be promoted by occupational therapy practitioners, such as adopting joint protection techniques, wearing a splint, adhering to a physician-suggested medication regimen, or regularly completing skin checks to prevent pressure sores.

As with most staged models, it is important to remember that not everyone will experience each stage, and often individuals may cycle between stages, reverting to an earlier stage and progressing again to a later stage. Individuals may also skip a stage altogether. With behavior change, such as ceasing substance abuse, stopping smoking, or beginning to exercise, several failed attempts to start or stop a behavior may be made before finally incorporating the new behavior in a habitual pattern. We might expect this same pattern with the adoption of new occupational behavior as well.

In the first stage, *precontemplation*, individuals are unaware or under-aware of a problem or the benefits of adopting a new behavior pattern, so there is no intention to change behavior in the foreseeable future. In the second stage, *contemplation*, people are aware that a problem exists and are seriously thinking about overcoming it, but have yet to make a commitment to action. In the third stage, *preparation*, intention is combined with behavioral criteria, so individuals are intending to take action in the next month or have unsuccessfully taken action in the recent past. In the fourth stage, *action*, individuals take steps to modify their behavior or seek experiences to modify their environment in order to overcome their problems. In the final stage, *maintenance*, individuals work to prevent relapse and consolidate the gains that they attained during action. The five stages of the TTM of Change are summarized in Box 15-3. Table 15-1 includes a selection of evidence on health behaviors in studies that used the TTM.

Although this model may appear relatively simple, the complexity of human behavior and the difficulty of altering behavior patterns must be recognized. As noted by Kielhofner (2007), habits resist change

---

BOX 15-3

The Transtheoretical Model of Change

- **Precontemplation:** Persons are unaware or under-aware of a health problem or the benefit of performing a health behavior.
- **Contemplation:** Persons are aware of a health problem and are considering taking action but have not committed to any specific action or begun performing a health behavior.
- **Preparation:** Intention to begin performance of a health behavior is combined with criteria for action that include a time frame to begin acting.
- **Action:** Individuals attempt to incorporate health behaviors into their routines.
- **Maintenance:** Health behaviors are successfully incorporated into daily routines so the behaviors become habitual.

---

because they are based on our most fundamental certainties about how the world is constructed. However, the construct of habits is critical to consider in regard to health behavior because habits organize our underlying performance capacities so that we can perform within our environments. Occupational therapists and occupational therapy assistants can play a crucial role in helping individuals to habituate health behaviors by incorporating those behaviors into their daily routines. Understanding the process of change can help the occupational therapy manager develop a program by incorporating elements to assist individuals at any stage of change and to move toward maintenance. Table 15-2 provides an example of how each stage of the TTM of Change can be incorporated into a program.

In the ESD Program case example presented later in this chapter, the health behavior addressed by the programming is a person living with HIV/AIDS adopting a strategy of carrying a day's supply of medications in his briefcase so that he does not find himself without access to his medications. This strategy improves his adherence to his physician-recommended medication regimen, a behavior that is critical to preventing the development of drug resistance.

TABLE 15-1

Summary of Selected Evidence Using the Transtheoretical Model (TTM) of Change

Author	Study Type	N (Sample Size)	Level of Evidence	Results
Blaney et al (2012)	Cross-sectional measure development	521 African American adults	Strong	Results support the use of TTM measures for tailored interventions to increase exercise in an at-risk population.
Riley, Toth, & Fava (2000)	Cross-sectional survey	9 women at risk and 10 HIV-infected women	Weak	The study supports use of the TTM to examine readiness to use stress management behavior in women regardless of their HIV serostatus.
Jammer, Wolitski, & Corby (1997)	Repeated cross-sectional sampling with matched intervention and comparison communities	3,081 injection drug users	Strong	77% of injection drug users in the intervention area reported being exposed to an intervention to increase condom carrying. Rates of condom carrying increased from 10% to 27% ($p < .001$). There was also an increase from 2.32 to 3.11 in mean stage of change for using condoms with other partners, while stage of change decreased in the comparison area ($p < .01$).
Galavotti et al (1995)	Cross-sectional questionnaire after intervention	296 women at high risk for HIV infection and transmission	Good	Results support the usefulness of the TTM for understanding and assessing contraceptive behavior among women at high risk for HIV infection and unintended pregnancy.
Glanz et al (1995)	Cross-sectional survey after intervention	17,121 employees participating in the Working Well Study	Good	The TTM proved useful in an intervention to reduce fat intake and increase fiber and fruit and vegetable intake. Stage of change was associated with fat, fiber, and fruit and vegetables intake in a stepwise manner as predicted.
Prochaska & DiClemente (1993)	Randomized assignment to one of four intervention conditions	756 smokers	Strong	Results suggest that providing smokers with interactive feedback about their stages of change, decisional balance, processes of change, self-efficacy, and temptation levels in critical smoking situations can produce greater success than just providing the best self-help manuals currently available.
Marcus et al (1992)	Correlational postintervention study	610 community members	Good	Most participants increased their stage of exercise adoption during a 6-week program designed using the TTM (62% of participants in contemplation became more active and 61% of participants in preparation became more active).

TABLE 15-2	
Application of the Transtheoretical Model (TTM) of Change Within a Program for Persons Living With HIV/AIDS	
Stage of Change	**Elements of Occupational Therapy Programming**
Precontemplation	Health education groups are conducted and include information on the definition of satisfactory medication adherence and the negative impact of missing medications and health problems associated with resistance to medications.
Contemplation	Activities to identify current adherence rate with physician-recommended medication regimens and causes for missing scheduled medications are undertaken.
Preparation	Information on strategies to improve medication adherence (e.g., carrying a full day's dose of medications in one's briefcase, backpack, or purse) is included in multiple venues, including support and educational groups, handouts, and planning in individual occupational therapy sessions. Activities are undertaken to assist the individual in identifying reasons for missing medication doses and selecting strategies to resolve those problems.
Action	The individual attempts to implement selected strategies with the support of the OT, other program staff, and peers. The expectation that attempts often initially fail is freely shared, and positive reinforcement is provided for successful implementation of strategies. The individual is an active partner with the OT in identifying strategies that are not a good match for his or her routine; dysfunctional strategies are dropped and alternatives are explored.
Maintenance	Occasional reassessment of adherence rates is included in group and individual occupational therapy sessions, positive reinforcement is provided often, and activities to help establish a positive view of a routine that includes the desired health behavior, such as having the individual mentor others, are incorporated.

The TTM of Change explains the process of change in regard to a discrete behavior. In other words, the model must be applied to each behavior that you wish an individual to consider starting, stopping, or continuing, or to avoid ever beginning. Therefore, the model may be applied to many aspects of the program (i.e., each behavior you want to change). Although this may appear confusing at first, it can be highlighted by the following simple example. If you stand outside of any health club, you will soon notice people emerge who have just invested considerable time and energy taking part in one "healthy" behavior, that of exercising. Some of these same individuals will immediately take part in the "unhealthy" behavior of lighting up a cigarette. Application of the TTM of Change to influence the health behavior of exercising will not automatically influence the health behavior of not smoking. Different interventions would need to be included in any program intended to influence both behaviors. Choices about health behaviors are complicated.

However, whereas some programs are targeted at improving health or quality of life by influencing multiple behaviors, you should recognize that often occupational therapy programming is targeted at incorporating discrete behaviors so that they become habits.

The Health Belief Model

The Health Belief Model (HBM) was originally developed in the 1950s through an initiative by the U.S. Public Health Service. The HBM describes the influence of individuals' beliefs in regard to a particular health behavior on whether the individuals are likely to adopt the behavior. The model posits that choices to behave or not behave in certain ways are influenced by four sets of *perceived beliefs*. These beliefs are *perceived susceptibility*, *perceived seriousness*, *perceived barriers*, and *perceived benefits*. In addition, a *cue to action* is thought to trigger behavior (acting or not acting).

Cues to action may be internal (such as pain or discomfort) or external (such as the presence of others involved in the behavior). An internal cue, such as fatigue or blurred vision, might cue a person with diabetes to check his or her blood sugar or take an insulin injection. An external cue, such as seeing a traveling partner put on a seat belt, might cue a person getting into a taxicab to put on his or her seat belt as well. These concepts were proposed as accounting for people's "readiness to act." An added concept, *cues to action*, would activate that readiness and stimulate overt behavior. A recent addition to the HBM is the concept of *self-efficacy*, or one's confidence in the ability to successfully perform an action. This concept was added by Rosenstock, Strecher, and Becker 1988 to help the HBM better fit the challenges of changing habitual unhealthy behaviors, such as being sedentary, smoking, or overeating (University of Twente, 2014).

It is also helpful to distinguish between the constructs of *knowledge* and *belief*; although both may influence behavior, different strategies may be required to change behavior depending upon the knowledge that an individual has, and what he or she believes. Knowledge is the condition of apprehending truth or fact. **Knowledge** entails the awareness that particular propositions or assertions are factual or true on the basis of some justification or evidence that sufficiently supports them. **Beliefs** are convictions or feelings that something is real or true. Belief systems rest at some point on a body of fundamental definitions or irreducible axiomatic principles whose truth is accepted a priori; they do not require, and may not be susceptible to, proof. Beliefs may be unassailable or closed propositions inaccessible to argument. *Belief* and *knowledge* are relative terms that are context dependent. We often have a tendency to claim our own worldview as knowledge and that of others as belief. For example, it might be reasonable to state that today most adults have the knowledge that a diet high in saturated fat and cholesterol may contribute to coronary artery disease. Such knowledge may be viewed as fact based on evidence presented through scientific trials. In contrast, some individuals believe that health status may be influenced by prayer. Although most would agree that, to date, such a belief has not been irrefutably proven by scientific inquiry, many hold a belief in a higher power that would make their belief in prayer impervious to argument.

It is worth noting that, in addition to using the HBM within a program to consider how to influence individual behaviors, the model can also be used to improve compliance with a program. Because this model spells out the factors that influence a person's acceptance and maintenance of the necessary steps to achieve change, it is often helpful in organizing a program in a way that will enhance compliance or participation in the program itself.

Table 15-3 provides examples of each of the four sets of beliefs of the HBM and an example of cues to action as they might influence the health behavior of wearing a bicycle helmet. Table 15-4 provides examples of selected evidence on the HBM.

TABLE 15-3	
The Health Belief Model Applied to the Health Behavior of Wearing a Bicycle Helmet	
Perceived Susceptibility	The beliefs that you are susceptible to a head injury if you fall while riding a bike, and that a fall is possible or likely, will increase the chances of wearing a helmet.
Perceived Seriousness	The belief that, if you fall and hit your head, the injury is likely to be serious will increase the chances of wearing a helmet.
Perceived Barriers	The beliefs that you might look silly, that helmets are hot, and that friends may make fun of you will decrease the chances of wearing a helmet.
Perceived Benefits	The beliefs that wearing a helmet will contribute to a sense of safety and well-being and set a good example for your children will increase the chances of wearing a helmet.
Cues to Action	A sense of guilt for getting on a bicycle in front of your children without a helmet and seeing your spouse put on a helmet may cue you to wear a helmet.

TABLE 15-4

Summary of Selected Evidence on the Health Belief Model (HBM)

Author	Study Type	N (Sample Size)	Level of Evidence	Results
Kim, Ahn, & No (2012)	Survey	251 students	Good	Perceived benefit of eating healthy food and perceived barrier for eating healthy food had significant effects on behavioral intentions and was a valid measurement to use to determine behavioral intentions.
Davis, Buchanan, & Green (2013)	Secondary analysis of cross-sectional survey	7,452 adults	Good	The constructs of self-efficacy, perceived benefits, and perceived susceptibility were significantly associated with race and ethnicity. The remaining three constructs were not statistically significant. Multivariate analysis revealed Hispanics were less likely to believe they could lower their chances of getting cancer than did African Americans and whites. Hispanics, Asians, and African Americans were more likely to believe they had a lower chance of getting cancer in the future than did whites.
Winfield & Whaley (2002)	Predictive	261 college students	Good	Perceived barriers were found to be a significant predictor of condom use.
Ali (2002)	Predictive	178 women	Good	Perceived susceptibility and perceived seriousness predicted coronary heart disease preventive behaviors.
Perkins (1999)	Predictive	144 adults	Strong	Patients who believe the risks of treatment outweigh the benefits are likely to discontinue their medication.
Sapp & Jensen (1998)	Cross-sectional survey	1,502 adults	Good	The HBM provided a good prediction of perceived dietary quality and moderate prediction of actual dietary quality.
Conrad, Cambell, Edington, & Faust (1996)	Quasi-experimental	310 smokers	Strong	Exposure to a worksite health-promoting environment as a cue to smoking reduction had a significant effect on posttest smoking.
Fischera & Frank (1995)	Descriptive	110 nurses	Weak	Found some support for the HBM, with noncompliers having significantly higher barrier scores.

Social Cognitive Theory

Originally presented by Bandura in the 1970s as Social Learning Theory, Social Cognitive Theory holds that behavior is determined by expectancies and incentives. Expectancies can be divided into three types: (1) expectancies about environmental cues, which are called environmental expectancies; (2) expectancies about the consequences of one's own behavior, which are called outcome expectancies; and (3) expectancies about one's competence to perform a behavior necessary to achieve a particular outcome, which are called efficacy expectations. Incentives (or reinforcements) are the value that an individual places on particular outcomes; these might include the praise or criticism of peers, improved perceived health, or financial impact (Rosenstock, Strecher, & Becker, 1988).

Expectancies and incentives influence behavior together. For example, a person who values the effects of beginning to exercise on a regular basis (incentives) will be more likely to attempt to exercise if he or she believes that (a) his or her current lack of exercise poses health threats (environmental cues), (b) exercising will decrease the threats and lead to improved health (outcome expectations), and (c) he or she is capable of adopting a new exercise regimen (efficacy expectations) (Bandura, 2012). Table 15-5 summarizes expectancies and incentives as they relate to adopting the health behavior of beginning to exercise.

Although all elements of Social Cognitive Theory are important and helpful to the occupational therapy manager who is planning a health-related program, the concept of how to impact clients' perceived self-efficacy is of particular importance. *Self-efficacy* relates to beliefs about performing *specific* behaviors in *particular situations*; it does not refer to a personality characteristic or a global trait that operates independently of contextual factors (Strecher et al, 1986).

In designing occupational therapy programming intended to foster changes in occupational behavior, it is important that we consider that efficacy expectations (the belief that one is capable of performing a certain behavior) are learned from primary sources; however, these sources are not of equal influence. These influences are described here and summarized in Box 15-4.

BOX 15-4

Four Sources of Learning for Efficacy Expectations (Perceived Self-Efficacy)

- **Performance accomplishments:** Learning by doing; providing a hands-on opportunity for a master experience.
- **Vicarious experience:** Learning by observation; best if the "model" is perceived as being like the client and to achieve mastery through effort rather than ease.
- **Verbal persuasion:** Learning by listening.
- **Physiological state:** One's level of arousal can affect one's readiness to attempt new occupational behavior.

TABLE 15-5

Social Cognitive Theory Applied to the Health Behavior of Beginning to Exercise

Environmental expectancies: what leads to what	Belief that not exercising poses threats to health may act as a cue to exercise.
Outcome expectancies: how behavior is likely to influence outcomes	Belief that exercising improves health and decreases threat supports exercise.
Efficacy expectations: confidence in the ability to perform a behavior	Belief that one is capable of incorporating exercise supports exercise.
Incentives: the value of an outcome	Valuing the praise of others for lost weight and lowered blood pressure supports exercise.

The first and most influential source refers to learning through experience or through *performance accomplishments*. Performance accomplishments are situations in which clients have the opportunity to achieve a sense of mastery through doing. An example of a performance accomplishment is when we provide a client with an opportunity to use an assistive device such as a sock assist to don a sock, and the client discovers that he or she can be successful in using the equipment.

The second source of learning is through observation of others involved in the behavior in question, or through *vicarious experiences*. A typical example of this might be when we show a client a videotape of a model using assistive equipment but don't necessarily allow the client hands-on time to practice. When using vicarious experiences, it is noteworthy that the use of models is more effective when the model is perceived to achieve mastery by overcoming difficulty rather than easily meeting the challenge presented. Therefore, if the model used in the videotape is a young occupational therapy fieldwork student who easily dons a sock using a sock assist, a client may perceive that the model is "not like me" and his or her sense of self-efficacy may not be impacted. The more closely the model resembles the client in age, level of function, and other characteristics, the more likely that the vicarious experience will affect perceived self-efficacy.

A third source of influence on perceived self-efficacy is that of *verbal persuasion*. Verbal persuasion is simply trying to convince a client to adopt a behavior; for example, trying to verbally convince a client who has undergone a total hip replacement to use a sock assist as part of his or her strategy post-surgery. Although this is a common method to try to convince occupational therapy clients to adopt new behavior, it is unfortunately much less effective than providing opportunities for performance accomplishment or to observe appropriate models.

Finally, a client's *physiological state* can influence his or her readiness to attempt a change in behavior and can affect his or her perceived self-efficacy. Clients who are overly aroused because they are nervous, fearful of pain or failure, or under the influence of sedatives or highly fatigued may not be well prepared to attempt to learn a new behavior. Remembering this and providing multiple opportunities, or returning to a client when he or she is more physiologically ready for intervention, may increase the likelihood of successfully influencing occupational behavior.

In providing health education or in attempting to convince clients to adopt new health-promoting occupational behavior, we must also consider the three following concepts in regard to perceived self-efficacy. Perceived self-efficacy may vary according to the *magnitude* or difficulty of the task. A client who has had hip replacement surgery may perceive that he or she can perform the simpler task of rising from a chair while following the recommendation not to flex the hip beyond 90 degrees, but may not perceive that he or she can perform the more difficult task of getting in or out of a car while following the same recommendation. Perceived self-efficacy may also vary according to the *strength* of the client's level of confidence for completing a particular task in a particular situation. Strength and magnitude may be closely related, but the strength of a person's conviction that he or she can complete a behavior may be influenced by factors beyond the task's magnitude or difficulty, such as prior experiences with similar tasks. Finally, we must consider the *generality*, or the degree to which expectations about a particular behavior in a particular situation will generalize to other situations. We often practice behaviors with clients only in medical settings, assuming that they will be able to generalize the behavior to the home or other settings in which they will need to perform a particular behavior.

Table 15-6 presents a summary of selected evidence on Social Cognitive Theory.

Choosing Conceptual Practice Models and Related Knowledge for the Development of Occupational Therapy Programming

A key issue in selecting a program's theoretical underpinning is the ability to identify the theoretical explanation for why a specific intervention results in a particular change. A key portion of this explanation is often referred to as **mechanisms of action**. A mechanism of action specifies what changes, how change proceeds, the conditions under which an intervention achieves beneficial results, and why a change may occur for certain groups of consumers and not others (Box 15-5) (Gitlin et al, 2000).

TABLE 15-6

Summary of Selected Evidence on Social Cognitive Theory

Author	Study Type	N (Sample Size)	Level of Evidence	Results
Dewar et al (2013)	Pre- and postintervention study using structural equation modeling	235 adolescent girls	Good	The model explained 28% and 34% of the variance in physical activity and intention, respectively. Only self-efficacy was associated with physical activity at 12 months. There was no support for intention or outcome expectations as proximal determinants of behavior. Self-efficacy was associated with outcome expectations and parental support; however, only outcome expectations predicted intention.
Anderson-Bill, Winett, Wojcik, & Williams (2011)	Analysis of questionnaires and activity logs	743 adults	Good	In a causal model, increases in self-efficacy at 7 months led to increased physical activity (PA) levels and, albeit marginally, weight loss at 16 months; increased PA was associated with greater weight loss.
Dilorio, Dudley, Soet, Watkins, & Maibach (2000)	Survey of a random sample of college students	1,380 students, 18 to 25 and single, who reported initiation of sexual intercourse	Good	Self-efficacy, the central variable in the theory, was related both directly and indirectly to condom use behaviors. The findings lend support to a condom use model based on Social Cognitive Theory and provide implications for HIV interventions.
Keller, Fleury, Gregor-Holt, & Thompson (1999)	Integrated literature review	Published research during the years 1990 to 1998 (N = 27 studies)	Weak	Descriptive studies found a statistically significant relationship between self-efficacy and exercise behavior. Intervention studies demonstrated that participation in an exercise program promoted self-efficacy, and programs designed to increase outcome expectations and self-efficacy significantly increased exercise behavior.
Langlois, Petosa, & Hallam (1999)	Nonequivalent comparison group design	Sixth-grade students: treatment group (N = 81); comparison group (N = 80)	Good	Students in the treatment group maintained a high level of confidence to refuse cigarette offers, whereas the confidence of the comparison group decreased significantly. They also increased their expectations for positive outcomes from refusing cigarette offers, whereas the expectations for positive outcomes of the comparison group decreased. The students' fear of negative outcomes was less impressionable and more stable. Behavioral capability to resist positive images of smoking was not affected by the program.
Kalichan & Nachimson (1999)	Cross-sectional survey	Sexually active HIV-positive persons (N = 266)	Good	Men who had not disclosed to partners indicated lower rates of condom use and scored significantly lower on a measure of self-efficacy for condom use compared with individuals who had disclosed. Women who had not disclosed reported the lowest disclosure self-efficacy. Building self-efficacy for serostatus disclosure should therefore become a high priority in interventions designed for people living with HIV or AIDS.
Sheeshka, Woolcott, & MacKinnon (1994)	Survey	White-collar employees (N = 490)	Weak	This study demonstrates that elements of Social Cognitive Theory may explain a substantial amount of the variance associated with intentions to adopt healthy eating practices.

Because satisfactory occupational functioning is dependent upon a wide range of occupational behaviors and because different theories or conceptual practice models are intended to address a range of phenomena, developing programming most often requires managers to use more than one practice model in combination. For example, MOHO seeks to explain the occupational nature of human beings and how we come to choose and participate in occupational forms. Although MOHO recognizes that occupational performance is dependent upon underlying capacities such as the ability to move one's arm or to sequence a series of actions in the appropriate order to complete daily activities, it does not address how to remediate or compensate for a decreased active range of motion or impaired cognition. Thus, when designing programming for someone who is likely to have both motor and cognitive deficits, such as an individual with a head injury, you must rely on multiple practice models to address all of the underlying mechanisms of action necessary to facilitate satisfactory occupational functioning.

Braveman et al (2002) identified four questions that can guide the selection of model(s) for program planning (Box 15-6). These questions may be used to evaluate the appropriateness of models in regard to the phenomena that they address so that various models may be effectively combined within a program. They also guide a manager in considering the pragmatic issues that arise in trying to implement programs within varied contexts, such as limitations in space, adequately trained personnel, or reimbursement. These questions are briefly explained and applied to the development of the occupational therapy components of a cardiac rehabilitation program in this section of the chapter.

Question 1: *Does the model specify the underlying mechanisms of action necessary to facilitate the desired type of change?*

Occupational therapists and occupational therapy assistants may be involved in a variety of types of interventions with a patient who is hospitalized after having a coronary artery bypass graft (CABG). These interventions may include activities of daily living, including self-care or home management; stress management, energy conservation, and work simplification techniques; environmental modification; and exploration of interests and hobbies that support a healthy lifestyle, such as exercise. The mechanisms of action that underlie a return to satisfactory occupational performance in each of these areas are different, and no single conceptual practice model addresses all the necessary mechanisms. Table 15-7 gives examples of areas of intervention, hypothesized mechanisms of action, and a proposed conceptual practice model that would be used to facilitate improved occupational performance. The table highlights the need to combine conceptual practice models to encompass all the key mechanisms of action to be addressed by a single occupational therapy program.

TABLE 15-7

Sample Areas of Intervention for a Patient Status Post-CABG, Hypothetical Mechanisms of Action to Explain Occupational Performance, and Related Conceptual Practice Models

Area of Intervention	Mechanisms of Action	Related Conceptual Practice Model
Exploration of new leisure interests	Interests influence choice and participation in occupational forms, and indirectly health status, by lowering stress and improving cardiovascular fitness and conditioning. Exposure to new interests may encourage occupational exploration and involvement in new occupational forms.	Model of Human Occupation
Self-care activities, including bathing and dressing	Involvement in everyday occupational forms, such as bathing while standing, can improve strength and endurance of persons who have become deconditioned secondary to illness or hospitalization.	Biomechanical Model (or frame of reference)
Environmental modifications and assistive and adaptive equipment to conserve energy and maximize safety	Adaptation of the environment can compensate for decreased performance capacity and increase independence.	Canadian Model of Occupational Performance

Question 2: *Is there sufficient evidence to support application of the model(s) to the consumer group and the type of change you wish to facilitate?*

As introduced in Chapter 1, the process of evaluating evidence requires the development of specific clinical questions. Assuming that the most important clinical question, "Is there evidence to support that cardiac rehabilitation is effective?" has been answered to the satisfaction of the program developer, the next step would be identifying the key components of effective programs.

At this point, the question that must be answered is whether there is a match between the underlying mechanisms of action thought to affect the desired occupational behavior, the key components of effective programming found in the literature (evidence), and the conceptual practice models chosen to guide program development. This matching process is an iterative one in which multiple comparisons and revisions to your thinking are likely to be made as you discover any type of mismatch between one component and another. Figure 15-2 represents the process

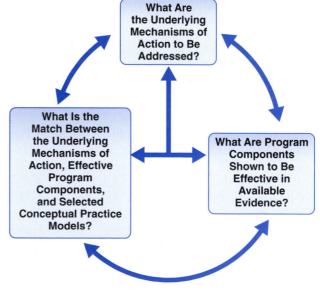

Figure ■ 15-2
Matching Mechanisms of Action, Evidence, and Conceptual Practice Models.

of evaluating the fit between the suspected mechanisms of action, the components of effective programming supported by evidence, and the phenomena addressed by conceptual practice models.

Question 3: Do the model(s) fit with the social, organizational, cultural, political, professional, and financial contexts in which the program must be implemented?

Many factors influence program development and implementation beyond just whether the program is theoretically sound and grounded in the most recent available evidence. Social, organizational, cultural, political, professional, and economic factors may also limit an occupational therapy manager's capacity to develop and implement a program in the exact manner that he or she wishes. For example, theory drawn from an occupational therapy conceptual practice model might suggest that exploration of leisure pursuits and interests as a mechanism for managing and reducing work-related stress is a valuable component of a cardiac rehabilitation program. However, the realities of staffing shortages, limits on the services that may be provided because of reimbursement mechanisms, or philosophical differences regarding the role of occupational therapy in an acute medical setting may force compromise or alterations in program design.

Considering the full range of factors that will influence how a conceptual practice model is used to guide program development can save valuable time by preventing investment of resources in program components that will be poorly received. It may also help the program developer consider ways in which the conceptual practice model (either in its entirety or its primary tenets) might be introduced to key stakeholders in the organization or delivery context so that program elements will be more likely to be accepted. For example, an in-service education program might be provided to physicians, nurses, and physical therapists (PTs) involved in the development of a cardiac rehabilitation program. This in-service might focus on the relationship between the pursuit of leisure interests and decreased stress, as well as

evidence to support addressing these issues in programming. Introduction to an occupational therapy conceptual practice model and possible interventions while acknowledging economic concerns could be included in such a presentation and be strengthened by linking the model to evidence on effective program components.

Question 4: Does implementation of the model have any special requirements for space, equipment, or personnel?

Although a theory supported by evidence might suggest a range of possible interventions, some interventions may require space, equipment, or personnel beyond the scope of the organization's resources. It is the program director's responsibility to plan for funding of staff salaries, training needs, new equipment, and space within available resources. Occupational therapists and occupational therapy assistants play different roles in different settings within the area of cardiac rehabilitation, ranging from involvement in only basic self-care intervention to much broader involvement in interventions, including stress management, energy conservation, and work simplification. In some settings, the occupational therapy practitioner may monitor physical activity. With the cardiac rehabilitation patient, involvement in any type of physical activity, from bathing to ambulation, typically requires monitoring the heart rate, blood pressure, and oxygen saturation; those occupational therapy personnel monitoring these functions should have undergone specific training and demonstrated specific competencies in these areas. The resource implications of involvement in such programming must be considered early in the process of program development.

The following section presents two case examples. The first program was developed and evaluated as a result of a federally funded project to promote persons living with HIV/AIDS to return to participation in productive occupational roles. The second case example describes the development of occupational therapy programming for people with cancer.

Developing an Occupational Therapy Program Using Evidence—The Enabling Self-Determination (ESD) for Persons Living With HIV/AIDS Program

The Enabling Self-Determination (ESD) for Persons Living With HIV/AIDS Program is an example of an occupational therapy program in which several program development models were utilized in conjunction with an occupational therapy conceptual practice model, as well as a number of theories and models from related knowledge. The ESD Program arose out of a prior occupational therapy program called the Employment Options (EO) Program. The EO Program was funded by a federal research and demonstration grant (Rehabilitation Services Administration Grant #H235A980170) and operated by the University of Illinois at Chicago Department of Occupational Therapy and the Howard Brown Health Center, a community-based health center serving Chicago's gay and lesbian population. The EO Program provided group educational services combined with vocationally focused occupational therapy to adults living with AIDS. The EO Program operated between 1998 and 2001 and enrolled 137 men and women living with AIDS in the Chicago area. At the completion of the project, 67% of participants had returned to work or were involved in a formal education effort (Braveman, Goldbaum, et al, 2001; Braveman, Sen, & Kielhofner, 2001; Braveman et al, 2002; Kielhofner et al, 2003).

At the completion of the EO Program, the subsequent ESD Program was initiated to further meet the needs of people living with AIDS who wished to explore a return to work and develop additional knowledge about how occupational therapy personnel could effectively work with this population. In this case, the population (persons with HIV or AIDS) and the problems of concern (return to work and independent living in the community) were identified before beginning to develop the program.

The next step in the process of moving forward was to delineate more specifically where and how an intervention would occur. The EO Program had primarily addressed the intrapersonal level according to the Ecological Model of Health Promotion by focusing on the participants' knowledge, attitudes, values, beliefs, and capacities. In planning the ESD Program, the planners decided that, in addition to intervention at the intrapersonal level, the program would seek to impact services at the interpersonal, organizational, and community levels in order to have a wider and sustained impact on the target population. Table 15-8 provides examples of the focus of interventions at each level of the Ecological Model of Health Promotion addressed in the ESD Program.

Once the decision was made to focus on a program that would have a wider and more sustained impact than the EO Program, and it was evident that the program would include interventions aimed at multiple levels of the environment, steps to plan a specific program model could begin. In the remainder of this section, each of the four steps of program development shown in Figure 15-1 and described earlier will be illustrated as they were applied to the development of the ESD Program.

Needs Assessment

During the first step, needs assessment, a program planner must describe the needs of the target population and identify resources available to him or her as well as the constraints and challenges faced. In the case of the ESD Program, the process of needs assessment required us to examine both the needs of the residents of supportive living facilities and, because the program included the goal of building the organizations' capacity to deliver services, the needs of the facility staff as well.

TABLE 15-8

Application of the Ecological Model of Health Promotion to the ESD Program

Level of the Ecological Model	Focus of Interventions in the ESD Program
Intrapersonal	Increase perceived self-efficacy in activities to support independent living in the community and return to work, such as budgeting, effective communication, and conflict management skills.
Interpersonal	Offer peer-led support groups or job clubs in which participants can discuss strategies, experiences, and frustrations related to returning to work or finding housing in the community.
Organizational	Work with facility leadership, peer educators, case managers, and transitional living staff to establish consistent expectations of behavior regarding involvement and attendance in programming.
Community	Work with nonprofit advocacy agencies, government-run "one-stop job centers," and transitional living facilities to develop effective and ongoing collaborative initiatives.

CASE EXAMPLE 1

The Needs of the Target Population: Residents of Supportive Living Facilities for Persons With HIV/AIDS

Although the EO Program had been largely successful with clients who had stable housing, many of the clients who resided in supportive living settings had dropped out of the program. Their situation was examined more closely by conducting key informant interviews with facility staff and by surveying 58 residents in five supportive living facilities in Chicago. Data from the survey highlighted that the residents of supportive living facilities closely resembled the nationally emerging population of people with AIDS. They were 20% female, 59% African American, and 15% Hispanic. More than 60% had a history of substance abuse and 50% had some form of mental illness. Most had lived chaotic lives characterized by unstable living situations or homelessness (68%), chronic unemployment (82%), hospitalization (84%), domestic violence (36%), and incarceration (41%). Half (50%) reported serious symptoms or medication side effects that complicated and interfered with

performing daily tasks. Many had limited education (15% lacked a high school diploma).

Further, the survey revealed that these individuals were in a complex dilemma about their lives, which had deteriorated so far that they required support for daily living. Most had come to the facilities following a period of serious illness or chaotic personal circumstances. They were aware that they would eventually be required to move beyond supportive living and expressed sincere wishes to do so, but their confidence about living on their own was severely shaken.

As a result of their experiences, these residents did not develop strong confidence in their vocational skills, and this affected their vocational interests and motivation. The vast majority (95%) had recently relied on public assistance. Most (75%) desired to both live on their own and find

Continued

CASE EXAMPLE 1

The Needs of the Target Population: Residents of Supportive Living Facilities for Persons With HIV/AIDS—cont'd

employment, but they reported uncertainty over whether they could handle the challenges involved. They were concerned about the impact of their prolonged absence from the work force and how peers and supervisors would respond to their illness. They also worried about the impact that working would have on their Social Security and health benefits, especially given the cost of their life-sustaining medications. Consequently, they lacked a clear and hopeful vision about how to become self-determining.

Most residents had experienced a near-total breakdown of everyday habits of living and were just beginning to reestablish routines that supported health and well-being. Like other persons with chronic illness, they had lost their ordinary involvements and were consumed with the routines of managing their own illnesses. Many expressed concern about overcoming the inertia of habitual inactivity and the challenges of instituting a daily life routine to support community living and working.

In addition, residents' stories reinforced that individuals with AIDS face very real environmental pressures to move beyond their current circumstances. The institutions in which they lived could only provide temporary, transitional housing. They faced limited access to public or governmental benefits, such as Social Security Disability Insurance or Medicaid, because of improved health and function. Living and participating in the community not only required that residents develop skills that many lacked for managing a home, but, because of the escalating costs and limited availability of affordable housing, community living frequently required that residents gain employment to increase their incomes.

However, the community and workplace presented attitudinal and other barriers to independence, integration, and work for a person with AIDS. For example, they legitimately worried over what would happen if they disclosed their HIV status to obtain services or request accommodations. By disclosing their status, they risked discrimination associated with AIDS. Alternatively, trying to "pass" in the workplace entailed difficulties (e.g., managing medication side effects such as fatigue and diarrhea without detection by others) that could, in turn, produce high levels of stress.

The Needs of Transitional Living Facilities for Persons Living With HIV/AIDS

At the time of program development, programs nationwide that were previously accustomed to serving clients with a terminal prognosis were struggling to make the transition to rehabilitative models of service delivery. Supportive living facilities for people with AIDS had been organized to provide care to meet basic needs such as housing, nutrition, basic case management, and often hospice care. The staff of these facilities simply lacked the knowledge, skills, and organizational structures for offering services to support self-determination.

Importantly, it was learned that residents were not accessing existing services in the community oriented to promoting independence in living or return to employment. This lack of utilization was because of several factors, including: (a) residents lacked the knowledge, skills, and habits to access services; (b) supportive living facilities' staff lacked the knowledge of agencies providing such services; and (c) agencies serving persons with disabilities did not actively target people with AIDS. Consequently, it became evident that an effective model of service must link people with AIDS to existing, relevant services.

CASE EXAMPLE 1

Choosing a Conceptual Practice Model

Two guiding frameworks were used to design the ESD Program. The first framework was the Social Model of Disability, which views disability as the result of a person's interaction with the environment (Charlton, 1998; Hahn, 2003; Oliver, 1996). This framework underscores how problems at the community or societal level, such as lack of housing and societal stereotypes, can impose disability on the individual and how eliminating social and physical barriers and creating proactive policies can reduce disability.

Complementing the Social Model of Disability, we used MOHO, which also emphasizes person–environment interaction and had been successfully used for two decades to design rehabilitation programs focused on supporting success in community living and employment. These programs had addressed groups that shared characteristics with our target population (e.g., people experiencing AIDS, homelessness, mental illness, and imprisonment) (Braveman et al, 2002; Kielhofner & Brinson, 1989; Pizzi, 1989; Salz, 1983).

Planning of the ESD Program capitalized on 15 years of experience and success in using this dual conceptual approach to design comprehensive programs focused on supporting self-determination in everyday life. In addition, the decision to utilize MOHO was based on the evolving evidence that supported the model. More than 80 studies had been published on MOHO, including basic research designed to test the theory and applied research that examined its utility in practice (Kielhofner & Iyenger, 2002).

Program Planning

In the second step, program planning, the focus of the program was identified as well as who must be involved in the planning to assure success (e.g., who were key decision-makers in the supportive living facilities who would have to approve the program). Goals and objectives for the program were established as well as methods to integrate the program into the existing systems and develop referral mechanisms.

The program was carefully designed to include a four-phase continuum of services. Each phase focused on supporting the development of personal skills, habits, and confidence as guided by the conceptual practice model upon which the program was based. Each program element was tied to the underlying mechanisms of action believed to facilitate residents' change in behavior and personal capacity. Equally important was addressing the environmental interventions and supports. People with disabilities in general face severe gaps in housing, education, transportation, jobs, and participation in many areas of life, along with discrimination and negative attitudinal barriers regarding disability. This was no less true for people with AIDS.

Ongoing research into factors that influence independence and employment success among persons with disabilities (including those with AIDS) indicated that self-determination involves transition through a process that can be conceptualized in four phases: (1) capacity for self-management, (2) identifying future goals and managing routines, (3) developing competence and vision, and (4) achieving success and satisfaction in everyday living and working (Barrett, Beer, & Kielhofner, 1999; Braveman & Helfrich, 2001; Kielhofner et al, 1999). Table 15-9 outlines the self-determination tasks expected to be accomplished in each phase of the program.

Continued

TABLE 15-9

Tasks Involved in Four Phases of Achieving Self-Determination

Capacity for Self-Maintenance	Developing Future Goals and Managing Routines	Developing Competence and Vision	Achieving Community Living and Work Success and Satisfaction
• Maintain positive health status (medication compliance, diet, and exercise). • Maintain sobriety and abstinence. • Manage fatigue and other symptoms while performing self-care and basic routines. • Explore alternatives for future independence and productivity. • Begin to identify and pursue short-term goals. • Build relationships with a peer group.	• Develop confidence and satisfaction in performance and plans for independence and productivity. • Identify goals related to independent self-manager, community participant, and worker roles. • Develop skills and basic habits for independence and productivity. • Continue positive health status, as well as sobriety and abstinence. • Identify and contribute to a peer group.	• Clarify a personal vision of desired life. • Identify and work as an active member within positive peer group(s). • Consistently work toward long-term goals. • Seek support to garner resources for goals attainment. • Enact values and interests; find satisfaction in daily life. • Take on roles (volunteer/ training). • Sustain patterns of independence, productivity, health, and sobriety.	• Sustain work performance. • Find work satisfaction. • Balance worker and other life roles. • Maintain routine that consolidates self-maintenance, community living, and productivity. • Actively advocate for personal needs and rights. • Identify and establish connections with relevant group(s) in the community.

CASE EXAMPLE 1

Program Planning—cont'd

The vocational components of the ESD Program also incorporated relevant elements from a "menu approach" and the Individual Placement and Support Model, two other areas of related knowledge for which we found sufficient evidence (Becker & Drake, 1994; Bond, 1998). These components included (a) early placement in actual work contexts, (b) integrated attention to vocational and mental health needs, (c) a consumer-focused "menu" of choices and paths, (d) continuous and comprehensive assessment, and (e) ongoing support as necessary for ultimate success.

The program sequence was designed to consider that a majority of the residents living in the transitional facilities would be managing recovery from substance abuse concurrently with their efforts to establish self-determination. Early phases of the program focused on self-management and establish-

ing routines and habits of self-management, including sobriety and medication adherence. The first two phases were of a length sufficient to allow for resolution of cognitive problems often present early in the recovery process. These "time-dependent results of abstinence" include marked improvement in memory, concentration, and problem-solving in the first months of abstinence, followed by gradual improvements over time (Goldman & Goodheim, 1988). Evidence found in the substance abuse literature to promote change guided decision-making about the program model. Emphasis on employment increased in phases 3 and 4 (the last 7 months of the program), consistent with the well-documented positive impact of vocational rehabilitation and employment on successful substance abuse recovery and reduced rates of relapse (Platt, 1995). The program elements of the ESD Program's four phases are summarized in Table 15-10.

TABLE 15-10

Overview of ESD Program Phases and Program Elements

Phase 1: Capacity for Self-Maintenance (1 Month)	Phase 2: Developing Future Goals and Managing Routine (3 Months)	Phase 3: Developing Competence and Vision (4 Months)	Phase 4: Achieving Community Living and Work Success Satisfaction (3 Months)
• Individual assessment and goal setting • Medication adherence • Nutrition and exercise program • Stress management • Orientation to local community • Development of positive support systems • Support groups led by peer mentors	• Home management and instrumental activities of daily living • Grooming and personal appearance • Interpersonal communication skills • Developing health interests and leisure pursuits • Household responsibilities • Facility-based jobs • Financial management skills • Support groups led by peer mentors	• Placement in volunteer positions or internships • Referral to the Office of Rehabilitation Services and one-stop job centers • Referrals to related training programs or schools • Job search preparation • Support groups led by peer mentors • Planning for transition to community living	• Job placement • Job coaching and peer mentoring • Managing benefits • Self-advocacy training • Obtaining community housing • Home visits and support in establishing and maintaining the home • Support groups led by peer mentors

CASE EXAMPLE 1

Program Implementation

During the third step, program implementation, the ESD Program was implemented according to our preestablished goals, objectives, and action plan. Actions taken were documented and results were communicated to key stakeholders. Program staff worked to coordinate and solve problems with facility staff and clients.

The program's plan was developed as part of a grant submitted for funding to the National Institute for Disability and Rehabilitation Research (NIDRR Grant H133G020217). This project was funded for 3 years, and implementation began in January 2003. Following the design of the ESD Program, implementation required developing the specifics of the program, hiring and training appropriate staff, integrating program services into the existing structures of the supportive living facilities that were participating in the program, and coordinating and documenting activities to facilitate program evaluation.

As the program was implemented, staff already familiar with the conceptual practice model upon which the program was planned (MOHO) were hired and provided with additional training in the assessments and tools to be used within the program. The program coordinator, who had developed and directed the prior EO Program, provided hands-on supervision and guidance to new project staff. Key to the project's success was the presence of existing facility staff such as case managers and life skill counselors. Program staff had to work carefully to introduce facility staff to concepts and strategies based on MOHO in lay terms. Continuous effort was made to include facility staff in day-to-day decision-making and to develop program materials with an eye to their long-term use by staff members who likely would not be OTs. As facility staff became more familiar with occupational therapy and with MOHO, they were able to provide helpful observations and insights about individual clients' interests, habits, and values, as well as the progress they were making toward reestablishing independent worker and self-management roles.

Continued

CASE EXAMPLE 1

Program Evaluation and Outcome Measures

During the last step, program evaluation, a plan was developed to measure the program's effects against the program goals. However, the program evaluation plan was really initiated at the beginning of the program development process when the program's desired outcomes were identified (the first step in program evaluation). Because this program, like the EO Program before it, had been funded to specifically identify and measure both processes and outcomes of the program, an extensive program evaluation system was developed.

The program evaluation system included both quantitative and qualitative strategies and was both formative (information was collected from all parties during program development to continuously improve the program) and summative (information was collected after implementation of the program on outcomes, effectiveness, and efficiency). Beginning in the earliest phase of the program, qualitative information was collected by conducting focus groups at each transitional living facility with both residents and staff. This approach was designed within a participatory action research (PAR) framework that called for all persons involved in research, including the subjects being studied, to be partners in the research process and to help guide the research process itself in addition to any interventions (Balcazar, Keys, Kaplan, & Suarez-Balcazar, 1998; Selener, 1997). Although PAR approaches are most often described in the context of research, they can be extremely useful in the formative stages of program development.

Multiple strategies were used to provide for the program's continuous quality improvement. These included obtaining feedback from residents after group and individual sessions, including residents when choosing topics for future intervention sessions, and meeting frequently with facility staff to discuss how program implementation could be improved. The program team met on a regular basis to discuss the challenges and successes they encountered during the program's implementation, and changes in strategies were made to accommodate the individual facilities' needs and cultures.

Quantitative elements of the program evaluation system focused on determining the program's end impact on residents. Therefore, two primary outcomes of the intervention were identified. The following outcome indicators were collected for all program participants 6 months after completing the program:

- The number of hours of paid employment per week
- The type of living situation that the resident was in (supported living or independent)

The funded portion of the program was completed and formal outcomes of the program were reported in 2008. Forty-six participants completed the formal study, which included a two-group nonrandomized control design. Participants were assigned to either the model program condition or standard care program. The model program included all the services previously mentioned, including individualized occupational therapy services, whereas the control program was limited to eight weekly educational groups. Data on productive participation were collected at 3, 6, and 9 months after completion of the model or standard program. Outcomes were compared at each time point. Participants in the two programs did not differ significantly on baseline demographic variables. Model program participants showed significantly higher levels of productive participation at all three time points ($p < .05$). Odds ratios were all greater than 3, reflecting that participants attending the model program were at least twice as likely to be productively engaged at all three time points (Kielhofner, Braveman, & Fogg, 2008).

CASE EXAMPLE 1

Program Evaluation and Outcome Measures—cont'd

This case example highlights how several theories and models related to the occupational therapy paradigm and derived from related knowledge were combined to guide development and implementation of a new program. Full outcome statistics on the program are not yet available; however, facility staff reports the following key changes:

- Increasing numbers of residents are accessing and utilizing state vocational rehabilitation services and services offered by nonprofit organizations related to educational and vocational preparedness.

- Increasing numbers of residents are seeking and finding paid employment.
- The percentage of residents who leave the facility in a planned manner on "good terms" and maintain contact with the facility is increasing, and the percentage who are asked to leave because of behavior problems is decreasing.
- The supportive living facility staff perceives dramatically increased levels of knowledge and skill to provide vocational readiness and independent living programming.

CASE EXAMPLE 2

Developing a Theory-Based Approach to Occupational Therapy Oncology Rehabilitation
(Courtesy of Lauro Munoz)

The University of Texas MD Anderson Cancer Center in Houston ranks as one of the world's most respected centers focused on cancer patient care, research, education, and prevention. It is one of only 41 comprehensive cancer centers designated by the National Cancer Institute. Since *U.S. News & World Report* began its annual Best Hospitals survey 25 years ago, MD Anderson has ranked No. 1 or No. 2 in cancer care every year. Since 1944, about 800,000 patients have turned to MD Anderson for research-driven care provided through a multidisciplinary approach pioneered at the institution. MD Anderson invests more than $500 million a year in research and ranks first in the number of grants awarded and total amount of grant dollars from the National Cancer Institute. During fiscal year (FY) 2014, MD Anderson provided cancer care for about 115,000 patients. Rehabilitation services at MD Anderson were initially established in 1952 as a section of the Division of Surgery, and became an independent department in

1967. Up until the mid-1990s there were fewer than 20 occupational therapy practitioners and physical therapy practitioners.

The demand for rehabilitation services progressively increased as the impact of rehabilitation on the quality of cancer patients' lives was more clearly recognized. Since 2008 the number of permanent staff in rehabilitation services has almost doubled, and today there are almost 140 full-time equivalent (FTE) staff, including occupational therapy practitioners, physical therapy practitioners, and support staff, including rehabilitation technicians, receptionists, and business staff. During FY 2015, the department treated nearly 20,000 patients and had gross revenue of more than $25 million.

During this expansive growth, the occupational therapy services provided at the University of Texas MD Anderson Cancer Center emphasized biomechanical assessments and interventions rather than

Continued

Developing a Theory-Based Approach to Occupational Therapy Oncology Rehabilitation—cont'd

the benefits of occupation and use of paradigmatic occupational therapy theories and knowledge with the oncology population. Concerns over increasing the emphasis of occupational therapy theory and conceptual practice models led to changes in practice that emphasized participation through occupation.

In an effort to enhance service provision and be theory driven, the outpatient supervisor and several new employees began introducing numerous theoretical models in the outpatient department. The group participated in training that offered theory-based interventions and assessments such as neurobehavioral assessment for cognition, executive dysfunction, visual adaptation, neurodevelopmental theory, fatigue assessment and management, lifestyle redesign, and pain management. These areas had not previously been consistently addressed and the supervisor identified that skill development in these areas would prove beneficial to clients. Also during this same time frame, the outpatient supervisor engaged in continuing education courses on MOHO and the use of the Model of Human

Occupation Screening Tool (MOHOST) and the Short Child Occupational Profile (SCOPE) (Bowyer et al, 2008; Kielhofner, 2007; Parkinson, Forsyth, & Kielhofner, 2008). Both of these assessments are MOHO-based, top down, client-centered evaluations.

In order to systematically determine the needs of the occupational therapy outpatient department, the outpatient supervisor chose to develop more formal programming and began with a needs assessment of the clients and the staff. Specifically, he examined the needs of the clients who were referred to physical therapy but who did not also receive a referral to occupational therapy. This needs assessment required the outpatient staff to examine the population's needs and identify the appropriate theory-based and evidence-based treatments to meet their needs. The needs assessment also examined the training needs of the outpatient occupational therapy staff and education that could be provided to the physical therapy staff in order to allow them to screen for potential occupational therapy needs in their clients.

Needs Assessment

The needs assessment showed that patients with neurological tumors were not consistently being referred to occupational therapy even though they exhibited impairments in cognition or vision. Patients with cancer-related fatigue or cancer-related pain were also not consitently being referred to occupational therapy. Furthermore, patients complaining of "chemo fog" or "chemo brain" were

not often referred to occupational therapy either. Another issue that began to arise was that clients were not engaging in purposeful occupations after returning home. The occupational therapy practitioners lacked the knowledge and skills required to deliver the desired services to the clients, and the PTs were unaware that these services could be provided by occupational therapy.

Program Planning and Staff Education and Training

Because there were a high number of patients with cognitive impairments either caused by lesions or chemo brain, the supervisor decided to begin

training in cognition. Occupational therapists were sent for A-ONE certification, which has been psychometrically validated as an assessment and

Program Planning and Staff Education and Training—cont'd

goal-setting tool for patients with cognitive impairments (Árnadóttir, 1990). The OTs became well versed in the Executive Function Performance Test. They explored treatment strategies, leading to training in "The Cognitive Orientation to Daily Occupational Performance (CO-OP)" programming, which has a developing body of evidence to support its use with patients experiencing cognitive impairments (Missiuna, Mandich, Polatajko, & Malloy-Miller, 2001). At this point, the physical therapy practitioners were also given a set of triggers for the referral to occupational therapy, which resulted in a response of "Wow, we did not know you all could do this."

Once visual impairments were identified as a need with the patient population, the staff used the Brain Injury Visual Assessment Battery for Adults (biVABA) as an assessment tool. Treatment strategies were then identified, resulting in the establishment of a standard of care (Warren, 2004). During this period, the staff researched assessment tools to measure fatigue, breathlessness, and pain, and identified several assessments for use. To provide a distinct way of measuring this symptomology, the staff decided that all assessments had to relate the symptom to performance of activities of daily living (ADLs) or instrumental activities of daily living (IADLs). Treatment strategies in lifestyle redesign were researched, with strategies identified.

Even though many evidence- or theory-based evaluations and treatments were identified, there was a lack of conceptual congruency between the assessments and models. The staff still needed a practice model to pull it all together and guide clinical reasoning. It was essential that treatment plans remained focused on the development of skills, return to habits and routines, and exploration of volition in this client population. MOHO was chosen as it provided the theoretical basis to assist in treatment planning and program development with a client-centered focus. MOHO also provides many psychometrically sound assessments and a large body of evidence to support its application. A sample of the assessments used with oncology patients at MD Anderson Cancer Center is included in Table 15-11. The use of MOHO also helped the staff focus on volition and client engagement in meaningful activity upon discharge from therapy services.

Continued

TABLE 15-11

Model of Human Occupation Assessments Used in Oncology Rehabilitation

Assessment	Description and Format	What Does This Assessment Provide the Therapist?
Model of Human Occupation Screening Tool (MOHOST)	Rating scale divided among six areas and 24 subsections	Highlights the impact of volition, habituation, skills, and the environment on occupational participation
Short Child Occupational Profile (SCOPE)	Rating scale divided among six areas and 24 subscales	Highlights the impact of volition, habituation, skills, and the environment on occupational participation
Occupational Circumstance Assessment-Interview and Rating Scale (OCAIRS)	A semistructured interview that takes about 20 to 30 minutes to administer	Provides a structure to the gathering, analyzing, and reporting of data on the extent and nature of an individual's occupational participation

CASE EXAMPLE 2

Program Implementation—cont'd

It must be noted that training and implementation of programs occurred simultaneously; in addition, newly researched assessments and treatments were implemented as they were needed. Formalized orientation was established for the physical therapy practitioners with triggers that would allow for referral to occupational therapy. The staff held meetings with physician groups such as physical medicine and rehabilitation in order to expose them to the new programming. Interestingly, the ophthalmology group began to read program documentation that included visual assessment and treatment, after which they requested an orientation with the occupational therapy practitioners. This led to the development of a vision clinic that included neuro-ophthalmology, optometry, and occupational therapy. Orientation also began among the inpatient clinicians in order to expose them to the outpatient programming, as well as encourage them to pull from the information that had been compiled by the practitioners.

Although the MOHOST and SCOPE were in use, there had been no formal training in MOHO

as a conceptual model. The department became engaged in a pilot study that included both the inpatient and outpatient staff. This pilot study, a 12-month training program in MOHO as a conceptual model, also provided the department's leadership with qualitative information on how training the entire staff in a conceptual model will affect practice, patient care, and outcomes. In this sense, staff were being trained through an evidence-based model to provide evidence to occupational therapy practitioners in developing a program using a conceptual model.

As a conceptual model, MOHO allowed the occupational therapy practitioners to pull from other theoretical bases in their treatment planning. As MOHO tools allowed individuals to drill down to specific factors that may have been impeding a client from engaging in occupation, the conceptual model then allowed them to pull from other theory bases for treatment and assessment, such as neurobehavior, the CO-OP, motor learning theory, and biomechanics. The contributions of various assessments and models are highlighted in Table 15-12.

Program Evaluation and Outcomes

The benefits of formally assessing both patient and staff needs and implementing an organized response were immediately evident. These benefits included (a) a common language among the therapists, (b) an overarching frame of thought guiding practitioners, (c) a feeling of being more unified in the department, and (d) patient goals that specifically look at a client's participation in occupation.

TABLE 15-12	
Contributions of Varied Assessments and Practice Models to the Oncology Program	
MOHO-Based Assessments	Highlights the impact of volition, habituation, skills, and the environment on occupational participation
Cognitive Models	Highlights the blatant and subtle changes that occur with a client who has an oncological diagnosis
Motor Learning Theory	Subtle to blatant motor changes that occur with oncological diagnosis can be assessed and treatment strategies selected
Biomechanical Model (or Frame of Reference)	Allows for orthotic fabrication, wheelchair and wheelchair cushion assessment and prescription, and simple musculoskeletal-strengthening programs

Chapter Summary

This chapter focused on the use of various types of theories and models to guide the development of occupational therapy programming. You were introduced to terminology including *theory, conceptual practice model, frame of reference, occupational therapy paradigm,* and *related knowledge*. The theme of using data, information, and other forms of evidence to guide practice was repeated, and this chapter demonstrated how an occupational therapy manager might use evidence to evaluate the applicability of various theories and models to guide program development.

You were introduced to the *mechanism of action* concept for change that specifies what changes, how change proceeds, the conditions under which an intervention achieves beneficial results, and why a change may occur for certain groups of consumers and not others. You were also provided four questions that can be used to help you choose which theories and models address the underlying mechanisms of action for the type of change you hope to promote through a given type of programming.

Numerous different examples were provided in this chapter to illustrate both how a model might be used to guide the steps of program development and how theories and conceptual practice models can be combined. The ESD Program and the oncology program at the University of Texas MD Anderson Cancer Center were presented as case examples of how occupational therapy programming can be developed by combining paradigmatic theory with related knowledge. These examples also illustrated how existing evidence was used to guide the development of a new program.

At the start of the chapter, you were introduced to David, an occupational therapy manager who was considering how the principles and strategies of evidence-based practice could be applied to his daily work as a manager. Specifically, he wondered about the connections between evidence-based practice and program development.

■ Real-Life Solutions

As David moved forward on working with his colleagues to develop a new day treatment program, he gave more thought to how he could utilize the strategies that he had just learned on finding and evaluating data, information, and other forms of evidence in his managerial responsibility for program development. David shared his questions with his colleagues who were managers in the disciplines of psychology, nursing, and social work, as well as with the psychiatrist with whom they worked. All of these managers noted that their disciplines were also promoting the principles of evidence-based practice and the strategies associated with its implementation.

Continued

■ **Real-Life Solutions—cont'd**

After consulting with peers who had experience in the area of program development, as well as searching the literature for descriptions of program development and examples of evidence-based programming, David decided to pursue the following activities:

- Read about and become familiar with key theories from related knowledge useful in program development, such as the TTM of Change, the HBM, Social Cognitive Theory, and theories related to the mechanisms of action that would underlie the challenges faced by the target population for the day treatment program.

- Adopt the use of a simple program development model to act as a guide for decision-making, to be supported by case examples using the model in occupational therapy or other professional literature.

- Become familiar with the primary occupational therapy conceptual practice models for which evidence exists so that he can make better informed decisions about choosing practice models in the future.

Study Questions

1. **A term used to describe the organization of knowledge that generates theory and the methods that are used by therapists in their everyday work to apply that theory, such as assessments and intervention strategies, is best called which of the following?**

   a. Frame of reference
   b. Paradigm
   c. Conceptual practice model
   d. Occupational therapy practice theory

2. **Knowledge that specifically addresses the identity and perspective of the occupational therapy profession is best called which of the following?**

   a. Sensory integrative frame of reference
   b. Occupational therapy paradigm
   c. MOHO conceptual practice model
   d. Occupational therapy practice theory

3. **A model or theory that helps you to understand where different prevention and health behavior interventions may occur is best called which of the following?**

   a. Health Belief Model
   b. Social Cognitive Theory
   c. Transtheoretical Stages of Change Theory
   d. Ecological Model of Health Promotion

4. **A model or theory that helps you understand how you can affect health behaviors by influencing four sets of beliefs is best called which of the following?**

   a. Health Belief Model
   b. Social Cognitive Theory
   c. Transtheoretical Stages of Change Theory
   d. Ecological Model of Health Promotion

5. **A model or theory that holds that behavior is determined by expectancies and incentives is best called which of the following?**

   a. Health Belief Model
   b. Social Cognitive Theory
   c. Transtheoretical Stages of Change Theory
   d. Ecological Model of Health Promotion

6. **A health-related concept that helps to indicate how change proceeds, designates the conditions under which an intervention achieves beneficial results, and suggests why change may occur for certain groups of consumers and not for others is best called which of the following?**

   a. Mechanism of action
   b. Health change indicator
   c. Predictive factor
   d. Performance accomplishment measure

7. **Which of the following best describes the relationship between theory and a program development model?**

   a. To be most effective and evidence-based, you should choose to use either an appropriate theory or a program development model.
   b. Most theories include a program development model, so a program development model is part of a theory.
   c. They are used in combination to guide decision-making about where, how, and when to intervene given a chosen problem or target population.
   d. Most program development models include a theory, so a theory is part of a program development model.

8. **Steps in the process of developing an evidence-based occupational therapy program include which of the following?**

   a. Program planning
   b. Needs assessment
   c. Evaluation of outcomes
   d. All of the above

Resources for Learning More About Developing Programs

Journals That Often Address Program Development

T & D Magazine

https://www.td.org/Publications/Magazines/TD

T & D Magazine is published by the American Society of Training and Development. The magazine's primary audience is training and development professionals and line managers who range from new practitioners to seasoned executives in business, government, academia, and consulting. The magazine provides practical information, advice and strategies, reports on new technologies and their application, and discussion of current and emerging best practices.

Journal of Organizational Behavior

http://onlinelibrary.wiley.com/journal/10.1002/(ISSN)1099-1379

The *Journal of Organizational Behavior* is dedicated to the study of how organizations impact people and how people shape organizations. It publishes worldwide work-related issues, including such topics as leadership and leadership development. The editorial staff encourages both theoretical and empirical inquiry from a diversity of perspectives, methods, and national cultures.

Associations That Are Concerned With Program Development

The American Society of Training and Development

http://www.astd.org/

The membership of the American Society of Training and Development (ASTD) includes over 70,000 individuals from various fields related to workplace learning and performance from over 100 countries. The ASTD's mission is to provide leadership to individuals, organizations, and society to achieve work-related competence, performance, and fulfillment.

The American Public Health Association

http://www.apha.org/

The American Public Health Association (APHA) is the oldest and largest organization of public health professionals in the world, representing more than 50,000 members from over 50 occupations of public health. The APHA is concerned with a broad set of issues affecting personal and environmental health, including federal and state funding for health programs, pollution control, programs and policies related to chronic and infectious diseases, a smoke-free society, and professional education in public health.

Useful Websites on Program Development

Program Development and Evaluation Unit, University of Wisconsin

http://www.uwex.edu/ces/pdande/index.html

The Program Development and Evaluation Unit provides training and technical assistance that enables cooperative extension campus and community-based faculty and staff to plan, implement, and evaluate high-quality educational programs. This website includes a program development model, as well as numerous .pdf files on "quick tips" related to aspects of program development and evaluation.

United Cerebral Palsy Association, Greater Utica (New York) Area Internet Resources for Nonprofits

http://www.ucp-utica.org/uwlinks/nonprofitlinks.htm

The United Cerebral Palsy Association of Greater Utica maintains a website with links to other websites on a wide range of topics related to developing and managing nonprofit organizations. The directory is organized by topic of interest and includes a section on outcome measurement and program evaluation that includes many topics of interest to those developing new programs. As with any website of this type, some of the links were not current, but this site has been well maintained and the majority of links are functional.

Reference List

Ali, N. S. (2002). Prediction of coronary heart disease preventive behaviors in women: A test of the Health Belief Model. *Women & Health, 35,* 83–96.

Anderson-Bill, E. S., Winett, R. A., Wojcik, J. R., & Williams, D. M. (2011). Aging and the social cognitive determinants of physical activity behavior and behavior change: Evidence from the Guide to Health Trial. *Journal of Aging Research, 2011*(Article ID 505928), 1–11.

Árnadóttir, G. (1990). *The brain and behavior: Assessing cortical function through activities of daily living.* Maryland Heights, MO: Mosby.

Balcazar, F. B., Keys, C. B., Kaplan, D. L., & Suarez-Balcazar, Y. (1998). Participatory action research and people with disabilities: Principles and challenges. *Canadian Journal of Rehabilitation, 12,* 105–112.

Bandura, A. (2012). Social Cognitive Theory. In P. A. M. Van Lange, A. W. Kruglanski, & E. T. Higgins (Eds.), *Handbook of theories and social psychology, volume one* (pp. 349–377). London, UK: Sage Publications.

Barrett, L., Beer, D., & Kielhofner, G. (1999). The importance of volitional narrative in treatment: An ethnographic case study in a work program. *Work, 12,* 79–92.

Becker, D. R., & Drake, R. E. (1994). Individual placement and support: A community mental health center approach to vocational rehabilitation. *Community Mental Health Journal, 34,* 71–82.

Blaney, C. L., Robbins, M. L., Palva, A. L., Redding, C. A, Rossi, J. S., Blissmer, B., . . . Oatley, K. (2012). Validation of the measures of the Transtheoretical Model for Exercise in an adult African-American sample. *Journal of Health Promotion, (26)*5, 317–326.

Bond, G. R. (1998). Principles of the Individual Placement and Support Model: Empirical support. *Psychiatric Rehabilitation Journal, 22,* 11–23.

Bowyer, P., Kramer, J., Poloszaj, A., Ross, M., Schwartz, O., Kielhofner, G., & Kramer, J. (2008). *The short child occupational profile, version 2.0.* Chicago, IL: Model of Human Occupation Clearing House—Department of Occupational Therapy, University of Illinois at Chicago.

Braveman, B., Goldbaum, L., Goldstein, K., Karlic, L., & Kielhofner, G. (2001). *Employment options: A program leading to the Employment of Persons Living With AIDS Program manual.* Chicago, IL: Model of Human Occupation Clearinghouse.

Braveman, B., & Helfrich, C. A. (2001). Occupational identity: Exploring the narratives of three men living with AIDS. *Journal of Occupational Science, 8,* 25–31.

Braveman, B., Kielhofner, G., Belanger, R., Llerena, V., & de las Heras, C. G. (2002). Program development. In G. Kielhofner (Ed.), *The Model of Human Occupation: Theory and application* (3rd ed.). Baltimore, MD: Williams & Wilkins.

Braveman, B., Sen, S., & Kielhofner, G. (2001). Community-based vocational rehabilitation programs. In M. Scaffa (Ed.), *Occupational therapy in community-based practice settings* (pp. 139–161). Philadelphia, PA: F. A. Davis.

Brownson, C. (2001). Program development for community health: Planning, implementation and evaluation strategies. In M. Scaffa (Ed.), *Occupational therapy in community-based practice settings* (pp. 95–116). Philadelphia, PA: F. A. Davis.

Buckley, P. (1996). *Essential papers on object relations.* New York, NY: New York University Press.

Charlton, J. (1998). *Nothing about us without us.* Berkeley, CA: University of California Press.

Cohn, E. S., & Coster, W. J. (2014). Unpacking our theoretical reasoning. In B. A. Boyt Schell, G. Gillen, & M. E. Scaffa (Eds.), *Willard and Spackman's occupational therapy* (p. 482). Philadelphia, PA: Lippincott, Williams & Wilkins.

Conrad, K. M., Cambell, R. T., Edington, D. W., & Faust, H. S. (1996). The worksite environment as a cue to smoking reduction. *Research in Nursing & Health, 19,* 21–31.

Crepeau, E. B., & Schell, B. A. B. (2003). Theory and practice in occupational therapy. In E. B. Crepeau, E. S. Cohn, & B. A. B. Schell (Eds.), *Willard and Spackman's occupational therapy* (10th ed., pp. 203–207). Philadelphia, PA: Lippincott, Williams & Wilkins.

Davis, J. L., Buchanan, K. L., & Green, B. L. (2013). Racial/ethnic differences in cancer prevention beliefs: Applying the Health Belief Model framework. *American Journal of Health Promotion, 27*(6), 384–389.

Dewar, D. L., Plotnlkoff, R. C., Morgan, P. J., Okely, A. D., Costigan, S. A., & Lubans, D. R. (2013). Testing Social Cognitive Theory to explain physical activity change in adolescent girls from low-income communities. *Research Quarterly for Exercise and Sport, 84*(4), 483–491.

Dilorio, C., Dudley, W. N., Soet, J., Watkins, J., & Maibach, E. (2000). A social cognitive-based model for condom use among college students. *Nursing Research, 49,* 208–214.

Fischera, S. D., & Frank, D. I. (1995). The Health Belief Model as a predictor of mammography screening. *Health Values, 18,* 3–9.

Galavotti, C., Cabral, R. J., Lansky, A., Grimley, D. M., Riley, G. E., & Prochaska, J. O. (1995). Validation of measures of condom and other contraceptive use among women at high risk for HIV infection and unintended pregnancy. *Health Psychology, 14,* 570–578.

Giles, G. M. (2011). Starting a new program, business or practice. In K. Jacobs & G. L. McCormack (Eds.), *The occupational therapy manager* (pp. 145–156). Bethesda, MD: AOTA Press.

Gitlin, L. N., Corcoran, M., Martindale-Adams, J., Malone, C., Stevens, A., & Winter, L. (2000). Identifying mechanisms of action: Why and how does intervention work? In R. Schulz (Ed.), *Handbook of dementia caregiving: Evidence-based interventions for family caregivers* (pp. 225–248). Philadelphia, PA: Springer.

Glanz, K., Patterson, R. E., Kristal, A. R., DiClemente, C., Heimendinger, J., Linnan, L., & McLerran, D. (1995). Stages of change in adopting healthy diets: Fat, fiber, and correlates of nutrient intake. *Health Education Quarterly, 21*(4), 499–519.

Goldman, R. S., & Goodheim, L. (1988). Experience-dependent cognitive recovery in alcoholics: A task component strategy. *Journal of Studies in Alcohol, 2,* 142–148.

Grossman, J., & Bortone, J. (1986). Program development. In S. C. Robertson (Ed.), *SCOPE: Strategies, concepts, and opportunities for program development and evaluation* (pp. 91–99). Bethesda, MD: American Occupational Therapy Association.

Hahn, H. (2003). Disability policy and the problem of discrimination. *Behavioral Scientist, 28,* 293–318.

Hooper, B., & Wood, W. (2014). The philosophy of occupational therapy. In B. A. Boyt Schell, G. Gillen, & M. Scaffa (Eds.), *Willard & Spackman's occupational therapy* (12th ed., pp. 35–46). Philadelphia, PA: Lippincott, Williams & Wilkins.

Jammer, M. S., Wolitski, R. J., & Corby, N. H. (1997). Impact of a longitudinal community HIV intervention targeting injecting drug users' stage of change for condom and bleach use. *American Journal of Health Promotion, 12*(1), 15–24.

Kalichan, S. C., & Nachimson, D. (1999). Self-efficacy and disclosure of HIV-positive serostatus to sex partners. *Health Psychology, 18,* 281–287.

Keller, C., Fleury, J., Gregor-Holt, N., & Thompson, T. (1999, January). Predictive ability of Social Cognitive Theory in exercise research: An integrated literature review. *Journal of Knowledge Synthesis in Nursing, 5,* 6–8.

Kielhofner, G. (2007). *The Model of Human Occupation: Theory and application* (4th ed.). Baltimore, MD: Williams & Wilkins.

Kielhofner, G. (2009). *Conceptual foundations of occupational therapy* (4th ed.). Philadelphia, PA: F. A. Davis.

Kielhofner, G., Baron, K., Braveman, B., Fisher, G. S., Hammel, J., & Littleton, M. (1999). The Model of Human Occupation: Understanding the worker who is ill or injured. *Work, 12,* 3–12.

Kielhofner, G., Braveman, B., Finlayson, M., Paul-Ward, A., Goldbaum, L., & Goldstein, K. (2003). Outcomes of a vocational rehabilitation program for people with AIDS. *American Journal of Occupational Therapy, 51,* 64–72.

Kielhofner, G., Braveman, B., & Fogg, L. (2008). A controlled study to enhance productive participation among people with HIV/AIDS. *American Journal of Occupational Therapy, 61,* 36–45.

Kielhofner, G., & Brinson, M. (1989). Development and evaluation of an aftercare program for young and chronic psychiatrically disabled adults. *Occupational Therapy in Mental Health, 9,* 53–74.

Kielhofner, G., & Iyenger, A. (2002). Research: Investigating MOHO. In *A Model of Human Occupation: Theory and application* (3rd ed., pp. 520–545). Baltimore, MD: Williams & Wilkins.

Kim, H. S., Ahn, J., & No, J. K. (2012). Applying the Health Belief Model to college students' health behavior. *Nutrition Research and Practice, 6,* 551–558.

Langlois, M. A., Petosa, R., & Hallam, J. S. (1999). Why do effective smoking prevention programs work? Student changes in Social Cognitive Theory constructs. *Journal of School Health, 69,* 326–331.

Lee, J. (2010). Achieving best practice: A review of evidence linked to occupation-focused practice models. *Occupational Therapy in Health Care, 24*(3), 206–222.

Marcus, B. H., Banspach, S. W., Lefebvre, C. R., Rossi, J. S., Carleton, R. A., & Abrams, D. B. (1992). Using the stages of change model to increase the adoption of physical activity among community participants. *American Journal of Health Promotion, 6,* 424–429.

McLeroy, K. R., Bibeau, D., Steckler, A., & Glanz, K. (1988). An ecological perspective on health promotion programs. *Health Education Quarterly, 25,* 351–377.

Missiuna, C., Mandich, A., Polatajko, H., & Malloy-Miller, T. (2001). Cognitive orientation to daily occupational performance (CO-OP): Part I—Theoretical foundations. *Physical and Occupational Therapy in Pediatrics, 20,* 69–81.

Oliver, M. (1996). *Understanding disability from theory to practice.* New York, NY: St. Martin's Press.

Parkinson, S., Forsyth, K., & Kielhofner, G. (2008). *The Model of Human Occupation Screening Tool.* Chicago, IL: Model of Human Occupation Clearinghouse, University of Illinois at Chicago Department of Occupational Therapy.

Perkins, D. O. (1999). Adherence to antipsychotic medications. *Journal of Clinical Psychiatry, 60,* 25–30.

Pizzi, M. A. (1989). The Model of Human Occupation and adults with HIV infection and AIDS. *American Journal of Occupational Therapy, 44,* 257–264.

Platt, J. J. (1995). Vocational rehabilitation of drug abusers. *Psychological Bulletin, 117,* 416–433.

Prochaska, J. O., & DiClemente, J. C. (1993). In search of how people change: Applications to addictive behavior. *American Psychologist, 47,* 1102–1114.

Prochaska, J. O., & Norcross, J. C. (2006). *Systems of psychotherapy: A transtheoretical analysis* (6th ed.). Pacific Grove, CA: Brooks-Cole.

Riley, T. A., Toth, J. M., & Fava, J. L. (2000). The Transtheoretical Model and stress management practices in women at risk for, or infected with HIV. *Journal of the Association of Nurses in AIDS Care, 11*(1), 67–77.

Rosenstock, I. M., Strecher, V. J., & Becker, M. H. (1988). Social Learning Theory and the Health Belief Model. *Health Education Quarterly, 15,* 175–183.

Sallis, J., Owen, N., & Fisher, E. (2008). Ecological Models of Health Behavior. In K. Glanz, B. K. Rimer, & K. Viswanath (Eds.), *Health behavior and health education: Theory, research, and practice* (3rd ed., pp. 462–484). San Francisco, CA: Jossey-Bass.

Salz, C. (1983). A theoretical approach to the treatment of work difficulties in borderline personalities. *Occupational Therapy in Mental Health, 3*, 33–46.

Sapp, S. G., & Jensen, H. H. (1998). An evaluation of the Health Belief Model for predicting perceived and actual dietary quality. *Journal of Applied Social Psychology, 28*, 235–248.

Scaffa, M. E. (2014). *Occupational therapy in community-based practice settings*. Philadelphia, PA: F. A. Davis.

Selener, D. (1997). *Participatory action research and social change*. Ithaca, NY: Cornell Participatory Action Research Network.

Sheeshka, J. D., Woolcott, D. M., & MacKinnon, N. J. (1994). An evaluation of a theory-based demonstration worksite nutrition promotion program. *American Journal of Health Promotion, 8*, 263–264.

Strecher, V. J., DeVillis, B. M., Becker, M. H., & Rosenstock, I. M. (1986). The role of self-efficacy in achieving health behavior change. *Health Education Quarterly, 13*, 73–91.

University of Twente. (2014). *Health Belief Model*. Retrieved from http://www.utwente.nl/cw/theorieenoverzicht/theory%20clusters/health%20communication/health_belief_model/.

Warren, M. (2004). The Brain Injury Visual Assessment Battery for Adults (biVABA). Hoover, AL: visAbilities Rehab Services.

Winfield, E. B., & Whaley, A. L. (2002). A comprehensive test of the Health Belief Model in the prediction of condom use among African American college students. *Journal of Black Psychology, 28*, 330–346.

Leading Evidence-Based Practice and Professional Considerations

CHAPTER 16

Introducing Others to Evidence-Based Practice

Marcia Finlayson, PhD, OT Reg (Ont), OTR
Brent Braveman, PhD, OTR/L, FAOTA

■ Real-Life Management

Angela is an occupational therapist (OT) with more than 20 years of experience. She has been a clinical supervisor for 12 years in an occupational therapy department in an acute rehabilitation hospital. She recently completed a postprofessional master's degree and conducted an evidence-based literature review for her master's project. After Angela presented her project to the staff as part of the departmental in-service program, Angela's boss, Lindsay, suggested that they might want to talk about ways to educate and train all the staff in evidence-based practice skills.

Although Angela was excited that her presentation was so well received, and that her boss valued her new skills enough to ask for her assistance, she was also unsure about exactly what she could recommend to Lindsay. Initially, Angela had found the process of finding and evaluating evidence overwhelming. Before her return to school, she had not been to a library for many years and only had basic word-processing and Internet skills. Like many persons, Angela had assumed that evidence-based practice was an approach that only persons who had skills in research and advanced statistical knowledge could apply. Through the process of completing her project, she had become more comfortable with conducting and documenting literature searches, reading journal articles, and using books, the Internet, her own clinical judgment, and her professional network to help her interpret the literature she found. She also now understood that, in addition to research evidence, therapists often have to learn to evaluate and make decisions using other types of evidence when research results are not yet available. However, even with her new skills and comfort level, she did not consider herself an expert. She found the idea of teaching others about evidence-based practice intimidating.

However, Angela was seldom one to back away from a challenge, so she decided to return to the library and to her network of peers to gather some information to prepare herself for her meeting with her boss. She could imagine some of the

Continued

■ Real-Life Management—cont'd

obstacles they would have to overcome, and she wanted to be able to offer solutions and strategies as well. Some of the obstacles that Angela identified included:

- How would they convince staff members that they had the time to participate in evidence-based practice activities?

- Did all staff members have to become equally skilled in finding and evaluating evidence, or could they work as a team?

- What resources existed that she and her boss could use to train and educate staff about evidence-based practice?

- How could Angela and her boss organize tools and aids to help staff members begin to incorporate evidence-based practice into their everyday work?

Critical Thinking Questions

As you read this chapter, consider the following questions:

- How can managers make both the time and the tools available to staff to facilitate the incorporation of evidence-based practice approaches into daily routines?

- How can managers help their staff become comfortable with using all valid forms of evidence, including clinical experience and judgment, websites, case studies, opinion of experts, qualitative reports, and various forms of experimental designs to guide practice?

- What are strategies that managers can use to create a culture in which evidence-based practice is valued?

- How can managers build structures within their department to support the adoption of an evidence-based approach?

Glossary

- **Critical appraisal:** process of judging the quality of a piece of information and determining its applicability to practice.
- **Critical appraisal matrix:** systematic method of summarizing a series of critical appraisals from individual articles to facilitate comparisons and decision-making.
- **Culture:** learned, shared set of basic assumptions or shared way of doing things that is based upon the underlying values and beliefs of the members of a particular society or members of a group.
- **Electronic bibliographic databases:** electronic compilations of published research, scholarly articles, books, government reports, newspaper articles, and other recognized sources of information.
- **Electronic table of contents alerts:** services provided by professional and scientific journals whereby alerts are e-mailed whenever articles that include key words you submit are published.
- **Knowledge transfer:** imparting of research knowledge from producers to potential users.
- **Levels of evidence:** criterion-referenced typology and classification system that provides guidance for evaluating the quality of a research

Glossary—cont'd

article; these levels are multilayered, typically including criteria for design, sample size, and internal and external validity.

- **Literature search:** systematic, explicit, and reproducible method for identifying, evaluating, and interpreting the existing body of recorded work produced by researchers, scholars, and practitioners.
- **Organizational structure:** the centralization of decision-making; formalization of rules, authority, communication, and compensation; standardization of work processes and skills; or control of output by acceptance of only adequate outcomes.
- **Sample size:** the number of participants in a study.

- **Translational research:** an effective translation of the new knowledge, mechanisms, and techniques generated by advances in basic science research into new approaches for prevention, diagnosis, and treatment of disease, which is essential for improving health.
- **Validity:** addresses whether or not a research design or a measurement tool was able to capture what it intended to capture (i.e., can the design answer the question posed; does the measurement tool measure what it says it does). There are two broad categories of validity: validity of methodology, which includes internal and external validity, and validity of measurement, which includes content, criterion, and construct validity.

Introduction

Learning the knowledge and skills, and adopting the values and ethical behavior, to make your own practice *evidence-based* is challenging, and can become more challenging when you are not in an environment or working alongside peers who are also seeking to incorporate the use of evidence into their practice. Supervising, teaching, and guiding others to base their practice upon evidence is a responsibility that often falls to occupational therapy managers. Accepting this responsibility can be even more challenging, especially when some of the staff members you are supervising have been practicing for some time without using evidence-based strategies. You must consider that introducing and supporting the use of evidence is a complex process and there are multiple factors that influence effective implementation of evidence-based guidelines including contextual factors (social, organizational, economic, and political) and individual factors (Heiwe et al, 2011). Ploeg, Davies, Edwards, Gifford, and Miller (2007) have shown that factors such as the learning process associated with the implementation of the evidence-based guidelines, the health-care providers' attitudes and beliefs, leadership support and integration of recommendations at an organizational level, resource constraints, collaboration, and established networks all affect the implementation process.

Throughout this book, you have learned the principles and strategies for finding and evaluating evidence, and you have been introduced to the wide range of occupational therapy and related knowledge that an occupational therapy manager might use in developing, implementing, and improving occupational therapy programming. Chapter 16 focuses on how you can use the information that you have learned and combine it with additional strategies to introduce others to evidence-based practice. We will begin by considering how managers can create an environment that supports evidence-based practice.

Creating an Environment to Support Evidence-Based Practice

The occupational therapy manager can play a pivotal role in helping evidence-based practice to become the accepted approach to practice within the department that he or she manages. The manager can take the lead in creating an environment in which both the process and the outcomes of evidence-based practice are valued. In Chapter 4, you learned that the term **culture** is widely accepted to mean a learned, shared set of basic assumptions or shared way of doing things that is based upon the underlying values and beliefs of the members of a particular society or members of a group. You also learned that shared values serve to influence the actions of an organization's members in several ways. Specifically, shared values

- Help turn commonplace, routine work into valued activities.
- Create a connection between the organization's mission and society's values.
- Provide a source of competitive advantage to the organization.

As a manager, if you wish others to come to value evidence-based practice, you must model that value in your own behavior and attitudes. This modeling means accepting the responsibilities that come with evidence-based practice and holding those individuals you supervise responsible as well. In Chapter 2, you were introduced to the responsibilities stemming from evidence-based practice, and they are presented again in Box 16-1.

By identifying and articulating the related *values* that are supported in the organization, the occupa-tional therapy manager can help make activities related to finding, evaluating, and incorporating evidence into practice both commonplace and valued routines. This is accomplished by connecting those activities to the department's and organization's mission and vision and supporting and rewarding staff for adopting such routines. Most importantly, a manager must find ways to allow staff members the time to learn, practice, and perform evidence-based practice activities. You must take care that you are not sending contradictory messages to staff members by asking them to adopt evidence-based practices but then structuring their jobs so that they do not have the time to perform the tasks related to finding and evaluating evidence or to communicate effectively with their patients and clients to involve them in decisions about how to use evidence in practice.

You must recognize that motivation and desire alone are not enough to carry the habits and practices of evidence-based practice into daily work. Although surveys of staff show that they generally have a positive outlook on using evidence-based practice, studies have also identified the multiple perceived barriers. For example, Upton, Stephens, Williams, and Scurlock-Evans (2014) completed a systematic review of published research on the attitudes, knowledge, and implementation of evidence-based practice. They reviewed research published between 2000 and 2012 and concluded that although OTs hold positive attitudes toward evidence-based practice they also identify a number of barriers, including those listed in Table 16-1.

BOX 16-1

Responsibilities Stemming From Evidence-Based Practice

- Staying up-to-date with the sources of information that may have an impact on the decisions you will make in practice
- Using sound judgment based on accepted practices and approaches about the information you have gathered by critically evaluating its quality
- Communicating with others about what you have learned from synthesizing information
- Recognizing that translating evidence into everyday practice will not be easy and will also require the application of evidence-based strategies

---

TABLE 16-1

Factors Perceived as Barriers to Evidence-Based Practice

• Workload pressures	• Relevance, applicability, availability, quality research evidence
• Time pressures	
• Insufficient staff	
• Lack of training and knowledge	• Communication
• Lack of skills	• Team functioning
• Lack of support	• Requiring too much motivation
	• Conflict with client-centered practice
	• Patient or provider safety treatments

One of the primary connections between organizational culture (e.g., shared values) and practice (what staff members do) that can facilitate evidence-based practice is the **organizational structure** that you put in place. Classically, organizational structure has been defined as the "centralization of decision-making, formalization of rules, authority, communication, and compensation, standardization of work processes and skills, and/or control of output by acceptance of only adequate outcomes" (Mintzberg, 1979). This practice sounds more complicated than it is; in fact, much of Chapter 17 is devoted to describing how managers create organizational structures and turn theory into practice. Such methods and strategies are at the very center of the manager's role. These methods include designing work processes that guide where and when work is performed, articulating the specifications for outputs or the work products that are considered acceptable, making the tools and resources available to support staff in work performance, and assuring that staff have the necessary skills (e.g., competencies) by providing the kinds of training required to perform the work.

The remainder of this chapter discusses ways that managers can build structures to create bridges from values to practice. We begin by examining how occupational therapy managers can facilitate the adoption of evidence-based practice strategies within the profession of occupational therapy by actively supporting fieldwork students during their entrée to the profession.

Fieldwork and Entry Into a Profession

Graduates from today's occupational therapy educational programs are entering practice with more sophisticated skills to support evidence-based practice than ever before. This is due in large part to the decision by the Accreditation Council for Occupational Therapy Education (ACOTE) to move requirements for entry-level education to the postbaccalaureate level in the United States with new accreditation standards effective in January of 2013 (ACOTE, 2015). Moreover, the creation of an accreditation process and standards for doctoral-entry programs (e.g., the OTD) added additional expectations for graduates from these programs. A side-by-side comparison of the accreditation standards

related to evidence-based practice and research shows some similar expectations for all levels of students, including occupational therapy students at both the master's and the doctoral level, as well as occupational therapy assistant (OTA) students. For example, Standard B.8.2 under Scholarship for the OTA reads:

Effectively locate and understand information including the quality of the source of the evidence. (ACOTE, 2015, p. 30)

This standard, which is slightly more advanced than the OTA guideline and is the same for both levels of occupational therapy students, reads:

Effectively locate, understand, critique, and evaluate information, including the quality of the evidence. (ACOTE, 2015, p. 30)

Standard B.8.4 in the same accreditation standards section of scholarship is similar for both levels of occupational therapy students but is more advanced at the doctoral level. For students at the master's level, the standard reads:

Demonstrate the skills necessary to design a scholarly proposal that includes the research question, relevant literature, sample, design, measurement, and data analysis. (ACOTE, 2015, p. 30)

For OT students at the doctoral level, the same standard includes the more advanced requirement of actually designing a scholarly proposal rather than demonstrating the skills necessary and reads:

Design a scholarly proposal that includes the research question, relevant literature, sample, design, measurement, and data analysis. (ACOTE, 2015, p. 30)

Educational programs for students entering the profession at the doctoral level must also meet the following standard, reflected in Standard 8.B.7 under the same section of the accreditation standards related to scholarship:

Implement a scholarly study that evaluates professional practice, service delivery, and/or professional issues (e.g. Scholarship of Integration, Scholarship of

Application, Scholarship of Teaching and Learning). (ACOTE, 2015, p. 30)

The expectations for Level I and Level II fieldwork experiences are the same for occupational therapy students at both the master's and the doctoral level. However, students entering the profession at the doctoral level have a significant additional experiential component, which must be a minimum of 16 weeks. The purpose of this experience is described in section C.2.0 of the accreditation standards (ACOTE, p. 36). The introduction to this section of standards reads:

> *The goal of the doctoral experiential component is to develop occupational therapists with advanced skills (those that are beyond a generalist level). The doctoral experiential component shall be an integral part of the program's curriculum design and shall include an in-depth experience in one or more of the following: clinical practice skills, research skills, administration, leadership, program and policy development, advocacy, education, or theory development. (ACOTE, 2015, p. 36)*

The fact that students are often entering practice settings as fieldwork students better prepared for evidence-based practice than their clinical fieldwork educators and their colleagues can be a challenge for the student, the fieldwork educator, and the fieldwork site. With conscious effort on the part of the occupational therapy manager, however, this challenge can be turned into an opportunity. It is important that managers prepare all current staff, including those who serve as clinical fieldwork educators, to become comfortable with the increasing focus on using evidence in practice. It is also important that managers recognize the potential gap in skills that some practitioners may have and treat it as they would any other skill set that must be learned. By using some creativity and ingenuity, and involving staff members themselves in choosing strategies that best fit your setting, you can use the influx of new skills that fieldwork students may bring as an advantage and an opportunity. A few examples of ways of doing this are included in Box 16-2.

Although leveraging the skills of recent graduates is important, it is also important to include strategies to support the application and retention of these skills. Morrison and Robertson (2011) summarized strategies to support new graduates to apply their

---

BOX 16-2

Strategies for Closing the Gap in Evidence-Based Practice Skills Between Existing Staff and Fieldwork Students and New Graduates

- Create an evidence-based library for staff members and fieldwork students in your department. Include examples of systematic reviews relevant to your setting, lists of useful websites, and examples of evidence-based review forms that they can use in their practice.
- Include an introduction to evidence-based resources, forms, tools, and expectations as part of the orientation process for both new staff members and fieldwork students.
- Encourage fieldwork students to contribute evidence-based resources and tools from their university program to the resources of your department.
- Pair fieldwork students who have more advanced computer skills for conducting formal literature searches with staff who have advanced clinical skills and judgment to find evidence related to a current clinical question.
- Collaborate with nursing, physical therapy, speech–language pathology, and other disciplines to have students work together in evidence-based practice assignments as a way of learning about teamwork and interdisciplinary practice.
- Have a staff member and a fieldwork student collaborate to present an in-service program to other staff and students on types of evidence, resources, and tools or to present a case in which they used evidence to guide decision-making.
- Include fieldwork students and staff members on a task force to develop a plan for incorporating evidence-based practice in your setting.

skills in evidence-based practice. These strategies include:

- An allocation of time to nonclinical tasks in the early stages of the transition period to search for evidence and critique research.
- Supervision and support groups to facilitate the transition of new graduates from students with skills in searching and appraising evidence to clinicians who are able to modify these skills to match the workplace resources.
- Clinical supervision to assist new graduates to use evidence judiciously to assist with problem-solving and to further develop their clinical reasoning within daily practice.
- Peer coaching to enhance and develop new graduates' understanding of clinical problems, which would allow them to restructure their knowledge in relation to evidence-based practice within a safe environment.

Technology and databases are frequently being modified or changed. It is important for new graduates to be able to access and utilize these resources. Familiarity with librarians and databases accessible to the workplace will assist in the search for evidence.

Evidence-Based Practice Competencies

In Chapter 12, you became familiar with the process of identifying and assessing competencies related to various aspects of practice. Including competencies on the knowledge, skills, attitudes, and critical and ethical reasoning necessary for evidence-based practice in your system for the assessment of competencies is a great example of building structures to support evidence-based practice. Furthermore, including competencies in the orientation process and in annual reviews allows you to identify and provide the training needed by staff as they are hired, and to send a clear message to staff about the value of evidence-based practice in your department. Once practitioners are caught up in their daily responsibilities and have the pressures of meeting productivity and quality expectations, it may be more difficult for them to spend time developing evidence-based practice competencies. Including such competency activities in orientation can be all the more important given this consideration.

Table 16-2 includes sample competencies related to evidence-based practice knowledge, skills, attitudes, and critical and ethical reasoning.

Teaching and Training Basics

Although much of what OTs and OTAs do with their patients and clients involves the teaching–learning process, occupational therapy practitioners learn relatively little about formal teaching strategies or how to respond to the learning needs of adult staff members in particular. Luckily, there are many easily accessible resources to guide these activities. Numerous Web pages provide hints and strategies on understanding adult learners, and ways to accommodate the fact that adults are typically motivated to learn for different reasons than children. In addition, these resources provide suggestions on ways to structure learning experiences for adults more effectively.

Much of today's information on adult learners continues to be based on the work and perspectives of Malcolm Knowles (1913–1997), a central figure in U.S. adult education in the second half of the 20th century. In the 1950s, he was the executive director of the Adult Education Association of the United States of America. He wrote the first major accounts of informal adult education and the history of adult education in the United States (Smith, 2004). The available knowledge about adults as learners and the fields of adult learning, training, and training design has grown considerably in the last few decades.

If you are a manager in a hospital or school system, undoubtedly there is someone within your organization or system familiar with the learning needs of adult workers who can assist you in designing effective training materials and approaches for educating your staff. It is likely that this individual has specialized knowledge in training design and delivery. If so, you are encouraged to take advantage of that resource. In addition, an introduction to the basic concepts to consider is provided next.

Knowles (1970) identified characteristics of adult learners that must be considered when designing training and learning experiences such as those often used to introduce new knowledge in the workplace. Although these assumptions have been criticized as not being universally applicable and as Eurocentric, they are still widely cited, including in the

TABLE 16-2

Sample Competencies to Support Evidence-Based Practice

Knowledge	Skills	Attitudes	Critical Reasoning	Ethical Reasoning
Knows occupational therapy conceptual practice models	Demonstrates use of relevant databases to find literature and evidence	Demonstrates appreciation of inclusion of patients in making intervention decisions based on evidence	Describes the process of decision-making when there is limited evidence related to an aspect of intervention	Identifies limits to his or her knowledge in relation to various aspects of occupational therapy practice
Identifies evidence-based practice resources	Formulates a clinical question that is sufficiently narrow to guide a search for evidence	Demonstrates an appreciation for lifelong learning and skill development	Describes the process of decision-making when there is contradictory evidence related to an aspect of intervention	Identifies steps to take if he or she is feeling unduly pressured into providing intervention that he or she feels is inappropriate or will be ineffective
Is familiar with relevant models in related fields	Selects and applies appropriate criteria to evaluate the specific form of evidence Evaluates and summarizes the evidence reviewed to answer the clinical question Describes summary of evidence using language and concepts appropriate to the audience (e.g., health-care team, consumer, payer)		Is able to give examples of how to combine clinical experience with evidence in order to deduce logical possible intervention options Demonstrates ability to generalize application of evidence from one clinical case to similar clinical cases	Demonstrates steps to incorporate evolving evidence into his or her professional development plan to maintain competence Demonstrates ability to balance clinical expertise, available evidence, and client goals to make a clinical decision

occupational therapy literature (Knecht-Sabres et al, 2013; Missiuana et al, 2012: Whitcombe, 2012). These assumptions include:

- Adults are autonomous and self-directed. Adults want to become active participants in the learning process and are often effective in guiding their own learning. Adult learners can assist you in identifying their learning needs and will often readily share their interests if asked, and these interests can be used to motivate learning.
- Adults bring their considerable life experiences and knowledge *from the workplace and other*

environments to the learning situation. Adults desire to connect new learning to prior experiences. Relating new knowledge, theories, and concepts to existing knowledge will help adults frame the learning experience and make more sense of it.

- Adults are goal-oriented. Adults enter a learning experience with particular goals and learning objectives in mind. Asking adults why they are taking part in learning can help you connect learning activities to these goals and increase learner satisfaction.
- Adults are relevancy-oriented. Adults want to understand *why* they are being taught something

and want to see the connection between learning activities and materials, as well as their goals, daily responsibilities, and future needs.

- Adults are practical. Adults typically prefer to learn what is of most interest and use to them and may not be interested in learning for learning's sake.

In addition, adults typically have motivations for learning that differ from those of children (Cantor, 2001). Understanding these motivations also helps in designing effective learning experiences for adult workers. These motivations include:

- To make or maintain social relationships
- To meet external expectations such as those mandated in the workplace or by accrediting or licensure bodies
- To learn to better serve others more effectively
- To achieve professional advancement and recognition
- To escape routine responsibilities or for intellectual stimulation
- For pure interest

It is not uncommon for the occupational therapy manager to develop and run educational sessions as part of department staff meetings alone or in conjunction with other managers or supervisors. Whenever possible, you are encouraged to take advantage of local subject matter experts and to be flexible about collaborating with other practitioners and managers in your local area. However, when you do find yourself responsible for leading a discussion or providing staff with instruction, keep in mind that instructors can help to motivate students via several means (Wlodkowski, 2011).

First, you should establish a friendly, open atmosphere that shows the participants that questions and participation are welcome. Setting a tone appropriate to the level of the objective's importance is essential. If the material has a high level of importance, a higher level of tension or stress should be established in the class to indicate the importance of what you are covering. However, people learn best under low to moderate stress; if the stress is too high, it becomes a barrier to learning. You must carefully consider the degree of difficulty of the materials you are covering as well. The degree of difficulty should be set high enough to challenge participants but not so high that they become frustrated by information overload. This balance is especially important when first introducing a topic such as evidence-based practice. It's better not to try to accomplish too much at one time. A good way to start is to identify long-term learning objectives (or the competencies you want staff to develop) and to break those objectives or competencies down into smaller units of learning that can be achieved within the time you have allotted for any given session.

In work settings, adults find themselves participating in learning experiences out of interest and desire to learn, but they are also highly likely to participate because they are instructed to do so by their supervisor. In deciding how to construct the learning experience, you should carefully consider how you present it to staff, as well as the attitude that your staff has toward the training. If staff members are hesitant because of a lack of confidence, because they cannot clearly see the value of training, or because they are pressured for time, you may want to start by providing low-stress and low-demand learning aimed primarily at introducing the value of the topic. Time pressures are among the major barriers reported in the literature to engaging in evidence-based practice. As a manager, you will have to create a structure that will support staff members to learn about evidence-based practice, and then later to apply what they have learned. You play a major role in minimizing these time pressures in the ways that you structure workloads and in-service and continuing education time.

A learner's affect, or emotional experience, while learning can influence the meaning and relevance he or she attaches to the learning. This does not mean that learning must always be "fun," but the introduction to learning about important topics such as evidence-based practice should be consciously and thoughtfully planned. If it is evident that your staff is nervous, distracted by other work responsibilities, or not invested in the learning experience, it will be important for you to resolve these issues before focusing on the specific learning objectives you have identified. Some ideas on different ways to resolve these issues are provided in Table 16-3.

Strategies for Teaching Each Step of the Evidence-Based Practice Process

In Chapter 2, you were introduced to the steps of the evidence-based practice process. These steps are

TABLE 16-3

Challenges and Potential Solutions to Introducing Your Staff to Evidence-Based Practice

Challenge	Potential Solutions
Staff members are nervous about evidence-based practice (EBP)	1. Start slowly, and use the steps of EBP to guide the development of your educational sessions. Break each step down, and think about how you can grade the skills within each step up and down. 2. Use worksheets, flowcharts, and other visual aids to guide staff along, step by step. 3. Emphasize the importance of clinical expertise in the EBP process, and build on the staff's confidence in this area to build confidence in the other areas of EBP. 4. Use small discussion and problem-solving groups so staff members can build and learn from each other's strengths.
Staff members are distracted by work responsibilities	1. Incorporate the EBP in-services and activities into the normal meetings in your department; ensure that they are not "add-on" activities. 2. Set up the EBP activities so that they are completed by teams of therapists so that the work can be shared. 3. Identify times of the month or year that have lower patient census, and organize EBP activities to correspond to these times. 4. Consider some type of workload incentive for EBP activity involvement.
Staff members are not invested in the learning experience	1. Bring in therapists from other local departments who are using EBP to talk about how and why EBP is useful. 2. Focus each EBP in-service on a specific patient problem that one of the therapists in the department is dealing with, using the in-service to help the therapist solve the problem. 3. Obtain the necessary certification to ensure that the EBP in-services will give the therapists continuing education credits for licensure, if relevant in your jurisdiction. 4. Consider some type of workload incentive for EBP activity involvement.

repeated in Box 16-3 and strategies for teaching each step are discussed in this section. Presenting the steps of this process to your staff and using them as a guide for organizing and structuring learning experiences is a helpful way of meeting the need that adult learners have for knowing *why* they are being asked to learn and *how* the new knowledge will be of help and use in their everyday lives.

The first step of the evidence-based practice process is to *frame a question related to a decision that needs to be made*. A great first exercise to help teach staff to frame (develop) a question is involving staff members in a group examination of their current practice. Reflecting on the current struggles and challenges that staff members are facing will help to make the relevance of the learning clear. Law (2008, p. 97) noted that well-built clinical questions include four elements: (1) a specific client group or population; (2) the assessment, treatment, or other clinical issues that you are

BOX 16-3

The Evidence-Based Practice Process

Step 1: *Frame* a question related to a decision that needs to be made.
Step 2: *Acquire* evidence that may contain information relevant to the question.
Step 3: *Assess* the evidence for accuracy, comprehensiveness, applicability, and actionability.
Step 4: *Present* the evidence to those who must act on it.
Step 5: *Apply* the evidence to the decision.
Step 6: *Evaluate* the results.

addressing; (3) the comparison; and (4) the outcome in which you are interested. This approach is also commonly referred to as P.I.C.O., or (P) patient or client (population), (I) intervention, (C) comparison, and (O) outcome.

One strategy for helping your staff members develop well-defined and well-built questions is to have them work in groups to begin this process. Perhaps you can start with a large-group activity, having staff brainstorm topics for clinical questions. Then the larger group can be broken down into smaller working groups to focus the questions and to prepare a well-built clinical question, using the three previously mentioned points to guide them. You may want to have these small groups share some common experiences—for example, they all work in particular service areas such as pediatrics or mental health, or they are all trying to select a new assessment tool for a particular client problem. You might also consider pairing within the small groups any OTs and OTAs who often collaborate.

Once the small groups have completed their questions, the teaching group can reconvene, share their work, and critique the questions identified by others. The critiques should focus on whether the questions contain the four components of a well-built question. Note that some questions may not require a comparison, and therefore will only contain three of the four components. Because the small groups are likely to have identified more than a single question, it may also be necessary for you to lead a discussion about which questions should be a priority to address in your setting. A worksheet for developing clinical questions is presented in Appendix 16-1 at the end of the chapter.

The second step in the evidence-based practice process is to *acquire evidence that may contain information relevant to the question*. An effective strategy for helping staff become more comfortable with locating resources to acquire evidence is to combine didactic instruction with experiential learning. Examples of brief workshops to help improve the comfort level and confidence in finding and using literature have been published (Sastre, Denny, McCoy, McCoy, & Spickard, 2011). You should begin by demonstrating and explaining resources to your staff members and then allow them time to experiment and practice on their own. Providing learners with "tip sheets" to guide their practice sessions is recommended. Such sheets may be ones that you develop on your own, or

they may come from one of many resources on evidence-based practice that are listed at the end of this chapter. Using the readily available online tutorials from the companies that run the major search databases is also an effective way of providing training in locating evidence; for example, access to online training programs and tutorials are available from the OVID website (http://www.ovid.com/) (OVID, 2004).

Another strategy for helping staff become more comfortable with locating resources to acquire evidence is to create a step-by-step example that they can replicate. That is, you can set your own clinical question and conduct a search to address it, keeping careful track of everything that you do and recording it in detail in a handout you can give to your staff to replicate. After they are finished, you can lead a discussion on what ideas they have for improving or refining the search, and then have them make these adaptations. This strategy is particularly useful for staff members who have very limited computer-searching experience, and need to develop their confidence in their ability to think through and conduct searches.

The third step in the evidence-based practice process is to *assess the evidence for accuracy, comprehensiveness, applicability, and actionability*. This is typically the step of the process that staff finds the most difficult, regardless of the type of resource that needs to be evaluated. Having staff members work in small groups is again recommended because it allows them to share their strengths, to see how others process information, to ask questions of others, and to provide and receive support to limit frustration. The use of journal clubs has been shown to be effective as a strategy for teaching clinical appraisal to medical students (Ahmadi et al, 2012). Providing structured forms to guide documentation of the evaluation of evidence is helpful. These forms should be easily accessible to your staff in hard copy, or they could be loaded on department computers to be filled out over a period of time. Either way, you want to make it easy for staff members to use the forms in a way that fits their work styles and workloads. Samples of questions to guide the development of such forms are provided throughout Chapter 2. In addition, sample appraisal forms that can be used for research articles and program descriptions, as well as a website, are presented in Appendices 16-2 through 16-5 at the end of this chapter. As your staff members' skills in evidence-based practice develop, you may want to encourage them to develop their own appraisal forms and customize them to focus on the types of information that are the most salient for their everyday practices.

The fourth step in the evidence-based practice process is to *present the evidence to those who must act on it*. This phase requires integration of the evidence into your practice setting and can be the most difficult if the information that has been located is contradictory or inconclusive. In order to help staff members think about *how* to evaluate and summarize information in order to present it, you may want to have them read some existing evidence-based reviews. For example, staff could read the evidence briefs series conducted by AOTA, or review a couple of relevant Cochrane reviews that are available online. Another resource is the Occupational Therapy Critically Appraised Topics website (http://www.otcats.com/). By reviewing existing evidence-based practice review summaries, staff members will be able to develop comfort with how such summaries are organized conceptually and how terminology is used. They will then be able to use these examples as a template for thinking about their own summaries for the information they have read.

Another strategy for helping staff members to evaluate and summarize the information they are gathering to prepare it for presentation is to provide them with a glossary of terms that they may be encountering during their reading. An example of such a glossary is provided in Box 16-4. Finally, choosing a standard "levels of evidence" typology for evaluating the literature (see Chapter 1) for use in your department may be helpful. You should use the typology consistently, and consider incorporating it into the forms that staff members will use during the process of appraising the literature they find. This will help staff members start to see the relationship between different types of evidence, and what each of these types can and cannot offer to their clinical decision-making processes.

After evaluating and summarizing the evidence, the next step in the evidence-based practice process is to *apply the evidence to the decision* whether it is a clinical or managerial question. Helping staff members to become proficient in this step of the evidence-based process involves getting them to connect their findings from the literature, their own clinical experience, and the goals of the client or clients to which the information they have gathered applies. Connecting all of these things can be complicated and may require a range of coordinated strategies that extend over time.

No one learns evidence-based practice in an afternoon. Rather, managers help staff learn to apply evidence-based practice by building structures to support its use. Emphasizing the value of evidence-based practice, and building it into the expectations and culture of your organization, will go a long way to incorporating it into the everyday work routines of employees. Using activities similar to those listed earlier in Box 16-2 will help you and your staff develop the *routines* of evidence-based practice. Additional examples of activities to assist with building and supporting evidence-based practice in the everyday routine of work are listed in Box 16-5.

A key part of the final step of evidence-based practice is to communicate the evidence that has been found to others to *evaluate the results as you* integrate and apply the evidence to actual practice. You and your staff will need to communicate evidence to your clients, your patients, or the consumers of occupational therapy. You will also need to communicate evidence to the other health professionals in your department and organization, as well as those individuals and companies that pay for your services. Communicating about the evidence is critical so key decision-makers (e.g., patients, family members, other care providers, payers) can be involved in deciding whether an intervention is warranted given what you know about the likelihood that it will be effective. More importantly, communicating about the evidence will increase the likelihood that these decisions are well informed, and based on more than just a guess about what might work. As the evidence is integrated and applied to your practice you must involve your clients, your patients, the consumers of occupational therapy, and other health professionals in evaluating the effectiveness and outcomes of your decision.

Because you and your staff will be communicating with different sorts of persons with varying interests and investment in the occupational therapy process, you will need to become comfortable with talking about the same evidence in different ways. Organizational leaders and managers from other departments will be concerned about resource utilization, including staff, space, equipment, and supplies. Payers will be concerned about costs to them and will want information such as the frequency and duration of intervention necessary to achieve desired outcomes. Patients will want to know whether the intervention is going to work, and how long it might take to see

BOX 16-4

Glossary of Evidence-Based Practice Terminology

- **Critical appraisal:** The process of judging the quality of a piece of information and determining its applicability to practice.
- **Critical appraisal matrix:** A systematic method of summarizing a series of critical appraisals from individual articles to facilitate comparisons and decision-making.
- **Electronic bibliographic database:** Electronic compilations of published research, scholarly articles, books, government reports, newspaper articles, and other recognized sources of information.
- **Electronic table of contents alerts:** A service provided by professional and scientific journals whereby alerts are e-mailed whenever articles that include key words you submit are published.
- **Levels of evidence:** A criterion-referenced typology and classification system that provides guidance for evaluating the quality of a research article; these levels are multilayered, typically including criteria for design, sample size, and internal and external validity.
- **Literature search:** A systematic, explicit, and reproducible method for identifying, evaluating, and interpreting the existing body of recorded work produced by researchers, scholars, and practitioners.
- **Sample size:** The number of participants in a study.
- **Validity:** There are two broad categories of validity: validity of methodology, which includes internal and external validity, and validity of measurement, which includes content, criterion, and construct validity. Ultimately, validity addresses whether or not a research design or a measurement tool was able to capture what it intended to capture (i.e., can the design answer the question posed; does the measurement tool measure what it says it does). Definitions of the different types of validity are as follows:

- *Internal validity:* addresses the question of whether or not there are other potential explanations for study findings that are a function of the study design (e.g., biases in sampling or measurement, history or maturation effects, testing effects).
- *External validity:* addresses the question of generalizability, and to whom the study findings can be applied. External validity is influenced primarily by the sampling method of the study, and whether or not there was differential dropout of participants.
- *Content validity:* a type of validity related to measurement that addresses the question of whether a particular instrument contains all relevant domains of content, given its intent.
- *Construct validity:* addresses the question of whether or not the instrument produces scores that demonstrate the expected relationships, based on theory, with other concepts and variables. Construct validity is population specific, and built over time through hypothesis testing. There are two types of construct validity: discriminate validity (hypothesize what your tool will *not* correspond with, and test this), and convergent validity (hypothesize what your tool *will* correspond with, and test this).
- *Criterion validity:* addresses the question of whether the instrument produces scores that approximate or correspond to an existing instrument that measures the same concept or construct, sometimes identified as the "gold standard." There are two types of criterion validity: concurrent validity (when the two instruments are administered at the same time and results compared) and predictive validity (when the current instrument is administered and then another one is used in the future; used when an instrument is being evaluated for its ability to identify characteristics or behaviors sooner than current tests allow).

BOX 16-5

Strategies for Building Evidence-Based Practice Into the Everyday Routines of Work

- Take advantage of skills and preferences. Not all staff will be skilled at conducting literature reviews or summarizing evidence. Create partnerships in which one staff member covers another's duties so that he or she may spend time in tasks specific to evidence-based practice.
- Train fieldwork students to learn and adopt evidence-based practice by building assignments into fieldwork experiences.
- Use volunteers; put specific requests into your volunteer office for students or others who might have skills in finding or preparing forms of evidence for review.
- Make evidence-based practice activities part of the work routine by scheduling article reviews and case discussions to generate clinical questions.
- Start a journal club to help staff develop skills in critical appraisal.
- Create partnerships with other local occupational therapy departments to share the work and benefits of conducting evidence-based practice reviews.
- Create, load, and maintain a list of evidence-based practice "favorite" Internet links on your department computers so that sites are easily found and accessed.
- Create interdisciplinary evidence-based practice *investigation teams* by having OTs, OTAs, physical therapists, nurses, and others work together to research and answer shared clinical questions.
- Encourage, recognize, and reward staff members who become *clinical resource experts* in a topic, in an area of intervention, or with diagnostic groups frequently seen in your practice setting.
- Create and maintain *reference sheets* that spell out the steps to find and evaluate evidence and put them everywhere (i.e., on all computers, on the wall near computers, etc.) so that staff members have easy access.

results. Law (2008) suggested that, regardless of whom you are communicating with, your message is more likely to be understood if it has the following attributes:

1. Nontechnical, simple, and concrete language with simple grammatical structure
2. Terms that cross cultures and perspectives
3. Brevity, with just enough detail for decision-making
4. Checks for confusion or lack of comprehension
5. Suggestions for concrete actions related to the information

Most importantly, you must keep in mind your responsibility to involve others in making decisions in a real way. Evidence-based practice *is not* a strategy for justifying to others what you have *already* decided to do, but rather a strategy for involving others in making decisions about what you *should* do in the future given what you know now.

As a second key part of the final step in the evidence-based practice process, it is critically important to ensure ongoing evaluation of the information being applied to practice. It is not enough to teach your staff members to find and evaluate evidence; you must also provide them guidance for evaluating whether the decisions they are making based on what they are learning are really making a difference. Tracking these changes may mean having to go back to the literature and reconsider assessment and outcome tools, as well as other systems for monitoring progress and change. Evidence-based practice is a cycle—one does not simply answer a question and move on. One must answer the question, evaluate the response, and perhaps refine the question or develop a new one. Evidence-based practice is an ongoing way of doing and improving practice.

Creating the Tools to Support Evidence-Based Practice

The following are examples of structures and tools that managers can put in place and use to support evidence-based practice becoming part of the everyday routines of work performed by the staff they supervise:

- *Worksheets for developing clinical questions:* Writing well-built clinical questions can be challenging. A worksheet can break down the components of a question, making it easier for clinicians to develop questions that are targeted and clear to follow.
- *Article review worksheets:* A written worksheet with predetermined questions can be useful to guide readers through the process of reviewing an article and assigning a level of evidence. Worksheets can be developed for different types of articles (quantitative, qualitative case reports, program descriptions, etc.) and kept in easily accessible files in hard copy or loaded onto computers. Worksheets can also be developed for websites, books, or any other type of resource commonly accessed for information in your department.
- *Critical appraisal matrices:* Charts can be constructed to summarize articles that are reviewed (see Appendix 16-6 at the end of the chapter). Matrices can be custom designed to capture the most salient information for your setting and your particular clinical problem. In a department, it would be possible to start a matrix on a computer, and have different therapists add to it as they find new literature.
- *Glossary of evidence-based practice terminology:* A list of definitions of commonly cited concepts, tools, and strategies used in evidence-based practice is also useful. Glossaries are simple ways of reinforcing key concepts as they are learned and help limit confusion among practitioners.
- *Evidence-based practice competencies:* Competencies are explicit statements that define specific areas of expertise and are related to effective or superior performance in a job. Competencies can relate to a point in an employee's employment or routine managerial processes, such as employee orientation or annual performance appraisals, or

to the intervention process, such as when learning a new skill.

Transferring Knowledge and Translating Research to Practice: A New Global Focus

The concepts of **knowledge transfer** and of **translational research** have had a global impact and are closely related to the concept of evidence-based practice. Although it may appear that these topics relate most directly to those who produce knowledge and research, they are terms that all occupational therapy practitioners should be familiar with. Managers with responsibility for developing programs as described in Chapter 15 will be especially concerned with helping staff transfer knowledge and apply evidence-based interventions in the practice setting.

Translational research is a priority of the National Institutes of Health and of the European Commission (Woolf, 2008). It has been defined as: "an effective translation of the new knowledge, mechanisms, and techniques generated by advances in basic science research into new approaches for prevention, diagnosis, and treatment of disease [which] is essential for improving health" (Fontanarosa & DeAngelis, 2002, p. 1728). A simple way of characterizing translational research is the descriptor "bench-to-bedside" or making sure that new treatments actually reach patients. Translational research most commonly refers to the development and translation of medically focused treatments such as the development and application of new medications.

Knowledge transfer is a term that may be more appropriately used when discussing the sharing and application of knowledge within occupational therapy and other health professions focused on habilitation and rehabilitation. Knowledge transfer can be described as a systematic approach to capture, collect, and share tacit knowledge in order to transfer it to become explicit knowledge. It also can be defined as simply "imparting of research knowledge from producers to potential users" (Kiefer et al, 2005, p. I-6; National Collaborating Centre for Methods and Tools, 2013).

The Johns Hopkins Quality and Safety Research Group has developed a model focused on translating evidence into practice and promoting knowledge transfer that has been applied to multiple types of interventions across disciplines (Pronovost, Beren-holtz, & Needham, 2008). The focus of the model includes:

- A focus on systems rather than care of individual patients
- Engagement of local interdisciplinary teams to assume ownership of the improvement project
- Creation of centralized support for the technical work
- Encouraging local adaptation of the intervention
- Creating a collaborative culture within the local unit and larger system

The model includes four steps that are briefly summarized next. Step one is to *summarize the evidence*, focusing on the identification of high payoff interventions with minimal barriers to implementation. Step two is to *identify local barriers to implementation*, which is achieved by observing the intervention performed by staff and identify roadblocks, bottlenecks, or places where the process may break down. Step three is to *measure performance* through the selection of process or outcome indicators, and fully piloting and developing ways to obtain accurate metrics of baseline performance. Step four is to implement what is referred to as the four E's, which are to (1) engage, (2) educate, (3) execute, and (4) evaluate. The four E's are similar to the PDSA process (plan, do, study, act) described in Chapter 13 in a continuous quality improvement (CQI) approach. The four E's are reflected in Figure 16-1.

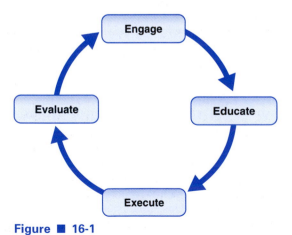

Figure ■ 16-1
The Four "E" Approach of Improving the Reliability of Knowledge Transfer.

To engage others, you must help them to understand why the intervention you are suggesting is important and what it will contribute to patient outcomes and the organization. You educate others by sharing the evidence to support the intervention using the strategies described throughout this chapter. During the third step (execute), you pilot the intervention. Pronovost, Berenholtz, and Needham (2008, p. 964) recommend developing an implementation toolkit that "provides a framework for redesigning care processes and includes three principles: standardize care processes, create independent checks (such as checklists), and learn from mistakes." To evaluate, measures of the key indicators are compared preintervention and postintervention. This model is applicable to inpatient and outpatient settings such as a safe surgery program in Michigan and programs in the emergency department and an outpatient diabetes service (Pronovost, Berenholtz, & Needham, 2008). The model has been applied successfully to interdisciplinary programs including occupational therapy to improve early mobility of patients in the intensive care unit (Friedman, 2014, personal communication; Lord et al, 2013).

Chapter Summary

This chapter focused on introducing evidence-based practice and the use of various forms of data, information, and other evidence used by managers to lead and direct occupational therapy services to others. Specifically, this chapter examined ways that managers can build organizational structures to help integrate evidence-based practice activities into the everyday work routines of occupational therapy practitioners.

Once a manager and the staff members he or she supervises adopt the values that underlie evidence-based practice and are ready to accept the corresponding responsibilities, they must also adopt new ways of working. Managers can facilitate this process by providing learning opportunities for staff, by making the tools to support evidence-based practice easily accessible, and by integrating the process of finding and evaluating evidence with other systems, such as a system for the assessment of competencies and reward structures.

It was stressed in this chapter that, as adults, staff members have characteristics and needs as learners that must be recognized if a manager is going to develop and deliver an effective educational experience. Fortunately, there are often resources available within larger organizations in which occupational therapy managers work to aid in the development and delivery of staff education and training. For managers who work in settings where this type of assistance is not available on-site, or for business owners who often must meet varied staff needs on their own, there are many easily accessible resources available on the Internet. Networking with other managers in your local area or through the use of some of the resources noted throughout this book, such as professional Listservs, are also strategies that can help managers effectively respond to the educational and training needs of staff.

Learning any complicated skill set can be a challenge, and evidence-based practice indeed requires that practitioners learn a varied set of skills that allow them to find, evaluate, communicate about, and integrate evidence into their service delivery. Managers face the challenge of learning not only to incorporate clinical evidence into their practice but also to recognize that evidence exists on a wide range of topics and issues, including organizational culture, leadership, supervision, program development, and communication, that can guide their practice as a manager. However, with the proliferation of books, articles, and Internet sites, and increased attention paid to evidence-based medicine and practice by accrediting bodies for educational programs and service delivery programs, it seems unlikely that this is a challenge that occupational therapy managers can avoid.

At the start of the chapter, you were introduced to Angela, who had recently learned more about the evidence-based practice process and had begun an endeavor to introduce others in her department to evidence-based practice and to facilitate their skill development.

■ Real-Life Solutions

As Angela began to search for information on teaching evidence-based practice to others, she noticed that much of what she initially encountered focused on evaluating the most advanced types of evidence, such as quantitative experimental investigations. It struck her that, for a novice, the mistaken idea that other forms of evidence, including qualitative research, program descriptions, case reports, expert opinions, and, most importantly, a practitioner's own clinical experience and judgment, were not valid might be reinforced. Angela also felt sure that one of the biggest obstacles to the other staff members in her department investing energy in learning about evidence-based practice would be helping them to find ways and time to integrate these new strategies into their daily work lives.

Angela decided to pull together some resources that could be used by the staff, including examples of critical appraisal questions and forms for different types of articles, information on free Internet-based tutorials on conducting searches in electronic bibliographic databases, and a list of Internet sites that included summaries of evidence, such as the evidence-based briefs series published by AOTA or the Cochrane Library. Although it was evident to Angela that making these resources readily available to the staff in paper or electronic formats would help, it also seemed clear that editing some of the forms to minimize the use of scientific language would make it easier for staff members to use the forms and to interpret and discuss with others the results of evidence-based analyses. Angela made a note to herself to start to draft a glossary of terms that staff members would commonly encounter so that they could refer to it and be less likely to feel overwhelmed.

When Angela met with her boss, Lindsay, to discuss what she had pulled together, she found that Lindsay had been busy as well. She had already reviewed some of the resources available on the Internet and had contacted a representative in the human resources and information management department to obtain assistance in designing training sessions on evidence-based practice and designing or purchasing tutorials on searching electronic bibliographic databases that could be accessed through the hospital's intranet. In addition, Lindsay had started to think about how the adoption of evidence-based practice could be supported and

Continued

■ **Real-Life Solutions—cont'd**

how she could communicate expectations as a manager by building activities related to evidence-based practice into existing departmental structures. For example, she had begun to consider the types of competencies that might be developed and that all staff would expect to be able to demonstrate.

As Angela and Lindsay continued to collaborate, they began to establish a network of other managers and clinicians who were also committed to promoting evidence-based practice. Through this network, they learned about some of the creative ways that other departments were having staff members work in groups to seek evidence to clinical questions they identified. Among other strategies, they found that some clinical departments were partnering with academicians, using volunteers, pairing fieldwork students with advanced clinicians, having weekly evidence-based practice brown-bag lunch seminars, and creating evidence-based practice teams composed of clinicians from multiple disciplines.

Angela and Lindsay both agreed that they would encounter resistance and roadblocks as

they worked to introduce evidence-based practice as an expectation for the department's staff. They knew that some staff members would think that it took too much time, other staff members would lack confidence in their skills to learn to search for evidence and evaluate it when found, and still others would be resistant to adopting the values and responsibilities related to including patients, families, and others in using evidence to make clinical decisions. However, Lindsay recounted the experience she had had just a few years earlier when the hospital introduced its computerized medical record system. She noted that, at first, most of the staff complained about having to spend time in trainings and how one member of the staff had simply stated that she was "too old of a dog to learn new tricks!" Yet, in less than a year, all of the staff members were routinely using the computer to document their interventions and she had not heard a complaint in months. Granted, it had taken extra effort by some of the staff members who were less comfortable with newer technology, but even they had eventually recognized the value of the new system. Lindsay was optimistic that it would be the same with evidence-based practice.

Study Questions

1. **Which of the following are benefits of shared values in the workplace?**

   a. They help turn commonplace, routine work into valued activities.
   b. They create a connection between the organization's mission and society's values.
   c. They provide a source of competitive advantage to the organization.
   d. All of the above.

2. **In regard to the research-related standards for accreditation in master's-entry and doctoral-entry educational programs for the OT, which of the following is true?**

   a. The research-related standards are the same in both types of entry-level programs.

   b. There are several research-related standards that are the same, several that are similar, and one standard for doctoral-entry programs requiring a research-related project not found in the master's-entry standards.
   c. Doctoral-entry standards differ only in the addition of expectations to evaluate qualitative research in addition to evaluating quantitative research.
   d. Doctoral-entry standards differ only in that they require doctoral students to teach evidence-based practice to others.

3. **Which of the following would best describe adult learners?**

   a. Adult learners learn in the same manner and for the same reasons as children.

b. Adult learners tend to be more dependent on others for motivation because they do not routinely participate in learning experiences.

c. Adult learners almost always are involved in learning only for financial gain such as a promotion.

d. Adult learners are self-directed, goal-oriented, and may have multiple internal and external motivations for learning.

4. Which of the following is not an element of a well-defined clinical question?

a. A specific client group or population

b. The assessment, treatment, or other clinical issues that you are addressing

c. The source where you are obtaining data

d. The outcome in which you are interested

5. Which of the following accurately represents P.I.C.O.?

a. (P) patient or client (population), (I) intervention, (C) comparison, and (O) outcome

b. (P) patient or client (population), (I) interviews, (C) comparison, and (O) outcome

c. (P) patient or client (population), (I) intervention, (C) critical appraisal, and (O) outcome

d. (P) patient or client (population), (I) intervention, (C) comparison, and (O) orientation

6. Which of the following is not a positive attribute of effective communication of a message on evidence-based practice for consumers or payers?

a. Nontechnical, simple, and concrete language with simple grammatical structure

b. Terms that cross cultures and perspectives

c. Specific detail providing in-depth explanation of all information that can be shared

d. Checks for confusion or lack of comprehension

7. Which of the following best describes knowledge transfer?

a. It is a systematic approach to capture, collect, and share tacit knowledge in order for its transfer to become explicit knowledge or imparting of research knowledge from producers to potential users.

b. It is an effective translation of the new knowledge, mechanisms, and techniques generated by advances in basic science research into new approaches for prevention, diagnosis, and treatment of disease, which is essential for improving health.

c. It is the evaluation of the effectiveness of original science or knowledge and the determination if additional research to help with application to the real world is appropriate.

d. It is the transfer of approved research protocols from one setting to another to help with validation of the research questions, study design, and data collection methodologies.

8. Which of the following is not one of the four E's presented to improve the reliability of knowledge transfer?

a. Engage

b. Educate

c. Encourage

d. Evaluate

Resources for Learning More About Introducing Others to Evidence-Based Practice

Journals That Are Likely to Include Evidence Relevant to Administration and Management of Health-Care Services

The Milbank Quarterly

http://onlinelibrary.wiley.com/journal/10.1111/%28ISSN%291468-0009

The Milbank Quarterly has been published for over seven decades and features peer-reviewed original research and articles that review health-care policy and provide analysis of current and evolving policy. Other content includes commentary from a range of professionals representing academicians, practitioners, researchers, and policy makers. Articles and commentary found in this journal represent multidisciplinary perspectives on empirical research as well as the application of research and policy in a variety of settings. Social, legal, and ethical issues are addressed.

Journal of Health Services Research & Policy

http://hsr.sagepub.com/

The *Journal of Health Services Research & Policy* includes articles presenting results of qualitative and quantitative multidisciplinary research from a wide variety of disciplines. In addition to the reporting of empirical results, articles also address current and evolving debates in the scientific, methodological, and empirical arenas.

Health Services Research

http://www.hsr.org/

The journal *Health Services Research* provides researchers, policy makers and analysts, and health-care administrators and managers with access to empirical findings as well as articles addressing policy and methodological issues. Readers interested in health-care financing, the organization or delivery of health services, or in the evaluation of health delivery outcomes will find *Health Services Research* a useful resource. The journal provides a forum for the exchange of practices related to individuals, health systems, and communities.

General Information on Finding and Evaluating the Literature

- Cochrane Collaboration and the Cochrane Library (http://www.cochrane.org/index0.htm)
- Health Information Research Unit at McMaster University (http://hiru.mcmaster.ca/)
- Database of Abstracts of Reviews of Effects (DARE) (http://www.crd.york.ac.uk/crdweb/

Occupational Therapy–Specific Resources on Evidence-Based Practice

- OTseeker (http://www.otseeker.com/)
- OT Critically Appraised Topics (http://www.otcats .com/)
- AOTA Evidence-Based Practice Project (http:// www.aota.org/)

- Center for Evidence-Based Rehabilitation at McMaster University (http://fw4.bluewirecs.ca/ ResearchResourcesnbsp/ResearchGroups/Centre forEvidenceBasedRehabilitation/tabid/543/ Default.aspx)

Professional Organizations Relevant to Administration and Management of Health-Care Services

American College of Healthcare Executives

http://www.ache.org/

The American College of Healthcare Executives (ACHE) is an international professional society of health-care executives working in a variety of settings, including hospitals, health-care systems, and other health-care organizations. The ACHE is known for its credentialing and educational programs. The annual Congress on Healthcare Management is a nationally recognized and widely attended event. The ACHE publishes the *Journal of Healthcare Management*, as well as a magazine titled *Healthcare Executive*.

Government-Related Websites and Documents

- Centers for Disease Control and Prevention (http:// www.cdc.gov/)
- National Center for Health Statistics (http://www .cdc.gov/nchs/)
- Agency for Health Care Research and Quality (http://www.ahcpr.gov/)
- Centers for Medicare and Medicaid Services (https://www.cms.gov/

Resources on Evaluating Information Found on Websites

- Beck, S. (1997). Evaluation criteria. *The good, the bad & the ugly: Or, why it's a good idea to evaluate Web sources.* Retrieved from http://lib.nmsu.edu/ instruction/evalcrit.html
- The University of California Berkeley Library. *Evaluating Web pages.* Retrieved from http://www. lib.berkeley.edu/TeachingLib/Guides/Internet/ Evaluate.html

Reference List

Accreditation Council for Occupational Therapy Education. (2015). *2011 ACOTE standards and interpretative guide*. Retrieved from http://www.aota.org/Education-Careers/Accreditation/StandardsReview.aspx.

Ahmadi, N., McKenzie, M. E., MacLean, A., Brown, C. J., Mastracci, T., & McLeod, R. S. (2012). Teaching evidence-based medicine to surgery residents: Is journal club the best format? A systematic review of the literature. *Journal of Surgical Education*, *61*(1), 91–100.

Cantor, J. (2001). *Delivering instruction to adult learners*. Toronto, Canada: Wall & Emerson.

Fontanarosa, P. B., & DeAngelis, C. D. (2002). Basic science and translational research in *JAMA*. *JAMA*, *287*(13), 1728.

Heiwe, S., Kajermo, K. N., Tyni-Lenne, R., Guidetti, S., Samuelsson, M., Andersson, I. L., & Wengstro, Y. (2011). Evidence-based practice: Attitudes, knowledge and behaviour among allied health care professionals. *International Journal for Quality in Health Care*, *23*(2), 198–209.

Kiefer, L., Frank, J., Di Ruggiero, E., Dobbins, M., Manuel, D., Gully, P. R., & Mowat, D. (2005). Fostering evidence-based decision-making in Canada: Examining the need for a Canadian population and public health evidence centre and research network. *Canadian Journal of Public Health/Revue Canadienne de Sante'e Publique*, I1–I19.

Knecht-Sabres, D. H. S., Lisa, J., Kovic, O. T. D., Wallingford, M. H. S., St Amand, M. P. H., & Ellen, L. (2013). Preparing occupational therapy students for the complexities of clinical practice. *The Open Journal of Occupational Therapy*, *1*(3), 4.

Knowles, M. (1970). *The modern practice of adult education: Andragogy vs. pedagogy*. New York, NY: Association Press.

Law, M. (2008). *Evidence-based rehabilitation: A guide to practice*. Thorofare, NJ: Slack.

Lord, R. K., Mayhew, C. R., Korupolu, R., Mantheiy, E. C., Friedman, M. A., Palmer, J. B., & Needham, D. M. (2013). ICU early physical rehabilitation programs: Financial modeling of cost savings. *Critical Care Medicine*, *41*(3), 717–724.

Mintzberg, H. (1979). *The structuring of organizations*. Englewood Cliffs, NJ: Prentice-Hall.

Missiuna, C. A., Pollock, N. A., Levac, D. E., Campbell, W. N., Whalen, S. D. S., Bennett, S. M., & Russell, D. J. (2012). Partnering for change: An innovative school-based occupational therapy service delivery model for children with developmental coordination disorder. *Canadian Journal of Occupational Therapy*, *79*(1), 41–50.

Morrison, T., & Robertson, L. (2011). The influences on new graduates' ability to implement evidence-based practice: A review of the literature. *New Zealand Journal of Occupational Therapy*, *58*(2), 37–40.

National Collaborating Centre for Methods and Tools. (2013). *Definitions and frameworks*. Retrieved from http://www.nccmt.ca/eiph/definitions_and_frameworks-eng.html.

OVID. (2004). OvidSP online training. Retrieved from http://www.ovid.com/webapp/wcs/stores/servlet/content_service_Training_13051_-1_13151.

Ploeg, J., Davies, B., Edwards, N., Gifford, W., & Miller, P. E. (2007). Factors influencing best-practice guidelines implementation: Lessons learned from administrators, nursing staff and project leaders. *Worldviews Evidence-Based Nursing*, *4*(4), 210–219.

Pronovost, P., Berenholtz, S., & Needham, D. (2008). Translating evidence into practice: A model for large-scale knowledge translation. *BMJ. British Medical Journal*, *337*(7676), 963–965.

Sastre, E. A., Denny, J. C., McCoy, J. A., McCoy, A. B., & Spickard, A. (2011). Teaching evidence-based medicine: Impact on students' literature use and inpatient clinical documentation. *Medical Teacher*, *33*(6), e306–e312.

Smith, M. K. (2004). Malcolm Knowles, informal adult education, self-direction and andragogy. In *The encyclopedia of informal education*. Retrieved from infed.org website: http://www.infed.org/thinkers/et-knowl.htm.

Upton, D., Stephens, D., Williams, B., & Scurlock-Evans, L. (2014). Occupational therapists' attitudes, knowledge, and implementation of evidence-based practice: A systematic review of published research. *British Journal of Occupational Therapy*, *77*(1), 24–38.

Whitcombe, S. W. (2012). Problem-based learning students' perceptions of professional knowledge and identity: Occupational therapists as "knowers." *British Journal of Occupational Therapy*, *75*(5), 1–7.

Wlodkowski, R. J. (2011). *Enhancing adult motivation to learn: A comprehensive guide for teaching all adults*. San Francisco, CA: John Wiley & Sons.

Woolf, S. H. (2008). The meaning of translational research and why it matters. *JAMA*, *299*(2), 211–213.

Appendix 16-1

Sample Worksheet for Developing Clinical Questions

Identify the client population:

Identify the outcome of interest:

Identify the intervention or exposure:

Using the information above, write your clinical question:

Identify the comparison intervention or exposure (if applicable):

Appendix 16-2

Sample Article Review Worksheet 1

Article Describing the Outcomes of an Intervention Using Quantitative Methods

Citation:

Study Purpose, Question, or Hypothesis:
• What was the guiding purpose, question, or hypothesis for this study?

Sampling:
What was the sampling procedure?
    Probability based (e.g., simple random sample)
    Nonprobability based (e.g., convenience sample, consecutive sample)

Sample:
• What is the average age of the sample?
• What is the gender distribution of the sample?
• What is the racial or ethnic distribution of the sample?
• What is the setting in which the sample is based (e.g., community, institution)?
• Based on the above information, is my patient similar to those described in the study?

Intervention:
• What was the experimental intervention used in the study?
• Was there a comparison intervention? If yes, what was it?
• Is there enough detail provided about the intervention that I could replicate it?
• Based on my interactions with my patient, would the experimental intervention be a good match?
• Would the experimental intervention be a good match for my time, resources, and capabilities or those of others in my setting?

Outcomes:
• What outcomes were expected from the experimental intervention?
• Are the outcomes consistent with the goals of my patient?
• Are the outcomes consistent with expectations of outcomes of third-party payers?
• What instruments were used to measure the outcomes?
• Were the reliability and validity of the measurement tools provided?

Results:
- Are the results of the study clearly stated?
- Was a prior hypothesis tested, or were the findings accidental?
- Is it clear how subjects were included in the analyses (i.e., can I account for all subjects in the study)?
- Is there a significant difference before and after the experimental intervention?
- Is there a significant difference between the experimental intervention group and the comparison group (if applicable) at the end of the study?
- If results were not statistically significant (either before, after, or between groups), are there other reasons to still consider the intervention?

Overall Appraisal:
- Are there biases that I believe influenced the quality and believability of the study? Consider sampling method, sample composition, consistency between the intervention and the outcome measures, assignment of subjects to groups, measurement process (i.e., use of blinding, if realistic), quality of analysis, and so forth.
- Based on my clinical experience, do the experimental intervention and the outcomes reported make sense?

Reasons to Adopt This Intervention (Benefits):
1.
2.
3.
4.

Reasons Not to Adopt This Intervention (Risks and Costs):
1.
2.
3.
4.

Decision and Rationale:

Based on the information at this time, I will make the following recommendation to my patient regarding the benefits, risks, costs, and alternatives of this intervention:

Appendix 16-3

Sample Article Review Worksheet 2

Article Describing Experiences of People or Phenomena of Interest Using Qualitative Methods

Citation:

Study Purpose, Question, or Hypothesis:
- What was the guiding purpose or question for this study?

Sampling:
- How were people recruited for this study?

- What are the potential limitations or biases inherent in this approach relative to the experiences being studied?

Sample:
- What is the average age of the sample?
- What is the gender distribution of the sample?
- What is the racial or ethnic distribution of the sample?
- What is the setting in which the sample is based (e.g., community, institution)?
- Based on the above information, is my patient similar to those described in the study?

Experiences or Phenomena of Interest:
- What was the experience or phenomenon that the researchers were trying to understand?
- How does understanding this experience or phenomenon relate to my practice?
- How did the researchers go about learning about these experiences or phenomena?
- What did the researchers learn? What were their key findings?
- Are the findings supported through the presentation of raw data (e.g., quotes, etc.)?

Overall Appraisal:
- Are there biases that I believe influenced the quality and believability of the study? Consider sampling method, sample composition, methods of data collection, characteristics of the data collector, methods of analysis, and so forth.
- Based on my clinical experience, do the findings make sense?

Reasons to Use the Findings (Benefits):
1.
2.
3.
4.

Reasons Not to Use the Findings (Risks and Costs):
1.
2.
3.
4.

Decision and Rationale:

Based on the information at this time, I will make the following recommendation to my patient regarding the benefits, risks, costs, and alternatives of the findings presented in this article:

Appendix 16-4

Sample Worksheet for Evaluating a Website

Web Address:

Web Developer:

Areas for Appraisal:
- Is the purpose of the website clear?
- Who is the target audience for the website?
- Does the website present information about a particular intervention or exposure (e.g., an assessment process)? If yes, does the website discuss outcomes of the intervention or exposure?
- What are the key points or messages presented on the website?
- How reliable are the key points or messages? Consider number, type, and age of citations; expertise of author(s); where material is published (e.g., peer-reviewed journal, professional magazine); consistency with other materials I have read.
- To what population or populations are the key points and messages relevant? Consider age, sex, setting, ethnicity or racial mix, diagnosis.
- What types of outcomes are addressed? Are these outcomes supported by data?

Overall Appraisal:
- Are there biases that I believe influenced the quality and believability of the information on the website? Consider age of material, authors of material, support for claims, and so forth.
- Based on my clinical experience, does the information make sense?

Reasons to Use the Information (Benefits):
1.
2.
3.
4.

Reasons Not to Use the Information (Risks and Costs):
1.
2.
3.
4.

Decision and Rationale:

Based on the information at this time, I will make the following recommendation to my patient regarding the benefits, risks, costs, and alternatives of the information presented in this website:

Appendix 16-5

Sample Worksheet for Evaluating a Program Description

Source of Program Description (i.e., colleague, book, journal article):

Areas for Appraisal:
- Is the purpose of the program clear?
- Who is the target population for the program?
- Does the target population match the types of patients I see?
- How are program participants identified and selected? Who performs this function?
- What exactly is the "program"? In other words, what are the parameters, interventions, and characteristics of the program?
- What are the intended outcomes of the program? Who evaluates the outcomes?
- What is the setting in which the program is delivered?
- Does this setting match mine?
- What are the staffing needs for the program?
- What are the other costs of the program?
- Are the resources needed by the program available in my setting?
- Is any evidence provided about the efficacy or effectiveness of the program?

Overall Appraisal:
- Based on my clinical experience, does the program make sense?

Reasons to Develop a Program Like This (Benefits):
1.
2.
3.
4.

Reasons Not to Develop a Program Like This (Risks and Costs):

1.
2.
3.
4.

Decision and Rationale:

Based on the information at this time, I will make the following recommendation to my patient regarding the benefits, risks, costs, and alternatives of a program like this:

Appendix 16-6

Sample Critical Appraisal Matrix

Citation	Question or Purpose	Sample	Intervention	Findings	Implications for Practice

Note: A critical appraisal matrix includes only the key information from individual critical appraisals of articles. By summarizing articles in a single table, a matrix facilitates comparisons between and across articles, and makes it easier to come to a conclusion about the evidence available.

CHAPTER 17

Turning Theory Into Practice: Managerial Strategies

Lauro Munoz, OTR, MOT, CHC
Patricia Bowyer, EdD, MS, OTR, FAOTA
Brent Braveman, PhD, OTR/L, FAOTA

■ Real-Life Management

At one point in his career, Lauro was promoted to a supervisory position in a large department of rehabilitation at an internationally recognized teaching and research oncology hospital. As the outpatient occupational therapy supervisor, Lauro was responsible for supervision of four staff occupational therapy practitioners. Outpatient occupational therapy was a newer area of practice at the hospital compared with other areas within the Department of Rehabilitation Services, which included both inpatient and outpatient occupational therapy and physical therapy. Many of the practitioners in the department were recent graduates. The practice in outpatient occupational therapy was limited to a focus on hand therapy and a pulmonary rehabilitation program. Although the physical therapy program had a broader focus, the physical therapy practitioners did not have an understanding of the potential services occupational therapy could provide. Lauro's major

challenge as the new supervisor was to develop and integrate current and cohesive occupational therapy approaches, which in turn would improve client outcomes and strengthen the recognition of the services occupational therapy had to offer.

Although there were many positive points about the staff and programs, there were also several challenges. For example, the physical therapy department was well established throughout the hospital and was the main driver and leader of rehabilitation services in the facility. As a result, physical therapy was well recognized and well utilized and occupational therapy was undervalued and underutilized. The limited scope of practice in outpatient occupational therapy was compounded by an inpatient occupational therapy team that sometimes limited its practice to a biomechanical approach. As a result, the nursing staff, physicians, and other potential referral sources did not recognize all that occupational therapy could offer in helping to attain client outcomes. Rather, occupational therapy was viewed as an extension of physical therapy or it was not considered at all. Major patient needs that the

Continued

occupational therapy practitioners could address were often overlooked. Two such examples were visual impairment and chemotherapy-induced neuropathy of the upper extremity. The idea that occupational therapy could effectively address cognitive and visual impairments of clients with brain lesions or help clients with issues related to mild cognitive impairments was novel to the entire rehabilitation team. Many of the interventions provided were limited to exercise and contrived tabletop activities with a goal of improving upper extremity function. Not surprisingly, the occupational therapy practitioners were insecure about the recognition of their contributions and their relative status as compared with physical therapy. On top of all this, there still was significant turnover, primarily because the job market was volatile as a result of the shortage of occupational therapy personnel. As Lauro began his new position, he had the following key questions:

1. How do I start to gain the trust of the staff, which will be necessary to build better practice?

2. How should we decide what constitutes *best practice*?

3. Once best practice is defined, how can we get (and keep) everyone on the same page?

4. What are the implications of changes in practice on staff roles, productivity, and billing?

5. How can we communicate the nature and value of our services to patients, physicians, and other members of the health-care team?

6. How will we know if all this is working for the patients as well as for the staff?

Critical Thinking Questions

As you read this chapter, consider the following questions:

- How do you integrate current theory and evidence on occupational therapy practice, management, and leadership to guide practice and develop effective policies for personnel management?

- How can current theory and relevant evidence guiding practice result in tangible tools and resources used to conduct and document occupational therapy?

- Are the personnel practices within the department, including staff selection, orientation, development, and performance appraisal, supporting and rewarding practices consistent with current theory?

- How do managers play a critical role in *leading* occupation-based and evidence-based practice in their settings?

Glossary

- **Community of practice:** group of people who share a concern, a set of problems, or a passion about a topic, and who deepen their knowledge and expertise in this area by interacting on an ongoing basis.

- **Domain of knowledge:** scope of knowledge that defines a set of issues.
- **Focus of intervention:** speaks to the degree to which a selected intervention is intended to fix an identified impairment versus helping the

Glossary—cont'd

person develop adaptations necessary to promote participation in desired occupations.

- **Job descriptions:** core personnel documents that serve to codify core duties and best practice and shape employee roles within communities of practice by communicating employee activities that will be valued.

- **Model of Human Occupation (MOHO):** widely used and recognized occupational therapy conceptual practice model.

- **Occupational Therapy Intervention Process Model:** framework for using occupation as a therapeutic intervention.

- **Shared practice:** practice that is developed by members of a community of practice to be effective in the application of their domain of knowledge.

Introduction

It is one thing to understand theory, research, and evidence, and to use them for planning and developing programs as described in Chapter 15. It is another thing to bring those programs to life and to create systems that support the people responsible for implementing the programs. The previous real-life management scenario portrays common challenges inherent in managing evidence-based practice that are faced by occupational therapy managers. Reflecting on the experiences and the actions that Lauro took in response, it can be said that Lauro's actions were designed to cultivate a **community of practice.** A community of practice can be defined as follows (Wenger, McDermott, & Snyder, 2002, p. 4):

Communities of practice are groups of people who share a concern, a set of problems, or a passion about a topic, and who deepen their knowledge and expertise in this area by interacting on an ongoing basis.

At first glance, it might seem odd to think about a *community* of practice. However, the concept and definition of what has been considered a community has varied widely in social science literature. Towns and cities have been called communities, but so have prisons and religious groups. Even corporations, factories, and trade unions have been referred to as

communities (Minar & Greer, 1969). Fellin (1993, 2001) described the useful concept that the persons we encounter may also have membership in nonplace, identificational communities. In this way, we might think about a group of occupational therapy practitioners who work in the same setting and share the same concerns as a community. The nature of the community may vary in size, in how homogeneous the members are, and in how long the community lasts. Table 17-1 provides examples of occupational therapy communities of practice, their focus, the participants, and the nature of their relationships. By seeking to understand the management task of building and maintaining a community of practice, managers can be sensitized to sociological as well as psychological issues that must be addressed.

Many communities of practice are not limited to a single department and are composed of individuals from different disciplines with different knowledge bases. Organizational consultants in private industry are advocating the support of such "knowledge communities" as a method of responding to globalization of companies and the rapidly changing configurations of teams and organizational units (Wenger et al, 2002). Skilled occupational therapy managers and supervisors can facilitate the creation and support of a community (or communities) of practice with the practitioners in their assigned area. In this chapter, we explore the specific leadership, management, and supervisory strategies that can be used to develop and support a community of practice.

TABLE 17-1

Communities of Practice in Occupational Therapy

Example	Focus	Participants	Nature of Relationships
Occupational therapy department	Delivery of effective service	Staff, supervisors, manager	Formal organizational hierarchy
Occupational therapy discipline group within a program management system	Mutual development and effective service	Staff assigned to programs	Informal or matrix relationships
Local pediatric special interest group—interdisciplinary	Advancement of knowledge and networking to improve service delivery across settings	Variety of therapists (i.e., occupational therapy, physical therapy, speech–language pathology) from varied settings	Informal, voluntary
American Occupational Therapy Association (AOTA) administrative and management special interest group	Sharing of knowledge and skills related to managing occupational therapy services	Members of AOTA who elect to join; generally people who are or want to become managers, supervisors, or administrators	Voluntary subset of professional society
International researchers looking at occupations and habits	Examination of cross-cultural aspects of human occupation and the implications for health	Faculty members and scholars in many countries interested in occupational science and occupational behavior	A mix of informal voluntary to formalized research relationships, some mentoring relationships

Communities of Practice Structures

Wenger et al (2002) suggested that there are three common aspects to the structure of communities of practice and that the combination of these structures is in part what makes each community of practice unique. These three common aspects are briefly discussed as applied to the experience of Lauro and his team.

- A **domain of knowledge** is the scope of knowledge that defines a set of issues. For instance, for Lauro and his team, there were some significant issues regarding the appropriate domain of knowledge for occupational therapy. By virtue of the way the department was organized, the scope of practice for outpatient occupational therapy was limited to the interests of the

previous outpatient supervisor and not by the needs of the population being served. Also, the focus on biomechanical approaches to intervention was a limiting factor for program growth and development. For example, the occupational performance areas assessed by practitioners on the neurology unit were exactly the same as on the leukemia unit. Reflective practice was not occurring on either unit. Rather, all areas of occupational therapy programming approached patient needs on a population basis and did not consider the needs of individual clients. There were few approaches to intervention that carried over from unit to unit, so that it was difficult to see the common core of occupational therapy services or even the unique contributions occupational therapy services could make to the various populations served.

- The community of practice concerned with the domain of knowledge included most of the individuals in the department—the occupational therapists (OTs) and occupational therapy assistants (OTAs). This community was nested within the larger community of the Department of Rehabilitation Services, which included physical therapy. The Department of Rehabilitation Services provided programming to different medical units and services that included health-care professionals such as physicians, physiatrists, nursing staff, speech–language pathologists, psychologists, and the administrative assistants. The community of practice was also part of the larger occupational therapy community within the city, the state, and the nation.
- The **shared practice** was the practice that Lauro and his team were developing to be effective in application of their domain of knowledge. McCormack, Jaffe, and Frey (2003) suggested that shared practice includes *roles*, such as what aspect of rehabilitation each team member attends to, or who reports at team meetings; *rules*, such as how soon initial evaluations need to be done and how vacation coverage is arranged; and *tools*, such as the actual assessment tools available and the forms used to document results.

The next section of this chapter focuses on the application of the roles, rules, and tools (many of which were introduced in Chapters 6 and 7) that must be addressed to support best practice.

Managing Practice: Roles, Rules, and Tools

As occupational therapy managers concerned about translating theory into evidence-based practice, we must ask ourselves, "What are the typical aspects of practice that must be addressed by managers?" McCormack (2011) noted that in contrast to the classic descriptions of management functions as planning, organizing and staffing, directing, and controlling, most managers have little time to reflect and are in fact "doers" whose planning is done in real time as the job demands are being addressed. If that is the case, it is all the more important that managers have a guiding idea or mental framework to use as the basis for making the myriad daily decisions that range from where to spend limited continuing education money to what to purchase for departmental equipment and supplies. Let's return to the key questions posed in the real-life management scenario at the beginning of this chapter and examine the strategies that Lauro used as he sought to shape practice and to develop a community of practice by attending to the structures that support practice.

How Do I Start to Gain the Trust of the Staff, Which Will Be Necessary to Build Better Practice?

Build Trust

You should start by building trust between yourself and the other members of the community of practice immediately. Whether you are a newly hired manager or promoted from within, you must understand what your staff members currently think and believe. A good example of how this can be done includes strategies implemented when a new director of the Department of Rehabilitation Services was hired. One of the first things the director did was to meet with every person in the department individually. This may sound overwhelming when persons are dealing with a large community of practice, but by limiting the meetings to 15 minutes he was able to connect personally with the entire staff in fewer than 2 months. The effort to connect with staff continues to this day. On a monthly basis, the director and each of the other members of the department's leadership team meet with individual staff members in sessions called "employee roundings." These sessions allow the leadership team members to have a chance to meet one-on-one with the staff to gain insight into their day-to-day practice, to continue to build upon the trust that was developed in the initial face-to-face interviews, and to have a structured meeting and communication time. Responses to a set of standard questions are tallied quarterly and the leadership team deals with any issues that require intervention. Changes based on the employee roundings are then shared with staff via a communication bulletin board.

The most effective format for interviews such as employee roundings is a semistructured interview. A

BOX 17-1

Questions for Getting to Know Your Staff

- What do you like about working here?
- What things are problems for you in working here?
- What would you like to see done to improve patient care?
- What would you like to see done to improve your ability to do your job?
- What things would you like to help with?
- What do you see as the strengths of the department?
- What resources currently assist you most to effectively perform your job?
- What do you need from me to support you in performing your job?

semistructured interview allows respondents the time and scope to talk about their opinions on a particular subject. The interviewer decides the focus of the interview and there may be areas the interviewer is interested in exploring. Examples of good questions to ask are provided in Box 17-1. Once you have obtained the answers, you can summarize them and feed them back to the group as a whole. This is an efficient way to demonstrate to staff members that you listened to them. It is preferable to do this in person at a staff meeting if at all possible because then you can ask for validation or clarification if needed.

Identify a Leadership Team

From these interviews, as well as the structure of your unit, you should identify a core leadership team to work with you on shaping the scope of practice. The director's strategy was to use the supervisory group within his department. Other strategies might be to use informal leaders or the more expert practitioners within a department. You can use this group as a sounding board and encourage its members to help you challenge current practices that may not be consistent with emerging evidence. It is important to find individuals who have sufficient competency to handle

the job's routine demands. These individuals are more likely to have the capacity to challenge their own thinking, in light of evidence that allows for continuous learning and improved practice performance (Christ, 2014).

Develop or Refresh the Unit's Mission, Vision, and Goals

You can use the information you learn from your staff and others about the quality of the services you provide and combine it with a thorough assessment of your department's strengths and areas for growth to complete a review of your department's mission, vision, and goals (see Chapter 6). Including a core group of leaders, supervisors, and staff in the process can help you to succeed. If your department does not have its own mission and vision statements, creating them with your staff can be an effective strategy for identifying the key things that bring them together as a community of practitioners. In addition to identifying what you have in common, this process also can identify differences in beliefs and understanding of which you may not be aware. Investigating these areas of differences can lead you to identify evidence-based questions to research as a group.

At the time that Lauro and his team began to examine their practice, the Department of Rehabilitation Services had not yet developed a mission and vision statement that truly reflected the department's goals. Because a current mission statement and vision statement did not exist, the director engaged the department in activities that would allow for interaction in order to get feedback from all staff members. The director used the feedback from the staff interviews and developed a department-wide activity in order to begin the development of mission and vision statements. Clustering the staff of almost 90 into groups of 10 and intentionally mixing staff and supervisors across various units streamlined the process. A team leader assigned to each group facilitated the generation of ideas by using the nominal group technique (described in Chapter 13). In addition to the strategic information provided by top management and the information from the individual interviews, the ideas formed the initial data on which the group based the departmental vision, as well as the operational objectives for the year.

How Should We Decide What Constitutes Best Practice?

By now you should have a good idea of the importance of keeping up with theory and emerging evidence as the cornerstone of shaping effective practice. The reality of keeping up with best practices is challenging for anyone, and this is particularly true for managers and supervisors who are often juggling multiple demands. Further, even if you and your staff try to keep up with the latest evidence, chances are that doing so on multiple fronts will create the additional challenge of a lack of consensus on shared practice expectations and standards for intervention.

Focusing your efforts and those of your staff can help and you can begin with your responsibilities. One way of focusing efforts is to lead your staff through the process of identifying departmental strengths and weaknesses in terms of skills and knowledge. You must prioritize the learning needs of the department and organize efforts to meet those needs first. There is no way around doing this. Incorporating theory and evidence into practice requires time to review and read the literature and to understand how to translate it into practice. Supporting each other in this process in an organized way, such as covering clients for an identified staff member who is conducting an evidence-based literature review related to a prioritized learning need, can make the process less daunting. You should focus your responsibilities in this process and show your team members that you are willing to support their efforts and that you value the process. Suggestions such as those provided in Chapter 16 can be utilized to support you in this process.

Embrace That Leading Practice Is Part of Your Job

Perhaps the most important strategy for the development of best practice is recognizing and embracing your responsibility as a leader and as a manager to shape practice as well as manage it. Managers sometimes choose to focus on the mechanics of management, such as budgeting or productivity, with the notion that they should let the staff take an eclectic approach. In fact, some managers seem to have developed the idea that there is something wrong with taking a role in *directing* the theoretical basis for practice in their setting. Although understandable, especially for new managers who are developing their leadership and managerial skills, avoiding this responsibility can result in very efficient therapists doing the wrong things well.

Leading practice may be particularly intimidating if you are accepting responsibility as a manager in an existing occupational therapy department where the culture of the department or "the way we do things around here" is well established. However, it is important to remember that changes in culture do not happen overnight and initial resistance to change is natural. One effective strategy would be to begin by introducing the principles of evidence-based practice to your staff so that, rather than being perceived as telling your staff that what they have been doing is wrong, you are questioning whether evidence supports a better approach. This strategy can result in both you and the staff learning something new because it forces you to examine your own assumptions while asking your staff to do the same.

You should make it your responsibility to keep up with emerging theories, research, and evidence. This may require that you place an equal priority on attending advanced theory presentations and on continuing education related to management and supervision. In particular, you should look for advances that may have implications across various specialties because these can often serve as unifying themes. You can be a role model by admitting that there are aspects of occupational therapy theory, research, and practice with which you struggle and that integrating these three is not always easy, even for you. Lauro used several resources that assisted him in moving toward unification of theory, research, and practice. Initially, he relied heavily on some key American Occupational Therapy Association (AOTA) documents, including those that defined the terminology most commonly used by occupational therapy personnel and sanctioned by AOTA to conceptualize the scope of the department's practice. His involvement with the AOTA special interest sections (SISs) allowed him to keep abreast of what was occurring with the profession on a clinical basis, such as what theoretical models were most investigated and any research articles that spoke of utilization of overlying theoretical frameworks in practice and for departments. Today, managers have a number of resources, including the AOTA

Occupational Therapy Practice Framework, Third Edition (AOTA, 2014) and *The Guide to Occupational Therapy Practice* (Moyers & Dale, 2007). Such documents generally reflect the current consensus on professional topics of interest such as the scope or domain of occupational therapy practice. They have credibility both within and outside of the profession because they represent a carefully generated and widely reviewed analysis. Another resource is the *Practice Guidelines* available from AOTA. These invaluable resources provide a template for best practice across a wide variety of practice settings and patient populations. Membership in an AOTA SIS and involvement through AOTA's social media site OTConnections© are other sources of information that can assist the manager with staying alert to practice trends and development of new evidence.

Attempts to operationalize the concepts represented in these documents will necessitate discussions with your leadership group and the staff, which in turn sets the stage for a more reflective stance toward current practice. Throughout this text, membership in both AOTA and your state occupational therapy association is emphasized as an effective strategy for networking and obtaining resources. Not only do resources such as the AOTA *Occupational Therapy Practice Framework* represent the work of top occupational therapy scholars, but it and other official documents are frequently reviewed and updated so that they can assist you in staying current with changes in thinking and terminology as you gain experience.

In addition to the utilization of AOTA official documents, Lauro began to incorporate the **Model of Human Occupation (MOHO)** because it seemed to hold some promise to unify the various disparate practices he supervised. Lauro had completed a short course through AOTA on using the Model of Human Occupation Screening Tool (MOHOST), which addresses a client's motivation for occupation, pattern of occupation, communication or interaction, process, and motor skills, as well as the environment (Model of Human Occupation Clearinghouse, 2014). Lauro believed that the tool and theory could develop into a beneficial synergy between theory and practice. However, he had not been exposed to the model in its entirety. Nonetheless, he had a sense that it held important potential for his practice setting. Even though he was not exactly sure where it would lead or what it meant for hands-on practice, Lauro committed to learn about MOHO and to pursue options for increasing contact with others who were familiar with and using the theory. The new director of rehabilitation services was also familiar with MOHO, which helped to create a synergy. This led Lauro to the next strategy.

Go to the Experts or Bring Them to You

One of the most critical functions a good leader and manager can perform is to support the development of clinical reasoning in his or her staff. Such development is supported by a blend of careful supervision combined with professional development activities. From a practical standpoint, managers need to think strategically about how they expend department travel and consulting funds, which are often limited if they exist at all. In addition to encouraging staff members to attend external continuing education events, a manager should carefully consider departmental priorities and balance offsite activities with onsite initiatives.

By tying continuing education experiences to established professional development plans (which correlate to the department's strategic plan), you can gradually build a synergistic pool of knowledge within your community of practice. Sometimes you can achieve a higher impact by bringing an expert on specific practice approaches to work with your staff directly. After working for several years as a manager, that is exactly what Lauro thought needed to happen. Lauro had begun to develop a research collaboration with a faculty member at a local university. Through the development of initial projects, Lauro began thinking about the need to introduce a unifying theory base to the staff to guide their practice. As a result of this realization, Lauro and his new research partner began to collaborate on a research study centered on clinical reasoning. A qualitative study was initiated to examine the effects of introduction of a unifying model for clinical reasoning on practitioners in a hospital-based unit. The unifying model chosen was MOHO.

Work Within Your System to Obtain Evidence That Will Support and Change Practice

Lauro initially took the lead by raising theory and practice issues with the staff, but over time he found he was having trouble keeping up with the literature and managing a complex team and set of services. A position as a rehabilitation regulatory specialist was created within the larger department, and Lauro decided that pursuing the positon would allow him to keep up with changes in practice and any regulatory issues that would affect the department, as well as focus more on the larger practice context within the department. The collaborative relationship he developed with local faculty also allowed for the introduction and development of new evidence. Supervisors in both occupational therapy and physical therapy were encouraged to teach at local universities and become involved in national association activities; this helped them to keep up with changes in clinical practice. Having a person dedicated to stay abreast of changes in practice and regulation can make knowledge acquisition easier and more efficient; however, there are many strategies that you may use that do not require extra funding or a person dedicated to this sole purpose. Among others, these strategies include:

- "Brown bag" informal lunch discussions of clients, daily dilemmas, clinical problems, or reports from continuing education events attended by staff
- "Journal clubs" in which staff members rotate responsibility for reading a journal article and leading discussions with other staff using a predetermined format
- Cotreating patients with your staff or at least occasionally treating patients in front of your staff so that you may role model the intervention approaches you are trying to promote
- Developing an active fieldwork education program and creating intentional fieldwork assignments that foster evidence-based review of literature and sharing of new knowledge between staff and students
- Case discussions that not only allow the presentation of clinical problems but also allow discussion and exploration of new strategies by involving the entire staff

Use Your Leadership Skills to Address Practice

Lauro and his research collaborator designed a 12-month staff development project focused on using MOHO (within an institutional review board [IRB]-approved research protocol) in which regular meetings were held with a group of practitioners. The practitioners participated in training sessions, completed assigned readings, and participated in discussion groups on implications for current practice. During the sessions, practitioners spent time analyzing current patients using some of the parameters that emerged from the readings and the experiences the clinicians were having while implementing MOHO into practice. Table 17-2 and Box 17-2 present a case study analysis guide used by the clinicians to apply MOHO based on an approach by Cubie and Kaplan (1982). This case study approach was conducted within compliance and privacy guidelines, using real and current patients at the rehabilitation facility, and provided a live laboratory with which to explore how new ideas might improve current practice. During the discussions, practitioners documented information and completed an analysis at the end of each discussion to seek implications for practice. A final analysis was completed at the end of the 12-month study. After the research study, staff were asked to spend time reflecting on what specific changes were needed in policies, forms, and other "roles, rules, and tools" to incorporate the new knowledge. This then became the basis for shifting a departmental practice from being a biomechanical or medical model to a more client-centered, occupation-based, and evidence-based approach.

Be Prepared for Resistance to Change and Even Some Staff Turnover

Probably the greatest concern of staff members during the 12-month staff development project process was that they would have to move away from utilizing the biomechanical frame of reference as part of the occupational therapy community of practice. What Lauro hoped would happen is that therapy techniques such as those exemplified by the underlying principles of neurodevelopmental treatment, biomechanical approaches, and contemporary task-oriented approaches would in fact be embedded within meaningful activities designed to help clients regain their desired life skills. Lauro and the occupational therapy supervisors played a key role by actively trying out the new concepts and modeling the blending of these new practice approaches with older established approaches. Ongoing personnel management strategies were effective in supporting the staff participants in the research

TABLE 17-2

Case Analysis Guide—Model of Human Occupation

MOHO Elements	Clinical Reasoning Question
Throughput Volition or Personal Causation	• Does the person anticipate success? • Does the person feel in control or controlled by others?
Values	• What is important to the person? • What goals does the person have?
Interests	• What does the person like to do?
Narrative	• What is this person's story? • How does the person's life story guide his or her values, interests, and sense of control? • What meaning do the person's performance abilities and limitations have for that person?
Habituation Roles	• What are this person's major occupational roles? • To what degree does the person feel he or she is meeting those role demands? • What expectations does the person have regarding roles, and how flexible are these? • How well balanced are the person's role behaviors?
Habits	• What is this person's typical routine? • How has this been changed? • How well organized are the habit patterns?

Performance Capacity	• Does the person have the necessary performance capacities needed for required occupational skills?
	  • Musculoskeletal
	  • Neurological
	  • Perceptual
	  • Cognitive
	• Have there been developmental, traumatic, or environmental stresses that limit skill acquisition?

Output	• Does the person participate in activities that are personally and socially significant?
	• Does the person use performance skills competently and consistently?
	  • Motor skills
	  • Process skills
	  • Communication or interaction skills
	• Is the person satisfied with current occupational performance and identity?
	• Is the person able to generate adaptive responses to challenges?

Environment	• What are the physical settings in which this person must perform? • What are the temporal expectations in the setting? • What are the social expectations for this person? • What cultural issues must be considered in the person's environment? • Overall, how would you characterize the importance of the person's occupational performance environments, relative to his or her opportunities, resources, demands, and constraints?

Feedback	• How does the physical environment support and limit desired occupational performance?
	  • Natural and built terrain
	  • Tools
	• How does the social environment support and limit desired occupational performance?
	  • Support systems
	  • Developmental expectations
	  • Cycle of illness or injury
	  • Role demands and flexibility
	• How will these factors impact the person's occupational identity, both now and in the future?

BOX 17-2

Reflective Questions for Case Analysis

Questions About the Case Itself
- What information do we have about each of the clinical reasoning questions in the case analysis?
- What is the quality of that information?
- Is that information considered in intervention planning and implementation?
- Is that information important to document?
- Is that information communicated to team members who might find it helpful?
- What information is lacking?
- Is there a practical way to obtain that information?
- Does anyone else on the team already collect that information?
- How might the information that is lacking influence intervention planning?

Questions About Departmental Practices That Arise From the Case Review
- Do we need to change our documentation forms or practices?
- Do we need to change our initial evaluations?
- Do we need to change our progress reports?

- Do we need to change our discharge summaries?
- Do we need to change our patient or client educational materials?
- Do we need to change our verbal reporting practices?
- Do we need to change our team meetings and rounds?
- Do we need to change our discharge planning?
- Do we need to change our patient or client educational sessions?
- Do we have the appropriate intervention resources?
- Do we have the furniture, tools, and other items available in our clinical areas to provide occupationally centered intervention?
- Do our policies support timely acquisition of resources needed to customize care?
- How can we gain better access to the person's natural environment?
- Are site visits or home visits possible?
- Can we obtain videotapes or photos?

---

in order to enact the desired changes. It was hoped that these trained staff members would then serve as champions for the entire occupational therapy department as the group would eventually move into one theory base of practice.

What Are Management Approaches to Maintain Gains After You Define Best Practices in Your Setting?

Because service delivery in occupational therapy is a staff-intensive process, it should be no surprise that both the departmental policies and the personnel management structures within the department need to be shaped to support effective practice. Once you have a general vision of how you believe best practice should occur within your unit, it is time to start operational-

izing those concepts into structures that support staff functioning and development.

Job Descriptions

The **job description** is perhaps the core personnel document that serves to codify best practice. It helps shape employee roles within communities of practice and serves to communicate valued employee activities. Key components of an effective job description are found in Box 17-3 and strategies for developing job descriptions are found in Box 17-4. A sample job description is provided at the end of this chapter (Appendix 17-1), as are resources for writing job descriptions.

Managers will find that they have varying levels of autonomy to create job descriptions in different organizations. If you are the owner of a private practice,

BOX 17-3

Key Elements of Job Descriptions

Job title: A brief two- to three-word phrase characterizing the job.
Example: Staff occupational therapist.

Job function: One or two sentences that capture the major purpose of the job.
Example: Provide comprehensive occupational therapy services, including assessment and evaluation; intervention planning and implementation in conjunction with assigned OTA; discharge planning; and documentation and administrative tasks associated with service delivery and assigned team roles.

Reporting relationships: Indicate to whom the person in this job reports to as well as whom he or she is responsible for supervising.
Example: Reports to occupational therapy manager; supervises assigned OTAs, aides, and fieldwork students.

Key performance expectations (also called major job duties): A listing of frequent and important job tasks that the person in this job must perform in order to meet the organization's expectations. These typically represent baseline expectations, rather than all the possibilities within the job. These may be subdivided into frequency of expectation, as shown in the example.
Example:
- Routine duties:
  - Responds to requests for services within 24 hours by screening clients relative to occupational performance concerns.

- Educates client and client's significant others on how to use adaptive strategies to perform desired occupational tasks.
- Periodic (or occasional) duties:
  - Completes monthly analysis of assigned quality improvement indicators and notifies supervisor of any areas not meeting expectations.
  - Serves as interim team supervisor to cover for short-term vacancies or absences of team supervisor.

Qualifications: A listing of required and preferred education, experience, and credentials required for the job.
Example:
- Licensed or licensure-eligible as an occupational therapist, registered, in the state of Georgia.
- Minimum 3 years of experience working with adults with physical disabilities.
- Excellent interpersonal skills.

Essential functions: Critical physical, cognitive, or emotional abilities that are required for job performance. Used to assist people with disabilities to identify whether they will require reasonable accommodation in order to perform the job.
Example:
- High tolerance for stress.
- Ability to lift 50 lbs. from knee to shoulder level.
- Judgment to appropriately implement departmental criteria to prioritize referrals.

then you may have complete control. Even so, you are cautioned to take the process of developing job descriptions very seriously. Job descriptions may be key documents in responding in a legal and responsible manner to situations, such as the request by an employee for a reasonable accommodation under the Americans with Disabilities Act (ADA). They are also critical elements of the performance appraisal and disciplinary processes described in Chapters 6 and 7. If you are part of a large health-care organization, community organization, or educational system, you may find that the job descriptions are standardized across the entire extended organization. If that is the case, you still may be able to develop addenda to these job descriptions to use within your own community of practice to further define expectations. Carefully developed and accurate job descriptions become the basis for supporting the community of practice. They

---

BOX 17-4

Developing Job Descriptions

Identify What the Job Consists Of
- Interview people currently in the job or who have similar jobs.
- If it is a totally new job, interview the people who will interact the most with employees in this position.
- Find out what tasks must be done in a typical day.
- Find out what additional tasks are done in a typical week.
- Find out what tasks recur with little frequency, such as monthly, quarterly, or annually.

Explore What Qualifications Are Needed
- Are there specific credentials required by legal or accrediting agencies?
- Are there experiences that are likely to best prepare the person for this role, or is no experience required beyond basic credentials?
- Is special knowledge or a set of specific skills needed?

- Are there standard expectations for all employees in this setting (i.e., ability to speak Spanish, religious preferences in faith-based institutions)?

Draft the Job Description for Review
- Using the key elements shown in Box 17-3, draft the job description.
- Refer to official documents or guides to ensure that the job description is adequately comprehensive and consistent with regional and national standards.
- Obtain feedback from critical reviewers, such as your supervisor, the human resources department, or peers outside your organization who have experience with this type of job.

Finalize the Job Description
- Format according to institutional requirements.
- Put date completed and initials of author in footnote.
- Place in appropriate reference manual or computer file for ready accessibility.

---

become one of those core documents that the busy manager uses as a reference when implementing all of the managerial functions, such as recruitment, orientation, and staff development.

Staff Development

Earlier in this chapter, we discussed the importance of strategically using resources for staff development. This is important not only during times of change but on an ongoing basis to assure that your management unit as a whole is systematically gaining and sharing new knowledge relevant to your practice goals. You should keep in mind that staff development requires more than just attendance at educational seminars or courses. Both OTs and OTAs need time to reflect on the ideas gained from such experiences and to discuss the possibilities for implementation. Many complex health-care groups have interdisciplinary (sometimes

now referred to as interprofessional) team activities, as well as discipline-specific time for staff development. These group times can be used as sounding boards for the potential implementation of new knowledge in that setting. These opportunities also provide support for each individual staff member as he or she seeks to meet professional obligations to maintain continuing competency (something else that can be explicitly stated in the job description).

Policies and Practices

In 1994, Barbara Schell observed that as simple as it seems, some of the greatest barriers to implementing effective practice often have to do with routine policies and practices such as the purchase of necessary supplies and equipment. Unfortunately, this is still true today. It is surprising how often occupational therapy managers will work to justify very sophisticated computerized equipment for assessing and intervening to improve performance capacity while neglecting much more mundane, inexpensive, but critical resources such as a good supply of the everyday objects used by their clients for work, leisure, and everyday life. Managers who want their staff members to exhibit evidence-based and occupation-based practices must take the time to make these practices convenient. This literally means taking a look at what supplies are available (and what are not).

In many occupational therapy departments you can easily find colored cones, pegboards, or Velcro checkerboards, although seldom do you observe anyone actually playing checkers or using the items in any type of daily occupation. In other settings, there may be hours of unstructured time during which clients drop in to the occupational therapy department to paint ceramic bowls or chess pieces, even though they may not have made the bowls or may never have played chess. The products often go unfinished or are left in the department after the client is discharged and are never used for their intended purpose. Often these items and activities have existed in the department for many years and continue to be used out of imitation by new staff members who observed more experienced staff members making use of them without questioning whether there was underlying theory and evidence to support their use.

Alternatively, in some occupational therapy departments you might observe clients who have had a stroke ironing a shirt using a real iron and ironing board, opening a can of cat food and putting it into a bowl, or making a picture frame as a niece or nephew's birthday present. You might even find someone practicing hanging a shirt or pair of pants in a *real* closet! Using real-life *occupations* in therapy is dependent upon having or being able to obtain the appropriate objects, however.

Because humans, as occupational beings, have such a great variety of interests and routines, supporting the type of intervention just described requires a careful look at purchasing policies and availability of support staff to quickly obtain important items for assessment and intervention. Mounting theory, evidence, and expert opinions suggest that the most effective assessments and interventions to improve performance capacity require that assessment and intervention occur in the context in which the performance occurs (Bodiam, 1999; Darragh, Sample, & Fisher, 1998; Gillen, 2013a; Mathiowetz & Bass-Haugen, 2002;

Park, Fisher, & Velozo, 1994; Pedretti & Umphred, 1996; Poole & Whitney, 2001).

For example, consider assessment and intervention related to motor performance. Table 17-3 shows a sample of selected evidence related to assessment and intervention to improve motor performance. A search was conducted in the PsycINFO, CINAHL, and Cochrane databases using the key words "functional assessment" and "motor learning." The search was limited to citations published in English since 1990 and limited to references to adults. This evidence generally supports assessment and intervention to improve motor performance in a naturalistic context. Moreover, studies support that such contextually based assessment and intervention does not require expensive equipment or simulated settings. Gathering and evaluating evidence such as that provided in Table 17-3 with your staff and identifying strategies to begin integrating such evidence in your setting is an example of *leading* practice as a manager.

As a manager, you soon realize that is not always possible to visit or to exactly reproduce the context in which a client typically performs an occupation. Even the best efforts to fill a clinic space with objects and furniture commonly found in homes or other settings will inherently fall short of perfectly duplicating the influences of a client's natural environment. However, whatever efforts you can take to make interventions more *naturalistic* may increase the likelihood that the occupational performance within interventions will hold increased meaning to your clients. You can do this by trying to have common items used among the clientele you serve, and also by asking clients to bring in objects they routinely use. Gathering, synthesizing, and presenting theory and evidence from the occupational therapy literature will help to frame approaches used by your staff. For example, several occupational therapy scholars have addressed the use of naturalistic occupation in key addresses to the profession.

In her 1998 Eleanor Clark Slagle Lecture, Anne Fisher provided a helpful framework for thinking about the relevance of the therapy process and how likely it is to harness the greatest therapeutic benefit (Fisher, 1998). In her lecture, Fisher examined the unique focus of occupational therapy on the use of purposeful and meaningful activity as a therapeutic agent. Further, she proposed that therapeutic occupation and adaptive occupation are the legitimate activities of occupational therapy. She also provided a model for intervention that she called the **Occupational**

TABLE 17-3
Sample Evidence on Assessing and Intervening to Improve Performance Capacity in Context

Author	Design	Strategies Investigated	N (Sample Size)	Level of Evidence	Results or Findings
Gilmore & Spaulding (2001)	Combined literature review	Treatment of individuals following stroke	N/A	Weak	Identified four factors contributing to motor learning (type of task, practice, feedback, and stages of learning).
Richardson (2000)	Randomized two-condition study	Compared application of motor learning principles in traditional clinic versus simulated (Easy Street) environment in older adults	80	Strong	Did not exclude benefits of contextually appropriate rehabilitation but found no benefit of expensive simulated environments over traditional settings.
Darragh et al (1998)	Comparison study	Household task performance versus unfamiliar clinic performance of persons with brain injury	20	Good	Significant positive difference in household task performance in process ability but not in motor ability during administration of the assessment of motor and process skills.
Park et al (1994)	Comparison study	Household performance versus clinic performance on IADL performance of older adults	20	Good	10 of 20 subjects performed significantly better in their homes, with process ability improving and motor ability remaining stable.

IADL, instrumental activities of daily living; N/A, not available.

Therapy Intervention Process Model. This model provides a framework for using occupation as a therapeutic intervention (Fisher, 1998). Table 17-4 builds on Fisher's work. This table can assist you in analyzing choices for intervention.

In his 2013 Eleanor Clark Slagle Lecture, Glen Gillen provided a guide and recommended a return to occupational therapy normalcy, allowing us to look at the ecological validly of testing, and stated that the ecological validity of testing can be extended by observing the patient's approach to tasks in the environment and observing the patient in his or her normal activity. He also stated that the evidence supports the use of task-specific, real-world activities (occupational therapy) having the potential to improve motor function and occupational performance, but also the potential to remodel and reorganize people's brains.

Furthermore, Gillen (2013a) presented evidence that showed occupational therapy practitioners were spending 66% of their treatment sessions in preparatory time and not engaged in occupation. According to Gillen (2013a), normalcy is occupation and is what occupational therapy personnel should strive to utilize as a driver in the occupational therapy process (assessment and intervention planning).

Focus of Intervention

The **focus of intervention** speaks to the degree to which a selected intervention is intended to fix an identified impairment versus helping the person develop adaptations necessary to promote participation in desired occupations. Within occupational

TABLE 17-4

Occupation as Therapy Intervention Choices

Activity Type	Framework Classification	Focus	Source of Meaning	Natural?	Examples
Exercise	Preparatory method	Remediation of impairments	Practitioner chosen	Contrived	Putty exercises, line drawing for eye–hand coordination
Contrived occupation	Purposeful activity	Remediation or skill development	Practitioner chosen	Contrived therapy using culturally common objects	Placing cones on a shelf and pretending they are dishes, throwing bean bags at a target
Therapeutic occupation: graded occupations to treat impairments, direct intervention of impairments in the context of occupation	Occupation-based intervention	Remediation or skill development	Chosen collaboratively for meaning to client and therapy potential	More naturalistic as it uses authentic aspects of occupation such as tools and context	Using a favorite card game to challenge attention, photographing flowers at different heights for a person who loves photography
Adaptive/compensatory occupation: assistive devices, teaching compensatory strategies, modifying physical or social environments	Occupation-based intervention	Improved occupational performance	Chosen collaboratively: therapy process selected to support performance	Naturalistic activity in natural context	Adapting morning routine to compensate for poor endurance Driving in a car after a stroke

therapy, various terms are used to describe types of interventions that fall along the continua of (a) activity type, (b) focus of therapy, (c) the source of meaning and purpose, (d) how real or natural an occupation is, and (5) OT practice framework classification. Gillen notes that current trends in the field suggest that occupation-based approaches are often most effective and proved a clearer external reflection of the occupational therapy profession's contribution to health care. Additionally, there may be a mix of activity types in order to minimize impairment and promote occupational functioning (Gillen, 2013b).

Exercise is a therapy choice that is contrived and initiated by the practitioner. The goal of this preparatory method is that the benefits of such exercise are transferred to occupational performance. The client is expected to comply, and you will find the practitioner spending much time explaining or convincing the client of the benefits of such activity. Activities of this sort don't typically occur in daily life but rather are invented as therapy routines. An example of a preparatory activity might be having a homemaker lift a cone from a chair to a shelf in a therapy gym while trying to convince the person it will help her to increase her strength and coordination. Research suggests that these approaches are less effective than ones that are more ecologically relevant and client-centered (Trombly, 1995).

Contrived occupation is a therapy choice that is primarily different from exercise because it is a more naturally occurring activity in daily life. Therefore, it is a bit more ecologically relevant but still has initial purpose and meaning coming from the practitioner. For instance, a practitioner might encourage a client to engage in a group activity in which everyone takes part in making a meal. Even if the person doesn't usually cook or prepare food, the practitioner might encourage the person's participation if the practitioner thinks this might be a good way to encourage socialization, help the person improve his or her ability to follow directions, and also help him or her to improve arm and hand coordination. Therefore, this activity is contrived and considered purposeful activity.

In contrast to exercise and contrived occupations, occupation-based interventions are more ecologically relevant or naturalistic and draw both their purpose and meaning from the client. The major difference between therapeutic occupation and compensatory occupation is the focus of the intervention. Therapeutic occupation is focused on remediating impairment, whereas compensatory occupation is focused on adaptive approaches to improving occupational performance. For instance, a therapeutic occupation might involve having a homemaker work on improving coordination by lifting dishes from the dishwasher to a kitchen cabinet, which is a much more naturalistic occupation, but one that requires her to move in a coordinated fashion. Alternatively, that same homemaker may be taught how to cook one-handed so that she can return to helping to care for her grandchildren, a role that brings with it great pride. That would be an example of compensatory occupation. The choice of focus depends on what is realistic, given the person's diagnostic condition, personal goals, and length of therapy.

Taking the challenge to lead practice so that it is most effective can be difficult. As mentioned earlier, you may encounter roadblocks that are tied to "how things have always been done." Table 17-5 lists some of the most common roadblocks encountered in many settings to changing and innovating practice, and provides suggestions grounded in policies, procedures, and simple managerial actions for overcoming them. These examples show how routine departmental poli-cies and practices can directly affect the practical ability of staff members to actually implement desired practice innovations.

What Are the Implications of Changes in Practice on Staff Roles, Productivity, and Billing?

One of the biggest challenges for managers and staff alike is to articulate appropriate role expectations and relate them to productivity expectations and billing procedures. Chapter 6 discussed approaches to measuring productivity. The relevant point for this chapter is that changes in approach to practice may affect both staffing patterns and productivity expectations. Consider the experience of one occupational therapy manager's approach to staffing to one that ended the delegation of activities of daily living (ADL) assessment and intervention solely to OTAs and required the OTs who were used to working only in the clinic to be involved in these staff activities. Although OTAs often contribute to the evaluation process by assessing ADL performance, the practice of overdelegation of ADL was no longer thought to be consistent with the developing understanding of occupational functioning. Occupational therapists and occupational therapy assistants were teamed and OTs assumed more responsibility for conducting ADL assessments personally. Occupational therapists started to use that time to obtain an occupational history related to self-care, as well as to observe how the individual's abilities to perform self-care tasks were affected by neurological impairments and environmental variables. As a result, patients received more customized care directed to their particular concerns, rather than a more standard approach based primarily on the person's diagnostic condition.

Productivity Expectations

Issues related to productivity expectations (expectations for the volume of billable services provided in a given period) will vary greatly from setting to setting and as the volume of referrals increases or decreases. As pressure to meet productivity standards increases, it can sometimes become difficult for staff members to feel that they have adequate control over the level and

TABLE 17-5

Roadblocks to Leading Occupation-Based and Evidence-Based Practice and Strategies for Overcoming the Obstacles

Roadblocks to Occupation-Based Assessment and Intervention	Strategies to Promote Occupation-Based Assessment and Intervention
Absence of items used in daily occupations, such as irons, pots and pans, or vacuums.	Have staff members develop a prioritized list of items they desire that can be purchased over time to support occupation-based assessment in context. Have clients bring in the items they are having difficulty using.
Staff members are resistant to giving up assessment of components.	Develop written clinical guidelines for how components can be assessed in context (e.g., you can evaluate functional range of motion by watching a patient put dishes away or reach into a refrigerator). Sequence initial evaluation forms so that client concerns and occupational performance issues are addressed first, along with performance context. Next, have only those impairments that appear to actually be affecting performance assessed in more detail. Point out how this increases efficiency because time is not wasted doing assessments that are not needed.
Staff members feel they first have to restore impairments, and then they can get to occupation.	Have supervisors or more expert clinicians model how to blend occupational and restorative techniques.
Forms, policies, and procedures do not support contextually based assessments.	Revise forms, policies, and procedures to cue staff to focus on occupational performance by focusing on occupations rather than components.
Staff members worry that they do not have the time to find and evaluate evidence.	Organize partnerships to facilitate literature reviews and interpretation of evidence by having other staff cover for some staff members, freeing them to search the literature or review and synthesize articles.
Physicians or other disciplines have set expectations that you focus on impairment-related issues or remediation of performance components rather than occupational performance.	Educate other staff to the use of therapeutic occupation through in-services, one-on-one meetings, Occupational Therapy Month activities, posters in lunchrooms, stories in newsletters, or sharing key articles or research emphasizing the value of occupation.

quality of care they wish to provide their clients. Helping to establish reasonable expectations and limits on what staff can hope to achieve within your setting is an important function for the occupational therapy manager. For example, managers in an acute care setting can often help staff problem-solve what they can most effectively address at that one point along the continuum of care. Reminding staff that many of their patients will continue to receive occupational therapy at the next point in the care continuum, such as a rehabilitation hospital, a skilled nursing facility, or at home, can help them to focus on occupation-based intervention even when treating patients in the context

of a length of stay that is often only a few days. As with many of the suggestions in this chapter, there are simple but important and effective ways to incorporate structures to support staff. For example, by simply adding one or two questions to the initial assessment form you can help staff to focus on occupation-based and client-centered goals appropriate for the setting. Examples of such questions include, "What is the patient's estimated length of stay?" and "What would the patient like to achieve in that length of time?"

In Lauro's department, productivity expectations were historically measured by service area and were established based on the historical productivity of a specific service area. This may sound easy but it was not. Language was changed from "productivity" or "productive time" to "billable time" as clinicians had become overly focused with the word *productivity* and over time had attached a negative connotation to it. Also, there were several interpretations of what billable time meant and ranges of time were given to the clinicians as opposed to specific targets. The result was that most clinicians found that meeting productivity requirements meant reaching the bottom end of the range. Educational sessions also had to be held in order to help define what time was billable with the patient and what was not. Although tools and requirements to guide billing, such as the use of *current procedural terminology (CPT) codes* discussed in Chapter 11, are available and widely used in billing, interpretation of what is billable and where it is coded can also be difficult. Clarity is required in these circumstances. In settings where you do not bill third parties for services provided, other systems will be used to determine productivity.

Billing and Reimbursement

As the occupational therapy staff identified improved practice approaches, Lauro had to make sure that the billing structure accurately reflected changes in practice. In general, the billing system should be kept very simple, allowing the staff maximum flexibility to perform assessments and interventions appropriate to the client's needs and the institution's mission. Exemplars of documentation were developed so that therapists could review documentation that reflected occupation-based therapy and would meet the requirements for reimbursement.

In medical-model settings, *coding* of services (e.g., assigning codes to charges based on diagnosis of the patient and the intervention performed within a treatment setting) is partly the responsibility of the occupational therapy practitioner and partly the responsibility of the occupational therapy manager. Often the codes associated with different types of interventions (CPT codes) are built into a charge system so that staff members indicate a type of occupational therapy intervention, such as "ADL" or "neuromuscular facilitation," and the appropriate CPT code is automatically attached in the electronic billing system. Although this makes submission of the correct CPT code more likely, it also distances the staff from

the process. It is easy for the staff and the occupational therapy manager to become complacent as a result of the automation. This complacency can lead to problems including denials for payment by payers such as Medicare when CPT codes do not match the diagnosis code (e.g., the *International Classification of Diseases*, 10th Edition [ICD–10] code). When rendered services do not clearly match the diagnosis (e.g., you make a splint for a patient living with AIDS who has upper extremity neuropathy, but the diagnosis code for AIDS is used rather than that for neuropathy) or when the same CPT code is used repeatedly (e.g., you bill for multiple sessions of home management rather than combining codes for self-care with those for cognition and neuromuscular facilitation), payment may be denied.

Working with staff to better understand how to code services to maximize reimbursement not only benefits the organization's financial health but can also sustain other efforts described in this chapter to support occupation-based and evidence-based practice. Proper coding requires staff members to apply the same logic to billing for services that they apply during occupational analysis when planning intervention. Just as we understand that an occupation such as unloading a dishwasher has not only the physical aspects of range of motion, strength, and coordination but also the cognitive aspects of planning and sequencing, we need to understand that payers wish to see that multiple factors are being addressed in treatment. By relating a daily activity such as deciding what charges to enter through an electronic health record or on a billing form to principles you are promoting within your community of practice, you can reinforce multiple concepts at the same time.

How Can We Communicate the Nature and Value of Our Services?

Because most of us function within a larger community of practice, it is important to consider how to communicate with this larger community about not only what we do on a daily basis but also about practice changes. Over time we must also communicate about how to reinforce new practice patterns and related expectations. Initially, as in any change process, key players must be informed and feedback opportunities provided. However, equally important is the recognition that it is in the everyday practices of team reporting, documentation, and communications with referring parties, payers, and the like that people form their opinion of the contributions of occupational therapy and their understanding of what we do. Appendix 17-2, provided at the end of this chapter, is an example of a matrix that poses some questions that can be used to assess how well such communications reflect occupation-based, client-centered, and evidence-based practice. Appendix 17-2 examines MOHO, but similar matrices could be developed for any conceptual practice model.

As managers, we can help staff members examine how *what* they say in everyday interactions can have dramatic effects on the understanding of others about occupational therapy in their practice setting. An example would be considering how staff members introduce themselves to new clients and how they explain to the client what it is that they do. When an OT or OTA explains occupational therapy to a patient who is in the hospital for a total hip replacement by saying "I'll work with you on things like bathing and dressing," he or she becomes, in the patient's mind, the "bathing and dressing therapist." Why would that patient explain that his or her biggest worries are how he or she is going to care for a pet and if he or she can still babysit for a grandchild to a bathing and dressing therapist?

Likewise, we can help staff reconsider everyday practices such as reporting on client progress in a team meeting. Rather than reporting changes in performance components such as stating that a child is "demonstrating improved hand coordination and manipulation skills," the same information might be conveyed by stating that the child "was able to pick up finger foods and small toys for the first time." In this manner, we not only communicate the same progress, but we also ground those to whom we are communicating solidly to our role with clients, thereby increasing the likelihood of continued and appropriate referrals. Integrating occupation-based and evidence-based practice does not always mean major shifts in what we do. Rather, the principles of occupation-based and evidence-based practice can be integrated into common everyday practices in simple ways such as how we explain what we do to others.

These examples are just a few of the ways that occupational therapy managers can turn theory into practice by integrating occupation-based and evidence-based practice in daily tasks. Other simple ways to integrate theory and evidence into communication and documentation include the following:

- Include terms such as *roles*, *occupation*, and *occupational performance* with examples so that others understand the terms found on paper forms and on drop-down menus in electronic documentation.
- Integrate occupational therapy terminology on referral forms (paper or electronic) by grouping common occupations together under headings such as *occupations of daily living*.
- Review discharge forms, patient education materials, and home programs and look for ways to replace language referencing performance components with language referencing occupations and "doing."

How Will We Know If All This Is Working for the Patients as Well as for the Staff?

This question takes us back to the whole notion of using evidence to guide practice. In responding to the real-life management scenario described at the beginning of the chapter, Lauro and the other members of the leadership team used several strategies, ranging from institutional to departmental practices:

- Staff evaluations routinely included an *upward appraisal* in which staff members identified personal, programmatic, and departmental strengths, weaknesses, and opportunities for improvement. Ongoing analyses of these factors provided trends.
- Staff morale was continually monitored with staff surveys on an annual basis and served to help develop committees that would help with issues such as communication or work–life balance.
- Staff members succeeded in being selected by peer groups (such as state and national conferences) to present their own clinical findings, clinical theory, and current trends in practice.

All of these provided information to allow the leadership group to make decisions that would improve morale and work–life balance.

Chapter Summary

Lauro's story demonstrates the priority that managers must place on advancing their knowledge as occupational therapy practitioners as well as managers. When they do this, they will be better positioned to challenge the system when evidence suggests that better outcomes can occur. Additionally, managers must be prepared to negotiate with administrators, staff, and payment sources to facilitate practical approaches to integrating best practices into the staff's day-to-day activities. Creating and supporting excellence in your community of practice is the essence of good management.

Finding, understanding, and evaluating evidence and information are the first steps of developing a community of practice focused on occupation-based and evidence-based practice. Managers need to take an active role in *leading* practice by becoming involved in these activities and further by supporting the staff members they supervise to become involved by creating structures and systems that support staff. Managers can use everyday structures such as documentation forms, billing forms, policies and procedures, meeting agendas, staff development plans, and purchasing systems to build communities of practice focused on the effective use of occupation and the most current evidence in practice.

■ Real-Life Solutions

Many changes have occurred within the department of rehabilitation since Lauro began his new role as supervisor with the outpatient team. Referrals for occupational therapy are being made specifically for mild cognitive impairment, vision, and fatigue; in addition, the outpatient team is implementing lifestyle redesign and programs to assist patients having issues with body image. The number of full-time equivalents (FTEs) in outpatient occupational therapy has now increased. The department continues to grow, and some of the practitioners have transferred to the inpatient service. As a result, the inpatient occupational therapy practitioners are acknowledging that their outpatient colleagues are using a different approach to practice. The inpatient practitioners are now asking for further training in different areas, but surprisingly they are asking for more workshops and training in

the use of MOHO as an overarching theory base to help unify practice.

This is not to say that all of the work is done for the team or the department. Newer graduates who are hired tend to be more familiar with the value of occupation-based and evidence-based intervention but require intensive mentoring in learning about oncology. Occupational therapy practitioners with experience in applying the occupational therapy process sometimes need guidance and mentoring in the application of occupation-based treatment and application of an overarching theory base. These more experienced practitioners can also struggle to move from a therapist-driven practice to a true client-centered practice. The various referral sources for the occupational therapy service continue to require education on the distinct contributions of occupational therapy. Most importantly, however, Lauro and his team are confident that they are not offering distinct occupational therapy service.

Study Questions

1. **Which of the following is a common aspect of the structure of a community of practice?**

   a. Domain of knowledge
   b. Community of people
   c. Shared practice
   d. All of the above

2. **As a manager, you should make it your business to keep up-to-date with which of the following?**

   a. Theories
   b. Research
   c. Evidence
   d. All of the above

3. **Which of the following is a term that refers to the scope of information about which a group is concerned and defines what the group members need to understand together?**

   a. Domain of practice
   b. Shared practice
   c. Domain of knowledge
   d. Paradigmatic knowledge

4. **Which of the following is the best example of a naturalistic occupation?**

   a. Placing Velcro checkers in a pattern on the back of a rolling mirror
   b. Challenging a patient's balance by having him or her reach to pick imaginary apples
   c. Having a patient put different-sized cups and plates into a cupboard
   d. Moving colored rings from one side of a "therapy arch" to the other

5. **Which of the following best describes the *focus of the intervention* as presented in this chapter?**

   a. The degree to which a selected intervention is intended to fix an identified impairment versus helping the person develop adaptations necessary to promote participation in desired occupations
   b. The degree to which a selected intervention is supported by current policies on billing
   c. The degree to which a selected intervention is consistent with the way other practitioners approach practice in the setting
   d. The degree to which a selected intervention is client-centered

6. **Which of the following is not a recommendation for assisting staff in staying abreast of changes in practice and regulation without the need for further funding?**

   a. Brown bag in-service presentations
   b. CE on CD (Continuing Ed on CD)
   c. Journal clubs
   d. Cotreating patients

7. **A management tool that helps to codify best practice in a setting by laying out staff responsibilities would best be called which of the following?**

   a. Job description
   b. Mission statement
   c. Vision statement
   d. Statement of operations

8. **Which of the following best characterizes occupation-based interventions?**

   a. Ecologically relevant
   b. Naturalistic
   c. Draw their purpose and meaning from the therapist
   d. Both a and b

Resources for Learning More About Turning Theory Into Practice

Journals That Often Address Occupation-Based Practice or Communities of Practice

OTJR: Occupation, Participation, and Health

http://www.healio.com/nursing/journals/otjr

The *OTJR: Occupation, Participation, and Health* is published by the American Occupational Therapy Foundation, Inc. Articles published in the journal include original research of interest to the occupational therapy personnel. In addition to reports of quantitative and qualitative research, the journal includes briefs, book reviews, letters to the editor, and commentaries.

Journal of Occupational Science

http://www.tandfonline.com/toc/rocc20/current#.VHnde75t5E4

The *Journal of Occupational Science* publishes articles by authors from around the world and promotes discussion of topics related to the emerging discipline of occupational science. The journal focuses on the unique experiences, concerns, and perspectives of the study of humans as occupational beings.

Organization Science

http://pubsonline.informs.org/journal/orsc

Organization Science publishes reports of research on the processes, structures, technologies, identities, capabilities, forms, and performance of organizations. This multidisciplinary journal addresses issues including organizational behavior and theory, strategic management, psychology, sociology, economics, political science, information systems, technology management, communication, and cognitive science. Research at different levels of analysis, including the organization, the groups or units that constitute organizations, and the networks in which organizations are embedded is published.

OD Practitioner (Journal of the Organization Development Network)

http://www.odnetwork.org/?Publications

This journal includes articles on a wide range of organizational development issues, including communities of practice.

Associations That Are Concerned With Occupation-Based Practice or Communities of Practice

The Organization Development Network

http://www.odnetwork.org/

Members of the Organization Development Network (OD Network) are practitioners representing a range of professional roles in a wide variety of organizations. The OD Network seeks to develop, support, and inspire practitioners and to enhance the body of knowledge in human organization and systems development. Members of the network are employed by private industry, nonprofit organizations, and government agencies or are private consultants, entrepreneurs, researchers, or academicians.

Other Resources

Jobdescriptions.com

http://www.jobdescriptions.com

This commercial website allows you to pay for a single use (under $20) or 1 year of unlimited service (approx-

imately $130). You can create single, customized job descriptions for your organization that meet the requirements of the Americans With Disabilities Act compliance. The site guides you through selection of a template selected from thousands of job descriptions and uses your responses to write a custom job description that reflects your unique situation. The site also helps you create an interview form that contains suggested interview questions from the competencies in the job description.

Management Assistance Programs for Nonprofits

www.mapfornonprofits.org/

The mission of the Management Assistance Programs for Nonprofits (MAP) is to build the capacity of nonprofit organizations to achieve mission-driven results. Since 1979, the group has provided quality, affordable management consulting and board recruitment services to thousands of nonprofit groups. MAP primarily works with nonprofit organizations in the greater Twin Cities metropolitan area of Minneapolis and St. Paul, Minnesota. However, this organization has an excellent website that has information on a large range of topics, including job descriptions, in its free management library, found at http://www.managementhelp.org/.

Reference List

American Occupational Therapy Association. (2014). Occupational therapy practice framework: Domain and process (3rd ed.). *American Journal of Occupational Therapy, 68*(Suppl.1), S1–S48.

Bodiam, C. (1999). The use of the Canadian Occupational Performance Measure for the assessment of outcome on a neurorehabilitation unit. *British Journal of Occupational Therapy, 62*, 123–126.

Christ, P. A. H. (2014). Competence and professional development. In In B. A. Boyt Schell, G. Gillen, & M. E. Scaffa (Eds.), *Willard and Spackman's occupational therapy* (pp. 989–1013). Philadelphia, PA: Lippincott, Williams and Wilkins.

Cubie, S. H., & Kaplan, K. (1982). A case analysis method for the Model of Human Occupation. *American Journal of Occupational Therapy, 36*, 646–648.

Darragh, A. R., Sample, P. L., & Fisher, A. G. (1998). Environment effect on functional task performance in adults with acquired brain injuries: Use of the assessment of motor and process skills. *Archives of Physical Medicine and Rehabilitation, 79*, 418–423.

Fellin, P. (1993). Reformulation of the context of community-based care. *Journal of Sociology and Social Welfare, 20*, 57–67.

Fellin, P. (2001). *The community and the social worker*. Pacific Grove, CA: Brooks/Cole Publishing Company.

Fisher, A. G. (1998). Uniting practice and theory in an occupational framework. *American Journal of Occupational Therapy, 52*, 509–522.

Gillen, G. (2013a). A fork in the road: An occupational hazard? *American Journal of Occupational Therapy, 67*(6), 641–652.

Gillen, G. (2013b). Occupational therapy interventions for individuals. In B. A. Boyt-Schell, G. Gillen, & M. Scaffa (Eds.), *Willard & Spackman's occupational therapy* (pp. 322–341). Philadelphia, PA: Wolters Kluwer Lippincott Williams & Wilkins.

Gilmore, P. E., & Spaulding, S. J. (2001). Motor control and motor learning: Implications for treatment of individuals post stroke. *Physical & Occupational Therapy in Geriatrics, 20*, 1–15.

Mathiowetz, V., & Bass-Haugen, J. (2002). Assessing abilities and capacities: Motor behavior. In C. A. Trombly & M. V. Radomski (Eds.), *Occupational therapy for physical dysfunction* (pp. 137–158). Philadelphia, PA: Lippincott, Williams & Wilkins.

McCormack, G. L. (2011). Common skill sets for occupational therapy managers and practitioners. In G. L. McCormack (Ed.), *The occupational therapy manager* (5th ed., p. 34). Bethesda, MD: AOTA Press.

McCormack, G. L., Jaffe, E. G., & Frey, W. F. (2003). New organizational perspectives. In G. L. McCormack, E. G. Jaffe, & M. Goodman-Lavey (Eds.), *The occupational therapy manager* (4th ed., pp. 85–126). Bethesda, MD: AOTA Press.

Minar, D., & Greer, S. (1969). *The concept of community: Readings with interpretation*. Chicago, IL: Aldine.

Model of Human Occupation Clearinghouse. (2014). *The Model of Human Occupation Screening Tool (MOHOST). Version 2.0*. Retrieved from http://www.cade.uic.edu/moho/productDetails.aspx?aid=4.

Moyers, P. A., & Dale, L. (2007). *The guide to occupational therapy practice* (2nd ed.). Bethesda, MD: AOTA Press.

Park, S., Fisher, A. G., & Velozo, C. A. (1994). Using the assessment of motor and process skills to compare occupational performance between clinic and home settings. *American Journal of Occupational Therapy, 48*, 697–709.

Pedretti, L. W., & Umphred, D. A. (1996). Motor learning and teaching activities in occupational therapy. In L. W. Pedretti (Ed.), *Occupational therapy: Practice skills for physical dysfunction* (4th ed., pp. 65–75). St. Louis, MO: Mosby–Year Book.

Poole, J. L., & Whitney, S. L. (2001). Assessments of motor function post stroke: A review. *Physical and Occupational Therapy in Geriatrics, 19*, 1–22.

Richardson, J. (2000). The use of a simulated environment (Easy Street) to retrain independent living skills in elderly persons: A randomized controlled trial. *Journals of Gerontology. Series A: Biological Sciences and Medical Sciences, 55*, 578–584.

Schell, B. A. B. (1994). *The effects of practice context on occupational therapists' clinical reasoning*. Doctoral Dissertation, University of Georgia, Dissertation Abstracts International.

Trombly, C. A. (1995). Occupation: Purposefulness and meaningfulness as therapeutic mechanisms. *American Journal of Occupational Therapy, 49*, 960–972.

Wenger, E., McDermott, R., & Snyder, W. M. (2002). *Cultivating communities of practice: A guide to managing knowledge*. Boston, MA: Harvard Business School Press.

Appendix 17-1

Sample Job Description

Title: Job Description for Occupational Therapist I

I. Function

To provide standard occupational therapy services to inpatients and outpatients as determined by the therapist's specific team assignment. To supervise fieldwork students assigned to the unit on which they work. To assist in administrative responsibilities, including patient record keeping, billing, daily and monthly team statistics, and maintenance and inventory of unit equipment and supplies.

II. Organizational Relationship

Reports directly to the team leader for the team to which she or he has been assigned as designated by the director of clinical services. Receives clinical supervision and patient assignment from the occupational therapist II and the team leader for the team on which she or he works.

III. Key Performance Expectations

A. *Patient Care*

1. Evaluates, under a physician's referral, patients of age ranges for which she or he has appropriate training and prior experience in regard to their need for occupational therapy services as assigned by the occupational therapist II or team leader on her or his team. Administers and interprets clinical and functional assessments to determine the patient's present level of physical, psychosocial, developmental, and functional status. Documents the results of these assessments appropriately. Orders and fabricates assistive and adaptive equipment.
2. Plans and implements individual and group patient treatments in accordance with strengths and deficits documented in clinical findings and appropriate to the age of the client based on principles and theories of occupational therapy.
3. Orients patients and families to objectives and functions of occupational therapy.
4. Schedules, plans, and carries out individual treatment of patients, with focus on prevention of ill effects of separation from home, hospitalization, and restoration of maximal occupational performance.
5. Provides indicated home programming and patient follow-up in conjunction with the interdisciplinary treatment team.
6. Communicates orally and in written form at the interdepartmental and intradepartmental levels regarding patient status and discharge planning. Attend rounds and conferences as assigned by the supervisor.
7. Participates in outpatient clinics as assigned by the supervisor to provide occupational therapy consultation, evaluation, treatment, and follow-up.
8. Functions as an integral member of the healthcare team and develops and maintains working relationships with peers and members of other disciplines within the medical center local communities as appropriate to his or her job responsibilities.
9. Coordinates treatment objectives and procedures with other disciplines, services, or agencies, both within and outside the hospital.
10. Assists other teams with patient care as necessary and assigned.
11. Participates in continuous quality improvement activities.

B. *Administration*

1. Patient related:
   a. Recommends the scheduling of patients for evaluation and treatment on a weekly basis, with awareness of the specific milieu of their team unit, to the occupational therapist II/team leader.

b. Records patient attendance and statistical data required by the unit and programs in which she or he works.

2. Unit related:
   a. Assists with inventory of supplies and equipment and other related duties as delegated by the supervisor.
   b. Assists in reporting of productivity or other statistics as delegated by the team leader.

C. Education

1. Provides supervision to occupational therapy and OTA students as assigned by the team leader.
2. Assists in undergraduate teaching (labs and lectures) as assigned.
3. Assists in the orientation of students and residents from other departments or representatives from interested community groups to occupational therapy as assigned by the team leader.

D. Professional

1. Participates in unit and departmental meetings and in-services.
2. Participates in patient-related meetings.
3. Participates in hospital and departmental committees as appropriate.
4. Participates in in-service education, workshops, and other continuing education experiences as appropriate to the ages and types of patients treated.

IV. Qualifications and Knowledge Required

To qualify for the position of occupational therapist I, an employee must be eligible for licensure by the State Department of Professional Regulation. No minimum period of experience is required. The employee is required to have a sound basic knowledge of occupational therapy theory, evaluation, and treatment with specific skills related to the patients treated by the team to which she or he is assigned. This includes familiarity with age-specific occupational roles and needs. Knowledge of departmental policies governing patient care, charting, billing, and confidentiality of patient-related information or records is necessary.

V. Supervision

A. Direct and Indirect Supervision Received

Work is assigned, reviewed, and approved by the team leader, or by the director of clinical services. After orientation and training, the employee is expected to complete routine work independently. Instructions are both oral and written (memos, departmental policies and procedures, physicians' orders).

B. Guidelines

Performance is guided by departmental protocol, patient care standards, university policies and procedures, and AOTA standards.

VI. Complexity

A. Employee Qualities

The employee is expected to become an integral member of the patient care–related team and the occupational therapy department. Initiation and independence are necessary qualities. The employee is expected to provide all aspects of patient care for those patients assigned to his or her care. The employee is expected to act as a role model for, and provide direct supervision to, occupational therapy and OTA students. Good interpersonal skills must be promoted to ensure proper patient care and a good working environment for both the employee and others.

B. Guidelines

Patient care services must be provided in accordance with all departmental and hospital guidelines to ensure comprehensive patient care. Administrative duties must be performed as assigned to permit the department to be properly recognized for its efforts.

VII. Contact With Others

Patients, staff, students, and visitors should interact within the Departments of Occupational Therapy, Physical Medicine and Rehabilitation, and Physical Therapy, and the University Medical Center.

VIII. Essential Functions and Environmental Demands

A. Physical Requirements

Refined motor skills in treatment techniques and general endurance for manual work beyond the sedentary level are necessary. Strength is needed to roll, lift, and transfer immobile patients. She or he must be able to perform all other essential physical, social, and cognitive aspects of occupational therapy treatment with patients of all ages treated by the team that she or he supervises.

B. Work Environment

1. There is frequent exposure to communicable diseases, such as active pulmonary tuberculosis, hepatitis, and respiratory infections, as well as to wound infections. There is exposure to patient secretions and drainage during the course of care.
2. There is increased risk for personal injury (shoulder, wrist, and back are common sites) when moving immobile patients and guarding against patient falls.

Appendix 17-2

Documentation and Reporting Matrix

Model of Human Occupation

Think about the typical documentation and reporting expectations in your practice. To what degree do they fit with current occupational therapy theories?

	Initial Evaluations	Progress Notes	Oral Reports	Discharge Summaries
Volitional Issues • Personal causation • Values • Interests • Life story				
Habituation • Roles • Routines				
Performance Capacity • Musculoskeletal • Neurological • Perceptual • Cognitive				
Environment • Physical • Social • Cultural				
Occupational Performance • Motor skills • Process skills • Communication and interaction skills				
Person–Environment Interaction • Skills and physical context • Skills and social context • Skills and cultural context				
Goals for Intervention • Client or patient generated • Focused on occupational outcomes				
Goal Attainment • Meaningful to client • Evaluated by client • Evaluated by therapist				

Responsible Participation in a Profession: Fostering Professionalism and Leading for Moral Action

Regina F. Doherty, OTD, OTR/L, FAOTA, FNAP
Elizabeth W. Peterson, PhD, OTR/L, FAOTA

■ Real-Life Management

Every day Ellyn and the occupational therapy staff with whom she works eat their lunch together and spend their lunchtime discussing a wide range of topics. Today the conversation turned to a letter that all occupational therapy practitioners in their state received from the state regulatory board informing them of changes to the state occupational therapy practice act. Some of Ellyn's coworkers were complaining about the addition of requirements for continuing education to the licensure act. They would now have to meet these requirements in order to renew their licenses to practice every other year. The staff members were voicing the concern that all of the benefits relating to continuing education provided by their employer had been eliminated and that they would now have to cover the cost of attending continuing education to satisfy the state's new requirements.

One of the staff, Carrie, expressed concern that the physical therapy state practice act had also been changed. It now included activities of daily living (ADLs) as part of the scope of practice definition for physical therapy. As Ellyn listened to the staff complain about the state of affairs, she became more and more frustrated. Ellyn became involved in her state occupational therapy association when she was a student and was elected as her class representative to the association. From that moment on, she had developed an intense interest in advocating for her profession and her clients at the local, state, and national legislative levels. She was still an active member of her state association as well as the American Occupational Therapy Association

Continued

■ **Real-Life Management—cont'd**

(AOTA). She volunteered on the state licensure committee and had even visited her congresswoman on Capitol Hill in Washington, DC, as part of AOTA's Capitol Hill Day.

Ellyn knew that few if any of the staff sitting at lunch were members of the state occupational therapy association and that less than half were members of AOTA. She found it frustrating that her peers complained about the outcomes of processes that they could have influenced but instead left to others. She decided that she needed to do something. Ellyn left lunch early to talk to her department director about how to most effectively engage her coworkers in discussions about the responsibilities of being a professional and how to implement strategies that would lead to enhanced professionalism in her department.

Critical Thinking Questions

As you read this chapter, consider the following questions:

- How does being an active participant in your state and national professional associations contribute to being a responsible occupational therapy service provider?

- What does a full understanding of how your professional association and other related bodies are structured, the functions they serve, and how you can become involved to influence the future of occupational therapy contribute to responsible participation in your profession?

- How can occupational therapy managers commit to ethical practice through an understanding of the resources and systems available to help their staff effectively identify, analyze, and resolve ethical issues that present in the professional practice environment?

Glossary

- **Interprofessional professionalism:** approach that focuses on the core values, competencies, and norms that multiple professions have identified as critical to the delivery of effective collaborative care.
- **Licensure:** approval of professional practice by a regulatory body, allowing an individual to practice with authority within a specific geographic region (e.g., state regulatory boards).
- **Profession:** term used to refer to an occupation whose core element is work based upon the mastery of a complex body of knowledge and skills and where members are governed by codes of ethics and profess a commitment to competence, integrity and morality, altruism, and the promotion of the public good within their domain, allowing autonomy in practice and the privilege of self-regulation.
- **Professional ethics:** principles or rules intended to express the particular values of a group of providers and that serve as guidelines for professional behavior.

Introduction

Throughout this book, membership in AOTA has been emphasized as an important strategy for finding useful resources related to data, information, and other forms of evidence. Additionally, it has been suggested that developing a network of peers at the local, state, and national levels can help you find and evaluate evidence and other resources to aid clinical and managerial decision-making. This theme will continue in Chapter 18; furthermore, it will be suggested that as a *professional* you have a responsibility to join and actively participate in both your state and national professional associations. Neither managers nor practitioners can fulfill their responsibilities that come with the adoption of an evidence-based approach to leadership, management, and practice without understanding the contexts in which practice occurs, and this requires a working knowledge of the key stakeholders that seek to influence the profession.

As an occupational therapy manager, you will not only have the responsibility of taking steps to play an active role in supporting and developing your chosen profession but will also play a vital role in encouraging the active participation of those you supervise. In order to be successful at both of these tasks, you must develop a working knowledge of the key organizations and bodies that are involved in shaping how practice occurs. Many of these bodies, such as AOTA, the National Board for Certification of Occupational Therapy, Inc. (NBCOT), state regulatory boards, and accreditation bodies, have been mentioned in other chapters. They are briefly discussed again in this chapter, focusing specifically on how a manager can become involved in or interact with each organization or body to obtain data, information, and other forms of evidence and to play a role in shaping the future of occupational therapy practice.

Finally, a key role of the occupational therapy manager is assuring that the occupational therapists (OTs), occupational therapy assistants (OTAs), occupational therapy fieldwork students, and others whom he or she supervises practice in an ethical and responsible manner. An introduction to ethics is therefore provided, including a compilation of common ethics theories, and supports for ethical practice both internal and external to occupational therapy practice environments are discussed.

What Does It Mean to Be a Professional?

Cruess, Johnston, and Cruess offer the following definition of a **profession**:

Profession: An occupation whose core element is work based upon the mastery of a complex body of knowledge and skills. . . . Its members are governed by codes of ethics and profess a commitment to competence, integrity and morality, altruism, and the promotion of the public good within their domain. These commitments form the basis of a social contract between a profession and society, which in return grants the profession a monopoly over the use of its knowledge base, the right to considerable autonomy in practice and the privilege of self-regulation. (2004, p. 76)

The practice of specialized expertise and the ethical obligations associated with said practice are two key factors that differentiate a profession from other occupations (Ozar, 2004). *Professional responsibility* is a dominant theme in professionalism. From an ethical point of view, this responsibility includes both accountability and responsiveness (Purtilo & Doherty, 2011).

As the notion of relationship-centered health care has evolved, so has the formation of collaborative interprofessional care teams (see Chapter 8). **Interprofessional professionalism** is a concept that has emerged from collaborative practice, education, and research. Interprofessional professionalism focuses on the competencies, core values, and norms that multiple professions have identified as critical to the delivery of collaborative care (Hammer et al, 2012; Holtman, Frost, Hammer, McGuinn, & Nunez, 2011). It underscores communication, collaboration, and negotiation across professional boundaries.

In the United States, the primary vehicle for a profession to have a unified influence to promote and develop its services to society is the *professional association*. Associations and bureaucracies and their relationship were discussed in Chapter 4. The implication for individual occupational therapy practitioners is clear. Being a responsible "professional" means one must join and sustain active membership in both his or her state occupational therapy association and AOTA. State associations not only provide a mechanism for interacting with our peers on a local level but typically also play critical roles in defining the nature of the profession's service at the state level through their influence on state regulatory bodies (e.g., licensure). As our national association, AOTA serves a range of critical functions related to the development and promotion of occupational therapy as a profession. The structure and function of these organizations and bodies are reviewed briefly in the next section of this chapter.

Occupational Therapy Professional Associations

The American Occupational Therapy Association (AOTA)

AOTA is the national professional association established in 1917 to represent the interests and concerns of occupational therapy practitioners and students of occupational therapy and to improve the quality of occupational therapy services (AOTA, 2014a). For occupational therapy practitioners, AOTA membership supports responsible participation in the profession for two important reasons. First, AOTA membership dues finance AOTA initiatives to assure the quality of occupational therapy services, educate the public, improve the quality of health care, and improve consumer access to health-care services. Second, AOTA provides a comprehensive array of professional development resources to members. Many of these resources are available to members on the AOTA website and include information specifically designed for occupational therapy practitioners to support evidence-based practice. AOTA members gain access to continuing education opportunities, subscriptions to the *American Journal of Occupational Therapy* and *OT Practice*, and online access to the *British Journal of Occupational Therapy* and the *Canadian Journal of Occupational Therapy*.

AOTA is governed by a structure that includes an executive director; as noted in Chapter 4, this paid employee is a professional experienced in running a nonprofit professional association. Often the executive director is not an occupational therapy practitioner but an expert in professional organization management. He or she is responsible for oversight of the activities of all paid staff and for collaborating with the volunteer sector of the association. The members of AOTA elect a group of volunteer officers, including a president, vice president, secretary, treasurer, and

directors, who serve on the association's board of directors. In addition to the board of directors, AOTA is led by a number of commissions, committees, and boards that are also often led by volunteers who are elected by the membership as a whole or a subset of the membership. One example of a subset of the membership includes the 11 special interest sections (SISs) that function to represent practice areas within the profession, such as administration and management (AMSIS), gerontology (GSIS), and education, among others. Each SIS elects a chairperson every 3 years. These chairpersons regularly meet as a group (the Special Interest Sections Council, or SISC) to advise the association on important matters, to develop products or resources to meet their members' needs, and to identify issues of importance that will affect practice. The primary bodies of AOTA are listed with brief descriptions in Box 18-1. The major functions of the association are listed in Box 18-2. AOTA's role in supporting ethical behavior among members is described later in this chapter.

The American Occupational Therapy Political Action Committee (AOTPAC)

AOTPAC is a voluntary, nonprofit, nonpartisan, unincorporated committee of members of AOTA that has been operational since 1978. The purpose of AOTPAC is to further the association's legislative aims by influencing or attempting to influence the selection, nomination, election, or appointment of any individual to any federal public office, and of any OT, OTA, or occupational therapy student member of AOTA seeking election to public office at any level. The committee is nonpartisan and is not affiliated with any political party (AOTA, 2014c).

Federal regulations prevent AOTA as an organization from making contributions to political candidates; however, as a separate nonprofit organization, a political action committee (PAC) is free to raise money and make donations to support the political campaigns of candidates with views that favor AOTA's agenda. AOTA is allowed to legally support the PAC by providing the operating expenses required for the PAC to fulfill its function.

AOTPAC is governed by a board of directors, with a chair and five directors representing each of five regions of the United States. In addition, there are nonvoting AOTA staff members who help to guide the

BOX 18-1

The Primary Governance Bodies of the American Occupational Therapy Association

- **Board of Directors:** The Board of Directors (Board) is composed of the elected officers of the association; directors are elected from the general membership and include at least one OTA and an appointed public member.
- **Representative Assembly (RA):** The RA, the policy-making body (e.g., congress) of AOTA, is made up of elected representatives from each state and Puerto Rico, chairpersons of advisory committees and commissions (e.g., the Special Interest Sections Council, the Commission on Practice, the Commission on Education), and a public member.

Standing Advisory Committees of the Board
- **Volunteer Leadership Development Committee (VLDC):** The VLDC is a standing advisory committee that promotes member participation and engagement, volunteer leadership development, and participation initiatives in AOTA. The VLDC recruits candidates, holds association elections, and coordinates professional awards of the association.
- **Special Interest Sections Council (SISC):** The SISC is a standing advisory committee organized to represent 11 specialty areas of practice and to meet the range of member needs related to practice in these areas.

Associated Advisory Councils of the Board
- **Accreditation Council for Occupational Therapy Education (ACOTE):** ACOTE is an associated advisory council of AOTA's Board of Directors and has the mission of fostering the development and accreditation of quality occupational therapy education programs. The chairperson is an organizational advisor to AOTA's Board of Directors. By establishing rigorous standards for occupational therapy education, ACOTE supports the preparation of competent occupational therapy practitioners.

Associated Bodies as Organizational Advisors to the Board
- **Affiliated State Association Presidents (ASAP):** ASAP is composed of state presidents from the 50 state occupational therapy associations (and Puerto Rico) affiliated with the AOTA; the chairperson is an organizational advisor to AOTA's Board of Directors.
- **Assembly of Student Delegates (ASD):** ASD is composed of student delegates from the membership and is an associated body of AOTA's Board of Directors. The chairperson acts as an organizational advisor to the Board. ASD provides a mechanism for the expression of student concerns, and offers a means whereby students can have effective input into the affairs of AOTA.

Advisory Commissions and Committees of the Representative Assembly
- **Ethics Commission (EC):** The EC is an advisory commission of the RA that is responsible for the development of the AOTA Code of Ethics and related ethics standards. The EC's primary role is ethics education; it reviews complaints and makes recommendations for discipline of AOTA members for ethical violations.
- **Commission on Practice (COP):** The COP is an advisory commission of the RA and serves AOTA by promoting the quality of occupational therapy practice and developing practice standards for OTs and OTAs relative to provider and consumer needs.
- **Commission on Education (COE):** The COE, an advisory commission of the RA, is a visionary group that identifies, analyzes, and anticipates issues in education. The COE generates education-related policy recommendations to the RA for deliberation. The COE works in conjunction with the Education Special Interest Section (EDSIS) and has interactions with the ACOTE.
- **Commission on Continuing Competence and Professional Development (CCCPD):** The CCCPD is a body of the RA that develops and maintains the standards for continued competence. The CCCPD develops tools to assist all members in the development and implementation of continuing competence plans.

BOX 18-2

Major Functions of the American Occupational Therapy Association

- Promote awareness of occupational therapy in society by keeping it visible and in demand
- Advocate for the profession at the national, state, and local legislative levels
- Provide for the continuing education and professional development needs of the membership
- Provide mechanisms and structures for the membership to interact with each other
- Support the provision of quality education for OTs and OTAs by developing and maintaining a process for accrediting educational programs
- Guide the membership in the delivery of ethical and responsible intervention
- Support the development of knowledge and scientific inquiry to develop evidence to guide occupational therapy practice
- Support the development of standards and guidelines to guide occupational therapy practice

PAC's activities. All of the money that supports the PAC's legislative activities comes from direct member contributions. AOTPAC provides a means for members to play an active role in the political process that influences payment and access to occupational therapy services.

Among others, AOTPAC cites three central criteria used in determining which candidates to support (AOTA, 2014c):

- Is the candidate sympathetic to the goals of the occupational therapy profession? Has the candidate supported specific proposals or policies advanced by the profession?
- If the candidate is incumbent, does the candidate hold a key position of responsibility (i.e., chair or member of an important committee or subcommittee; member of the majority or minority leadership)?

- If the candidate is a nonincumbent, will the candidate pursue assignment to a key committee or subcommittee, or be likely to be in a position to assist the profession?

The American Occupational Therapy Foundation (AOTF)

The American Occupational Therapy Foundation (AOTF) is a 501(c)(3) charitable, scientific, and educational organization founded in 1965. AOTF's mission is to "advance research, education and public awareness for occupational therapy so that all people may participate fully in life regardless of their physical, social, mental or developmental circumstances" (AOTF, 2014a, n.p.). AOTF operationalizes its mission through grant and scholarship programs, publications (e.g., *OTJR: Occupation, Participation and Health*), and through the Wilma L. West Library, which houses an extensive collection of literature and resources on occupational therapy and related subject areas.

AOTF often works in partnership with AOTA to develop and deliver programming to support the profession. The AOTF/AOTA Intervention Research Grant Program, which supports intervention research, is an important example of the AOTF and AOTA collaborative efforts. Likewise, the AOTF Institute for the Study of Occupation and Health, which is the chief programmatic arm of the foundation, often works with AOTA to advance education, leadership, and research in the field. AOTA and AOTF jointly sponsor both the Leadership Mentoring Program and Research Advisory Panel (RAP). The RAP:

> . . . advises the AOTA and AOTF boards of directors in several matters, including the translation of research to education and practice, and the review of the research agenda of the profession and its alignment with national research priorities and emerging social and technology issues. The panel also fosters critical analyses of issues related to the delivery of services, evolution of theories, and the overall body of knowledge relevant to occupational therapy. (AOTF, 2014b, n.p.)

AOTF raises public awareness of the link between everyday living and health through programming and activities ranging from Wilma L. West Library–based initiatives and press releases to its awards program. AOTF also sponsors the Academy of Research in

Occupational Therapy. The Academy, which was established in 1983, is made up of a distinguished body of researchers who have made important contributions toward the science of occupational therapy.

The Fund to Promote Awareness of Occupational Therapy

The Fund to Promote Awareness of Occupational Therapy (The Fund) was founded in 2002 as a separate 501(c)(3) nonprofit organization as part of a long-term strategy to raise awareness of occupational therapy. The Fund runs promotional campaigns and activities with the goal of achieving "greater understanding, availability and use of occupational therapy and to promote the profession's contributions to health, wellness, participation, productivity and quality of life in society" (AOTA, 2014b, n.p.).

Examples of projects created and directed by the Fund include increasing awareness of back injury in children caused by carrying overloaded backpacks, and research undertaken to better understand how messages about occupational therapy can most effectively reach various audiences and build a lasting identity for the profession. The Fund's promotional materials such as the "Promote OT Toolkit" are available at http://www.promoteot.org/PG_ProfessionalsGuide.html for use by managers and all occupational therapy practitioners who want to improve understanding and use of occupational therapy in their local communities.

The National Board for Certification of Occupational Therapy, Inc. (NBCOT®)

NBCOT is a nonprofit credentialing agency that provides certification for the occupational therapy profession. As the credentialing agency for the profession of occupational therapy, NBCOT serves to assure the public that persons practicing as occupational therapy practitioners have entry-level competence.

Only graduates of accredited or approved occupational therapy and OTA programs are eligible to sit for the national certification examinations administered by NBCOT. NBCOT administers two examinations: the COTA Examination and the OTR Examination. NBCOT conducts practice analyses every 5 years, and the questions on the certification examinations are derived from the results of those studies (NBCOT, 2013). Before sitting for an NBCOT certification examination, certification candidates must agree to abide by the NBCOT Code of Conduct. In its Candidate/Certificant Code of Conduct, NBCOT defines and clarifies the professional responsibilities:

> *As certified professionals in the field of occupational therapy, NBCOT certificants will at all times act with integrity and adhere to high standards for personal and professional conduct, accept responsibility for their actions, both personally and professionally, continually seek to enhance their professional capabilities, practice with fairness and honesty, abide by all federal, state, and local laws and regulations, and encourage others to act in a professional manner consistent with the certification standards and responsibilities set forth below. (NBCOT, 2014b, n.p.)*

NBCOT's role in regulation of occupational therapy practice is described later in this chapter.

After successfully completing the national certification examination for the OTA, a graduate of an OTA program is designated as "certified occupational therapy assistant" (COTA). After successfully completing the certification examination for the OT, a graduate of an occupational therapy program is designated as "occupational therapist registered" (OTR). Most states require licensure to practice, and state licenses are usually based on the results of the NBCOT certification examination.

NBCOT certification is granted for a 3-year period. Although initial certification is required for occupational therapy practitioners, recertification is voluntary. Because there is a professional development unit (PDU) requirement associated with recertification, practitioners who are recertified are demonstrating not only their pledge to the NBCOT Code of Conduct, but also their commitment to professional competency. Occupational therapy assistants who choose not to recertify can no longer use the "COTA" credential, and OTs who choose not to recertify can no longer use the "OTR" credential.

In addition to the development and administration of the certification examination, and overseeing the recertification process, the NBCOT fulfills several other functions. NBCOT provides many competency resources for occupational therapy practitioners. For example, NBCOT offers a professional development log to help practitioners track the 36 PDUs needed to maintain current certification status. NBCOT also offers a professional development provider registry to support practitioners' recertification efforts. NBCOT has developed self-assessment tools, which are available at http://www.nbcot.org. These tools create a means by which OTs and OTAs can reflect on their professional competence and continuing education needs.

State Occupational Therapy Associations

State occupational therapy associations serve many of the same functions for occupational therapy professionals on a state level that AOTA performs on a national level. In addition to being a mechanism to develop and maintain a network of peers, state associations serve the following functions:

- Providing opportunities for continuing education and professional development through state association conferences, publications, and sponsored events
- Advocating for the profession at the state level through political action and lobbying to influence outcomes of processes such as licensure and other forms of regulatory control
- Increasing public awareness of occupational therapy
- Providing a vehicle for occupational therapy practitioners to develop networks of peers to support professional development and practice
- Providing an opportunity for members to develop skills in leadership, interpersonal communication, management, and other personal and professional skills

Interprofessional Associations

Recognizing that health-care issues are characteristically broad and complex, and that they must be examined from many perspectives, a number of organizations now serve to support interprofessional education and practice. Some of these associations include the National Academies of Practice, the Interprofessional Education Collaborative, the Interprofessional Professionalism Collaborative, and the American Interprofessional Health Collaborative. These organizations promote common goals on important interprofessional health-care topics reflecting current and future issues in practice, education, policy, and research. They share their work with discipline-specific professional organizations, health-care planners, public agencies, and other interested parties. Many hold national conferences and disseminate scholarly work via resources, policy statements, and journals dedicated to interprofessional health-care topics. See the resources at the end of this chapter for sample interprofessional associations.

Ethics

Being a responsible professional, whether your primary role is as a practitioner, manager, educator, or researcher, includes having an understanding of ethics as a discipline and the systems in place to help occupational therapy service providers recognize, analyze, and resolve the ethical problems that they encounter in professional practice. Leadership and management today involve motivating staff to achieve best practices, and best practices are enhanced by ethical reflection. When leaders demonstrate, mentor, and endorse ethical decision-making, their staff members are more likely to focus on their own moral reasoning (Newton, 2013). In order to best understand ethics in practice, we must familiarize ourselves with ethics theory and terminology.

What Is Ethics?

Ethics is a branch of philosophy that guides ways of understanding and examining a moral life (Beauchamp & Childress, 2009). When a practitioner or manager asks "What is the morally correct action to take for this case or situation?" he or she calls upon moral reasoning. Moral reasoning is a mode of professional reasoning that requires the practitioner to recognize and apply ethics knowledge and skills to achieve best practice. Several ethics theories, approaches, and decision-making models help to guide clinicians and managers with the ethical dimensions of professional practice.

Ethics theories and approaches attempt to identify and justify existing norms (Beauchamp & Childress,

2009). In a pluralistic society with divergent moralities, no single unifying ethics theory or vision of morality prevails. A debate over which theory is "right" and which theory is "wrong" is really beside the point. Ethics experts encourage us to focus on acceptable features in different theories, often with attention to how ethical decisions are justified, without having to choose one over the other (Beauchamp & Childress, 2009; Kornblau & Burkhardt, 2012; Purtilo & Doherty, 2011). Understanding the different theories adds depth to ethical thought and action.

Professional ethics are principles or rules intended to express the particular values of a group of providers and that serve as guidelines for professional behavior. They help to explain the profession to people served, and serve as a code of conduct. As Corbett (1993) explained, our professional ethics within occupational therapy are the rules we use to make certain that each therapist is operating in a fashion that protects the integrity of our profession, and hence the viability of all occupational therapy practitioners. These rules ensure our clients' best interests and protect the profession itself and its position in the public mind. Although professional codes of ethics are also a means of establishing trust between the professional and society, codes are only one element of professional behavior, and they do not automatically create the desired professional practice (Scanlon & Glover, 1995).

Selected basic terms related to ethics principles and concepts are presented in Box 18-3. Terms related to ethics theories are presented in Box 18-4.

Applying Ethics Knowledge and Skills

Ethical Problems

Understanding ethics theories and debating their application may seem like a philosophical exercise; in reality, however, ethics theories and principles are highly relevant to daily life—especially the life of a health-care provider. The complex and ever-changing nature of health-care delivery systems and advances in health technologies are two trends that have led to an increased prevalence of ethical questions in occupational therapy practice. Many of these ethical issues present as moral distress. Moral distress is a type of ethical problem that occurs when practitioners know the right thing to do, but cannot achieve it because of internal constraints, external barriers, or uncertainty. As a result, practitioners may experience cognitive or emotional discomfort because they are prevented from being the kind of professionals they know they *should* be (Purtilo & Doherty, 2011). Topics that cause moral distress in occupational therapy practice with high frequency include those surrounding reimbursement, maintaining confidentiality, addressing conflicts around goal setting, and balancing institutional needs versus what is best for the client (Doherty, Dellinger, Gately, Pullo, & Sullivan, 2012; Foye, Kirschner, Brady-Wagner, Stocking, & Siegler, 2002; Slater & Brandt, 2011). Managers are often the first line of defense for practitioners facing moral distress. Managers must answer the "ethical call" to ensure effective quality and safety outcomes for the client (Piper, 2011).

By definition, an ethical dilemma is a choice between two equally compelling alternatives. It is a situation marked by conflict between ethical beliefs that involves choices between alternatives that appear equally morally acceptable (Kornblau & Burkhardt, 2012). These "right versus right" decisions are more challenging; as Barbara Wells puts it, they "pit our values against each other and require ethical fitness, which, like physical fitness, must be methodically developed over time through consistent and repetitive application" (Wells, 2003, p. 6). The nature and scope of occupational therapy practice provide plenty of fuel for ethical dilemmas. An example would be the OT or OTA working in acute care who constantly has to decide how to ration her time spent with patients in order to provide services to as many clients as possible, or the school-based therapist who is beginning to suspect that one of the students he is following is the victim of neglect, but is concerned about angering the parents and possibly placing the child in greater harm. Ethics aids everyone in the evaluation of morality, conduct, and social practices.

Ethical Decision-Making Models

Occupational therapy service providers can draw from the work of several authors to learn strategies that can be used to analyze ethical problems in a structured and systematic way (Bailey & Schwartzberg, 2003;

BOX 18-3

Ethics Principles and Related Terminology

- **Autonomy:** A norm of respecting one's capacity to act on decisions freely and independently; often called the principle of self-determination (Beauchamp & Childress, 2009).
- **Beneficence:** Principle of doing good.
- **Bioethics:** Branch of ethics devoted to the study of problems surrounding medical practice, health-care delivery, and medical and biological research (Bailey & Schwartzberg, 2003).
- **Compassion:** Desire to identify with or sense something of another's experience—a precursor of caring (Hack, 2005).
- **Competence:** Having the cognitive and psychological ability to make decisions that others judge to be rational; to be judged competent, it is necessary for the individual to be able to communicate these decisions to others (Hansen, 2003).
- **Confidentiality:** Practice of keeping privileged patient information within proper bounds. Confidentiality always involves a relationship, whereas privacy does not (Purtilo & Doherty, 2011).
- **Conflict of interest:** Conflict between the private interests and the public obligations of a person in an official position (*American Heritage College Dictionary*, 1993).
- **Conscientiousness:** Intending to do what is right; trying with due diligence to determine what is right (Beauchamp & Childress, 2009).
- **Discernment:** Ability to make a good decision without being unduly influenced by extraneous considerations, personal biases, fears, and undue influences of others (Pozgar, 2005).
- **Distributive justice:** Method of determining how to dispense or allocate resources (e.g., equal shares for all; first come, first served; the greatest good for the greatest number) (Hansen, 2003).
- **Duty:** Act or course of action required by custom, law, or religion (*American Heritage College Dictionary*, 1993). The position of "OT" brings with it a number of duties outlined by the law and the profession.
- **Ethical dilemma:** Situation marked by conflict between ethical beliefs and involving choice between alternatives that appear to be equally morally acceptable (Kornblau & Burkhardt, 2012).
- **Fidelity:** Faithfulness; being true to commitments and obligations.

- **Informed consent:** Client's right to full disclosure of what is to be expected in terms of plan of care and the known risks and benefits associated with such a plan (Slater, 2011).
- **Integrity:** Person's awareness of and commitment to doing the morally right thing (Purtilo & Doherty, 2011).
- **Justice:** Principle of fairness; a group of norms for distributing benefits, risks, and costs fairly (Beauchamp & Childress, 2009). Three types of justice commonly used in ethics are distributive (social), compensatory, and procedural.
- **Nonmaleficence:** Fundamental duty that instructs us to avoid inflicting harm.
- **Paternalism:** Intentional overriding of one person's known preferences or actions by another person, wherein the person who overrides justifies the action by the goal of benefiting or avoiding harm to the person whose preferences or actions are overridden (Beauchamp & Childress, 2009).
- **Principle:** Basic truth, law, or assumption that may serve to act as a standard for behavior. Principles may be general in nature and may rely upon rules to guide specific action.
- **Rights:** Justified claims that individuals and groups can make upon other individuals or upon society; to have a right is to be in a position to determine, by one's choices, what others should do or need not do (Beauchamp & Childress, 2009).
- **Shared decision-making:** Process in which information is exchanged between the client and the provider or the care team. Shared decision-making is the basis of informed consent.
- **Substituted judgment:** Means of decision-making invoked by a surrogate decision-maker who makes a decision for an incompetent person based on what the person would have wanted when competent (Purtilo & Doherty, 2011).
- **Trust:** Confident belief in and reliance upon the moral character and competence of another person (Beauchamp & Childress, 2009).
- **Veracity:** Duty to truthfulness.
- **Virtue:** Character trait and an internal disposition to seek moral perfection, to live one's life in accord with this moral law, and to attain a balance between noble intention and just action (Pellegrino, 1995).

BOX 18-4

Common Ethics Theories and Approaches

- **Care-based ethics:** Based on the assumption that a caring relationship is an ethics-based framework within which to examine ethical issues. Moral reasoning involves the intertwining of emotion, cognition, and action (Benjamin & Curtis, 2001).
- **Casuistry or case-based ethics:** An approach to analyzing moral issues or problems based on a formal and systematic method of closely examining cases. Casuists hold that ultimately you can find common moral themes among cases (Beauchamp & Childress, 2009).
- **Character or virtue-based ethics:** An ethics theory where the emphasis is on the agent or the person. The standard is the good person, whom one can rely on to be good and to do good under all circumstances.
- **Communitarianism or community-based theory:** Theories that consider benefit to the community as a whole as the standard by which to make correct moral judgment.
- **Consequentialism (teleological theory):** This theory focuses on consequences and outcomes of a deed or action as the standard by which to make correct moral judgments. Utilitarianism is a teleological theory (Kornblau & Burkhardt, 2012).
- **Deontological theories:** "Duty-driven" theories that focus on one's duties and rights in order to evaluate an ethical course of action and its outcomes (Purtilo & Doherty, 2011).

- **Liberal individualism or rights-based theory:** Theories that focus on a person's individual rights (civil, political, legal) in order to determine an ethical course of action. These rights protect the individual from societal intrusions (Beauchamp & Childress, 2009).
- **Narrative approaches:** Asserts that good moral judgment relies on the analysis and consideration of many voices and accounts of the story before interpreting it for moral significance (Hunter, 2004).
- **Principle-based approach:** Relies on ordinary shared moral beliefs to provide a basis for the evaluation and criticism of actions. General norms guide actions that often leave room for judgment, because principles are "prima facie," meaning one can trump the other (e.g., beneficence, nonmaleficence) (Beauchamp & Childress, 2009).
- **Utilitarianism:** An ethical theory that states the right action is one that maximizes utility (the greater good for the greatest number) and results in the best consequences for all (Slater, 2011).
- **Virtue theory:** A theory that concerns itself with the types of virtues, integrity, or character traits one should display. This theory examines the roles one plays and behavioral expectations each role encourages or requires (Kornblau & Burkhardt, 2012; Sim, 1997).

Gervais, 2005; Hansen & Kyler-Hutchison, 1989; Kornblau & Burkhardt, 2012; Purtilo & Doherty, 2011; Scanlon & Glover, 1995; Swisher, Arslanian, & Davis, 2005). Purtilo and Doherty (2011) have identified the six-step process of ethical decision-making. This decision-making tool was introduced in 1981 and has been used across the health professions and in a variety of settings to help practitioners recognize, critically reason, act, and (perhaps most importantly) reflect on ethical aspects of practice. The six-step process is outlined in Box 18-5. Occupational therapy managers can apply this decision-making model to cases that arise in their practice settings. Through systematic case analysis, practitioners are able to become more aware of their own decision-making and deliver client-centered care with an emphasis on moral conduct.

BOX 18-5

The Six-Step Process of Ethical Decision-Making (Purtilo & Doherty, 2011)

Step 1: Gather Relevant Information
Gathering as much relevant information as possible is essential. Consider the clinical indications, the known (versus believed) facts in the case, the stakeholders, the preference of the client and/or family, and the contextual factors.

Step 2: Identify the Type of Ethical Problem
There may be confounding legal or clinical problems that also apply to the case, but the goal here is to focus on the *moral* ones. Identify if the problem is a moral distress or an ethical dilemma.

Step 3: Use Ethics Theories or Approaches to Analyze the Problem(s)
Which ethics theories or principles apply to the case or situation and why?

Step 4: Explore the Practical Alternative
What is the range of options? Which ethical theories or principles support each alternative? Is one alternative better than another?

Step 5: Complete the Action
The goal of the analysis is to act. Because moral agents are held accountable for their actions, they must call upon their moral courage to complete this crucial step.

Step 6: Evaluate the Process and Outcome
Reflect on the situation to better prepare for the future. What went well? What would you do differently if faced with the same situation again? What were the most challenging aspects of the situation? Reflection on action fosters continued learning.

(With permission from Purtilo, R. B., & Doherty, R. F. (2011). Ethical dimensions in the health professions [5th ed.] Elsevier.)

CASE EXAMPLE 1

Erin, Ray, and Cross-Coverage Competency

Erin is an OT working in a 200-bed acute inpatient rehabilitation hospital. She has over 5 years of clinical experience in rehabilitation with a focus on clients with complex medical needs. Erin is covering a client, Ingrid, for her colleague, Ray. Ingrid is recovering from cardiac bypass complicated by postoperative renal failure and ICU neuropathy. Upon treating the client, Erin notes that she has been prescribed the incorrect splint. She is currently wearing a cock-up wrist splint, but requires a resting hand splint given her level of motor involvement and muscle shortening because of the prolonged ICU stay. Erin also notes that this is a pattern with Ray. She immediately recalls a client whom she covered last month who was in a similar situation.

The next day when Ray returns, Erin talks to him about the client whom she covered. She relays her concern that Ingrid was prescribed the wrong device and reviews with Ray her opinion regarding the insufficient clinical (and research) evidence to support the existing plan. She emphasizes to Ray that the client will not achieve the best outcome from this splint, and may actually be set back by its use. She urges Ray to follow up to ensure best practice standards are met. Ray thanks Erin, saying, "Oh, thanks for covering her. I knew it wasn't the best splint but it is the only one I know how to make. Cindy [the occupational therapy manager] keeps telling me I need to learn more splinting, but I just don't have the time right now. We are so busy."

Erin, Ray, and Cross-Coverage Competency—cont'd

Erin finds herself frustrated by Ray's response. She wraps up the conversation by telling him, "That's not really an option, Ray. We need to make sure our clients get the treatment they need. Ask for help if you need to but just make sure you follow up." The next week Ray is out sick. Erin is once again assigned to cover Ray's client, Ingrid. She reads through the notes and is disappointed and upset to find that the positioning program has not been revised. She realizes she has an ethical problem on her hands and begins to think about her own actions thus far and the options moving forward.

- Does Erin have an ethical problem and, if so, what type?

- What are her professional responsibilities in this case? What types of supports are available to her?
- You are the manager supervising *both* practitioners and have become aware of the situation.
  - What steps should you take to address the issue(s) now that it is brought to your attention?
  - How do competencies, virtues, and abilities relate to the care outcomes of quality and safety?
  - How will you use this situation to inform the ethical culture in your department?

Why Do Managers Need to Learn About Ethics?

In their efforts to support delivery of high-quality services within a given occupational therapy department, managers are well served to recognize that "best practice" and "ethical practice" are inextricably linked. As noted by Christiansen and Lou (2001), ethical issues are part of every health-care encounter, and moral principles such as truth, fairness, doing the right thing, avoiding harm, and respecting autonomy lie at the heart of these ethical concerns. In her 1983 Eleanor Clarke Slagle Lecture, Joan Rogers eloquently articulated the ethics question that clinicians are challenged to answer: "What among the many things that could be done for this patient, ought to be done?" (Rogers, 1983, p. 602). Because the answer to this question involves a *judgment*, influenced by both facts and the client's values, the professional reasoning process terminates in an ethical decision, rather than a scientific one. Thus, the quality of the services provided is directly impacted by a clinician's ability to negotiate the ethics questions experienced in practice.

Occupational therapy practitioners have a legal and ethical responsibility to be competent in the services they are delivering. Concerns related to provider competency can be quite diverse, and range from administering an assessment without proper credentialing to failing to use proper safety precautions during treatment. At the heart of all concerns related to provider competency is the recognition that failure to provide service with competence can result in harm to the patient (maleficence). Failure to act when we know a better way to serve the patient is unethical (Piper, 2011). Although each practitioner is responsible for knowing the laws that regulate practice, the supervisory nature of many managerial positions places increased responsibility on the individual running a department. Occupational therapy managers often evaluate the competency of students entering the field or occupational therapy practitioners working in a new setting (e.g., the neonatal intensive care unit). Ultimately, it is often the occupational therapy manager who is held accountable for both the accomplishments and mistakes occurring within a department. In addition to failing to support best practices within his or her department, a manager who neglects supervisory responsibilities associated with establishing and monitoring provider

Continued

CASE EXAMPLE 1

Why Do Managers Need to Learn About Ethics?—cont'd

competency can be the subject of legal and ethical conduct violations, and may face disciplinary action.

Changes in health-care regulation occur frequently, and often lead practitioners into unfamiliar territory where the luxury of drawing from prior experience is absent. In such situations, ethical problem-solving skills become all the more valuable. National trends impact occupational therapy practice; in some cases, these trends have converged to increase the likelihood of encountering ethical dilemmas in practice. Such trends include new health-care policy, regulations, and delivery systems; expanding cultural diversity; genomics; medical and informational technology advances (including the information explosion and social media); and the issues related to meeting the needs of our aging population. Even the trend of evidence-based practice and outcomes-based care brings with it a number of serious ethical considerations. Christiansen and Lou (2001) described evidence-based practice as a "gift that comes in ethical wrapping." They advised that, from a moral and professional standpoint, the dangers of not attending to the evidence are just as significant as the ethical issues attending to its application.

The overview of national trends provided here is intended to highlight the heightened need for occupational therapy managers to be prepared to address ethical dimensions of practice. Although dealing with moral distress and ethical dilemmas is recognized as a stressful aspect of practice, managers are in strategic positions to support staff and patients who may be confronted with these issues in the care delivery setting.

How Can Managers Actively Support Ethical Practice Within a Department?

Supporting Ethical Behavior

Ethical leadership behaviors have a distinct impact on patient outcomes. Leaders with more complex moral reasoning are more likely to value goals that go beyond immediate self-interest and to foresee the benefits of actions that serve the collective good (Turner, Barling, Epitropaki, Butcher, & Milner, 2002). By helping their staff members examine how their own values are translated into practice, they can evaluate the effectiveness of decisions, actions, and outcomes in a timely manner (Doucette, 2013; Russell, Fitzgerald, Williamson, Manor, & Whybrow, 2002). Kyler (1999) has drawn from previous work (Kanny & Kyler, 1999) to provide a number of suggestions to individuals teaching ethics within occupational therapy curricula. Because the manager's role in supporting ethical practice within a department often parallels the role of an occupational therapy educator, a number of these strategies can be used by managers to support ethical practice within an occupational therapy department. Practical strategies and suggestions for supporting ethical practice (Delany, Edwards, Jensen, & Skinner, 2010; Foglia, Pearlman, Bottrell, Altemose & Fox, 2013; Kanny & Kyler, 1999; Kyler, 1999; Wells, 2003) are presented in Box 18-6.

It is important to note that the process of supporting ethical practice among staff members begins with the creation of a moral culture and a *milieu* that supports staff members' involvement in identification and resolution of ethical problems. Within a supportive environment, an occupational therapy manager can help staff members gain an awareness of values shared by the entire health-care team, including those that may or may not be shared by clients and their families.

In the end, the positive outcomes yielded by fostering attention to, and resolution of, ethical problems

BOX 18-6

Supporting Ethical Practice Within Occupational Therapy Departments: Suggestions for Managers

- Recognize that supporting ethical practice within a department requires managers to first explore their own values and develop their own ethical reasoning skills in order to be comfortable with the topic.
- Model appropriate sensitivity to ethical issues. Share and explain your decisions on ethical issues as they arise.
- Communicate clear expectations for ethical practice. Anticipate the barriers your staff may face in meeting these expectations.
- Examine ethics theories, principles, and related concepts, and incorporate discussion of ethics theories and principles into conversations about patient care to make these connections.
- Identify formal and informal avenues to improve cultural competence.
- Help staff members recognize the ethical significance of their values, employer policies, individual decisions, and group decisions.
- Identify the channels that the recipient of services or health-care practitioner may utilize to resolve a problem or serve as a resource.
- Understand the formal and informal ethics dispute resolution systems that have jurisdiction over occupational therapy practice.
- Be able to quickly access resources (including internal, institution-specific documents and AOTA documents) that can be used to guide behavior, and know the content of those documents.
- Support the ethics program or committee in your institution.
- Help clinicians realize that their own positions cannot simply be a matter of opinion.
- Support discussions of explanations and professional reasoning.
- Actively listen to others and help staff recognize that listening to others is vitally important to the formulation of cogent arguments and decisions. Listen actively, think reflectively, and reason critically.
- Facilitate the formulation of questions that arise out of ethically stressful situations.
- Appreciate the "messiness." Humans are complex, so there are no easy answers. There are often convincing arguments on both sides of an ethical issue.
- Recognize that reorganization disrupts the flow of care delivery. Anticipate with staff any ethical implications of change processes.

Source: Foglia, Pearlman, Bottrell, Altemose, and Fox (2013); Delany, Edwards, Jensen, and Skinner (2010); Wells (2003); Kyler (1999); and Kanny and Kyler (1999).

among staff are many. In addition to being better able to manage ethical problems, staff members who learn skills associated with analyzing moral distress and ethical dilemmas will be capable of more thoughtful decision-making in treatment, which should influence the quality of care provided. Additionally, those clinicians will be better prepared to manage the day-to-day stress associated with patient care, and may be better equipped to avoid the "burn out" experienced by so many health professionals. When faced with difficult ethical decisions, the manager must be ever-present in the discussion, employ active listening, and ask clarify-

ing questions. It is helpful for managers to compassionately acknowledge both the clinician's and the client's feelings and emotions. Managers can recognize that it may not be possible to provide answers to all questions. However, it is helpful to be honest and to display a willingness to further explore issues.

Ethics Committees

When strategies to support application of ethics in professional practice are examined, it is important to discuss the role of institution-based ethics committees. Occupational therapy managers who ensure occupational therapy representation on organization-wide ethics committees are taking highly visible and productive steps toward bringing core values into sharper focus and enhancing practice. Ethics committees are vital internal supports to all health-care organizations. Whether at the discipline-specific level or the hospital or organization level, it is essential that OTs and OTAs are prepared to participate on these committees.

Ethics committees provide an environment for safe and open discussion of moral questions that can range from basic to complex. Ethics committees are interprofessional; in this way, topics and cases can be reviewed and analyzed from many different perspectives. Morality is a culture, and ethics committees promote this culture by helping staff members with different beliefs, cultures, and professional codes observe and explore important issues. It is important to remember that different staff groups within the same institution, or even the same profession, may speak different clinical languages and be bound by different codes of ethics; hence, the interprofessional approach to ethics is rich in debate and analysis. For example, an OT may be bound by his or her code of ethics to discharge a patient who is making no gains in therapy and no longer has a need for services based on his or her functional status. The nurse for the same patient is bound by her code of ethics to never desert this patient as long as he or she remains in need of care.

Ideally, interprofessional ethics committees include representation from each clinical discipline. A typical committee includes a physician, nurse, social worker, OT, physical therapist (PT), case manager, speech–language pathologist, chaplain, respiratory therapist, pharmacist, administrator, and patient advocate or community representative. Ethics committees in different institutions have different charges. Most serve to consult, educate, and assist with policy review and development. They empower staff members as they provide a process to handle difficult ethical issues and ease the potential emotional responses of staff. Ethics committees serve to encourage decisions in accordance with ethical institutional policies. They are also able to provide the institution with case histories so that trends and decisions can be monitored at the organizational level.

Ethics Consultation

In addition to ethics committees, many institutions may have an ethicist or ethics consultant on staff. When a care team requests ethics consultation, also known as an "ethics consult," it may be answered by an individual or committee. The overarching goal of ethics consultation is to facilitate resolution of conflicts in a respectful atmosphere with attention to the interests, rights, and responsibilities of those involved. In 2011, the American Society for Bioethics and Humanities (ASBH) published its second edition of the *Core Competencies for Health Care Ethics Consultation* (ASBH, 2011). This work built on previous work in the field that identified the following skills required for ethics consultation: ethics assessment skills, process skills, and interpersonal skills (Aulisio, Arnold, & Younger, 2000). Ethics assessment skills are necessary to distinguish the ethical dimensions of the case and identify morally acceptable options and their associated consequences. This includes core knowledge in moral reasoning and common ethics domains. Process skills are needed to resolve values uncertainty or conflict. Interpersonal skills are necessary so active listening and communication that is respectful, supportive, and empathetic to all parties involved occurs. Consultants today also require competency in evaluative and quality improvement skills as they relate to ethics consultation and care delivery. They must effectively facilitate and document mediation processes and recommendations to the patient care team and other stakeholders.

Occupational therapy practitioners are a natural fit for institutional and organizational ethics committees. Ethics encompasses values clarification, shared decision-making, meaningful participation, and narrative reasoning—all skills that occupational therapy professionals are highly knowledgeable in. Occupational therapy practitioners have unique training in understanding and applying meaningful occupation. They typically follow clients throughout the life span and bring a broad spectrum of knowledge to ethics committees. Occupational therapy practitioners are also skilled facilitators and understand group dynamics, which is always needed when debating heated moral issues.

Managers who support their occupational therapy staff's participation on ethics committees will find that committee membership brings with it many benefits to their occupational therapy department. The ethics committee member undergoes intense education and training in ethics. He or she then brings this expanded knowledge base to the occupational therapy department and assists in the departmental facilitation of "difficult discussions." The committee member serves as a resource to both other disciplines in the hospital and the occupational therapy staff to promote values clarification and mentor less experienced staff in applying ethical reasoning to their professional practice. In a study of PTs and OTs, Barnitt (1998) found that dealing with ethical dilemmas was a skilled and stressful aspect of practice. The study also found that one of the positive influences on this stress was support from peers. The occupational therapy representative on the ethics committee is able to provide this support. This in turn leads to improved coping skills among staff and an environment that supports moral courage and ethical practice.

In the event that you manage an occupational therapy department or service in an organization that does not have a facility-wide ethics committee, there are other resources to turn to. The facility's partnering or umbrella organization may have a broader-based committee that serves to address the ethics. Other internal facility resources include the advocacy office (or an ombudsman service), the social services department, chaplaincy services, the human resources department, and the institutional review board as related to research activities. It is important to remember that ethics resources should always be readily accessible, and that staff members need to know that their occupational therapy administration is on the front line when it comes to dealing with ethics questions that arise in professional practice. A supportive administration promotes reflective practitioners.

CASE EXAMPLE 2

Linda and the Not-So-Smart Smartphone

Barbara is the director of rehabilitation services at The Kaplan Family Group Home. Barbara received a call from Susan Brenner, the home's director, who told her that she needed to see her in the administrative offices immediately. Susan subsequently told Barbara that they received a complaint from a family member this morning regarding the actions of Linda, a COTA who has worked at the home for over 13 years. Linda was working with Thomas, a resident with severe development delay, when the two found themselves in a peculiar situation. Linda was attempting to help Thomas transfer out of his chair in the dining room to get to the group room when they realized he was literally stuck between the two arms of the chair. Thomas roared with laughter, saying, "I guess I ate too much." Linda tried to make light of the situation and said to Thomas, "If you could only see yourself." She then took out her smartphone, took a picture of Thomas, and showed it to him. After some quick thinking, the two of them managed to safely wiggle the rear side of the chair arm free and transfer Thomas out

of the chair. Later that evening Linda was out to dinner with friends. She checked the time on her smartphone and it was then she found the picture, saying to her friends, "Look at this—the funniest thing happened to me and one of my favorite patients today." She showed her friends the picture of Thomas and they laughed, sharing stories of odd things in the workplace.

Thomas's cousin happened to be the waitress waiting on Linda and her friends at the restaurant. Thomas's mother told Susan that in addition to filing a complaint with The Kaplan Family Group Home, she was also planning on filing with the State Licensure Board and that she expected "swift action" on this violation of her son's rights. Barbara has known Linda for 7 years and trusts that she would never intentionally harm Thomas or any of her clients; however, she is extremely disappointed and knows that she must take steps to address the situation.

Continued

CASE EXAMPLE 2

Linda and the Not-So-Smart Smartphone—cont'd

- Linda failed to uphold her legal and ethical obligation of maintaining the confidentiality and privacy of her patients at all times. What ethical principle does this violate?
- Barbara is faced with an ethical problem. What type of problem is it? Is this a moral distress or an ethical dilemma?
- There is a confounding legal problem in this case as well. Describe the nature of the legal problem for both Linda as a licensed individual and The Kaplan Family Group Home as an organization.
- What resources are available to Barbara as a manager? If you were in her shoes, what actions would you take to resolve this situation and prevent similar situations from happening in the future?

How Does the Profession Support Ethical Behavior?

A number of strategies that department managers can use to support ethical practice among staff members have been presented. This discussion of external supports and regulations focuses on the following groups: accreditation bodies, NBCOT, our professional membership organization (AOTA), and bodies responsible for state regulation of occupational therapy. These bodies assist occupational therapy practitioners in understanding their responsibilities to practice both ethically and legally. They also act as resources to the public and provide vehicles for filing complaints when it is believed that rules have been violated.

Accreditation

Accreditation is a process by which an institution or organization seeks to demonstrate to an accrediting agency that it complies with generally accepted standards set forth by appropriate professional organizations. Accreditation status is awarded to an organization that demonstrates compliance with standards established by the accrediting body. Accreditation may be voluntary (e.g., Commission on Accreditation of Rehabilitation Facilities), mandatory at a state level

(e.g., licensure to operate), or required in practicality (e.g., The Joint Commission accreditation is tied to reimbursement). Accreditation signifies to consumers of services that agencies have met predetermined, generally recognized standards. Accreditation is relevant to initiatives to develop and maintain ethical practices because many accrediting agencies require accredited institutions to have policies (e.g., patient nondiscrimination policy) and processes (e.g., case consultation) that support ethical practice. For example, The Joint Commission requires that all health-care organizations have a process to address ethical issues related to patient care and organizational ethics. The Joint Commission rules specifically require that institutions must have a process to examine ethical issues in marketing, admissions, discharges, billing, and relationships with third-party payers.

A single health-care institution may be accredited by more than one accreditation body. It is important for managers to know which accreditation bodies their organization is accredited by (and accreditation goals set by their organization), the expectation guidelines set forth by each accrediting agency, and how their department-specific accreditation activities fit in with their organization's overall accreditation policies and activities. Often hospitalwide accreditation activities complement, and can build upon, the accreditation activities going on within individual departments.

Regulation of Occupational Therapy Practice

Occupational therapists and occupational therapy assistants are typically regulated by both state regulatory boards (SRBs) and NBCOT. These regulatory agencies share the function of protecting the public; however, they perform this function in different ways.

State Regulatory Boards

Occupational therapy is regulated in all 50 states and three U.S. territories, but the level of regulation varies significantly. Most states have determined that **licensure** is the most effective approach to regulating occupational therapy practitioners. All 53 jurisdictions in the United States (50 states, the District of Columbia, Guam, and Puerto Rico) have licensure laws for OTs and OTAs. Collectively known as SRBs, these regulatory bodies serve, safeguard, and promote the public welfare by ensuring that qualifications and standards for professional practice are properly evaluated, accurately applied, and vigorously enforced. In some states, SRBs protect the public by prohibiting practice by unlicensed OTs or OTAs.

It is important to appreciate the distinction between licensure and other forms of regulation. Generally, unlike certification, registration, and trademark laws, a licensure law defines a lawful scope of practice for practitioners. Defining a scope of practice legally articulates the domain of practice and provides guidance to facilities, providers, consumers, and major public and private health and education facilities on the appropriate use of services and practitioners. Defining practice can further ensure important *patient protections* by offering guidance on appropriate care, particularly in the investigation and resolution of consumer complaints involving fraudulent or negligent delivery of services.

The SRBs have the authority provided by state law to discipline occupational therapy practitioners who violate regulations. States that include codes of ethics (or statements describing the ethical conduct expected by occupational therapy practitioners) in their laws can discipline practitioners who violate those codes. Drawing on the example of provider competency used earlier in this chapter, working outside a scope of practice often raises serious concerns regarding provider competency and increases risk of harm to the patient, and thus is one example of a violation that represents both legal and ethical misconduct.

Although state procedures for processing complaints are not uniform, the process used in Illinois is provided as an example of how a state might process a complaint. After an initial review within the Illinois Department of Professional Regulation, a complaint is assigned to a department investigator. The investigator is responsible for determining whether or not there has been a potential violation of a licensing law or department rules and regulations. After developing the facts in cases in which there appears to be a violation, the investigator refers the case to a prosecuting attorney. If the staff attorney concludes that the matter has been sufficiently investigated and there is evidence supporting the complaint, formal charges are filed. Disciplinary actions imposed by states range from censure (a formal expression of disapproval that is publicly announced) to temporary suspension of practice privileges (the loss of certification for a certain duration, after which the individual may be required to apply for reinstatement) or permanent prohibition from practice in the state.

The National Board for Certification in Occupational Therapy

The overarching functions of NBCOT were described earlier in this chapter. It is essential for every occupational therapy practitioner to understand the central role that NBCOT has in the regulation of occupational therapy practice. NBCOT has jurisdiction over all individuals who are certified by it, as well as those individuals who have applied to take the certification examinations. NBCOT is centrally concerned with "safe, proficient and/or competent practice in occupational therapy practice" (NBCOT, 2014a, n.p.). To that end, the NBCOT Code of Conduct contains many principles that reflect expectations of ethical practice.

NBCOT investigates complaints against occupational therapy practitioners as a means of protecting the public. The Disciplinary Action Information Exchange Network (DAIEN) contains a listing of final disciplinary actions and nondisciplinary actions taken by NBCOT, as well as disciplinary actions taken by state regulatory entities. Actions are posted to the DAIEN on a quarterly basis and removed after 1 year.

Although NBCOT's disciplinary actions are independent of SRBs or AOTA's EC, NBCOT communicates with other bodies that serve disciplinary functions, including state regulatory agencies.

NBCOT's disciplinary actions (reprimand, ineligibility for certification, censure, probation, suspension, and revocation of certification) are overseen by the NBCOT's Qualifications and Compliance Review Committee. An explanation of the NBCOT's disciplinary action program is easily accessed via its website (http://www.nbcot.org).

Any manager who has concerns about unethical conduct can call NBCOT and discuss those concerns with staff involved in the disciplinary action program. NBCOT staff members are available to offer direction on filing a complaint with NBCOT, as well as other areas where it may be appropriate to file a complaint (such as with an SRB or AOTA). In addition, NBCOT staff would convey information about NBCOT's disciplinary action process, direct the manager to the NBCOT Web page for additional information on the disciplinary process, and offer other possible options that an administrator may want to consider given the concerns conveyed.

The AOTA and Ethics

AOTA is committed to both educating practitioners about ethical occupational therapy practice and enforcing the ethical standards of the profession. As a voluntary professional organization, AOTA has no direct authority over occupational therapy personnel who are not members. It does, however, have limited authority over members regardless of their role (e.g., practitioner, educator, consultant, researcher, or scholar). In contrast, other bodies that regulate occupational therapy are primarily concerned with the actions of practitioners.

The Ethics Commission (EC), which is one of the bodies of the Representative Assembly (RA) of AOTA, leads AOTA in its ethics education and enforcement initiatives. The EC is made up of nine members, including two public members and AOTA's legal counsel. The EC can be contacted via e-mail at ethics@aota.org for assistance and resources to resolve ethical concerns.

The EC has produced numerous resources to describe, define, and support the values to which those within the profession should aspire. Key among these resources is the Occupational Therapy Code of Ethics (AOTA, 2015), which includes core values, principles, and standards of conduct. Additional resources written by EC members include the *Reference Guide to the Occupational Therapy Code of Ethics and Ethics Standards* (Slater, 2011); advisory opinions and articles appearing in *OT Practice*, which is the clinical and professional magazine of AOTA; and the enforcement procedures for the Occupational Therapy Code of Ethics (available at http://www.aota.org/en/Practice/Ethics/EC). The latter provides specific information about the EC's disciplinary process. The AOTA website features links to frequently requested documents that support the professional community, advisory opinions that cover a variety of topics with ethical implications, and a link to a page featuring frequently asked questions about ethics. Descriptions of disciplinary actions that can be taken by AOTA (i.e., reprimand, censure, probation, suspension of membership, and permanent revocation of membership) and a listing of disciplinary actions taken can be found in the ethics section of the AOTA website.

CASE EXAMPLE 3

Miguel—An Ounce of Prevention

Miguel has been employed by Seven Winds, a company that owns four large skilled nursing facilities in Illinois, for 11 years. Miguel moved into a managerial role 3 years ago and now supervises six OTRs and seven COTAs. These OTRs and COTAs work across the four skilled nursing facilities owned by Seven Winds. Miguel, like all members of the rehabilitation team, is a member of AOTA. Last week, at a meeting led by top administrators within Seven Winds, Miguel learned that the company was

CASE EXAMPLE 3

Miguel—An Ounce of Prevention—cont'd

in trouble financially and that it was likely that at least one-fourth of the rehabilitation division would be cut if the financial picture did not improve in the next 6 months. Additionally, the administrators disclosed that there was a real possibility that one of the four skilled nursing facilities would be closed. Miguel was very concerned about this because the staff and residents of the facility at highest risk for closure had created a strong community. Miguel knew that many of the people who lived there were long-time residents who considered the skilled nursing facility their home. The administrators, none of whom were occupational therapy practitioners, listed a number of strategies to increase revenues. Providing more group-based occupational therapy and physical therapy interventions was discussed at length and described as an "optimal strategy." The administrators also made it clear that they expected to see at least a 20% increase in rehabilitation revenues over the next 6 months. In a private conversation, one of the administrators told Miguel that scheduling therapy appointments "creatively" so there was overlap between patients seen and individual charges would be encouraged

to generate more revenue. Miguel recognized that if communicated to the staff as such, the imperative to increase rehabilitation revenues, combined with the administrators' suggested strategies and views on how to increase those revenues, may tempt the OTRs and COTAs to charge patients for individual treatment, when they actually received group-based services. Miguel knew he had to be proactive to prevent this situation from occurring.

- Miguel's goal is to be proactive and prevent a breach of professional conduct. How can he best explain to administration his concern regarding the proposed billing strategy?
- What ethical theories and principles help support Miguel in his decision-making?
- Is Miguel faced with an ethical problem? If so, what is it?
- What resources are available to Miguel?
- How do the AOTA Code of Ethics, the NBCOT Code of Conduct, and the State of Illinois Licensure Act serve as supporting resources to Miguel?

Some Final Thoughts on Occupational Therapy Managers and Ethics

Occupational therapists, occupational therapy assistants, and occupational therapy fieldwork students are holistic practitioners who interact with diverse individuals, organizations, and health-care teams in the ever-changing field of professional practice. Occupational therapy managers need to be comfortable responding to ethical issues on a case-by-case basis. They must use their skills in moral reasoning and ethical analysis to effectively lead and mentor their staff, addressing ethics quality gaps on both the individual and systems levels. Creating a supportive workplace environment that facilitates the exploration of

values and ethics resources promotes best practice. In an ethical culture and environment, employee "burnout" can be minimized and professionalism can be fostered in a collaborative fashion. In summary, supporting ethical programs and fostering ethical reasoning among practitioners is an inherent part of good occupational therapy practice and administration.

Chapter Summary

This chapter introduced you to common characterizations of a *profession* and what it means to be a *professional*. Being a member of a profession carries with it associated responsibilities, including joining and sustaining membership in your state occupational therapy association and in AOTA. AOTA's purpose and structure, as well as the purpose of other related organizations and bodies, were reviewed.

A primary focus of this chapter was an introduction to ethics as a discipline and branch of philosophy that the occupational therapy manager can use to guide practice and to respond to the common ethical concerns that managers and practitioners encounter. Terminology related to ethics principles and concepts was defined and numerous ethics theories were listed. Supports for the manager to guide ethical practice both internal and external to the profession were provided, and case examples illustrated some of the common dilemmas that managers and the staff members they supervise face.

Occupational therapists, occupational therapy assistants, occupational therapy fieldwork students, and especially occupational therapy managers must understand the professional systems in which they operate if they hope to have an influence on the contexts in which they practice. There are numerous ways that we can support our profession, ranging from joining and sustaining membership in professional organizations to volunteering for a wide variety of leadership roles available at both the state and national levels. If we choose not to be active participants and responsible professionals, we also abdicate our right to complain about the system in which we practice.

At the start of the chapter, you were introduced to Ellyn, who had become frustrated with some of the staff members with whom she worked because they complained about events occurring within their profession but did not have membership in their state occupational therapy association or AOTA. Ellyn worked with her manager and coworkers to create a plan to enhance the professionalism in her department. As the leader of her department, Ellen's manager will be an important influence on the effectiveness of this plan.

■ Real-Life Solutions

The director of the department in which Ellyn worked agreed that an in-service education presentation on becoming "responsible professionals" was a good start to their "professionalism" initiative. To prepare, Ellyn gathered information on AOTA, her state occupational therapy association, and other related organizations and bodies that influenced the practice of occupational therapy in her state. As she did this, she realized that there was much that she did not know about the structure of these bodies and the many volunteer opportunities that were available. She was particularly interested in the process that the RA used to make decisions and to charge various AOTA committees and commissions with doing work on behalf of the association.

Initially, Ellyn had felt quite angry at her coworkers about the attitude they had adopted. To her, it seemed that they were blaming others for developments when they had not accepted responsibility for participating in the process. As she began to prepare her presentation, however, it struck her that, without understanding how the various bodies were organized and how they completed their business, it might be easy to assume that an individual could have little impact on the end results. Ellyn decided to focus her presentation on the organization of AOTA and related bodies, such as AOTF, AOTPAC, her state association, NBCOT, and the state regulatory board, and on the many ways that individuals could participate in the process of influencing the service provided to society by the occupational therapy profession.

Study Questions

1. **Which of the following is a professional body incorporated in 1917 to represent the interests and concerns of occupational therapy practitioners and students of occupational therapy and to improve the quality of occupational therapy services?**

   a. National Board for Certification of Occupational Therapy, Inc.
   b. American Occupational Therapy Association
   c. Fund to Promote Occupational Therapy
   d. American Occupational Therapy Political Action Committee

2. **Which of the following best describes the purpose of the AOTA code of ethics?**

   a. To guide members toward ethical courses of action in professional and volunteer roles
   b. To outline the standard of conduct the public can expect
   c. To delineate enforceable principles and standards of conduct that apply to AOTA members
   d. All of the above

3. **Which of the following best describes an ethical dilemma?**

   a. A conflict between ethical beliefs involving choices between alternatives that appear equally morally acceptable
   b. A conflict in which there is a clear moral choice and a clear immoral choice (the right versus wrong scenario)
   c. A conflict in which there is no true moral option (the lesser of the two evils scenario)
   d. A conflict between approaches to distribution of available resources and rewards

4. **Which of the following is true regarding the American Occupational Therapy Political Action Committee (AOTPAC)?**

   a. AOTPAC only provides contributions to candidates from the ruling majority party.
   b. The purpose of AOTPAC is to further the legislative aims of AOTA by attempting to influence the selection, nomination, election, or appointment of persons to elected office.
   c. AOTPAC is a committee of the Association under direct authority of the AOTA Board of Directors.
   d. AOTPAC raises money through solicitation of donations and selling advocacy-related continuing education and products.

5. **Which of the following is true regarding state regulatory boards?**

   a. The role of state regulatory boards is to enforce rules established to define and regulate occupational therapy, which are established at a national level.
   b. Less than half of the states in the United States have a state regulatory board responsible for oversight of some aspect of occupational therapy practice.
   c. State regulatory boards refer all issues related to ethical breaches or other disciplinary matters to AOTA for review and determination.
   d. None of the above is true.

6. **Which of the following is accurate regarding the governance structure of AOTA?**

   a. AOTA is governed by a single governing body responsible for the association's policy, finances, and promotional activities.
   b. All members of the governing bodies of AOTA are paid professionals hired to carry out their roles and responsibilities.
   c. The executive director of AOTA must be an OT with at least 10 years of experience as defined in the bylaws of the association.
   d. The Representative Assembly is AOTA's "congress" and is responsible for oversight of professional policy as one of the association's two main governing bodies.

7. **Which of the following is concerned with ethics and ethical practice?**

   a. National Board for Certification in Occupational Therapy
   b. American Occupational Therapy Association
   c. State regulatory boards
   d. All of the above

8. **The process of ethical decision making is often as important as the outcome. The *first* step in the ethical decision making process is:**

   a. Gather relevant information.
   b. Consult the ethics committee.
   c. Explore practical alternatives.
   d. Use ethics theories to analyze the problem.

Resources for Learning More About Participating in a Profession

Journals That Often Include Articles About Professionalism and Ethics

Cambridge Quarterly of Health Care Ethics

http://journals.cambridge.org/action/
displayJournal?jid=CQH

The *Cambridge Quarterly of Health Care Ethics* is designed to meet the needs of professionals serving on health-care ethics committees in hospitals, nursing homes, hospices, and rehabilitation centers. The aim of the journal is to serve as the international forum for the wide range of serious and urgent issues faced by members of health-care ethics committees, physicians, nurses, social workers, clergy, lawyers, and community representatives.

The Journal of Clinical Ethics

http://www.clinicalethics.com/

The Journal of Clinical Ethics is a leading peer-reviewed journal written for and by physicians, nurses, attorneys, clergy, ethicists, and others whose decisions directly affect patients. It is a partner journal of *American Society of Bioethics and Humanities*.

American Journal of Bioethics

http://www.tandfonline.com/loi/uajb20#
.VfM957U09NI

The American Journal of Bioethics provides readers with peer-reviewed scholarship about ethical issues in medicine and the biomedical sciences. Journal content includes many disciplines, including health care, medicine, public health, philosophy, biomedical science, religion, law, health services research, and social work.

Journal of Interprofessional Care

http://www.tandfonline.com/loi/ijic20#.VfM-CrU09NI

The *Journal of Interprofessional Care* is an international journal that disseminates research and new developments in the field of interprofessional education and practice. Contributions contain an explicit interpro-fessional focus, and involve a range of settings, professions, and fields.

Professional Organizations Concerned With the Profession of Occupational Therapy

The American Occupational Therapy Association

http://www.aota.org/

The mission of AOTA advances the quality, availability, use, and support of occupational therapy through standard setting, advocacy, education, and research on behalf of its members and the public. AOTA provides its members with a variety of resources and supports to promote responsible participation in the profession of occupational therapy. AOTA promotes awareness on the part of the general public of occupational therapy, advocates at the national and state legislative levels, supports state occupational therapy associations, and provides members and managers with resources for dealing with ethical dilemmas.

The American Occupational Therapy Foundation

http://www.aotf.org/

Through the use of fiscal and human resources, AOTF expands and refines the body of knowledge of occupational therapy and promotes understanding of the value of occupation in the interest of the public good. AOTF promotes a society in which individuals, regardless of age or ability, may participate in occupations of their choice that give meaning to their lives, and foster health and well-being. The goals of AOTF include securing contributions and managing assets, promoting scientific inquiry, and supporting excellence in education about occupation and occupational therapy.

The American Occupational Therapy Political Action Committee

http://www.aota.org/advocacy-policy/aotpac.aspx

AOTPAC is a voluntary, nonprofit, unincorporated committee of members of AOTA. AOTPAC was authorized by the RA in 1976 and has been operational since the spring of 1978. The purpose of AOTPAC is to further the legislative aims of AOTA by influencing or attempting to influence the selection, nomination, election, or appointment of any individual to any federal public office, and of any OT, OTA, or occupational therapy student member of AOTA seeking election to public office at any level.

The National Board for Certification in Occupational Therapy, Inc. (NBCOT)

http://www.nbcot.org/

NBCOT is a nonprofit credentialing agency responsible for certification for the occupational therapy profession. NBCOT develops, administers, and continually reviews a certification process that reflects current standards of entry-level practice in occupational therapy. NBCOT also works with state regulatory authorities, providing information on credentials, disciplinary actions, and regulatory and certification renewal issues. NBCOT is responsible for establishing initial competency through its certification examination and has requirements for maintaining certification related to continuing education to promote continued competency.

Professional Organizations Concerned With Interprofessional Collaboration and Education

The American Interprofessional Health Collaborative (AIHC)

http://www.aihc-us.org/

The AIHC aims to transcend boundaries and transform learning, policies, practices, and scholarship toward an improved system of health and wellness for individual patients, communities, and populations. The American Interprofessional Health Collaborative believes educating those entrusted with the health of individuals, communities, and populations to value and respect each other's unique expertise and skills and to work together is fundamental to care that is effective, safe, of high quality, and efficient in terms of cost, resources, and time. AIHC is composed of individuals

and organizations committed to assuring health in all policies and systems impacting health and care delivery.

The National Center for Interprofessional Practice and Education

https://nexusipe.org

The National Center for Interprofessional Practice and Education (Nexus) leads, coordinates, and studies the advancement of collaborative, team-based health professions education and patient care as an efficient model for improving quality, outcomes, and cost. Housed at the University of Minnesota, it is a public–private partnership created in 2012 through a cooperative agreement with the U.S. Health Resources and Services Administration and three private foundations.

The National Academies of Practice (NAP)

https://www.napractice.org/eweb/startpage.aspx

NAP is a nonprofit organization founded in 1981 to advise governmental bodies on our health-care system. Distinguished practitioners and scholars are elected by their peers from 10 different health professions to join the only interprofessional group of health-care practitioners and scholars dedicated to supporting affordable, accessible, coordinated quality health care for all. NAP believes that health care should encompass physical, behavioral, and social health and include prevention as a core strategy. NAP holds national forums and publishes policy papers on important interprofessional health-care topics reflecting current and future issues about practice, education, policy, and research.

The Interprofessional Education Collaborative

https://ipecollaborative.org/

The Interprofessional Education Collaborative (IPEC) was formed in 2009 by six national education associations of schools in the health professions. IPEC serves to "promote and encourage constituent efforts that would advance substantive interprofessional learning experiences to help prepare future clinicians for team-based care of patients." IPEC has published several high-quality, peer-reviewed, competency-based resources and learning modules for interprofessional health education and collaborative practice.

Useful Resources on Ethics

The National Center for Ethics in Healthcare

http://www.ethics.va.gov

The National Center for Ethics in Healthcare (NCEHC) serves as the VA's authoritative resource for addressing complex ethical issues that arise in patient care, health-care management, and research. In an effort to establish a national, standardized, comprehensive, systematic, integrated approach to ethics in health care, the VA launched the Integrated Ethics Program in 2008. This innovative model is based on established methods for achieving performance excellence, principles of continuous quality improvement, and proven strategies for organizational change.

The Integrated Ethics Web Page

http://www.ethics.va.gov/integratedethics

The Integrated Ethics Web page provides comprehensive resources for promoting, measuring, and improving performance relating to ethics. These include a focus on ethical leadership with tools in ethical leadership self-assessment, ethical decision-making tools, and other ethics activities that can be used in various health-care delivery settings.

The Hastings Center

http://www.thehastingscenter.org

The Hastings Center is an independent, nonpartisan, and nonprofit bioethics research institute founded in 1969. Its mission is "to address fundamental ethical issues in the areas of health, medicine, and the environment as they affect individuals, communities, and societies." The Hastings Center has identified the following five broad areas where the nation and global community face serious challenges and where bioethics can help: health and health care; children and families; aging, chronic illness, and care near the end of life; emerging science and conceptions of the self; and

human impact on the natural world. The Hastings Center publishes several reports and resources, including BioEthics Forum (http://www.thehastingscenter.org/BioethicsForum), a blog for diverse commentary on issues in bioethics.

The Ethics Resource Center (ERC)

http://www.ethics.org

The ERC is a nonprofit, nonpartisan educational organization devoted to independent research and the advancement of high ethical standards and practices in public and private institutions. Founded in 1922, the ERC's mission is to strengthen ethical leadership worldwide by providing leading-edge expertise and services through research, education, and partnerships. The ERC has a stated vision of promoting a world in which individuals and organizations act with integrity. ERC researchers analyze current and emerging issues and produce new ideas and benchmarks that matter for the public trust. They publish national surveys and resources, including webinars and ethics toolkits with practical guides that support organizational ethics.

Reference List

American Heritage College Dictionary (3rd ed.). (1993). Boston, MA: Houghton Mifflin.

American Occupational Therapy Association. (2015). Occupational Therapy Code of Ethics (2015. *American Journal of Occupational Therapy, 69*(Suppl. 3).

American Occupational Therapy Association. (2014a). *About AOTA*. Retrieved from http:// www.aota.org.

American Occupational Therapy Association. (2014b). *About the fund to promote awareness of occupational therapy*. Retrieved from http://www.promoteot.org/AF_AboutTheFund.html.

American Occupational Therapy Association. (2014c). *AOTPAC fact sheet*. Retrieved from http://www.aota.org.

American Occupational Therapy Foundation. (2014a). *American Occupational Therapy Foundation mission*. Retrieved from http:// www.aotf.org/aboutaotf/visionmissiongoals

American Occupational Therapy Foundation. (2014b). *AOTA/ AOTF Research Advisory Panel*. Retrieved from http://www.aotf.org/programspartnerships/jointinitiativeswithaota/aotaaotfresearchadvisorypanel.aspx.

American Society for Bioethics and Humanities' Core Competencies Update Task Force. (2011). *Core competencies for health care ethics consultation: The report of the American Society for Bioethics and Humanities* (2nd ed.). Glenview, IL: American Society for Bioethics and Humanities.

Aulisio, M. P., Arnold, R. M., & Younger, S. J. (2000). Health care ethics consultation: Nature, goals and competencies. A position paper from the Society for Health and Human Values–Society for Bioethics Consultation Task Force on Standards for Bioethics Consultation. *Annals of Internal Medicine, 133*, 59–69.

Bailey, D. M., & Schwartzberg, S. L. (2003). *Ethical and legal dilemmas*. Philadelphia, PA: F. A. Davis.

Barnitt, R. (1998). Ethical dilemmas in occupational therapy and physical therapy: A survey of practitioners in the UK National Health Service. *Journal of Medical Ethics, 24*, 193–199.

Beauchamp, T. L., & Childress, J. F. (2009). *Principles of biomedical ethics* (6th ed.). New York, NY: Oxford University Press.

Benjamin, M., & Curtis, J. (2001). *Ethics in nursing*. New York, NY: Oxford University Press.

Christiansen, C., & Lou, J. Q. (2001). Evidence-based practice forum: Ethical considerations related to evidence-based practice. *The American Journal of Occupational Therapy, 55*, 345–349.

Corbett, K. (1993). Ethics in occupational therapy practice. *Canadian Journal of Occupational Therapy, 60*, 115–119.

Cruess, S. R., Johnston, S., & Cruess, R. L. (2004). "Profession": A working definition for medical educators. *Teaching and Learning in Medicine, 16*(1), 74–76.

Delany, C. M., Edwards, I., Jensen, G. M., & Skinner, E. (2010). Closing the gap between ethics knowledge and practice through active engagement: An applied model of physical therapy ethics. *Physical Therapy, 90*(7), 1068–1078.

Diffendal, J. (2002). The rules: Knowing laws and ethics makes good OT practice. *Advance for Occupational Therapy Practitioners, 18*(4), 9–11.

Doherty, R. F., Dellinger, A., Gately, M., Pullo, R., & Sullivan, S. (2012). *Ethical issues in occupational therapy: A survey of practitioners*. Poster presented at the American Occupational Therapy Association 2012 Annual Conference, Indianapolis, IN.

Doucette, J. N. (2013). Decision making through the ethics lens. *Nursing Management, 44*(9), 46–50.

Foglia, M. B., Pearlman, R. A., Bottrell, M., Altemose, J. K., & Fox, E. (2009). Ethical challenges within Veterans Administration Healthcare Facilities: Perspectives of managers, clinicians, patients, and ethics committee chairpersons. *The American Journal of Bioethics, 9*(4), 28–36.

Foye, S. J., Kirschner, K. L., Brady-Wagner, L. C., Stocking, C., & Siegler, M. (2002). Ethical issues in rehabilitation: A qualitative analysis of dilemmas identified by occupational therapists. *Topics in Stroke Rehabilitation, 9*, 89–101.

Gervais, K. G. (2005). A model for ethical decision making to inform the ethics education of future professionals. In R. Purtilo, G. M. Jensen, & C. B. Royeen (Eds.), *Educating for moral action: A sourcebook in health and rehabilitation ethics* (pp. 185–190). Philadelphia, PA: F. A. Davis.

Hack, L. M. (2005). Disparity in practice: Healing the breach. In R. Purtilo, G. M. Jensen, & C. B. Royeen (Eds.), *Educating for moral action: A sourcebook in health and rehabilitation ethics* (pp. 121–130). Philadelphia, PA: F. A. Davis.

Hammer, D., Anderson, M. B., Brunson, W. D., Grus, C., Huen, L., Holtman, M., . . . Gandy Frost, J. (2012). Defining and measuring construct of interprofessional professionalism. *Journal of Allied Health, 41*(2), e49–e53.

Hansen, R., & Kyler-Hutchison, P. (1989, April). *Light at the end of the tunnel*. Workshop presented at the Annual Conference of the American Occupational Therapy Association, Baltimore, MD.

Hansen, R. A. (2003). Ethics in occupational therapy. In E. B. Crepeau, E. S. Cohn, & B. A. B. Schell (Eds.), *Willard & Spackman's occupational therapy* (10th ed., pp. 953–961). Philadelphia, PA: Lippincott, Williams & Wilkins.

Holtman, M. S., Frost, J. S., Hammer, D. P., McGuinn, K., & Nunez, L. M. (2011). Interprofessional professionalism: Linking professionalism and interprofessional care. *Journal of Interprofessional Care, 25*, 383–385.

Hunter, K. (2004). Narrative. In S. G. Post (Ed.), *Encyclopedia of bioethics* (3rd ed., pp. 1875–1876). New York, NY: Macmillan.

Kanny, E. M., & Kyler, P. L. (1999). Are faculty prepared to address ethical issues in education? *American Journal of Occupational Therapy, 53*, 72–74.

Kornblau, B. A., & Burkhardt, A. (2012). *Ethics in rehabilitation: A clinical perspective* (2nd ed.). Thorofare, NJ: Slack.

Kyler, P. L. (1999). *Teaching ethics*. Bethesda, MD: American Occupational Therapy Association.

National Board for Certification in Occupational Therapy, Inc. (2013). *2012 Practice analysis of the occupational therapist registered: Executive summary*. Retrieved from http://www.nbcot.org/assets/candidate-pdfs/2012-practice-analysis-executive-otr

National Board for Certification in Occupational Therapy, Inc. (2014a). *About us: Principles and mission*. Retrieved from http://www.nbcot.org.

National Board for Certification in Occupational Therapy, Inc. (2014b). *NBCOT Code of Conduct*. Retrieved from http://www.nbcot.org/code-of-conduct

Newton, L. (2013). Ethical leadership means empowering your followers. *Alberta RN, 69*(1), 30–31.

Ozar, D. T. (2004). Profession and professional ethics. In S. G. Post, (Ed.), *Encyclopedia of bioethics* (3rd ed., pp. 2158–2169). New York, NY: Macmillan References.

Pelligrino, E. D. (1995). Toward a virtue-based normative ethics for the health professions. *Kennedy Institute of Ethics Journal, 5*, 253–277.

Piper, L. E. (2011). The ethical leadership challenge: Creating a culture of patient- and family-centered care in the hospital setting. *The Health Care Manager, 30*(2), 125–132.

Pozgar, G. D. (2005). *Legal and ethical issues for health professionals*. Sudbury, MA: Jones and Bartlett.

Purtilo, R., & Doherty, R. (2011). *Ethical dimensions in the health professions* (5th ed.). St. Louis, MO: Elsevier.

Rogers, J. (1983). Clinical reasoning: The ethics, science and art. 1983 Eleanor Clarke Slagle Lecture. *American Journal of Occupational Therapy, 37*, 601–616.

Russell, C., Fitzgerald, M. H., Williamson, P., Manor, D., & Whybrow, S. (2002). Independence as a practice issue in occupational therapy: The safety clause. *American Journal of Occupational Therapy, 56*, 369–379.

Scanlon, C., & Glover, J. (1995). Ethical issues. A professional code of ethics: Providing a moral compass for turbulent times. *ONF, 22*, 1515–1521.

Sim, J. (1997). *Ethical decision making in practice*. Oxford, UK: Butterworth Heinemann.

Slater, D. Y. (2011). *Reference guide to the code of ethics & ethics standards* (2010 ed.). Bethesda, MD: American Occupational Therapy Association.

Slater, D. Y., & Brandt, L. C. (2011). Combating moral distress. In D. Y. Slater (Ed.), *Reference guide to the occupational therapy code of ethics and ethics standards* (2010 ed., pp. 107–113). Bethesda, MD: AOTA Press.

Swisher, L., Arslanian, L. E., & Davis, C. M. (2005). The Realm–Individual–Process–Situation (RIPS) model of ethical decision making. *HPA Resource—Official Publication of the American Physical Therapy Association Section on Health Policy and Administration*, *5*(3), 1, 3–18.

Turner, N., Barling, J., Epitropaki, O., Butcher, V., & Milner, C. (2002). Transformational leadership and moral reasoning. *Journal of Applied Psychology*, *87*(2), 304–311. PMID: 12002958

Wells, B. G. (2003). Leadership for ethical decision-making. *American Journal of Pharmaceutical Education*, *67*(1), 5–8.

Answer Key to Chapter Study Questions

Section I: Introduction to Leadership and Evidence-Based Management

Chapter 1: Leadership: The Art, Science, and Evidence

1. b
2. c
3. d
4. d
5. a
6. a
7. b
8. c

Chapter 2: Engaging in Evidence-Based Management

1. d
2. b
3. a
4. d
5. c
6. b
7. a
8. b

Section II: Leading and Managing in Context

Chapter 3: Understanding Health-Care Systems and Practice Contexts

1. d
2. b
3. d
4. b
5. d
6. a
7. c
8. a

Chapter 4: Understanding and Working Within Organizations

1. d
2. b
3. c
4. a
5. b
6. d
7. a
8. b

Chapter 5: Communicating Effectively in Complex Environments

1. d		**5.** b
2. a		**6.** c
3. d		**7.** d
4. a		**8.** c

Chapter 6: Roles and Functions of Managers: Planning, Organizing and Staffing, Directing, and Controlling

1. c		**5.** d
2. a		**6.** b
3. d		**7.** c
4. a		**8.** b

Chapter 7: Roles and Functions of Supervisors

1. c		**5.** c
2. a		**6.** a
3. b		**7.** d
4. b		**8.** d

Chapter 8: Professional Teams, Interprofessional Education, and Collaborative Practice

1. c		**5.** a
2. b		**6.** b
3. b		**7.** d
4. d		**8.** c

Section III: Managerial Skills, Responsibilities, and Competencies

Chapter 9: Strategic Planning

1. b		**5.** d
2. c		**6.** a
3. d		**7.** d
4. b		**8.** d

Chapter 10: Managing Change and Solving Problems

1. d		**5.** b
2. c		**6.** d
3. b		**7.** c
4. a		**8.** b

Chapter 11: Financial Planning, Management, and Budgeting

1. d		**5.** d
2. a		**6.** c
3. c		**7.** b
4. a		**8.** c

Chapter 12: Assessing and Promoting Clinical and Managerial Competency

1. c		**5.** a
2. d		**6.** b
3. a		**7.** d
4. b		**8.** b

Chapter 13: Continuous Quality Improvement

1. d		**5.** d
2. a		**6.** a
3. c		**7.** c
4. b		**8.** b

Chapter 14: Marketing Occupational Therapy Services

1. a		**5.** a
2. b		**6.** a
3. b		**7.** c
4. c		**8.** d

Chapter 15: Developing Evidence-Based Occupational Therapy Programming

1. c		**5.** b
2. b		**6.** a
3. d		**7.** c
4. b		**8.** d

Section IV: Leading Evidence-Based Practice and Professional Considerations

Chapter 16: Introducing Others to Evidence-Based Practice

1. d   5. a
2. b   6. c
3. d   7. a
4. c   8. c

Chapter 17: Turning Theory Into Practice: Managerial Strategies

1. d   5. a
2. d   6. b
3. c   7. a
4. c   8. d

Chapter 18: Responsible Participation in a Profession: Fostering Professionalism and Leading for Moral Action

1. b   5. d
2. d   6. d
3. a   7. d
4. b   8. a

Index

Note: The letter b indicates a boxed feature on the page. The letter f indicates a figure. The letter t indicates a table.

Occupational Therapy Intervention Process Model, 441, 452–453, 454t

The Occupational Therapy Manager, 8

Occupational therapy paradigm, 377, 378

Occupational therapy professional associations, 470–474

Occupational therapy service delivery settings, 63–67
evidence-based management and, 39–41

Occupation-based interventions, 455, 456t

Occupation-based practice, 460–461

ODEP. *See* Office of Disability Employment Policy

OD Network. *See* Organization Development Network

OD Practitioner (Journal of the Organization Development Network), 461

Office of Disability Employment Policy (ODEP), 88

Office of Inspector General (OIG), 69

Office of Minority Health Resource Center, 90

OIG. *See* Office of Inspector General

Oncology rehabilitation
MOHO and, 403, 403t
theory-based approach occupational therapy, case study, 401–404
theory-based approach to case study, 401–404
contributions of assessments and practice models to, 404, 405t
needs assessment, 402
program evaluation and outcomes for, 404
program implementation for, 404
program planning, staff education and training, 402–403

Open systems, 94, 97–98, 99b
individual as, 258, 258f

Operating margin, 278, 284b

Operating plan, 236, 238

Operational definitions, 103

Operationalizing, 342

Operational planning, 162–168
strategic planning *versus*, 237–238

Operations improvement, 116–118

Opportunity costs, 362

Organizational assessment, 358
marketing and, 361–362
strategies for, 362, 362b

Organizational behavior, trends in, 116–119

Organizational charts, 94, 112

Organizational climate, 105b

Organizational culture, 103–106
levels of analysis for understanding, 104, 105f
observable phenomena related to, 105b
practice and, 417

Organizational development, 116–119

Organizational environments
external, 101–103
internal, 103–106

Organizational function, trends in, 116–119

Organizational learning, 118–119
CQI and, 329–330
evidence on, 119, 120t
managers' role in, 119

Organizational life, 98–99

Organizational mission, 102

Organizational mission and values, strategic planning and reviewing of, 243–246

Organizational profile, 236, 240
developing, 241b

Organizational structure, 112–116, 415, 417
advantages and disadvantages of, 115, 115t
purposes of, 112–113, 112b

Organizational theory, 95–97, 97t

Organization Development Network (OD Network), 461

Organizations. *See also specific types of organizations*
change in, 102b, 261, 261b, 267–268
classifying, 63
competency and, 300
assessment of, 321
CQI and, 116, 354
critical thinking questions, 94
external change and adaptation of, 102b
financial planning, management, and budgeting-related, 295
history of, 95–97
interprofessional collaboration and education-concerned, 491
journals related to, 122–123
layers of, 100, 100f
leadership theories within, 8
learning, 118–119
marketing occupational therapy services-related, 374
open systems applied to, 99b
operations improvement, 116–118
private business, 108–111
process reengineering, 116–118
professional organizations and associations concerned with study of, 123–124
professional team-related, 231
profession of occupational therapy and concerned, 490–491
real-life management and, 93
real-life solutions and, 121
resources on, 122–123
by social sector, 111–112
society and, 96
study of, 96
subsystems, 100
as systems, 97–100
types of, 106–108
understanding and working within, 93–124